CURRENT
DIAGNOSIS &
TREATMENT

A QUICK Reference for the Clinician

CURRENT DIAGNOSIS & TREATMENT

Edited by
Roy Pounder   Mark Hamilton

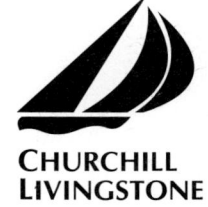
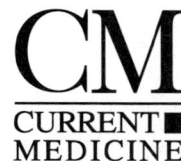

A QUICK Reference for the Clinician

© Copyright 1995 by Current Medicine, Inc.
34-42 Cleveland Street
London W1P 6LB, UK

Distributed by Churchill Livingstone
Robert Stevenson House
1-3 Baxter's Place
Leith Walk
Edinburgh EH1 3AF, UK

All rights reserved. No part of this publication may be reproduced, stored in a retrieval system or transmitted in any form or by any means electronic, mechanical, photocopying, recording or otherwise without the prior written permission of the copyright holder.

British Library Cataloguing-in-Publication Data. A catalogue record for this book is available from the British Library.

ISBN 0-443-05599-8 (Churchill Livingstone)

Although every effort has been made to ensure that drug doses and other information are presented accurately in this publication, the ultimate responsibility rests with the prescribing physician. Neither the publishers nor the authors can be held responsible for errors or for any consequences arising from the use of the information contained herein. Any product mentioned in this publication should be used in accordance with the prescribing information prepared by the manufacturers. No claims or endorsements are made for any drug or compound at present under clinical investigation.

Project editor: Sara Black
Illustrators: Paul Bernson, Stuart Molloy, Yaron Tracz
Designer: Mark Riches
Typesetters: Simon Banister, Claire Huntley, Sylvia Purnell
Production: Adrienne Hanratty
Indexer: Judith Field

Printed in Hong Kong

Contents

ix Preface
x Figure acknowledgements
xi How to use this book
xii Abbreviations

1 AIDS

Contributors
1 Contents
2 AIDS
4 AIDS-related lymphoma
6 Candidiasis, buccal and oesophageal in AIDS
8 Cytomegalovirus infection in AIDS
10 Diarrhoea and HIV infection
12 Kaposi's sarcoma in AIDS
14 Meningitis, cryptococcal in AIDS
16 Mycobacterium avium intracellulare infection in AIDS
18 Pneumocystis carinii pneumonia in AIDS
20 Pulmonary complications of immunosuppression
22 Toxoplasmosis in AIDS
24 Index

2 CARDIOLOGY

Contributors
1 Contents
2 Angina pectoris
4 Angina, unstable
6 Aortic dissection
8 Aortic regurgitation
10 Aortic stenosis
12 Atrial septal defect
14 Cardiac failure and dilated cardiomyopathy
16 Cardiopulmonary resuscitation
18 Dyslipoproteinaemia
20 Eisenmenger complex
22 Endocarditis
24 Heart block
26 Hypertension
28 Hypertrophic cardiomyopathy
30 Mitral regurgitation
32 Mitral stenosis
34 Myocardial infarction
36 Pericarditis and tamponade
38 Pulmonary embolism
40 Restrictive cardiomyopathy and constrictive pericarditis

Cardiology *cont.*
42 Shock, acute hypotensive
44 Tachycardia, supraventricular
46 Tachycardia, ventricular
48 Wolff–Parkinson–White syndrome
50 Index

3 DERMATOLOGY

Contributors
1 Contents
2 Acne
4 Alopecia
6 Bullous disorders
8 Eczema
10 Fungal nail infections
12 Psoriasis
14 Urticaria
16 Vasculitis, skin manifestations
18 Viral warts
20 Index

4 ENDOCRINOLOGY & METABOLIC DISORDERS

Contributors
1 Contents
2 Acromegaly
4 Addison's disease
6 Cushing's syndrome
8 Diabetes insipidus
10 Diabetes mellitus, insulin-dependent
12 Diabetes mellitus, non-insulin-dependent
14 Diabetic management in children
16 Diabetic management in pregnancy
18 Diabetic management in surgery
20 Female hypergonadotrophic hypogonadism
22 Female hypogonadotrophic hypogonadism
24 Growth abnormalities, short stature
26 Growth abnormalities, tall stature
28 Hypercalcaemia
30 Hyperglycaemic emergencies
32 Hyperprolactinaemia
34 Hyperthyroidism
36 Hypocalcaemia

Contents

Endocrinology & metabolic disorders *cont.*
- 38 Hypoglycaemia
- 40 Hypopituitarism
- 42 Hypothyroidism
- 44 Obesity
- 46 Phaeochromocytoma
- 48 Polycystic ovarian disease
- 50 Pubertal abnormalities
- 52 Syndrome of inappropriate antidiuresis
- 54 Testicular disorders
- 56 Thyroid carcinoma
- 58 Index

5 GASTROENTEROLOGY

Contributors
- 1 Contents
- 2 Achalasia
- 4 Anaemia, pernicious
- 6 Bacterial overgrowth of the small intestine
- 8 Coeliac disease
- 10 Colorectal cancer
- 12 Crohn's disease
- 14 Diverticular disease of the colon
- 16 Duodenal ulcer
- 18 Enteric infections
- 20 Gallstones, cholesterol
- 22 Gastric cancer
- 24 Gastric ulceration
- 26 Gastrointestinal bleeding
- 28 Irritable bowel syndrome
- 30 Oesophageal carcinoma
- 32 Oesophagitis and hiatus hernia
- 34 Pancreatic cancer
- 36 Pancreatitis, acute
- 38 Pancreatitis, chronic
- 40 Ulcerative colitis
- 42 Zollinger–Ellison syndrome
- 44 Index

6 HAEMATOLOGY

Contributors
- 1 Contents
- 2 Anaemia, aplastic
- 4 Anaemia, megaloblastic
- 6 Disseminated intravascular coagulation
- 8 Haemophilia and von Willebrand's disease
- 10 Hodgkin's disease
- 12 Infections in haematological malignancy
- 14 Leukaemia, acute lymphoblastic in adults
- 16 Leukaemia, acute lymphoblastic in children
- 18 Leukaemia, acute myeloid
- 20 Leukaemia, chronic lymphocytic
- 22 Leukaemia, hairy cell
- 24 Multiple myeloma
- 26 Myeloproliferative disorders
- 28 Non-Hodgkin's lymphoma
- 30 Platelet disorders
- 32 Platelet disorders
- 34 Sickle cell disease
- 36 Thalassaemia
- 38 Transfusion medicine
- 40 Waldenström's macroglobulinaemia
- 42 Index

7 HEPATOLOGY

Contributors
- 1 Contents
- 2 Ascites
- 4 Cholangitis, primary sclerosing
- 6 Cirrhosis, primary biliary
- 8 Hepatic encephalopathy
- 10 Hepatitis, acute
- 12 Hepatitis, chronic
- 14 Hepatocellular carcinoma
- 16 Liver failure, fulminant
- 18 Variceal bleeding
- 20 Index

8 INFECTIOUS DISEASES

Contributors
1 Contents
2 Chronic fatigue syndrome
4 Erythema multiforme and Stevens–Johnson syndrome
6 Erythema nodosum
8 Fungal infections, invasive
10 Gram-negative septicaemia
12 Henoch-Schönlein purpura
14 Herpes simplex infection
16 Herpes zoster and varicella
18 Leptospirosis
20 Lyme disease
22 Malaria
24 Measles
26 Parvovirus B19 infection
28 Pharyngitis
30 Rheumatic fever, acute
32 Rubella (German measles)
34 Skin infection
36 Toxic shock syndrome
38 Tuberculosis, extrapulmonary
40 Typhoid and paratyphoid fevers
42 Index

9 NEPHROLOGY

Contributors
1 Contents
2 Dialysis
4 Glomerulonephritis
6 Haemolytic uraemic syndrome
8 Hyperkalaemia and hypokalaemia
10 Hypernatraemia and hyponatraemia
12 Nephropathies, tubulointerstitial
14 Polycystic kidney disease, autosomal-dominant
16 Renal artery stenosis
18 Renal failure, acute
20 Renal failure, chronic
22 Renal transplantation
24 Renal tubular acidosis
26 Urinary tract infection
28 Index

10 NEUROLOGY

Contributors
1 Contents
2 Cerebral tumour
4 Coma
6 Cranial arteritis
8 Dementia
10 Encephalitis
12 Epilepsy
14 Facial pain, atypical
16 Guillain–Barré syndrome
18 Idiopathic polymyositis
20 Intracerebral haemorrhage
22 Meningitis, bacterial
24 Migraine
26 Motor neurone disease
28 Multiple sclerosis
30 Myasthenia gravis
32 Neuralgia, postherpetic
34 Neuralgia, trigeminal
36 Neuropathy, peripheral
38 Parkinson's disease
40 Sleep disorders
42 Spinal cord and cauda equina compression
44 Stroke
46 Transient ischaemic attacks
48 Tremor
50 Index

11 PSYCHIATRY

Contributors
1 Contents
2 Alcohol withdrawal syndrome
4 Attempted suicide
6 Bulimia nervosa
8 Depression and mania
10 Obsessive compulsive disorder
12 Panic and generalized anxiety disorder
14 Personality disorders
16 Postnatal mental illness
18 Schizophrenia
20 Index

12 RESPIRATORY DISORDERS

Contributors
1 Contents
2 Adult respiratory distress syndrome
4 Asthma
6 Asthma, occupational
8 Bronchiectasis and cystic fibrosis
10 Chronic obstructive airway disease
12 Fibrosing alveolitis
14 Granulomatoses
(16) Lung cancer
18 Pleural effusion
20 Pneumonia
22 Sarcoidosis
24 Sleep apnoea, central, hypoventilation, periodic breathing
26 Sleep apnoea, obstructive
28 Tuberculosis, pulmonary
30 Index

13 RHEUMATOLOGY & MUSCULAR DISORDERS

Contributors
1 Contents
2 Acute crystal synovitis
4 Ankylosing spondylitis
6 Arthritis, psoriatic
8 Arthritis, rheumatoid
10 Arthritis, septic
12 Gout
14 Myositis, inflammatory
16 Osteoarthritis
18 Polymyalgia rheumatica and giant-cell arteritis
20 Systemic lupus erythematosus
22 Systemic sclerosis
24 Vasculitis, systemic
26 Index

Preface

Current Diagnosis and Treatment is a book that has been prepared for the active doctor. It provides up-to-date authoritative clinical information about most major medical problems. There is little space for explanation – the book provides reminders for the qualified doctor, who needs to be 'brought up to speed' about the modern diagnosis and management of a clinical problem that is outside his or her area of normal clinical activity.

Readers will become familiar with the standard format: symptoms, signs, investigations, complications, differential diagnosis, aetiology, and epidemiology on the left-hand page; diet and lifestyle, pharmacological treatment, occasional surgical treatment, management issues, prognosis, and the latest references on the right-hand page.

The layout caused major problems in the preparation of this first edition. We provided each author with detailed instructions and a sample layout. The 214 contributions had to be transformed into the pages that you read. This process demanded enormous skill and perseverance by, particularly, Sara Black and her colleagues at Current Science. The authors have been wonderfully tolerant. Like good wine, we anticipate that *Current Diagnosis and Treatment* will improve over the years. We plan to bring out a revised edition annually. In the spirit of competitive writing, I am sure the book will get better and better!

Current Diagnosis and Treatment has one unusual feature for a textbook – not only are the individual contributions written by the very best UK experts, but each contribution has been subjected to editorial scrutiny by one of the 13 section editors, and each contribution has also been peer-reviewed by two experts. Our thanks go to the 220 colleagues who have acted as authors, editors, and referees.

This book is full of information. We have tried very hard to eliminate any errors, but readers are advised that they must confirm recommended dosages in the drug data sheets before prescribing any drug regimen. If errors are detected, or if there are suggestions for improvement – for example, useful topics that are not covered – please write to us and we will make amends. Our policy is continuous improvement!

Roy Pounder Mark Hamilton

London, 1995

Figure acknowledgements

We gratefully acknowledge the publishers and individuals who allowed us to use the following illustrations.

AIDS

Page 6. Adapted with permission from Smith DE *et al.*: Itraconazole versus ketoconazole in the treatment of oral and oesophageal candidosis in patients infected with HIV. *AIDS* 1991, **5**:1367–1371.

Page 16. Reproduced with permission from Scolar A, French P, Miller R: *Mycobacterium avium intracellulare* infection in the acquired immunodeficiency syndrome. *Br J Hosp Med* 1991, **46**:295–300.

Cardiology

Page 28. Reproduced with permission from Slade AKB, Saumarel RC, McKenna WJ: The arrythmogenic substrate – diagnostic and therapeutic implications: hypertrophic cardiomyopathy. *Eur Heart J* 1993, **14**:84–90.

Endocrinology

Page 16. Adapted with permission from *Clinical Diabetes: An Illustrated Text*, by GM Besser, HJ Bodansky, AG Cudworth, Mosby–Wolfe an imprint of Times Mirror International Publishers Ltd., London, UK, 1995

Page 32. Courtesy of Professor A Grossman, Department of Endocrinology, St Bartholomew's Hospital, London, UK.

Page 38. Adapted with permission from Frier BM, Fisher M (eds): *Hypoglycaemia and Diabetes*. London: Edward Arnold.

Page 44. Adapted with permission from Garrow J: *Obesity and Related Diseases*. Edinburgh: Churchill Livingstone, 1988.

Gastroenterology

Page 20. Adapted with permission from Northfield TC, Jazrawi RP: Non-surgical treatment of gallstones: overall strategy. In *Bile Acids in Health and Disease*. Dodrecht: Kluwer Academic Publications, 1988, pp 205–213.

Page 34. Adapted with permission from Tsuchiya R: Resection of cancer of the pancreas – the Japanese experience. *Baillières Clin Gastroenterol* 1990, **4**:431–434.

Page 56. Reproduced with permission from Franklyn JA, Sheppard MC: Thyroid nodules and thyroid cancer – diagnostic aspects. *Baillières Clin Endocrinol Metab* 1988, **2**:767.

Haematology

Page 22. Courtesy of Dr John Smith, Director, Wessex Regional Immunology Service Tenovus Laboratory, Southampton General Hospital.

Infectious diseases

Page 2. Adapted with permission from Ho-Yen DO: The epidemiology of post viral fatigue syndrome. *Scott Med J* 1988, **33**:368–369.

Page 22. Adapted with permission from Bradley D et al.: Malaria imported into the United Kingdom in 1992 and 1993. *Communicable Diseases Report* 1994, **4**:R169–R172.

Page 24. Adapted with permission from Ramsay M *et al.*: The epidemiology of measles in England and Wales. *Communicable Diseases Report* 1994, **4**:R141–R145.

Page 28. Adapted with permission from Gay NJ *et al.*: Age specific antibody prevalence to parvovirus B19: how many women are infected in pregnancy? *Communicable Diseases Report* 1994, **4**:R104–R107.

Page 34. Adapted with permission from Miller E *et al.*: Rubella surveillance to June 1994. *Communicable Diseases Report* 1994, **4**:R146–R152.

Page 38. Adapted from *MMWR Morb Mortal Wkly Rep* 1992, **41**:58.

Page 38. Adapted from *MMWR Morb Mortal Wkly Rep* 1990, **39**:421–423.

Page 40. Reproduced with permission from Kennedy DH: Extrapulmonary tuberculosis. *Update* 1983, **27**:671–684.

Nephrology

Page 12. Adapted with permission from Sweny P *et al.*: *The Kidney and its Disorders*. Oxford: Blackwell Scientific Publications, 1989.

Page 16. Reproduced with permission from Stansby G *et al.*: Atherosclerotic renal artery stenosis. *Br J Hosp Med* 1993, **49**:388.

Neurology

Page 4. Adapted with permission from Swash M, Oxberry J (eds): *Clinical Neurology*. Edinburgh: Churchill Livingstone, 1991, p 191.

Psychiatry

Page 9. Adapted with permission from Kupfer DJ: Lessons to be learned from long-term treatment of affective disorder. *J Clin Psychiatry* 1991, **52 (suppl)**:12–16. Copyright 1991, Physicians Postgraduate Press.

Respiratory disorders

Page 15. Adapted with permission from Hoffman GS *et al.*: Wegener granulomatosis: an analysis of 158 patients. *Ann Intern Med* 1992, **116**:488–498.

How to use this book

Current Diagnosis and Treatment provides current expert recommendations on the diagnosis and treatment of all major disorders throughout medicine in the form of tabular summaries. Essential guidelines on each of the topics have been condensed into two pages of vital information, summarizing the main procedures in diagnosis and management of each disorder to provide a quick and easy reference.

Each disorder is presented as a 'spread' of two facing pages: the main procedures in diagnosis on the left and treatment options on the right.

Listed in the main column of the **Diagnosis** page are the common symptoms, signs, and complications of the disorder, with brief notes explaining their significance and probability of occurrence, together with details of investigations that can be used to aid diagnosis.

The pink side column contains information to help the reader evaluate the probability that an individual patient has the disorder. It may also include other information that could be useful in making a diagnosis (e.g. classification or grading systems, comparison of different diagnostic methods).

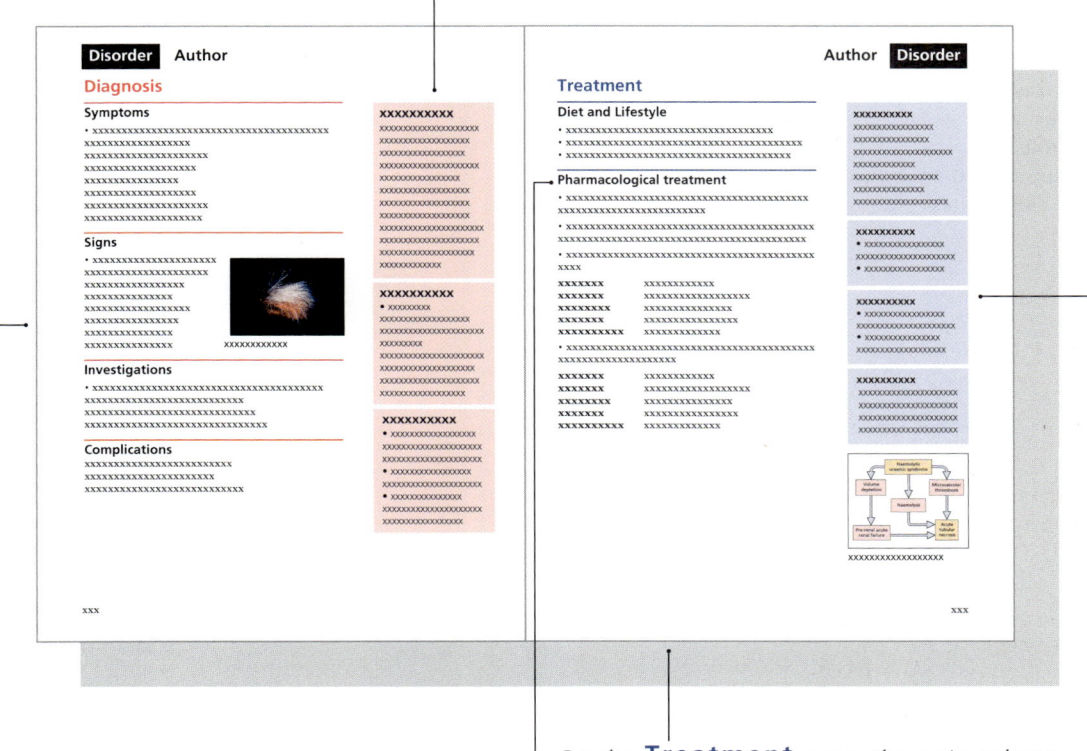

On the **Treatment** page, the main column contains information on lifestyle management and nonspecialist medical therapy of the disorder, with general information on specialist management when this is the main treatment.

Whenever possible under 'Pharmacological treatment', guidelines are given on the standard dosage for commonly used drugs, with details of contraindications and precautions, main drug interactions, and main side effects. In each case, however, the manufacturer's drug data sheet should be consulted before any regimen is prescribed.

The main goals of treatment (e.g. to cure, to palliate, to prevent), prognosis after treatment, precautions that the physician should take during and after treatment, and any other information that could help the clinician to make treatment decisions (e.g. other non-pharmacological treatment options, special situations or groups of patients) are given in the blue side column. The key references at the end of this column provide the reader with further practical information.

xi

Abbreviations

AIDS, acquired immunodeficiency syndrome
CNS, central nervous system
CRP, C-reactive protein
CSF, cerebrospinal fluid
CT, computed tomography
DNA, deoxyribonucleic acid
ECG, electrocardiography
EEG, electroencephalography
ESR, erythrocyte sedimentation rate
GP, general practitioner
H_2, histamine
HIV, human immunodeficiency virus
HLA, human leucocyte antigen
5-HT, 5-hydroxytryptamine (serotonin)
IgA, IgG, IgM, immunoglobulin A, G, M
i.m., intramuscular
INR, international normalized ratio
i.t., intrathecal
i.v., intravenous
MRI, magnetic resonance imaging
NSAID, nonsteroidal anti-inflammatory drug
RNA, ribonucleic acid
s.c., subcutaneous
SLE, systemic lupus erythematosus
U&E, urea and electrolytes

CURRENT DIAGNOSIS & TREATMENT

in

AIDS

Edited by
Brian Gazzard

Series editors
Roy Pounder
Mark Hamilton

A QUICK Reference for the Clinician

Contributors

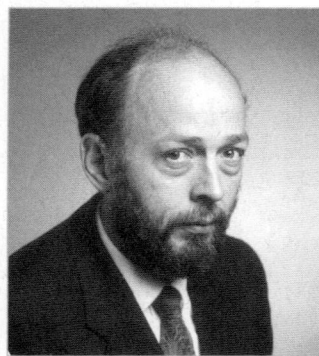

EDITOR
Brian Gazzard

Dr Brian Gazzard is Clinical Director of the HIV/GUM Unit at Chelsea and Westminster Hospital, London. His research interests are clinical trials of antiretroviral agents in HIV infection and the pathogenesis and clinical manifestations of gut disease in infected patients.

REFEREES
Dr Caroline Bradbeer
Department of Genitourinary Medicine
St Thomas' Hospital
London, UK

Dr Anton Pozniak
Department of Genitourinary Medicine
King's Healthcare
London, UK

AUTHORS

AIDS
Dr Brian Gazzard
HIV/GUM Unit
Chelsea and Westminster Hospital
London, UK

AIDS-related lymphoma
Dr Margaret Spittle
Meyerstein Institute of Clinical Oncology
Middlesex Hospital
London, UK

Candidiasis, buccal and oesophageal in AIDS
Dr Don Smith
Community HIV Research Network
St Vincent's Hospital Medical Centre
Sydney, Australia

Cytomegalovirus infection in AIDS
Dr Christine Katlama
Departement des Maladies Infectieuses
Groupe Hospitalier Pitie-Salpetriere
Paris, France

Diarrhoea and HIV infection
Dr Brian Gazzard
HIV/GUM Unit
Chelsea and Westminster Hospital
London, UK

Kaposi's sarcoma in AIDS
Dr Fiona Boag
St Stephen's Centre
Chelsea and Westminster Hospital
London, UK

Meningitis cryptococcal in AIDS
Dr Roberto J Guiloff
Regional Neurosciences Centre
Charing Cross Hospital
London, UK

Mycobacterium avium intracellulare infection in AIDS
Dr Robert F Miller
Department of Medicine
University College Hospital
London, UK

Pneumocystis carinii pneumonia in AIDS
Dr Simon Barton
HIV/GUM Unit
Chelsea and Westminster Hospital
London, UK

Toxoplasmosis AIDS
Dr Giovanna Mallucci
Prion Disease Group
St Mary's Hospital
London, UK

Dr Margaret Johnson
Department of Thoracic Medicine
Royal Free Hospital
London, UK

Contents

2 AIDS

4 AIDS-related lymphoma

6 Candidiasis, buccal and oesophageal in AIDS

8 Cytomegalovirus infection in AIDS

10 Diarrhoea and HIV infection

12 Kaposi's sarcoma in AIDS
   gastrointestinal Kaposi's sarcoma
   lymphatic Kaposi's sarcoma
   mucocutaneous Kaposi's sarcoma
   pulmonary Kaposi's sarcoma

14 Meningitis, cryptococcal in AIDS

16 *Mycobacterium avium intracellulare* infection in AIDS

18 *Pneumocystis carinii* pneumonia in AIDS

20 Pulmonary complications of immunosuppression

22 Toxoplasmosis in AIDS

24 Index

AIDS B.G. Gazzard

Diagnosis

Definition
- AIDS is defined by progressive immunodeficiency without another cause, manifest by various conditions, including the following:

Opportunistic infections
Viral: cytomegalovirus.

Bacterial: *Mycobacterium avium intracellulare,* disseminated *M. tuberculosis,* recurrent *Salmonella* spp.

Fungal: *Candida albicans, Cryptococcus neoformans, Histoplasma capsulatum.*

Protozoan: *Pneumocystis carinii,* cryptosporidia, microsporidia, isospora (not diagnostic of AIDS).

Unusual tumours
Kaposi's sarcoma.

Non-T-cell lymphoma.

Invasive cervical carcinoma.

Neurological manifestations
AIDS dementia complex.

Vacuolar myelopathy.

Progressive multifocal leukoencephalopathy.

Symptoms
- Several minor symptoms, especially skin rashes (particularly caused by herpes zoster infection), occur during the asymptomatic period of 10 years or more after seroconversion.

Meningism, skin rash, temperature, lymphadenopathy (seroconversion illness): in 50% of patients.

Unexplained diarrhoea, fever, marked asthenia, minor opportunistic infections: particularly buccal candidiasis and oral hairy leucoplakia; in 'pre-AIDS'.

Signs
Skin rash, meningism: in seroconversion.

Lymphadenopathy, skin conditions: in asymptomatic stage.

Buccal candidiasis, oral hairy leucoplakia: in pre-AIDS.

Opportunistic infection: in AIDS.

Investigations
- The symptom complex is usually strongly suggestive of HIV infection.
- In the asymptomatic phase, the diagnosis can be made only by HIV testing.

HIV test: antibodies to HIV (usually occurring within 3 months of exposure) measured by enzyme-linked immunosorbent assay, usually confirmed by second test or, less often, Western blot analysis to check pattern of antibody response.

CD4 lymphocyte count: used to assess immune function; normal value $\sim 800 \times 10^6$/L; patients with $<500 \times 10^6$/L will probably progress eventually; patients with $<200 \times 10^6$/L are liable to various opportunistic infections.

HIV p24 antigen analysis: presence of antigen in circulation implies active replication and carries poor prognosis; this test will probably be superseded by direct measurement of viral load using polymerase chain reaction.

Complications
Not applicable.

Differential diagnosis
Congenital immunodeficiency.

Iatrogenic immunodeficiency: e.g. after bone-marrow transplantation.

HIV-antibody-negative CD4 lymphopenia: rare; different epidemiology from HIV infection.

Aetiology
- AIDS is caused by infection by HIV.
- HIV leads to a progressive fall in T-helper (CD4) cells and a failure of T-cell proliferation after antigenic stimulation, even by T cells uninfected by HIV.

Epidemiology
- Geographically, three patterns of disease are seen:

North America and Western Europe
- Transmission is mainly among men having sex with men and among intravenous drug users, with only limited transmission vertically or among recipients of blood products (patients with haemophilia who received blood products between 1975 and 1984).
- In the UK, the peak transmission among men having sex with men was in the early 1980s. The number of heterosexual people and intravenous drug users infected remains small, but the potential for exponential increase remains.

Sub-Saharan Africa
- The disease is predominantly a heterosexual epidemic, with major transmission vertically and through blood products.

Asia
- Transmission is sporadic, with introduction of the epidemic through blood products and visitors; although the disease is not widespread in these countries, an explosive increase in numbers is occurring, mainly by heterosexual transmission.

Treatment

Diet and lifestyle
- A high-energy diet is advised to reduce weight loss.
- Gentle exercise should be encouraged, and smoking and stress reduced.

Pharmacological treatment
- The following drugs are only weakly antiretroviral *in vivo*, with a modest fall seen in viral load.
- Zidovudine (azidothymidine, AZT) is the only drug shown in controlled studies to prolong life when given to symptomatic patients.
- The time at which treatment should be initiated and the use of combinations of the drugs remain controversial.

AZT
Standard dosage	AZT 200 mg 3 times daily.
Contraindications	Bone-marrow suppression.
Special points	Only licensed for symptomatic disease.
Main drug interactions	Drugs with similar toxic profile.
Main side effects	Bone-marrow suppression, occasionally myopathy.

Didanosine
Standard dosage	Didanosine 200 mg twice daily.
Contraindications	Previous pancreatitis.
Special points	Only licensed for AZT-intolerant or failing patients.
Main drug interactions	Given in alkaline buffer, which may reduce absorption of compounds needing acidification in the stomach.
Main side effects	Severe pancreatitis in advanced immunosuppression, possible peripheral neuropathy.

Dideoxycytosine
Standard dosage	Dideoxycytosine 0.75 mg 3 times daily.
Contraindications	Pre-existing peripheral neuropathy.
Special points	Licensed for AZT-intolerant patients.
Main drug interactions	None known.
Main side effects	Peripheral neuropathy, stomatitis.

Treatment aims
To eradicate the virus.
To restore immunocompetence.
To prolong life.
To improve quality of life.

Prognosis
- 60% of patients progress to AIDS within 10 years of seroconversion.
- 10% remain well, with no evidence of immunological deterioration at this time; whether they remain well in the long term remains unclear.
- The median survival from AIDS diagnosis is 2 years.

Follow-up and management
- Asymptomatic patients are reviewed once or twice a year, when a CD4 count should be done.
- Patients with low CD4 counts ($<200 \times 10^6$/L) should be reviewed every 3 months to allow possible antiretroviral treatment and prophylactic treatment against opportunistic infections to be considered.

Key references
Alderson T: New directions for the antiretroviral chemotherapy of AIDS – a basis for a pharmacological approach to treatment. *Biol Rev* 1993, **68**:265–289.

Hoth DF *et al.*: HIV vaccine development: a progress report. *Ann Intern Med* 1994, **121**:603–611.

Pinching AJ: Immunological consequences of human immunodeficiency virus infection. *Rev Med Microbiol* 1990, **1**:83–91.

Sheppard HW, Ascher MS: The natural history and pathogenesis of HIV infection. *Annu Rev Microbiol* 1992, **460**:533–564.

Weissman IL: AIDS: the whole body view. *Curr Biol* 1993, **30**:766–769.

AIDS-related lymphoma — M.F. Spittle

Diagnosis

Symptoms
- Lymphoma B symptoms may be difficult to differentiate from other symptoms of HIV infection and AIDS.

Persistent nodal enlargement: in 50% of patients.

Cough, shortness of breath.

Abdominal pain, haematemesis.

Headaches, fits, focal neurological deficits, drowsiness.

Painful and ulcerated tonsils.

Localized indurated skin nodule.

Weakness, weight loss, night sweats, fever.

Signs
Enlarged discrete rubbery nodes in neck, axillae, or groins.

Hepatosplenomegaly.

Infiltrated subcutaneous mass.

Abdominal mass: may cause obstruction.

Palpable rectal mass.

Raised intracranial pressure, papilloedema, focal neurological signs.

Mass involving unusual site: e.g. heart.

Anaemia, pyrexia, petechiae.

Investigations
Fine-needle aspiration: can give diagnosis but cannot type lymphoma satisfactorily.

Biopsy: to type lymphoma.

Full blood count and ESR measurement: baseline for treatment.

CT of chest, abdomen, and pelvis.

Lumbar puncture: high incidence of CSF involvement.

MRI, CT, CT-guided biopsy: to detect cerebral lymphoma; histology may not be obtainable; diagnosis is made *post mortem* in 50% of patients.

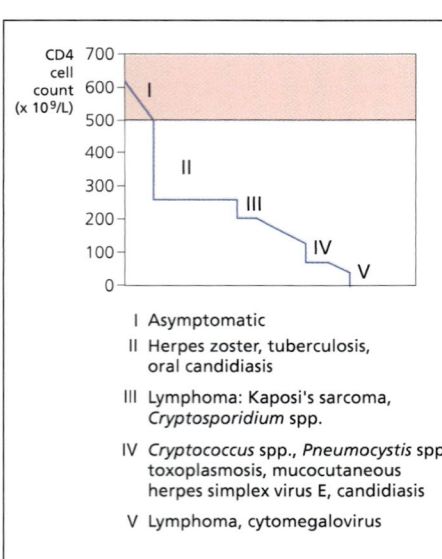

I Asymptomatic
II Herpes zoster, tuberculosis, oral candidiasis
III Lymphoma: Kaposi's sarcoma, *Cryptosporidium* spp.
IV *Cryptococcus* spp., *Pneumocystis* spp., toxoplasmosis, mucocutaneous herpes simplex virus E, candidiasis
V Lymphoma, cytomegalovirus

Relationship of CD4 cell count to clinical condition.

Complications
Poor bone-marrow reserve: because of infections or drugs.

Many opportunist infections.

Differential diagnosis
Nodal
Persistent generalized lymphadenopathy.

Extranodal
Nonspecific tonsillar ulcers, Kaposi's sarcoma. Cerebral toxoplasmosis, demyelination.

Systemic
Pyrexia of unknown origin, *Mycobacterium avium intracellulare* or *M. tuberculosis* infection, HIV infection, drug reactions.

Aetiology
Non-Hodgkin's lymphoma
- HIV-related immunosuppression may allow lymphoproliferation driven by Epstein–Barr virus or other cytokines.
- Non-Hodgkin's lymphoma is seen in other immunosuppressed states: Wiskott–Aldrich syndrome (congenital), organ-transplant recipients.

Epidemiology
- Non-Hodgkin's lymphoma accounts for 3% of AIDS-defining diagnoses in HIV-positive patients; it is the AIDS-defining diagnosis in 60% of those in whom it occurs.
- It usually occurs with a falling CD4 count ($<200 \times 10^6$/L) but rarely with a high count; CNS lymphoma occurs when the CD4 count is very low ($<30 \times 10^6$/L).
- It is seen equally in all risk groups.
- It is the most common AIDS-related malignancy in heterosexuals.

Pathology
B-cell non-Hodgkin's lymphoma
High grade: 90% small, non-cleaved cells (65% immunoblastic, 25% Burkitt).
Low grade: occasionally, not related to AIDS.

Treatment

Diet and lifestyle
- No special precautions are necessary.

Pharmacological treatment
- Specialist supervision is needed.
- Discussion of treatment options with the patient is vital.
- Patients with good performance status and high CD4 counts are treated by conventional CHOP chemotherapy (cyclophosphamide, vincristine, adriamycin, prednisolone) or short-course high-dose multiple-agent regimens; traditional non-AIDS regimens may cause worsening of prognosis in poor-risk AIDS patients.
- Patients with poor performance status, low CD4 counts ($<100 \times 10^6$/L), and previous AIDS-defining diagnoses can receive low-dose CHOP or vincristine and bleomycin with steroids.
- CNS prophylaxis with intrathecal methotrexate is important because CNS involvement is frequent.
- All chemotherapy is immunosuppressive, depresses bone-marrow function, and may precipitate infection.

Treatment aims
To avoid overwhelming infection in good-risk patients receiving high-dose chemotherapy. To maintain quality of life.

Other treatments

Radiotherapy
- This is useful in palliative treatment of nodal masses unresponsive to chemotherapy or when chemotherapy is not possible. External beam radiotherapy for localized extranodal sites: e.g. lymphoma of tonsil. Whole-brain radiotherapy for cerebral lymphoma.

Bone-marrow support
With colony-stimulating factors.

Prognosis
- The median survival is <6 months (worse than for non-HIV-related non-Hodgkin's lymphoma, stage for stage).
- Factors associated with poor prognosis include having AIDS before diagnosis of lymphoma, poor performance status (<70% Karnofsky), having a CD4 count <10×10^6/L.
- 50% of patients die of non-Hodgkin's lymphoma, 50% of AIDS-related problems.
- Burkitt's lymphoma responds better to chemotherapy than immunoblastic lymphoma does.
- The median survival for cerebral lymphoma is 4–8 weeks.

Follow-up and management
- Patients should be provided with psychological support and continuing care.

Key references

Ioachim HL et al.: Acquired immunodeficiency syndrome associated lymphomas. Clinical, pathologic, immunologic, and viral characteristics of 111 cases. *Hum Pathol* 1991, **22**:659–673.

Levine AM et al.: Human immunodeficiency virus-related lymphoma. Prognostic factors predictive of survival. *Cancer* 1991, **68**:2466–2472.

Levine AM et al.: Low dose chemotherapy with central nervous system prophylaxis and zidovudine maintenance in AIDS related lymphoma. A prospective multi-institutional trial. *JAMA* 1991, **266**:84–88.

Candidiasis, buccal and oesophageal in AIDS — D. Smith

Diagnosis

Symptoms
- 30% of patients are asymptomatic.

Altered taste sensation.

Oral discomfort or pain.

Coated mouth or tongue.

Dysphagia: especially with acidic orange drinks or dry toast.

Odynophagia.

Loss of appetite.

Signs
Angular cheilitis.

Intraoral removable white plaques, with erythematous underlying mucosa.

Intraoral mucosal ulceration or erythema.

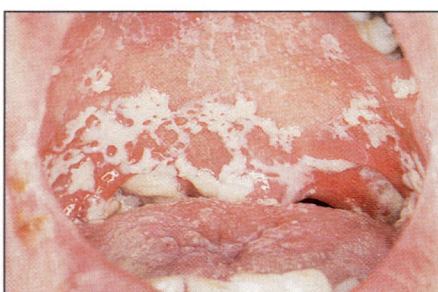 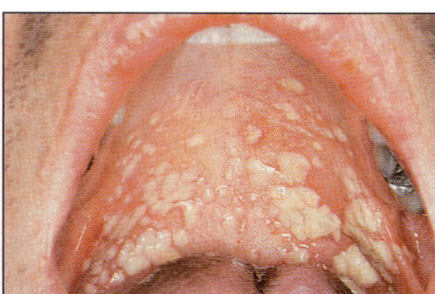

Curdish white plaques of pseudomembranous candidiasis.

Investigations

Buccal candidiasis
- The diagnosis is usually obvious without further investigation.

Direct microscopy: direct staining of mouth scraping with hydrogen peroxide or Gram stain rapidly confirms presence of fungal hyphae.

Mouth swab or washings: to determine sensitivity of *Candida* spp.

Oesophageal candidiasis

Fibreoptic endoscopy: allows direct visualization of oesophageal involvement, with biopsy confirming diagnosis; should be considered gold standard.

Barium-swallow radiography: can highlight linear filling defects but detects only 50% of cases.

Complications
Oral ulceration.

Weight loss: secondary to depressed appetite.

Oesophageal obstruction: rarely, secondary to overgrowth of *Candida* spp. (systemic dissemination unusual).

Differential diagnosis
Oral hairy leukoplakia.

HIV-related gingivitis, peridontitis, herpes simplex, or giant aphthous ulcers.

Cytomegalovirus ulceration of the oesophagus, acid reflux, Kaposi's sarcoma, or lymphoma.

Aetiology
- Candidiasis is the overgrowth and invasion of mucosal surfaces by *Candida albicans* or occasionally other *Candida* spp. The emergence of clinical disease is related to the loss of cell-mediated immunity and not to the presence of more virulent *Candida* strains.
- In HIV infection, buccal candidiasis is often seen when the number of circulating CD4 lymphocytes is $<350 \times 10^6/L$, and oesophageal candidiasis is seen when CD4 cells are $<250 \times 10^6/L$.

Epidemiology
- *Candida albicans* is a normal commensal of the mouth and can be cultured from 30% of the population.
- Although both buccal and oesophageal candidiasis have been described during acute primary infection with HIV, they are generally associated with moderate to severe immunodeficiency 4–10 years after initial infection.
- 90% of HIV-infected patients develop candidiasis at some stage of their illness.
- Oesophageal, bronchopulmonary, or invasive candidiasis is classified as an AIDS-defining opportunistic infection.

Treatment

Diet and lifestyle
- 'Candida-free' or acidophilus diets are of no benefit; avoiding snack foods rich in glucose, however, appears to reduce the severity of episodes.

Pharmacological treatment

Topical antifungals
- Amphotericin, nystatin, and clotrimazole are all of benefit in mild cases of buccal candidiasis; they become less effective, however, as the patient's immune status deteriorates and do not treat any oesophageal involvement.
- They are also occasionally useful in suppressing relapses.

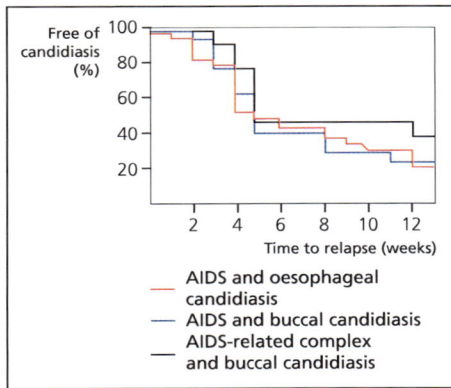

Patients free of relapse after clinical and mycological clearance.

Ketoconazole
- Ketoconazole is effective for buccal and oesophageal disease, with improvement in symptoms occurring within 3 days.

Standard dosage	Ketoconazole doses greater than given on data sheet (200 mg twice daily) often needed in AIDS patients because of reduced absorption (secondary to achlorhydria).
Contraindications	Liver disease, azole hypersensitivity.
Main drug interactions	Decreased absorption with antacids, cimetidine, or omeprazole; increased metabolism with rifampicin, rifabutin, or phenytoin.
Main side effects	Rash, nausea, altered liver function tests.

Itraconazole
- Itraconazole is equally effective (70% response rates at 1 week and 90% at 1 month) but less hepatotoxic than ketoconazole.

Standard dosage	Itraconazole 200 mg daily for 1–4 weeks.
Contraindications	Azole hypersensitivity.
Special points	An oral suspension is available in some countries on a compassionate basis, with better absorption features.
Main drug interactions	Decreased absorption with antacids, cimetidine, or omeprazole; increased metabolism with rifampicin, rifabutin, or phenytoin.
Main side effects	Rash, nausea.

Fluconazole
- Fluconazole is as effective as other azoles, but it is predominantly renally excreted so the patient does not suffer from hepatic metabolism problems.

Standard dosage	Fluconazole 50–400 mg daily for 1–4 weeks.
Contraindications	Azole hypersensitivity.
Special points	Reduced dose in patients with renal impairment.
Main drug interactions	Pentamidine, amphotericin-induced nephrotoxicity may impair renal excretion.
Main side effects	Abnormalities in liver function (higher doses), rashes.

Treatment aims
To suppress *Candida albicans* overgrowth.

Prognosis
- 59% of patients with pseudomembranous candidiasis develop an AIDS diagnosis within 3 months.
- ~80% of patients with acute *Pneumocystis carinii* pneumonia also have buccal candidiasis.
- 80% of patients with a successfully treated episode of buccal or oesophageal candidiasis relapse within 3 months.

Follow-up and management
- Patients often relapse after treatment, so detecting relapses early is important; they are often mild and easily treated over time.
- As immunodeficiency worsens, episodes become more frequent and less responsive to treatment; occasionally, continuous suppressive doses of an azole or courses of intravenous amphotericin are needed.

Causes of treatment failure
Poor drug absorption.
Increased metabolism or excretion from other drugs.
Candida albicans developing drug resistance.
Non-albicans species or dual infection.
Immunodeficiency too severe for drug treatment alone to work.

Key references
Klein RS *et al.*: Oral candidiasis in high risk patients as the initial manifestation of the acquired immunodeficiency syndrome. *N Engl J Med* 1984, **311**:354-358.

Laine L *et al.*: Fluconazole compared with ketoconazole for the treatment of *Candida* esophagitis in AIDS. A randomized trial. *Ann Intern Med* 1992, **117**:655–660.

Miyasaki SH *et al.*: The identification and tracking of *Candida albicans* isolates from oral lesions in HIV-seropositive individuals. *J Acquir Immun Defic Syndr* 1992, **5**:1039–1046.

Smith DE *et al.*: Itraconazole versus ketoconazole in the treatment of oral and oesophageal candidosis in patients infected with HIV. *AIDS* 1991, **5**:1367–1371.

Cytomegalovirus infection in AIDS
C. Katlama

Diagnosis

Symptoms

Loss of vision, floaters, decrease in visual acuity, unexplained fever: indicating retinitis (asymptomatic at early stage).

Fever, anorexia, weight loss, diarrhoea, pain, cramps: indicating gastrointestinal tract infection (oesophagitis, gastritis, colitis).

Fever, motor deficit, headaches, seizures, somnolence: indicating myelitis.

Motor or sensitive deficit, incontinence: indicating myelitis.

Fever, cough, dyspnoea: indicating pneumonitis.

Signs

Fever: in 60–80% of patients with cytomegalovirus disseminated infection.

Decreased visual acuity: indicating retinitis.

Weight loss, abdominal tenderness, haemorrhages: indicating gastrointestinal tract infections.

Neurological deficit, lethargy, coma: indicating CNS complications.

Increase of respiratory rate, minimal findings at auscultation: indicating pneumonitis.

Investigations

- The disease is caused by recrudescence of a latent infection, so serological tests are of limited value.

Fundoscopy: in retinitis, shows haemorrhagic exudates and necrotic areas.

Endoscopy: in gastrointestinal tract infection, shows submucosal haemorrhages, ulceration; each level of tract may be involved, e.g. oesophagus, stomach, duodenum, small intestine, or colon.

Ultrasonography: in cholangitis, shows dilatation of biliary tract.

Biopsy: in cholangitis, shows cytomegalovirus inclusions.

CSF culture: in encephalitis or myelitis, shows increased cells (nonspecific), presence of cytomegalovirus (unusual) in culture or polymerase chain reaction.

CT or MRI: in encephalitis or myelitis, shows ventriculitis or ependymitis, using contrast enhancement.

Bronchoalveolar lavage or biopsy: in pneumonitis, shows cytomegalovirus inclusions.

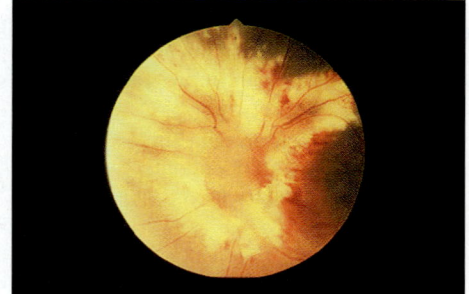

Fundoscopic appearance of cytomegalovirus retinitis.

Complications

Loss of vision, retinal detachment, acute retinal necrosis.

Gastrointestinal tract perforation, haemorrhages.

Respiratory failure.

Coma or death.

Differential diagnosis

Retinitis
Cotton-wool spot.
Toxoplasmosis.
Herpes simplex or varicella–zoster virus.
Acute retinal necrosis.
Syphilis.
Pneumocystis carinii choroiditis.

Gastrointestinal tract
Cryptosporidiosis or microsporidiosis.
Giardia, *Entamoeba*, *Shigella*, or *Campylobacter* spp. infection.
Lymphoma.
Kaposi's sarcoma.

Encephalitis or myelitis
HIV encephalopathy or myelopathy.
Progressive multifocal leukoencephalopathy.
Aseptic meningitis.
Herpes virus encephalitis.

Pneumonitis
Pneumocystis carinii infection.
Mycobacteria infection.

Aetiology

- Reactivation of latent cytomegalovirus infection due to underlying immune deficiency may be a cause.
- Cytomegalovirus infection is a potential cofactor of HIV disease.

Epidemiology

- >90% of homosexual or bisexual men have latent cytomegalovirus infection.
- Cytomegalovirus disease is found in 20–40% of AIDS patients.
- End-stage opportunistic infection occurs in 90% of patients with CD4 counts of $<50 \times 10^6$/L (median, 25×10^6/L).

Treatment

Diet and lifestyle
- During the acute phase of any gastrointestinal tract localization, spicy food should be avoided and alcohol or aspirin consumption restricted.

Pharmacological treatment

Choice of treatment
- Systemic treatment is indicated in acute visceral localization. Foscarnet and ganciclovir have similar efficacy: 90% in retinitis, 80–95% in gastrointestinal tract disorder, 60–80% in pneumonitis.
- Maintenance treatment is indicated for retinitis and gastrointestinal tract involvement (non-systematically). Foscarnet and ganciclovir have similar efficacy: 50% relapse within 4 months.

Foscarnet
- Foscarnet is active against all herpes viruses, including cytomegalovirus, and HIV.
- Advantages include absence of haemotoxicity and anti-HIV effect; disadvantages include the long infusion time.

Standard dosage	*Acute:* foscarnet 90–100 mg/kg in 0.75–1 L saline isotonic solution i.v. twice daily 90 min infusion for 2–3 weeks. *Maintenance:* foscarnet 90–100 mg/kg 0.75–1 L saline isotonic solution i.v. once daily, 90–120 min infusion.
Contraindications	Renal impairment, concomitant nephrotoxic drugs.
Main drug interactions	Amphotericin B, i.v. pentamidine.
Main side effects	Nephrotoxicity, hypocalcaemia, nausea, genital ulcer.

Ganciclovir
- Ganciclovir is more practical than foscarnet.
- It is used for systemic therapy.
- It is active against cytomegalovirus and herpes virus.
- Disadvantages include haemotoxicity and resistance in some strains of cytomegalovirus.

Standard dosage	*Acute:* ganciclovir 5 mg/kg i.v. twice daily, 20 min infusion for 2–3 weeks. *Maintenance:* ganciclovir 5 mg/kg i.v. once daily long term.
Contraindications	Neutropenia, anaemia, resistant strains.
Main drug interactions	Zidovudine and other haemotoxic drugs.
Main side effects	Neutropenia, thrombocytopenia (frequent); rash-convulsion (unusual).

- Recently, oral ganciclovir 3 g daily has been shown to reduce progression after i.v. induction. Prophylaxis with this drug for patients with CD4 counts $<100 \times 10^6$/L reduces the rate of subsequent cytomegalovirus disease.

Treatment aims
To prevent replication of cytomegalovirus. To halt progress of disease.

Prognosis
- The incidence of recurrent visceral manifestations of cytomegalovirus is high.
- Medium survival is 12–18 months.
- Without maintenance treatment, the relapse rate is 90% in retinitis.

Follow-up and management
- Patients having acute treatment should be followed up every week.
- Patients having maintenance treatment must be followed up every 2–3 weeks.

Key references

Dieterich D: Cytomegalovirus colitis in AIDS. *J Acquir Immune Defic Syndr* 1991 **Suppl 1**:529–535.

Jabs D, SOCA group: Mortality in patients with acquired immunodeficiency syndrome treated with either foscarnet or ganciclovir for cytomegalovirus retinitis. *N Engl J Med* 1992, **326**:213–220.

Katlama C *et al.*: Foscarnet induction therapy from CMV retinitis in AIDS. Comparison of twice daily and three times daily regimens. *J Acquir Immune Defic Syndr* 1992, **5**:518–524.

Diarrhoea and HIV infection — B.G. Gazzard

Diagnosis

Symptoms
Watery, large-volume diarrhoea: >400 ml daily.
Little abdominal pain.
Little vomiting.

Signs
Prominent weight loss and dehydration: possibly.

Investigations
Stool staining and microscopy: possibly with concentration of stools; Ziehl–Neelsen stain for cryptosporidia and *Isospora* spp.; trichome or florescent stain for microsporidia; microscopy of fresh stool for amoeba and cysts of *Giardia* spp.

Small-intestinal biopsy: electron microscopy gold standard for diagnosis of microsporidia, although these are seen by stool staining or light microscopy; histological diagnosis of *Giardia* spp., *Isospora* spp., and cryptosporidia made in ~10% of patients without parasites detected in stools.

Rectal biopsy: microsporidia not seen; evidence of cryptosporidia or amoebae unsuspected in stool analysis occasionally found.

Tests of malabsorption: protozoan infection associated with partial villus atrophy and malabsorption, particularly of vitamin B_{12} (Schilling test).

Complications
Toxic dilatation: unusual.

Right upper quadrant pain, cholangeographic appearances of 'AIDS-related sclerosing cholangitis'.

Gross wasting, inanition, death.

Differential diagnosis
Viral diarrhoea: cytomegalovirus infection may be bloody and associated with abdominal pain.

Bacterial diarrhoea: *Shigella*, *Salmonella*, and *Campylobacter* spp. cause acute diarrhoea with systemic symptoms; opportunistic bacterial infection by *Mycobacterium avium intracellulare* causes watery diarrhoea in patients with severely reduced CD4 counts ($<100 \times 10^6$/L).

'Pathogen-negative diarrhoea': after complete investigation, large-volume diarrhoea with no cause is rare; low-volume irritable-bowel diarrhoea is more common in patients with CD4 counts $>200 \times 10^6$/L.

Aetiology
- Causes include the following:
Cryptosporidia infection.
Microsporidia infection (at least two species: *Septata intestinalis* and *Enterocytozoon bienusi*).
Isospora spp. infection.
Entamoeba spp. infection.
Giardia spp. infection.

Epidemiology
- Cryptosporidiosis occurs in animal handlers and is associated with sexual transmission; water-borne outbreaks are known.
- Microsporidiosis only occurs in severely immunosuppressed patients (CD4 lymphocyte count $<100 \times 10^6$/L).
- *Isospora* infection is common in South Americans and Africans; it occasionally occurs in travellers to these continents.
- Infection by *Entamoeba* spp. is common in homosexual men, although these strains are usually not pathogenic.
- *Giardia* infection is common in homosexual men (possible sexual transmission); it is more common in HIV-seropositive men.

Treatment

Diet and lifestyle
- Safe sexual practices reduce sexual transmission.
- Immunosuppressed patients with a CD4 count $<200 \times 10^6$/L should boil drinking water.
- Care must be taken when gardening or handling pets or domestic animals.

Pharmacological treatment

General treatment
Rehydration, usually with oral rehydration fluids.

Stool volume reduction with antimotility agents (e.g. codeine phosphate 30–80 mg daily) or stronger opiates.

Specific vitamin supplementation for malabsorption.

Transient stool volume reduction during treatment by somatostatin analogues (e.g. octreotide 50–200 µg 2–3 times daily).

For cryptosporidiosis
- No standard treatment is of proven value.

Standard dosage	Paromomycin 500 mg 4 times daily (most successful). Alternatively, erythromycin 500 mg 4 times daily, spiramycin 1 g 3–4 times daily, or azithromycin up to 1.5 g daily.
Contraindications	None.
Special points	*Paromomycin:* stool volumes reduced by 50%, but cryptosporidia not eradicated.
Main drug interactions	None known.
Main side effects	None known.

For microsporidiosis
- No standard treatment is of proven value.

Standard dosage	Albendazole 400 mg twice daily or metronidazole 400 mg 3 times daily.
Contraindications	None.
Special points	*Albendazole:* eradicates *Septata intestinalis*, less effect on *Enterocytozoon bienusi*. *Metronidazole:* may produce symptomatic benefit.
Main drug interactions	*Metronidazole:* alcohol.
Main side effects	*Metronidazole:* nausea.

For *Entamoeba histolytica* infection
- Metronidazole 400 mg 3 times daily for 1 week is usually given, although the pathogenesis of the organism is often uncertain.

For giardiasis
- Patients can be given metronidazole 1.2–2 g daily for 3 days, tinidazole 2 g initially, repeated if necessary, or mepacrine 100 mg 3 times daily for 5–7 days, repeated after 2 weeks if necessary.

Treatment aims
To resolve diarrhoea.

To eradicate organism.

To promote weight gain or prevent weight loss.

Prognosis

Cryptosporidiosis
- In patients with CD4 counts $>200 \times 10^6$/L, the diarrhoea resolves eventually.
- In patients with CD4 counts $<200 \times 10^6$/L, the diarrhoea may be chronic.
- Diarrhoea usually continues despite treatment.
- In patients with CD4 counts $>200 \times 10^6$/L, the prognosis depends on the CD4 count, rather than on the diarrhoea.
- In patients with CD4 counts $<200 \times 10^6$/L, median survival is 1 year.

Microsporidiosis
- Diarrhoea usually continues despite treatment.
- Median survival is <1 year.

Other infections
- Diarrhoea usually resolves with treatment, but patients may relapse after treatment has stopped.
- The prognosis depends on the underlying CD4 count, rather than on the diarrhoea.

Follow-up and management
- Eradication of organism must be checked.
- Continuing diarrhoea leads to wasting due to severe anorexia; therefore, the need for supplements, elemental diets, or nasogastric or gastrostomy feeding must be reviewed.

Key references
Blanchard C *et al.*: Cryptosporidiosis in HIV-seropositive patients. *Q J Med* 1992, **85**:813–823.

Dietrich DT, Rahmin M: Cytomegalovirus colitis in AIDS. *J Acquir Immun Defic Syndr* 1991, **4 (suppl 1)**: S29–S35.

Orenstein J *et al.*: Intestinal microsporidiosis as a cause of diarrhoea in human immunodeficiency virus-infected patients. *Hum Pathol* 1991, **21**:475–481.

Kaposi's sarcoma in AIDS F. Boag

Diagnosis

Symptoms

Mucocutaneous
Psychosocial problems.
Pain, restricted movement: due to flexion contractures and bulk of tumour; late-stage.

Lymphatic
Painful lymphadenopathy and oedema.

Pulmonary
- 20–50% of patients are asymptomatic; the disease is found *post mortem*.

Dyspnoea, haemoptysis, chest pain (pleuritic or dull ache).

Gastrointestinal
- Up to 50% of patients are asymptomatic; the disease is found *post mortem*.

Anorexia, abdominal pain, haematemesis, melaena.

Signs

Mucocutaneous
Pink, violacious, purple, brown, or black macule, plaque, or nodule.
Surrounding purple/yellow halo.

Lymphatic
Firm or indurated lymphadenopathy.
Oedema of dependent limbs.
Compression of adjacent structures.

Pulmonary
Chest clear or with effusion or scattered crepitations.
Respiratory failure.

Gastrointestinal
Signs of intermittent or acute bowel obstruction.
Palpable mass.

Other signs
Organomegaly.

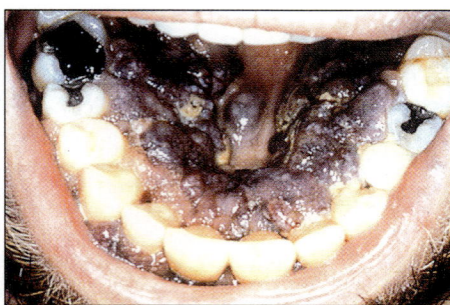
Oral Kaposi's sarcoma in HIV disease

Investigations

General
Lymphocyte subset analysis: Kaposi's sarcoma can occur at any stage; tends to be more aggressive in immunosuppressed patients (CD4 count <200 × 10^6/L).
Full blood count: to assess anaemia; neutrophil and platelet count needed before chemotherapy.
Skin biopsy: for confirmation.

Pulmonary
Chest radiography: may be normal or reveal infiltrates, nodules, or pleural effusion.
Fibreoptic bronchoscopy: for visualization and biopsy.

Gastrointestinal
Fibreoptic endoscopy or sigmoidoscopy: for visualization and biopsy.
Ultrasonography or CT: with guided biopsy, if disease is not seen by endoscopy.
Laparoscopy or laparotomy: for intermittent or acute bowel obstruction, to relieve obstruction and obtain biopsy.

Complications

Ulceration, infection, immobilization oedema.
Gastrointestinal obstruction, haemorrhage.
Respiratory failure.

Differential diagnosis
Purpura, haematoma, angioma, naevus.
Bacillary angiomatosis, dermatofibroma, melanoma.

Aetiology
- The cause is unknown, but the following may have a role:

Genetic predisposition (elderly men from eastern Europe and Africa).
Immunosuppression.
HIV infection.
Growth factors and cytokines promoting growth of Kaposi's sarcoma.
Possibly, a transmitted cofactor (perhaps sexually transmitted).
Possibly, a new human herpes virus.

Epidemiology
- Kaposi's sarcoma occurs in up to 48% of homosexual men with AIDS.
- It is increasing in heterosexual Africans with AIDS, in women who have acquired HIV from bisexual men, and in other risk groups.
- It is rare in children with AIDS.
- It is rarely seen in haemophiliac patients with AIDS.

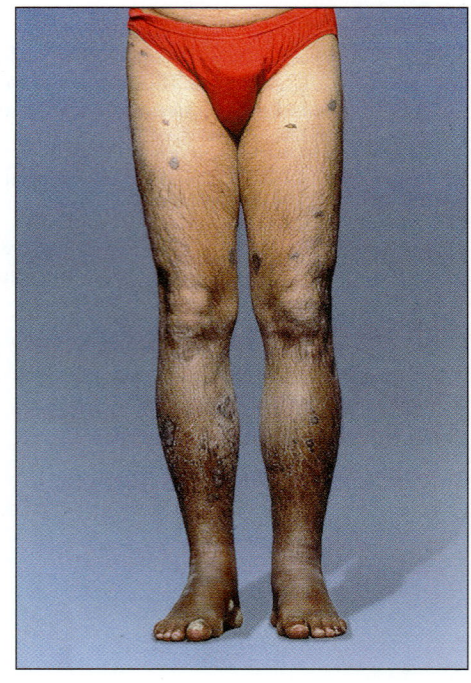
Generalized cutaneous Kaposi's sarcoma.

Treatment

Diet and lifestyle
- Energy intake should be sufficient to maintain weight; vitamin and micronutrient intake must be adequate.
- Safe sex is recommended.

Pharmacological treatment
- All treatment must be given under specialist supervision.

Intralesional chemotherapy
- Intralesional chemotherapy is indicated for limited mucocutaneous disease.

Standard dosage	Vinblastine into lesion until blanching occurs.
Contraindications	Infection at site.
Main drug interactions	None of importance.
Main side effects	Local pain and ulceration.

Interferons
- Interferons are indicated for good-prognosis Kaposi's sarcoma.

Standard dosage	Interferon-α i.m. or s.c. daily, possibly with zidovudine.
Contraindications	Bone-marrow suppression, renal or hepatic impairment.
Special points	Lesions may recur after treatment stops.
Main drug interactions	None of importance.
Main side effects	Influenza-like symptoms, neutropenia, anaemia.

Bleomycin and vincristine
- These are the first-line chemotherapy in the UK, for patients with rapidly progressive disease.

Standard dosage	Vincristine (or vinblastine if neuropathy develops) and bleomycin every 2 weeks, with hydrocortisone.
Contraindications	Pregnancy and lactation (all), severe lung impairment (bleomycin); caution if patient has a neuropathy.
Main drug interactions	Increased phenytoin concentrations.
Main side effects	*Bleomycin*: rashes, increased skin pigmentation, Raynaud's phenomenon, hypersensitivity reaction, dose-related progressive pulmonary fibrosis. *Vincristine*: alopecia, peripheral and autonomic neuropathy. *Vinblastine*: myelotoxicity, neurotoxic (less than vincristine).

Etoposide or epirubicin
- Etoposide or epirubicin is used if standard chemotherapy fails.

Standard dosage	Etoposide for 3 days every 21 days or orally for 14 days every 28 days. Epirubicin weekly.
Contraindications	Significant new motor weakness, pregnancy or lactation; caution in cardiac disease (epirubicin).
Main drug interactions	None of importance.
Main side effects	*Etoposide*: myelotoxicity, alopecia, nausea, vomiting. *Epirubicin*: cardiomyopathy, skin irritation.

Liposomal daunorubicin and doxorubicin
- Liposomal daunorubicin and doxorubicin are currently available within clinical trials or for compassionate use only; they are fairly widely used in the UK.

Treatment aims
To achieve cosmetic improvement (limited disease).
To control new lesion development and to treat existing lesions (advancing disease).
To reduce tumour bulk and to treat pain, immobility, and infection (advanced disease).

Other treatments
- Radiotherapy under specialist supervision is the treatment of choice unless control of new lesion is required; it is often combined with chemotherapy.
- It is very sensitive and so must be used with extreme caution.
- Side effects include erythema, increased pigmentation, and oropharynx.

Prognosis
- Prognosis is extremely variable; survival may be for months or years.
- Death is often due to other AIDS-defining illnesses.
- Factors indicating poor prognosis include the following:

CD4 count $<200 \times 10^6$/L.
Previous opportunistic infections.
'B' symptoms.
Tumour-associated oedema.
Non-nodal visceral Kaposi's sarcoma.

Follow-up and management
- Full blood count must be monitored.
- Patients with limited disease must be followed up every 3 months.
- Patients with extensive disease must be followed up every 1–2 weeks.

Key references
Cohen J: Is a new virus the cause of KS? *Science* 1994, **266**:1803–1804.

Lilenbaum RC, Ratner L: Systemic treatment of Kaposi's sarcoma: current status and future directions. *AIDS* 1994, **8**:141–151.

Milliken S, Boyle M: Update on HIV and neoplastic disease. *AIDS* 1993, **7 (suppl 1)**: 203–209.

Meningitis, cryptococcal in AIDS — R.J. Guiloff

Diagnosis

Symptoms

Immunosuppression: with CD4 counts $<100 \times 10^9$/L.

Short history: usually <3 weeks but can be acute (~24 h).

Headache: in 81% of patients.

Fever: in 77%.

Nausea or vomiting: in 44%.

Photophobia: in 27%.

Seizures: in 5%; can be the presenting feature.

Signs

- No signs are reported in >50% of patients, depending much on the experience of the examiner.

Abnormal mental state: in 28%.

Focal neurological signs and papilloedema: rare; if present, space-occupying lesions such as toxoplasmosis or cerebral lymphoma should be suspected.

Extraneural involvement: in 20%, with pulmonary infiltrates and, occasionally, skin lesions.

Investigations

- Cryptococcal antigen in blood is nearly always positive.

CT or MRI: must be performed before lumbar puncture to exclude a mass lesion; usually shows no abnormality or cerebral atrophy; communicating hydrocephalus infrequent; low-density lesions, scattered and symmetrical, sometimes seen, attributed to dilatation of the Virchow–Robin perivascular spaces by collections of cryptococci or to infarcts.

CSF culture: to establish diagnosis; usually shows mononuclear pleocytosis (<700/ml) and raised protein; glucose may be low, sometimes the only abnormality; india-ink preparation can suggest cryptococci in 75% of patients; cryptococcal antigen usually positive; cryptococcus can be cultured from other sites (sputum, blood, faeces, bone marrow) in 65%.

Other investigations: abnormal liver function, low albumin concentration, or hyponatraemia in 20%; lymphopenia common in peripheral blood.

Complications

Death: during the acute illness despite treatment (up to 30% of patients); sometimes due to other overwhelming systemic infections or progression of the meningitis with seizures, cranial nerve palsies, stupor, and coma.

Cerebral cryptococcomas: i.e. cryptococcal abscesses; rare.

Differential diagnosis

Viral and tuberculous meningitis.
Cerebral toxoplasmosis.
Cerebral lymphoma.
Benign headaches (migraine, tension, depression).
Other causes of fever.

Aetiology

- Cryptococcus is a yeast present in high quantities in the excreta from pigeons.
- Infection is acquired by inhalation.
- The spread to the CNS is haematogenous.

Epidemiology

- Most cases of cryptococcal meningitis are AIDS-related.
- Cryptococcal meningitis is found in 2–12% of AIDS patients in different clinical series and in 3–11% on post-mortem examination.
- It is the presentation of AIDS or the AIDS-defining illness in 46% of HIV-seropositive patients who have it.
- It is the most frequent cause of meningitis and the third most common opportunistic infection, after cytomegalovirus and *T. gondii* in AIDS patients.

Treatment

Diet and lifestyle
- No special precautions are necessary.

Pharmacological treatment

Initial treatment
- The established initial treatment is by amphotericin B and flucytosine.
- Treatment of the first episode fails in 15–30% of patients.
- Two successive negative cultures of CSF, blood, and urine obtained at least 1 week apart are a good criterion for improvement.

Standard dosage	Amphotericin B 0.25 mg/kg i.v. daily, increasing to 1–1.5 mg/kg over 3 days, and flucytosine 50 mg/kg daily. Usual course is 6 weeks; some give amphotericin B alone for 2–6 weeks, depending on improvement.
Contraindications	Renal failure, pregnancy, breast-feeding, old age.
Special points	Hepatic and renal function, blood count, electrolytes, and drug concentrations must be monitored.
Main drug interactions	*Amphotericin B:* increased risk of nephrotoxicity with cyclosporin, aminoglycosides; antagonizes miconazole.
Main side effects	*Amphotericin B:* nausea, vomiting, fever, nephrotoxicity. *Flucytosine:* diarrhoea, bone-marrow suppression.

Maintenance treatment
- ~50% of HIV-seropositive patients with cryptococcal meningitis relapse without maintenance treatment.
- The usual reason for a prophylactic antifungal such as fluconazole is to protect against *Candida* infection and cryptococcal meningitis.

Standard dosage	Fluconazole 200–400 mg orally daily for life.
Contraindications	Possibly breast-feeding, pregnancy, children.
Special points	Can be used for initial treatment i.v. or orally at 400 mg daily in mildly ill patients who are not obtunded. Itraconazole is a useful alternative.
Main drug interactions	Enhances warfarin, phenytoin, theophylline, cyclosporin, sulphonylureas; reduces rifampicin.
Main side effects	Diarrhoea, bone-marrow suppression.

Treatment aims
To eradicate cryptococcal infection.

Prognosis
- 30–50% of patients do not respond to treatment.

Follow-up and management
- Patients should be closely followed, particularly for the first year when relapses are more common.

Key references
Bozzette SA et al.: A placebo controlled trial of maintenance therapy with fluconazole after treatment of cryptococcal meningitis in the acquired immmunodeficiency syndrome. California Collaborative Treatment Group. *N Engl J Med* 1991, **324**:580–584.

Chuck SL, Sande MA: Infections with *Cryptococcus neoformans* in the acquired immunodeficiency syndrome. *N Engl J Med* 1989, **321**:794–799.

Saag MS et al.: Comparison of amphotericin B with fluconazole in the treatment of acute AIDS-associated cryptococcal meningitis. *N Engl J Med* 1992, **326**:83–89.

Weinke T et al.: Cryptococcosis in AIDS patients: observations concerning CNS involvement. *J Neurol* 1989, **236**:38–42.

Mycobacterium avium intracellulare infection in AIDS — R.F. Miller

Diagnosis

Symptoms
- Symptoms of disseminated *Mycobacterium avium* or *M. intracellulare* infection may be difficult to distinguish from those of HIV infection.
- Disseminated infection may be asymptomatic.

Systemic
Fever: with or without sweats.
Anorexia and malaise.
Weight loss: often associated with anaemia and neutropenia.

Gastrointestinal
Chronic diarrhoea and abdominal pain: resulting from *M. avium intracellulare* invasion of the colon or small bowel or bulky retroperitoneal lymph nodes infected by *M. avium intracellulare*.
Chronic malabsorption: similar to Whipple's disease.
Extrabiliary obstructive jaundice: secondary to periportal lymphadenopathy.

Signs
Weight loss, oral candidiasis, cutaneous Kaposi's sarcoma: evidence of underlying HIV infection and other HIV-associated complications.

Weight loss, anaemia, hepato(spleno)megaly: indicating disseminated disease.

Localized or cutaneous abscesses, endophthalmitis, arthritis, localized pneumonia: rare; tend to occur in patients with CD4 counts $>100 \times 10^6$/L.

Investigations
Biopsy: diagnosis of disseminated *M. avium intracellulare* infection made by isolation or culture from any normally sterile site (blood, bone-marrow, lymph-node, and liver biopsy best); negative blood cultures unusual with positive histology from lymph-node, liver, or bone-marrow biopsy; stains may show acid and alcohol-fast bacilli before blood cultures become positive, thus suggesting diagnosis.

Blood culture: using lysis/centrifugation or radiometric technique, yield increased (from 60% to almost 100%); 5–50 days needed for blood cultures to become positive.

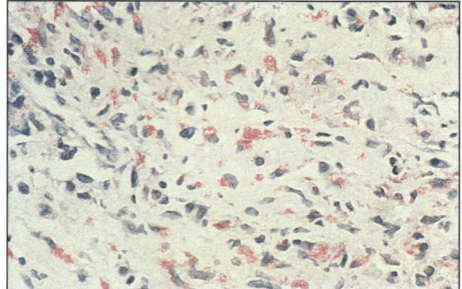

Lymph node biopsy. Numerous clumps of acid-fast bacilli are seen within the tissue. There is no granulamatous response. Magnification × 400.

- Isolation of *M. avium intracellulare* from sputum, bronchoalveolar lavage, and urine is frequent but is not diagnostic of disseminated infection.

Complications
None.

Differential diagnosis
Progression of HIV or other systemic opportunistic infection.

Aetiology
- Two closely related species, *Mycobacterium avium* and *M. intracellulare*, known as *M. avium intracellulare*, cause widely disseminated infection in AIDS patients: up to 30% have disseminated infection diagnosed before death, and about 50% are found to have it at post-mortem examination.
- Disseminated infection occurs exclusively in patients with advanced HIV disease and CD4 counts $<100 \times 10^6$/L.
- The host defect in AIDS patients allowing dissemination is probably macrophage dysfunction.
- The source of invasion in AIDS patients may be gastrointestinal or respiratory: large numbers of mycobacteria within macrophages of the small bowel lamina propria suggest that the bowel is the portal of entry; respiratory isolation of *M. avium intracellulare* (not diagnostic of disseminated infection) frequently precedes disseminated infection, suggesting that infection may also begin in the lungs.

Epidemiology
- *M. avium intracellulare* is ubiquitous in the environment, being found in water, soil, animals, and dairy products.

Pathogenesis and pathology
- Almost all AIDS patients with disseminated *M. avium intracellulare* have positive blood cultures (in contrast to those with stool, urine, or respiratory secretion colonization).
- Mycobacteraemia usually ranges from 10^1 to 10^4 colony-forming units/ml blood.
- In patients with disseminated infection, the liver, spleen, and lymph nodes are found at post-mortem examination to contain up to 10^{10} colony-forming units/g tissue.
- Histology of involved organs reveals absent or poorly formed granulomata and mycobacteria within macrophages. Little tissue destruction is seen, despite heavy mycobacterial load.

Treatment

Diet and lifestyle
- No special precautions are necessary.

Pharmacological treatment
- *Mycobacterium avium intracellulare* is resistant to most antituberculous drugs at concentrations achievable in plasma, yet >50% of strains can be inhibited by achievable concentrations of amikacin, azithromycin, ciprofloxacin, clarithromycin, clofazimine, cycloserine, ethambutol, ethionamide, or rifabutin.
- Single-agent treatment (e.g. by clarithromycin) is of temporary benefit only: fever, anorexia, and mycobacteraemia return rapidly; combination therapy is more effective.

Standard dosage	Rifabutin 300–600 mg orally once daily and ethambutol 15 mg/kg orally once daily, with clarithromycin 500–1000 mg orally twice daily. Ciprofloxacin 500 mg orally twice daily and clofazimine 100 mg orally once daily can be used in cases of intolerance, although benefit is limited. Amikacin 7.5 mg/kg i.v. once daily may be added for patients with refractory fever or anorexia. Treatment is given for 2–4 weeks.
Contraindications	Previous drug hypersensitivity. *Rifabutin*: jaundice, porphyria. *Ethambutol*: renal impairment, optic neuritis. *Clarithromycin*: porphyria, hepatic or renal failure.
Special points	Drug levels must be monitored. Palliative glucocorticoids (oral prednisolone 1–2 mg/kg daily) may be given to patients with very advanced HIV disease who have profound anorexia and weight loss, without adversely affecting prognosis.
Main drug interactions	*Rifabutin:* induces hepatic microsome enzyme activity and so increases metabolism of azole drugs; interacts with fluconazole or clarithromycin to produce uveitis in 30% of patients if >300 mg of rifabutin are given daily. If steroids are given with an antibacterial regimen containing rifampicin or rifabutin, the dose should be doubled to take account of the hepatic microsome-inducing effects of the drugs.
Main side effects	*Rifabutin*: nausea and vomiting, diarrhoea, anorexia; body fluids become orange-red. *Ethambutol*: optic neuritis, red–green colour blindness, peripheral neuritis. *Ciprofloxacin*: nausea and vomiting, abdominal pain, diarrhoea, headache, photosensitivity, arthralgia, myalgia. *Clarithromycin*: nausea and vomiting, abdominal pain, diarrhoea. *Clofazimine*: nausea, giddiness, headache, diarrhoea; skin and urine coloured terracotta red.

- Recent studies have shown that long-term rifabutin 300 mg orally once daily given as primary prophylaxis to patients with AIDS and CD4 counts 200 × 10^6/L reduces the risk of developing *M. avium intracellulare* bacteraemia by half but does not improve survival.

Treatment aims
To reduce mycobacteraemia or fever and transfusion requirements.
- Cure is not achievable.

Prognosis
- Survival in AIDS patients with disseminated *Mycobacterium avium intracellulare* infection is shorter (median, 4.1 months) than in comparable patients (with similar CD4 counts) without disseminated infection (median, 11 months).
- The presence of *M. avium intracellulare* in respiratory secretions strongly predicts the subsequent development of disseminated infection.

Follow-up and management
- Treatment is for life.

Key references
Jacobson MA: Mycobacterial disease. In *The Medical Management of AIDS* edn 3. Edited by Sande MA, Volberding PA. Philadelphia: WB Saunders, 1992, pp 284–296.

Masur H: Recommendations on prophylaxis and therapy for disseminated *Mycobacterium avium* complex disease in patients infected with the human immuno-deficiency virus. *N Engl J Med* 1993, **329**:898-904.

Scoular A, French P, Miller RF: *Mycobacterium avium intracellulare* infection in the acquired immunodeficiency syndrome. *Br J Hosp Med* 1991, **46**:295–300.

Pneumocystis carinii pneumonia in AIDS — S.E. Barton

Diagnosis

Symptoms

Fever, fatigue, weight loss: for weeks or months before respiratory symptoms develop.

Non-productive cough, shortness of breath: initially on exertion, then at rest with disease progression.

- The absence of symptoms does not exclude *Pneumocystis carinii* pneumonia, especially in patients who are receiving prophylaxis or who have had previous episodes of infection.

Signs

Wasting, fever, diffuse lymphadenopathy, oral candidiasis, hairy leukoplakia, cutaneous Kaposi's sarcoma: general signs of immunosuppression secondary to HIV infection.

Tachypnoea, dry rales: revealed by auscultation, but often no chest signs.

Splenomegaly, fundal abnormalities: rare extrapulmonary signs of infection.

Investigations

- An HIV antibody test is not necessary in patients not known to be previously infected by HIV but who have evident immunosuppression leading to a diagnosis of AIDS. More significant is a CD4 lymphocyte cell count: *Pneumocystis carinii* pneumonia is more probable if the count is $<200 \times 10^6/L$.

Full blood count: to exclude anaemia.

Plain chest radiography: may show diffuse interstitial infiltration, sensitive but non-specific indicator of disease; various other appearances, including lobar shadowing, occur.

Arterial oxygen tension measurement: hypoxia common in advanced disease, but its absence does not exclude diagnosis, and it is present with many other respiratory conditions.

Exercise oximetry: a useful noninvasive test; positive result defined as fall in arterial oxygen tension to <90% during 10 min exercise on an exercise cycle set to standard resistance and speed.

Sputum analysis: obviates need for routine bronchoscopy if laboratory is experienced; sputum induced by inhaled nebulized hypertonic saline solution; samples stained by Grocott and immunofluorescent stains.

Baseline U&E measurement, liver function tests: useful for evaluating response to and possible side effects of treatment.

Fibreoptic bronchoscopy: reserved for patients who do not respond to treatment after 5 days or whose test results are either inconclusive or suggest separate or additional disorder.

Complications

Pneumothorax.

Restrictive lung disease.

Non-pulmonary disseminated *Pneumocystis carinii* infection.

Adult respiratory distress syndrome.

Differential diagnosis

Bacterial chest infection.
Pulmonary Kaposi's sarcoma.
Pulmonary tuberculosis.
Bronchial candidiasis.
Lymphoma.
Symptomatic anaemia.
Asthma.
Cytomegalovirus pneumonitis.
Septicaemia.
Histoplasmosis.
Disseminated blastomycosis.

Aetiology

- The pneumonia is caused by infection by *Pneumocystis carinii* (possibly a fungus or protozoan).
- Acquisition may be common early in life (and controlled by the immune system) or occur shortly before the disease develops.

Epidemiology

- Most children have serological evidence of previous *Pneumocystis carinii* infection by the age of 4 years; the disease was first recognised because of epidemics in orphanages after World War II.
- The disease is the most common AIDS opportunistic infection in people with HIV-induced immunosuppression, with no difference between sex or race, although it occurs significantly less often in many developing countries.

Treatment

Diet and lifestyle
- Special attention to nutrition and supplementation of diet is needed during and after *Pneumocystis carinii* pneumonia.

Pharmacological treatment

Treatment of the disease
- Most treatment is based on inhibition of folic acid metabolism.
- The most effective agent is co-trimoxazole; in less severely ill patients, oral treatment may be used.
- Unfortunately, up to 40% of patients fail to complete a treatment course because of allergic or toxic side effects.
- Alternative treatment includes atovoquone, clindamycin and primaquine, trimethoprim and dapsone or pentamidine either i.v. or inhaled.
- Corticosteroids have been shown to reduce mortality and the risk of respiratory failure in patients presenting with partial arterial oxygen pressure <8 kPa. The subsequent use of antiretrovirals has been shown to improve survival.

Standard dosage	Co-trimoxazole 40 ml (960 mg/10 ml) in 5% dextrose 500 ml i.v. over 1–3 h twice daily for 14 days.
Contraindications	Hypersensitivity.
Special points	Full blood count, U&E monitoring, and liver function tests must be done.
Main drug interactions	None.
Main side effects	Nausea and vomiting (antiemetic can be given), skin rash, leucopenia, thrombocytopenia, raised liver function tests.

Prophylaxis
- Primary prophylaxis is recommended in patients with clinical evidence of immunosuppression (e.g. buccal candidiasis) or other opportunistic infections or laboratory evidence (CD4 count $<200 \times 10^6$/L).
- Secondary prophylaxis should be offered to patients who have had previous episodes of *Pneumocystis carinii* pneumonia.

Standard dosage	Co-trimoxazole 2 tablets 3 times weekly or 1 tablet daily. Alternatively, dapsone 100 mg daily or pentamidine 300 mg inhaled fortnightly.
Contraindications	Allergy to sulphonamides or trimethoprim.
Special points	Co-trimoxazole may also reduce the incidence of subsequent toxoplasmosis and bacterial infection.
Main drug interactions	None.
Main side effects	Skin rash, nausea and vomiting, leucopenia, thrombocytopenia, raised liver function tests.

Treatment aims
To treat pneumonia.
To return patient's quality of life.
To suppress future infection.

Prognosis
- Mortality for the first episode of *Pneumocystis carinii* pneumonia is <10% but is higher for subsequent attacks.

Follow-up and management
- Full blood count should be done after treatment because anaemia is common.
- Patients should be followed up at least monthly.

Key references
Masur H: Prevention and treatment of *Pneumocystis* pneumonia. *N Engl J Med* 1992, **327**:1853–1860.

Miller RF, Mitchell DM: AIDS and the lung: update. 1992. 1. *Pneumocystis carinii* pneumonia. *Thorax* 1992, **47**:305–314.

Moe AA, Hardy WD: *Pneumocystis carinii* infection in the HIV-seropositive patient. *Infect Dis Clin North Am* 1994, **8**:331–364.

Pulmonary complications of immunosuppression — A. Millar

Diagnosis

Symptoms
- Symptoms may be minimal.

Breathlessness, cough, sputum production, haemoptysis, chest pain, weight loss, general malaise.

- The combination of symptoms is important in differential diagnosis; for example, haemoptysis with chest pain suggests Kaposi's sarcoma in AIDS but pneumonia in other forms of immunosuppression.

Signs
- Possibly no signs are manifest.

Tachypnoea.
Cyanosis: indicating respiratory failure.
Consolidation: suggesting bacterial infection.
Collapse: suggesting infection or neoplasia.
Pleural effusion: suggesting mycobacterial infection or neoplasia.

Investigations
- The choice of investigation depends on the physical signs and symptoms and the degree of immunosuppression.

To assess degree of immunosuppression
Immunoglobulin measurement, leucocyte function assessment: in patients with suspected congenital immunosuppression.

Full blood count, differential leucocyte count: in patients with acquired immunosuppression, e.g. to assess neutropenia, after organ transplantation.

Immunoglobulin measurement, CD4 count: in patients with acquired immunosuppression; normal CD4 count in early stages of HIV infection, bacterial infection common; low CD4 count in late stages of HIV infection, opportunistic infection or neoplasia more likely.

To assess pulmonary complications of immunosuppression
Chest radiography: to identify focal or generalized abnormality.

CT: to assess pulmonary abnormalities in more detail (e.g. intrathoracic lymph nodes).

Gallium scan: to identify areas of abnormality in lung in patients with general malaise and nonspecific symptoms.

DTPA (diethylenetriaminepentaacetic acid) clearance measurement: to identify abnormalities in patients with breathlessness but few other symptoms, to show need for invasive investigation.

Oximetry or arterial blood gas measurement: at rest or exercise, essential for early detection of respiratory failure.

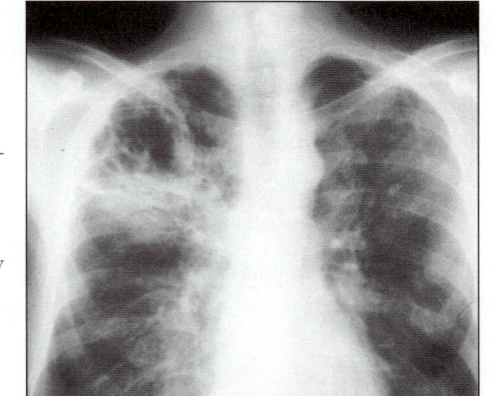

Chest radiograph showing cavitating aspergilloma.

Sputum culture and cytology: in patients with unproductive coughs, sputum may be induced by inhalation of 3% nebulized saline solution.

Bronchoscopy, bronchoalveolar lavage, transbronchial biopsy, open lung biopsy: for tissue diagnosis.

Mediastinoscopy: if mediastinal lymph-node disease has been identified.

Complications
Respiratory failure.
Disseminated infection.
Disseminated secondary malignancy.

Differential diagnosis
- The diagnosis depends on the course, stage, and degree of immunosuppression, in addition to local pathogenic load, which may differ in community, hospital, or geographical location.

Pneumocystis carinii pneumonia (see *Pneumocystis carinii* pneumonia in AIDS for details).
Bacterial infection (including mycobacteria).
Viral infection (e.g. cytomegalovirus).
Fungal infection (e.g. aspergillus, candida).
Parasitic infection.
Kaposi's sarcoma.
Secondary B cell lymphoma.
Secondary carcinoma.
Lymphocytic interstitial pneumonitis.
Graft-versus-host disease or rejection episodes in transplant recipients.

Aetiology

Congenital causes
Genetically determined absence or reduction in immune response, e.g. X-linked infantile hypogammaglobulinaemia (Bruton type).

Acquired causes
HIV infection.
Organ transplantation.
Drug treatment, e.g. steroids, azathiaprine, cyclosporin A (used in rheumatoid arthritis, asthma, ulcerative colitis).

Causes of relative immunosuppression
Diabetes.
Old age.

Epidemiology
- 1 in 100 000 people suffers from congenital immunosuppression.
- The incidence of acquired immunosuppression is increasing with the use of immunosuppressive drugs, organ transplantation, and HIV infection.

Treatment

Diet and lifestyle
- Excessive alcohol consumption and poor diet should be avoided because they can directly produce relative immunosuppression.
- Cigarette smoking should be stopped because of the increased incidence of pulmonary complications in immunosuppressed patients who smoke.

Pharmacological treatment
- Treatment depends on diagnosis, which should be as accurate as possible.
- In deteriorating patients, treatment must be started empirically, depending on the most probable cause or agent; this is determined by the combination of symptoms, signs, degree of immunocompromise, stage of immunocompromise, and local pathogenic load.

Antibiotics
- If a specific organism is not detected, broad-spectrum cover should be used, with microbiological advice about local pathogens, e.g. imipinem 1–2 g i.v. daily in divided doses.

Antituberculous drugs
- Conventional quadruple treatment (ethambutol, rifampicin, pyrazinamide, isoniazid) is recommended until sensitivity is available.

Antiviral agents
Ganciclovir 6 mg/kg twice daily initially, then maintenance dose depending on response.
Foscarnet 90 mg/kg continuous infusion over 90 min twice daily depending on renal function.
- Renal function and leucocyte count must be monitored.

Antifungal agents
Amphotericin B 0.25 mg i.v., increasing to 1 mg/kg daily, depending on renal function.
Liposomal amphotericin 1 mg/kg i.v. daily, increasing to 3 mg/kg daily, depending on renal function.
Itraconazole 200 mg daily.

Chemotherapy
- Chemotherapy may be used in certain patients with Kaposi's sarcoma or secondary B cell lymphoma or carcinoma.
- The choice of treatment is determined locally, and the use of chemotherapy combined with radiotherapy for symptomatic treatment must be considered.

Steroids
- Steroids may be used to reduce inflammatory response and to provide short-term symptomatic relief (e.g. of general malaise).

Zidovudine (AZT)
- Zidovudine may be used to treat processes thought to be related directly to HIV infection, e.g. lymphocytic interstitial pneumonitis.
- The dose should be 500–600 mg daily, depending on response, renal function, and bone-marrow function.

Treatment aims
- Treatment aims depend on the nature of the immunosuppression and the form of pulmonary complication; the following are examples.
To eradicate infection and to prevent recurrence.
To relieve symptoms of secondary neoplasia or Kaposi's sarcoma.

Other treatments
Controlled oxygen therapy.
Continuous positive airways pressure.
Mechanical ventilation: needs careful consideration, ideally with the patient or a relative, before commencement.

Prognosis
- Prognosis depends on the cause of immunosuppression and the form of pulmonary complication.
- Mortality is 10–20% in transiently neutropenic patients with bacterial infection.
- Mortality is ultimately 100% in patients with HIV infection and secondary neoplasia.
- If the immunosuppression is reversible, recurrence is unlikely after the patient has recovered from an acute event.

Follow-up and management
- In continuing immunosuppression, follow-up and management depend on the specific diagnosis: for example, patients may need prolonged prophylactic treatment against recurrence of mycobacterial disease.

Key references
Dichter JR, Levine SJ, Shelhamer JH: Approach to the immunocompromised host with pulmonary symptoms. *Hematol Oncol Clin North Am* 1993, **7**:887–912.
Murray JF, Mills J: Pulmonary infectious complications of human immunodeficiency virus infection. Part I and Part II. *Am Rev Respir Dis* 1990, **141**:1356–1372, 1582–1589.
Verra F et al.: Bronchoalveolar lavage in immunocompromised patients: clinical and functional consequences. *Chest* 1992, **101**:1215–1220.

Toxoplasmosis in AIDS
G. Mallucci and M. Johnson

Diagnosis

Symptoms

Primary infection
Fever, lymphadenopathy, glandular fever-like illness.

Secondary infection
Reactivation of tachyzoites: in cysts in any tissue, particularly brain, also eye, heart, and lung; symptoms are due to focal brain abscess, possibly with diffuse meningoencephalitis.

Focal symptoms
- These occur in 70% of patients with cerebral abscess.
- Initially, they may be subtle or transient, evolving to persistent focal neurological deficits, including the following:

Hemiparesis, hemisensory loss, movement disorders, ataxia, visual field deficits, cranial nerve palsies, aphasia.

Severe localized headaches: in 45% of patients.

Focal and secondarily generalized seizures: in 38%.

Non-focal symptoms
- These may predominate in up to 40% of patients.

Fever and malaise (variable), disorientation, psychosis, neck stiffness (in 5%), increasing confusion and coma.

Signs
- Focal signs, e.g. cerebellar tremor, extrapyramidal signs, and hemiplegia, are common; they indicate multiple or focal CNS lesions.
- Signs of infection (fever, meningism) are unreliable and inconsistent.

Investigations

Toxoplasma serology: initial investigation; IgG reflects chronic infection; IgM, acute seroconversion; negative test does not exclude diagnosis.

CT of brain with contrast: urgent; in 70–80% of patients, shows single or multiple ring-enhancing lesions with oedema (mainly in basal ganglia and bilaterally at corticomedullary junction).

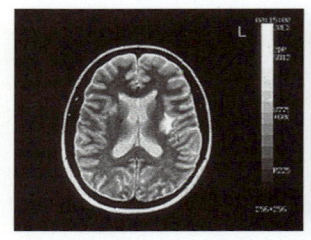

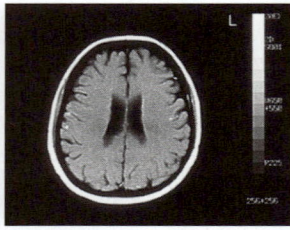

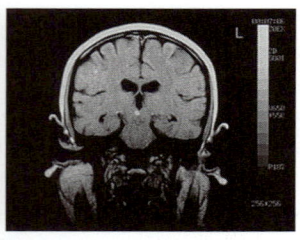

MRI of a patient with cerebral toxoplasmosis. Transverse section before (left) and after contrast (middle) shows multiple lesions; coronal section (right) shows several cortical lesions and one brainstem lesion.

MRI of brain: as alternative to CT scanning or for patients with single or no lesions on CT (20–30%); increases sensitivity for multiple lesions and may reveal lesions accessible to biopsy; demonstration of single lesion strongly suggests cause other than toxoplasmosis.

Lumbar puncture: in absence of cerebral oedema on brain scan; to detect intrathecal toxoplasma antibody production; CSF cellularity, protein, and glucose nonspecific in HIV.

Brain biopsy: indicated for single lesions on MRI or for non-responders to treatment.

Complications

Fitting, coning, or hydrocephalus.

Panhypopituitarism, inappropriate antidiuretic hormone secretion.

Diffuse encephalitis, death.

Differential diagnosis

Focal neurological dysfunction
Primary CNS lymphoma, metastatic non-Hodgkin's lymphoma, progressive multifocal leukodystrophy (common).

Cytomegalovirus, herpes simplex virus, herpes zoster virus, cryptococcal meningitis, abcesses (*Tuberculosis, Nocardia, Candida* spp.), cerebrovascular disease (rare).

Diffuse encephalitis
AIDS encephalitis, AIDS dementia syndrome, cytomegalovirus or herpes simplex encephalitis.

Aetiology
- Toxoplasmosis is caused by infection with *Toxoplasma gondii*; spread is by the faeco-oral route.
- Silent chronic infection is characterized by tachyzoites in tissue cysts throughout the body.
- Acute reactivation involves cyst rupture, causing an encephalitis and a focal necrotizing vasculitic process.

Epidemiology
- Toxoplasmosis is ubiquitous in human populations.
- The incidence reflects the background seroprevalence in a given group: 20% of adults in the UK are seropositive (90% in France).
- Up to 30% of HIV-infected people who are seropositive for *Toxoplasma gondii* develop cerebral toxoplasmosis, usually with CD4 counts $<100 \times 10^6$/L.
- Overall, toxoplasma accounts for 40% of known CNS infection and 33% of intracerebral lesions in AIDS patients.

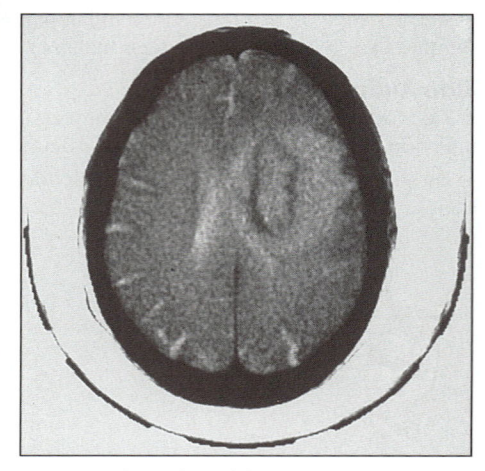

Contrast-enhanced CT of the same patient shows a single lesion in the left temporal lobe.

Treatment

Diet and lifestyle
- No special precautions are necessary.

Pharmacological treatment
- Treatment is commenced empirically for a presumptive diagnosis of toxoplasma encephalitis based on clinical presentation and CT or MRI evidence (usually) of focal or multifocal encephalitis.
- The main regimen is pyrimethamine and folinic acid with either sulphadiazine or clindamycin; expert advice is essential.

Standard dosage	Pyrimethamine 75 mg to load (or 100–200 mg), then 50–75 mg orally daily. Folinic acid 15 mg daily to prevent myelosuppression. Sulphadiazine 4–6 g daily in divided doses. Clindamycin 2400 mg daily in divided doses.
Contraindications	*Pyrimethamine:* hepatic or renal impairment. *Sulphadiazine:* pregnancy, renal or hepatic failure, jaundice, porphyria. *Clindamycin:* diarrhoeal states.
Special points	Careful monitoring of neurological condition and repeat CT or MRI to check for improvement in the first 14 days of treatment are imperative. With clinical and radiographic improvement, treatment is normally continued for 4–6 weeks; if no improvement occurs in the first 14 days, stereotactic brain biopsy should be considered. *Pyrimethamine, sulphadiazine:* disrupt folic acid metabolism; blood count must be monitored weekly. *Clindamycin:* liver function and blood count must be monitored.
Main drug interactions	*Pyrimethamine:* increased antifolate effect with phenytoin and trimethoprim. *Sulphadiazine:* warfarin, phenytoin, pyrimethamine, cyclosporin. *Clindamycin:* neostigmine, tubocurarine.
Main side effects	*Pyrimethamine:* nausea, vomiting, myelosuppression (folate). *Folinic acid:* pyrexia. *Sulphadiazine:* nausea, vomiting, rashes, blood dyscrasias (treatment must be stopped immediately), nephrotoxicity, headache, hepatitis (rare); adverse reaction rate 40%. *Clindamycin:* nausea, vomiting, rash, diarrhoea (rare but serious pseudomembranous colitis; treatment must be stopped immediately).

- In patients with significant mass effect or decreased consciousness level, steroids are indicated, e.g. high-dose dexamethasone 8 mg orally or i.v. 4 times daily.
- Steroids may complicate the interpretation of clinical improvement and CT or MRI resolution during empirical antitoxoplasma treatment.
- They should be reduced and withdrawn as soon as is reasonable, and repeat scans performed to check for exacerbation.

Treatment aims
To cure acute illness.
To prevent relapse.

Prognosis
- 90% of patients, including those in coma, respond to antitoxoplasma chemotherapy in 14–21 days, often sooner, but one-third have residual neurological defect.
- The relapse rate is up to 50%.

Follow-up and management
- Maintenance treatment must be lifelong because of the presence of cysts, against which chemotherapy is ineffective.
- Pyrimethamine 25–50 mg daily, sulphadiazine 2–4 g daily (or clindamycin), and folinic acid 10 mg on alternate days must be continued indefinitely.

Key references
Mariuz P, Luft BJ: Toxoplasmic encephalitis. In *AIDS Clinical Review*. Edited by Volberding and Jacobson, 1992.

Porter SB, Sande MA: Toxoplasmosis of the central nervous system in the acquired immune deficiency syndrome. *N Eng J Med* 1992, **327**:1643–1647.

Index

A

abscess 16
  Candida 22
  cerebral 22
  cryptococcal 14
  Nocardia 22
  Tuberculosis 22

acquired immune deficiency syndrome *see* AIDS

adult respiratory distress syndrome 18

AIDS 2
  dementia 2, 22
  encephalitis 22

AIDS-related lymphoma 4

albendazole for microsporidiosis 11

amikacin for *Mycobacterium avium intracellulare* infection 17

amphotericin B
  for candidiasis 7
  for cryptococcal meningitis 15
  for pulmonary complications of immunosuppression 21

antibiotics for pulmonary complications of immunosuppression 21

antifungal agents
  for candidiasis 7
  for cryptococcal meningitis 15
  for pulmonary complications of immunosuppression 21

antimotility agents for diarrhoea 11

antiretroviral agents for *Pneumocystis carinii* pneumonia 19

antituberculous agents for pulmonary complications of immunosuppression 21

antiviral agents for pulmonary complications of immunosuppression 21

Aspergillus infections 20

atovoquone for *Pneumocystis carinii* pneumonia 19

azidothymidine *see* zidovudine

azithromycin
  for cryptosporidiosis 11
  for *Mycobacterium avium intracellulare* infection 17

AZT *see* zidovudine

B

bacterial
  diarrhoea 10
  infection 2, 18, 20

blastomycosis, disseminated 18

bleomycin
  for AIDS-related lymphoma 5
  for Kaposi's sarcoma 13

brain *see* cerebral

C

Campylobacter infection 8, 10

Candida
  abscess 22
  infection 2, 20 *see also* candidiasis

candidiasis *see also Candida* infection
  bronchial 18
  buccal 2, 6
  oesophageal 6
  oral 16, 18

cerebral
  abscess 22
  cryptococcoma 14
  demyelination 4
  lymphoma 14
  toxoplasmosis 4, 14

cervical carcinoma 2

cheilitis, angular 6

cholangitis, sclerosing 10

CHOP (cyclophosphamide, vincristine, adriamycin, prednisolone) for AIDS-related lymphoma 5

choroiditis, *Pneumocystis carinii* 8

ciprofloxacin for *Mycobacterium avium intracellulare* infection 17

clarithromcyin for *Mycobacterium avium intracellulare* infection 17

clindamycin
  for *Pneumocystis carinii* pneumonia 19
  for toxoplasmosis 23

clofazimine for *Mycobacterium avium intracellulare* infection 17

clotrimazole for candidiasis 7

CNS
  lesions 22
  lymphoma 22

codeine phosphate for diarrhoea 11

colitis 8

continuous positive airways pressure for pulmonary complications of immunosuppression 21

corticosteroids
  for AIDS-related lymphoma 5
  for *Pneumocystis carinii* pneumonia 19
  for pulmonary complications of immunosuppression 21
  for toxoplasmosis 23

co-trimoxazole for *Pneumocystis carinii* pneumonia 19

cotton-wool spot 8

cranial nerve palsy 14

cryptococcal
  abscess 14
  infection 2
  meningitis 14, 22

cryptococcoma, cerebral 14

cryptosporidiosis 2, 8, 11

cycloserine for *Mycobacterium avium intracellulare* infection 17

cytomegalovirus
  infection 2, 6, 8, 10, 20, 22
  pneumonitis 18

D

dapsone for *Pneumocystis carinii* pneumonia 19

daunorubicin for Kaposi's sarcoma 13

demyelination, cerebral 4

dermatofibroma 12

dexamethasone for toxoplasmosis 23

diarrhoea
  and HIV infection 10
  bacterial 10
  pathogen-negative 10
  viral 10

didanosine for AIDS 3

dideoxycytosine for AIDS 3

dilatation, toxic 10

doxorubicin for Kaposi's sarcoma 13

E

effusion, pleural 20

encephalitis 22
  AIDS 22
  herpes 8, 22

encephalopathy, HIV 8

Entamoeba infection 8, 11

epirubicin for Kaposi's sarcoma 13

erythromycin for cryptosporidiosis 11

ethambutol
  for *Mycobacterium avium intracellulare* infection 17
  for pulmonary complications of immunosuppression 21

ethionamide for *Mycobacterium avium intracellulare* infection 17

etoposide for Kaposi's sarcoma 13

Index

F

fluconazole
    for candidiasis 7
    for cryptococcal meningitis 15

flucytosine for cryptococcal meningitis 15

folinic acid for toxoplasmosis 23

foscarnet
    for cytomegalovirus infection 9
    for pulmonary complications of immuno-suppression 21

fungal infection 2, 20

G

ganciclovir
    for cytomegalovirus infection 9
    for pulmonary complications of immuno-suppression 21

gastritis 8

gastrointestinal
    haemorrhage 8, 12
    infection 8
    obstruction 12
    perforation 8

Giardia infection 8

gingivitis 6

graft-versus-host disease 20

H

haematoma 12

haemorrhage, gastrointestinal 8, 12

herpes
    encephalitis 8, 22
    simplex infection 6, 8, 22
    zoster infection 22

histoplasmosis 2, 18

HIV
    antibody-negative CD4 lymphopenia 2
    encephalopathy 8
    infection 4
        and diarrhoea 10
    myelopathy 8
    progression 16

HTLV-III
    infections *see* HIV infection
    LAV infection *see* HIV infection

human T-lymphotrophic virus type III infections *see* HIV infection

hydrocephalus 22

hydrocortisone for Kaposi's sarcoma 13

I

imipinem for pulmonary complications of immunosuppression 21

immobilization oedema 12

immunoblastoma *see* lymphoma

immunodeficiency 2
    acquired *see* AIDS
    congenital 2
    iatrogenic 2

immunosuppression, pulmonary complications of 20

inappropriate antidiuretic hormone secretion 22

infection
    Aspergillus 20
    bacterial 2, 18, 20
    Campylobacter 8, 10
    Candida 2, 20 *see also* candidiasis
    Cryptococcus 2
    cryptosporidia 2
    cytomegalovirus 2, 6, 8, 10, 20, 22
    Entamoeba 8, 11
    fungal 2, 20
    gastrointestinal 8
    Giardia 8
    herpes
        simplex 6, 8, 22
        zoster 22
    Histoplasma 2, 18
    HIV 4
        and diarrhoea 10
    isospora 2
    Lamblia see Giardia infection
    microsporidia 2, 8, 11
    Monilia see Candida infection, candidiasis
    mycobacterial 8, 20
    Mycobacterium
        avium intracellulare 2, 4, 10, 16
        tuberculosis 2, 4
    parasitic 20
    Pneumocystis carinii 2, 8
    protozoan 2
    Salmonella 2, 10
    Shigella 8, 10
    varicella–zoster 8
    viral 2, 20

interferon-α for Kaposi's sarcoma 13

isoniazid for pulmonary complications of immunosuppression 21

isospora infection 2

itraconazole
    for candidiasis 7
    for cryptococcal meningitis 15
    for pulmonary complications of immuno-suppression 21

K

Kaposi's sarcoma 2, 4, 6, 8, 12, 20
    cutaneous 16, 18
    gastrointestinal 12
    lymphatic 12
    mucocutaneous 12
    pulmonary 12, 18

ketoconazole for candidiasis 7

L

Lamblia infection *see Giardia* infection

lesions, CNS 22

leukodystrophy, progressive multifocal 22

leukoencephalopathy, progressive multifocal 2, 8

leukoplakia, oral hairy 2, 6, 18

lymphoma
    AIDS-related 4
    B cell 20
    cerebral 14
    CNS 22
    non-Hodgkin's 22
    non-T-cell 2

M

mechanical ventilation for pulmonary complications of immunosuppression 21

melanoma 12

meningitis
    aseptic 8
    cryptococcal 14, 22
    tuberculous 14
    viral 14

meningoencephalitis 22

mepacrine for giardiasis 11

methotrexate for AIDS-related lymphoma 5

metronidazole
    for *Entamoeba* infection 11
    for giardiasis 11
    for microsporidiosis 11

microsporidiosis 2, 8, 11

Monilia see Candida, candidiasis

mycobacterial infection 8, 20

Mycobacterium
    avium intracellulare infection 2, 4, 10, 16
    tuberculosis infection 2, 4

myelitis 8

myelopathy
    HIV 8
    vacuolar 2

Index

N

naevus 12
necrosis, acute retinal 8
Nocardia abscess 22
non-Hodgkin's lymphoma 22
nystatin for candidiasis 7

O

obstruction
    gastrointestinal 12
    oesophageal 6
octreotide for diarrhoea 11
oedema, immobilization 12
oesophageal
    candidiasis 6
    obstruction 6
    ulceration 6
oesophagitis 8
opiates for diarrhoea 11
oxygen therapy, controlled, for pulmonary complications of immunosuppression 21

P

palsy, cranial nerve 14
panhypopituitarism 22
parasitic infection 20
paromomycin for cryptosporidiosis 11
pentamidine
    for *Pneumocystis carinii* pneumonia 19
perforation, gastrointestinal 8
peridontitis 6
pleural effusion 20
Pneumocystis carinii
    choroiditis 8
    infection 2, 8
    pneumonia 18, 20
pneumonia 16, 20
    Pneumocystis carinii 18, 20
pneumonitis 8
    cytomegalovirus 18
    lymphocytic interstitial 20
pneumothorax 18
primaquine for *Pneumocystis carinii* pneumonia 19
protozoan infection 2
pulmonary
    complications of immunosuppression 20
    Kaposi's sarcoma 12, 18
    tuberculosis 18
purpura 12
pyrazinamide for pulmonary complications of immunosuppression 21
pyrimethamine for toxoplasmosis 23

R

radiotherapy
    for AIDS-related lymphoma
        external beam 5
        whole-body 5
    for Kaposi's sarcoma 13
reflux, acid 6
rehydration for diarrhoea 11
rejection of transplant 20
respiratory
    distress syndrome, adult 18
    failure 8, 12, 20
retinal
    detachment 8
    necrosis, acute 8
retinitis 8
rifabutin for *Mycobacterium avium intracellulare* infection 17
rifampicin for pulmonary complications of immunosuppression 21

S

salivary gland disease *see* cytomegalovirus infections
Salmonella infection 2, 10
sarcoma, Kaposi's 2, 4, 6, 8, 12, 20
    cutaneous 16, 18
    gastrointestinal 12
    lymphatic 12
    mucocutaneous 12
    pulmonary 12, 18
Shigella infection 8, 10
somatostatin analogues for diarrhoea 11
spiramycin for cryptosporidiosis 11
steroids *see* corticosteroids
sulphadiazine for toxoplasmosis 23

T

tinidazole for giardiasis 11
tonsillar ulcers 4
toxic dilatation 10
toxoplasmosis 8, 22
    cerebral 4, 14
transplant rejection 20
trans-sphenoidal surgery for cytomegalovirus infection 91
tremor, cerebellar 22
trimethoprim for *Pneumocystis carinii* pneumonia 19
tuberculosis, pulmonary 18
Tuberculosis abscess 22
tuberculous meningitis 14

U

ulceration 12
    giant aphthous 6
    oesophageal 6
    oral 6
    tonsillar 4

V

varicella–zoster infection 8
ventilation, mechanical, for pulmonary complications of immunosuppression 21
vinblastine for Kaposi's sarcoma 13
vincristine
    for AIDS-related lymphoma 5
    for Kaposi's sarcoma 13
viral
    diarrhoea 10
    infections 2, 20
    meningitis 14
vision, loss of 8
vitamin supplements for diarrhoea 11

Z

zidovudine
    for AIDS 3
    for Kaposi's sarcoma 13
    for pulmonary complications of immunosuppression 21

CURRENT DIAGNOSIS & TREATMENT

in

Cardiology

Edited by
Nigel Buller

Series editors
Roy Pounder
Mark Hamilton

A QUICK Reference for the Clinician

Contributors

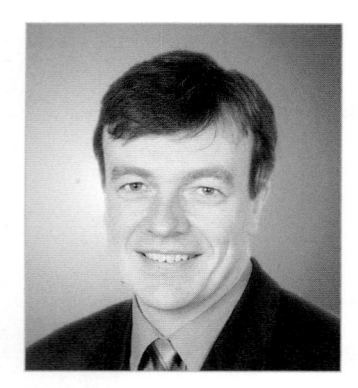

EDITOR

N BULLER

Dr Nigel Buller is Consultant Cardiologist at the Queen Elizabeth Hospital, Birmingham. His special interests are the management of ischaemic heart disease, including primary and secondary prevention, interventional cardi-ology, and the development of coronary artery stents.

REFEREES

Dr Roger Hall
Department of Cardiology
University Hospital of Wales
Cardiff, UK

Dr Paul Oldershaw
Department of Cardiology
Royal Brompton Hospital
London, UK

AUTHORS

ANGINA PECTORIS
Dr Sara Thorne
Neonatal Unit
Hammersmith Hospital
London, UK

Dr Nigel Buller
Department of Cardiology
Queen Elizabeth Hospital
Birmingham, UK

ANGINA, UNSTABLE
Dr Sara Thorne
Neonatal Unit
Hammersmith Hospital
London, UK

Dr Nigel Buller
Department of Cardiology
Queen Elizabeth Hospital
Birmingham, UK

AORTIC DISSECTION
Dr Iain A Simpson
Wessex Cardiac Unit
Southampton University Hospital
Southampton, UK

AORTIC REGURGITATION
Dr Jonathan Clague
Department of Cardiology
St George's Hospital
London, UK

AORTIC STENOSIS
Dr Jonathan Clague
Department of Cardiology
St George's Hospital
London, UK

ATRIAL SEPTAL DEFECT
Dr Stephen JD Brecker
Department of Cardiology
London Chest Hospital
London, UK

CARDIAC FAILURE AND DILATED CARDIOMYOPATHY
Dr Andrew JS Coats
Department of Cardiac Medicine
National Heart and Lung Institute
London, UK

CARDIOPULMONARY RESUSCITATION
Dr Geralyn Wynne
Resuscitation Unit
Royal Free Hospital
London, UK

Dr Nicholas Chronos
Department of Invasive Cardiology
Royal Brompton Hospital
London, UK

DYSLIPOPROTEINAEMIA
Professor Anthony Winder
Department of Chemical and Human Metabolism
Royal Free Hospital
London, UK

EISENMENGER COMPLEX
Dr Stephen JD Brecker
Department of Cardiology
London Chest Hospital
London, UK

ENDOCARDITIS
Dr Jim Hall
Cardiothoracic Unit
South Cleveland Hospital
Middlesborough, UK

HEART BLOCK
Dr Stephen JD Brecker
Department of Cardiology
London Chest Hospital
London, UK

HYPERTENSION
Dr Andrew JS Coats
Department of Cardiac Medicine
National Heart and Lung Institute
London, UK

HYPERTROPHIC CARDIOMYOPATHY
Professor William J McKenna
Department of Cardiological Sciences
St George's Hospital
London, UK

Dr Aris Anastasakis
Department of Cardiological Sciences
St George's Hospital
London, UK

MITRAL REGURGITATION
Dr Michael Norell
Department of Cardiology
Hull Royal Infirmary
Hull, UK

MITRAL STENOSIS
Dr Michael Norell
Department of Cardiology
Hull Royal Infirmary
Hull, UK

MYOCARDIAL INFARCTION
Dr Stephen RM Holmberg
Department of Cardiology
Royal Sussex County Hospital
Brighton, UK

PERICARDITIS AND TAMPONADE
Dr Tony Gershlick
Department of Cardiology
Leicester Royal Infirmary
Leicester, UK

PULMONARY EMBOLISM
Dr Kim Priestley
Consultant Cardiologist
Solihull Hospital
Solihull, UK

Dr Simon P Hanley
Chest Directorate
North Manchester General Hospital
Manchester, UK

RESTRICTIVE CARDIOMYOPATHY AND CONSTRICTIVE PERICARDITIS
Dr Iain A Simpson
Wessex Cardiac Unit
Southampton University Hospital
Southampton, UK

SHOCK, ACUTE HYPOTENSIVE
Dr Andrew Pitkin
Department of Cardiology
Royal Devon and Exeter Hospital
Exeter, UK

Dr David Smith
Department of Cardiology
Royal Devon and Exeter Hospital
Exeter, UK

TACHYCARDIA, SUPRAVENTRICULAR
Dr Cliff Garratt
Department of Cardiology
Leicester Royal Infirmary
Leicester, UK

TACHYCARDIA, VENTRICULAR
Dr David Ward
Department of Cardiology
St George's Hospital
London, UK

WOLFF–PARKINSON–WHITE SYNDROME
Dr John Morgan
Wessex Cardiothoracic Unit
Southampton University Hospital
Southampton, UK

Contents

2 Angina pectoris

4 Angina, unstable

6 Aortic dissection
   distal dissection
   proximal dissection

8 Aortic regurgitation

10 Aortic stenosis

12 Atrial septal defect
   ostium primum defect
   ostium secundum defect

14 Cardiac failure and dilated cardiomyopathy

16 Cardiopulmonary resuscitation
   asystole
   electromechanical dissociation
   pulseless ventricular fibrillation
   ventricular tachycardia

18 Dyslipoproteinaemia

20 Eisenmenger complex

22 Endocarditis
   acute endocarditis
   culture-negative endocarditis
   marantic endocarditis
   noninfective endocarditis
   subacute endocarditis

24 Heart block
   first-degree atrioventricular block
   second-degree (Mobitz types I and II) atrioventricular block
   third-degree (complete) atrioventricular block

26 Hypertension

28 Hypertrophic cardiomyopathy

30 Mitral regurgitation

32 Mitral stenosis

34 Myocardial infarction

36 Pericarditis and tamponade

38 Pulmonary embolism

40 Restrictive cardiomyopathy and constrictive pericarditis

42 Shock, acute hypotensive

44 Tachycardia, supraventricular
   atrioventricular nodal re-entrant tachycardia
   atrioventricular re-entrant tachycardia

46 Tachycardia, ventricular

48 Wolff–Parkinson–White syndrome

50 Index

Angina pectoris   S. Thorne and N. Buller

Diagnosis

Symptoms
Chest discomfort: brought on by physical exertion or emotions, e.g. anger, excitement; repeatable in onset, rapid resolution with rest, worse in cold weather and after meals; heavy, constricting, crushing, not sharp, often described as unpleasant rather than painful; may radiate down inner aspects of arms or into neck or jaw, rarely radiates into epigastrium or back.

Signs
- Typically no signs are manifest, but patients should be examined for evidence of the following:

Hyperlipidaemia.
Hypertension.
Left ventricular outflow obstruction: i.e. aortic stenosis, hypertrophic cardiomyopathy.
Diabetes.
Previous myocardial damage.

Investigations
Full blood count: anaemia aggravates angina.
Resting ECG: to detect left ventricular hypertrophy or past myocardial infarction.
Chest radiography: to check heart size and pulmonary vasculature.
Exercise stress test: to precipitate symptoms, to document workload at onset, and to record any associated ECG abnormality (planar ST segment depression or arrhythmia).
Thallium myocardial perfusion imaging: mainly used when conventional exercise stress test cannot be done or when ECG cannot be interpreted (e.g. left bundle branch block); thallium administered during exercise or pharmacological stress test delineates an area of myocardial hypoperfusion; re-imaging after rest shows redistribution unless infarction has occurred.
Coronary angiography: gold standard; provides detailed anatomical information about site and severity of luminal narrowing but does not show atherosclerosis itself; prerequisite for consideration of angioplasty or surgery.

Complications
Unstable angina.
Acute myocardial infarction.
Arrhythmias.

Differential diagnosis

Cardiac
Pericarditis.
Myocardial infarction.
Aortic dissection.

Non-cardiac
Oesophageal spasm.
Reflux oesophagitis.
Peptic ulceration.
Musculoskeletal pain.
Cervical spondylosis.
Da Costa's syndrome.

Aetiology

Causes
Coronary atherosclerosis in 99% of patients.
Aortic stenosis.
Hypertrophic cardiomyopathy.
Arteritis.

Risk factors
Family history.
Smoking.
Diabetes.
Hypertension.
Hyperlipidaemia.
Obesity.

Epidemiology

- Coronary atherosclerosis is endemic in industrialized countries, but the incidence is decreasing.
- In England and Wales, ischaemic heart disease accounts for 150 000 deaths annually (26% of all deaths).
- No accurate figures are available for the prevalence of angina pectoris, but, in people aged >30 years, it is >2.6%.

Treatment

Diet and lifestyle
- Exercise should be encouraged, obesity corrected, and cigarette smoking stopped.

Pharmacological treatment
- All patients should be screened for hyperlipidaemia and treated as appropriate, including dietary and drug treatment as indicated.
- Hypertension and diabetes should be managed aggressively.
- An individual patient may, at different stages, need medical treatment, percutaneous transluminal coronary angioplasty, and coronary artery bypass grafting.

Nitrates
- For patients with mild symptoms, short-acting sublingual nitrates may be sufficient (including prophylactic use).
- With long-acting oral nitrates, tolerance is common, so a nitrate-free period should be provided.

Standard dosage	Sublingual or oral nitrates or nitrate patches, dose depends on agent.
Contraindications	Hypotension.
Special points	Glyceryl trinitrate tablets have a limited shelf life.
Main drug interactions	Reduced effect of sublingual preparations with drugs causing dry mouth (e.g. disopyramide, tricyclic antidepressants, atropine); hypotension with other vasodilators; reduced heparin effect with glyceryl trinitrate.
Main side effects	Headache, postural hypotension.

Beta blockers
- Beta blockers are the mainstay of regular anti-anginal treatment.

Standard dosage	Depends on agent.
Contraindications	Atrioventricular conduction defects, heart failure, asthma; caution in diabetes (masks symptoms of hypoglycaemia), peripheral vascular disease.
Special points	May be usefully combined with short- and long-acting nitrates and calcium antagonists.
Main drug interactions	Increased risk of hypotension, bradycardia, and atrioventricular block with many agents.
Main side effects	Lethargy, impotence, bronchospasm, cold extremities.

Calcium antagonists
- Calcium antagonists are useful in patients in whom beta blockers are contraindicated or who cannot tolerate beta blockers; in such cases, a calcium antagonist with negative chronotropic action should be prescribed (e.g. diltiazem, verapamil).
- If used in the setting of an impaired ventricle, a calcium antagonist without negative inotropic activity should be prescribed (e.g. amlodipine).

Standard dosage	Depends on agent.
Contraindications	Depend on chronotropic and inotropic effect.
Main drug interactions	Increased hypotensive effect with many agents; increased risk of atrioventricular block when negatively chronotropic agents combined with many agents (e.g. beta blockers); increased effect of some antiepileptics (e.g. phenytoin, carbamazepine).
Main side effects	Headache, oedema, flushing.

Antiplatelet agents
- Aspirin has no proven role in primary prevention, but all patients with obstructive arterial disease benefit from long-term medium doses, so aspirin should only be omitted if strongly contraindicated.

Treatment aims
To control symptoms and restore normal exercise tolerance.
To prevent disease progression.
To improve prognosis.

Other treatments

Percutaneous transluminal coronary angioplasty
- This is complementary to drug treatment and surgery, but no improvement in prognosis has been shown.
- Best results are achieved in discrete single-vessel coronary artery disease.
- The restenosis rate is ~30% at 6 months.

Coronary artery bypass grafting
- This has prognostic value in patients with left main-stem coronary stenosis or three-vessel coronary artery disease and impaired left ventricular function.
- The risk of surgery is largely related to the degree of impairment of left ventricular function.

Prognosis
- 14% of patients with newly diagnosed angina pectoris progress to unstable angina, myocardial infarction, or death within 1 year.
- Mortality at coronary artery bypass grafting with normal ventricular function is 1%.

Follow-up and management
- Atherosclerosis is a progressive disease with no cure, so follow-up is important.
- Risk factor modification is an essential part of management.

Key references
Antiplatelet Trialists' Collaboration: Collaborative overview of randomised trials of antiplatelet therapy. I: Prevention of death, myocardial infarction, and stroke by prolonged antiplatelet therapy in various categories of patients. *BMJ* 1994, **308**:81–106.

Working Party of the Joint Audit Committee of the British Cardiac Society and the Royal College of Physicians of London: The investigation and management of stable angina. *J R Coll Physicians Lond* 1993, **27**:267–273.

Angina, unstable
S. Thorne and N. Buller

Diagnosis

Symptoms
Angina occurring at rest or on trivial provocation.

Signs
- During pain, autonomic manifestations may occur, e.g. the following:

Sweating.
Pallor.
Tachycardia.

Investigations
Full blood count: anaemia aggravates angina; leucocytosis suggests infarction.

Cardiac enzyme measurement: to exclude infarction, creatine kinase MB preferable.

ECG: at rest and during pain to document phasic change, typically ST segment depression.

Chest radiography: to assess heart size and pulmonary vasculature.

Echocardiography: to assess ventricular function and to exclude differential diagnosis, e.g. aortic stenosis.

Coronary angiography: if pain does not settle with bed-rest, to assess for further treatment (coronary artery bypass grafting or percutaneous transluminal coronary angiography); usually identifies 'culprit' lesion.

Complications
Myocardial infarction.
Ventricular tachycardia, ventricular fibrillation.

Differential diagnosis

Cardiac
Myocardial infarction.
Aortic dissection.
Pericarditis.

Non-cardiac
Pulmonary embolism.

Aetiology
- Unstable angina is caused by rupture of a lipid-laden, macrophage-rich, atherosclerotic plaque; rupture occurs when circumferential tension exceeds the tensile strength of the fibrous cap.
- Exposure of blood to the ruptured plaque leads to activation of platelets and coagulation system, with consequent thrombosis and coronary artery spasm; in the setting of unstable angina, vessel occlusion is either transient or incomplete.

Epidemiology
- 14% of patients with newly diagnosed stable angina progress to unstable angina, myocardial infarction, or death within 1 year.

Treatment

Diet and lifestyle
- Patients should be hospitalized, with strict bed-rest, possibly with sedation.

Pharmacological treatment
- Patients should be admitted to a high-dependency or coronary care unit and have continuous ECG monitoring.

Antiplatelet agents
Standard dosage	Aspirin 300 mg initially, 75 mg daily maintenance.
Contraindications	Hypersensitivity.
Special points	Dipyridamole should be used if patient is allergic to aspirin.
Main drug interactions	Warfarin.
Main side effects	Gastric erosion.

Anticoagulants
Standard dosage	Heparin i.v. continuous infusion, dose adjusted according to activated partial thromboplastin time.
Contraindications	Gastrointestinal bleeding, recent major surgery, haemorrhagic stroke.
Main drug interactions	Reduced effect with glyceryl trinitrate.
Main side effects	Bleeding, rarely thrombocytopenia.

Nitrates
- Nitrates are used to reduce coronary artery spasm at the site of plaque rupture.

Standard dosage	Nitroglycerine or isosorbide i.v. infusion, starting at 20–30 µg/min, adjusted according to symptoms.
Contraindications	Severe symptomatic hypotension.
Special points	Patients may develop drug tolerance.
Main drug interactions	Reduced heparin effect.
Main side effects	Hypotension, headache.

Beta blockers
Standard dosage	Depends on agent.
Contraindications	Atrioventricular conduction defects, heart failure, asthma; caution in diabetes (masks symptoms of hypoglycaemia), peripheral vascular disease.
Special points	May be usefully combined with short- and long-acting nitrates.
Main drug interactions	Increased risk of hypotension, bradycardia, and atrioventricular block with many agents.
Main side effects	Lethargy, impotence, bronchospasm, cold extremities.

Calcium antagonists
- Calcium antagonists are useful in patients in whom beta blockers are contraindicated or who cannot tolerate beta blockers; in such cases, a calcium antagonist with negative chronotropic action should be prescribed (e.g. diltiazem).
- If used in the setting of an impaired ventricle, a calcium antagonist without negative inotropic activity should be prescribed (e.g. amlodipine).

Standard dosage	Depends on agent.
Contraindications	Depend on chronotropic and inotropic effect.
Main drug interactions	Increased hypotensive effect with many agents; increased risk of atrioventricular block when negatively chronotropic agents combined with many agents (e.g. beta blockers); increased effect of some antiepileptics (e.g. phenytoin, carbamazepine).
Main side effects	Headache, oedema, flushing.

Treatment aims
To prevent complications, while allowing healing of the ruptured plaque.

Other treatments

Revascularization
- Unstable angina is a medical emergency: patients whose symptoms do not resolve rapidly on full medical treatment should be transferred to a cardiothoracic centre for coronary angiography with a view to revascularization.
- The choice between percutaneous transluminal coronary angiography and coronary artery bypass surgery depends on the anatomical substrate of the unstable plaque and the presence or absence of additional disease. Both procedures carry an increased risk if performed in the setting of unstable symptoms.

Prognosis
- In hospital, the mortality is 1%; non-fatal myocardial infarction is 8%.

Follow-up and management
- After the ruptured plaque has healed, the patient's symptoms depend on the degree of fixed luminal obstruction; the patient should be investigated and managed as for angina pectoris.

Key references
MacIsaac IA, Thomas JD, Topol EJ: Toward the quiescent coronary plaque. *J Am Coll Cardiol* 1993, **22**:1228–1241.

McMurray J, Rankin A: Treatment of myocardial infarction, unstable angina and angina pectoris. *BMJ* 1994, **309**:1343–1350.

Aortic dissection — I.A. Simpson

Diagnosis

Symptoms
Severe back or chest pain: tearing quality; sudden onset; back pain associated with dissection of descending thoracic aorta.
Neck or jaw pain: may indicate involvement of aortic arch.
Nausea, vomiting, sweating.
Syncope.
Dyspnoea: resulting from pulmonary oedema.
Paraplegia.
Abdominal pain.

Signs
General
Hypertension.
Mild pyrexia.

Proximal dissection
Loss of upper limb pulses or differential limb blood pressure.
Aortic regurgitation.
Cardiac tamponade.
Neurological deficit.
Hypotension: often associated with cardiac tamponade.

Distal dissection
Lower limb ischaemia.
Oliguria or anuria.

- The distinction between proximal and distal dissection should not be based solely on clinical criteria.

Investigations
ECG: to detect acute myocardial infarction and hypertensive changes.
Chest radiography: for widening of mediastinum, pleural effusion, pericardial effusion.
Echocardiography: to detect flap in ascending aorta, presence of aortic regurgitation, and pericardial effusion.
Transoesophageal echocardiography: to detect presence and extent of intimal flap in thoracic aorta, relationship to coronary ostia, pericardial effusion, presence of aortic regurgitation.
Advantages: rapid diagnosis; can be performed in intensive care unit.
Disadvantages: needs sedation; may precipitate hypertensive reaction; proximal aortic arch not well visualized.
CT or MRI: to detect presence and extent of intimal flap, pericardial effusion, extension of dissection to abdominal aorta.
Advantages: visualization of entire aorta; identification of visceral jeopardy; noninvasive.
Disadvantages: time-consuming; unsuitable for unstable patients who must be moved from intensive care.
Contrast angiography: largely superseded by above investigations, although some centres still prefer coronary angiography before surgical intervention.

Complications
Death.
Aortic rupture.
Stroke.
Paraplegia.
Ischaemic bowel.
Renal infarction.
Limb ischaemia.
Acute myocardial infarction.

Differential diagnosis
Acute myocardial infarction.
Acute myocardial ischaemia.
Acute aortic regurgitation.
Thoracic aortic aneurysm.
Musculoskeletal chest pain.
Pulmonary embolism.
Pericarditis.

Aetiology
- The underlying disease process is cystic medial necrosis of the aorta.
- Causes include the following:
Hypertension (in most patients).
Marfan syndrome.
Atheroma.
Pregnancy.

Epidemiology
- The annual incidence of acute aortic dissection is ~5–10 in one million population.
- 80–90% of patients are >60 years old.

Classification
DeBakey classification
Type I: tear in ascending aorta, with dissection extending into arch and descending aorta.
Type II: tear and dissection localized to ascending aorta.
Type III: originates in descending aorta, usually propagating distally for a variable distance.

Stanford classification
Type A: includes all proximal dissections and distal dissections that extend proximally to involve the arch and ascending aorta.
Type B: all other distal dissections without proximal extension.

Treatment

Diet and lifestyle
- After surgical repair, patients are generally advised to avoid circumstances that cause an acute rise in blood pressure, e.g. lifting or carrying heavy objects or weights.

Pharmacological treatment
- Treatment for patients with type A dissections is primarily surgical.
- Pharmacological treatment is usually reserved for patients with type B dissections.

Emergency treatment
- In addition to bed-rest and arterial blood pressure monitoring, patients should be treated by oral beta blockade to reduce the rate of blood pressure rise and sodium nitroprusside to maintain systolic blood pressure at 100–120 mmHg.

Subsequent treatment
- Long-term management of hypertension is necessary, with medication (oral beta blockade, calcium antagonism, angiotensin-converting enzyme inhibition) to reduce blood pressure and the rate of rise of blood pressure; systolic blood pressure of 130–140 mmHg or less is the aim. See Hypertension *for details*.

Non-pharmacological treatment

Indications for surgery
Type A dissection.
Type B dissection: limb ischaemia, renal compromise, aortic rupture, extension of dissection to proximal aorta.

Types of surgery
Excision of intimal tear.
Obliteration of proximal false lumen.
Resuturing of aorta, possibly with interposition graft.
Resuspension of aortic valve in patients with aortic regurgitation secondary to proximal extent of dissection.
Aortic valve replacement.
Composite aortic graft (with attached mechanical aortic valve replacement) and re-implantation of coronary arteries; operation of choice in patients with Marfan syndrome.
Interposition aortic graft to descending aorta (vital organ perfusion may arise from false lumen, which may need to be left open at its proximal or distal end).

Complications of surgery
Death.
Bleeding.
Infection.
Renal failure.
Spinal-cord ischaemia with paraplegia.
Progressive aortic regurgitation.
Aneurysm formation.
Redissection.
Acute myocardial infarction.

Treatment aims
To provide analgesia and sedation.
To stabilize dissection flap.
To treat underlying condition, usually systemic hypertension.

Prognosis
- Prognostic data from patients with untreated aortic dissection are sparse.
- In patients with type A dissection, mortality is ~60% after nonsurgical treatment (inpatient: 1 month) and 15–30% after surgical treatment.
- In patients with type B dissection, 1-month mortality is <10% after non-surgical treatment.

Follow-up and management
- Follow-up should be under the supervision of a cardiologist.
- Regular MRI or transoesophageal echocardiography is advised.

Key references
Guilmet D *et al.*: Aortic dissection: anatomic types and surgical approaches. *J Cardiovasc Surg Torino* 1993, **34**:23–32.

Nienaber CA *et al.*: The diagnosis of thoracic aortic dissection by noninvasive imaging procedures. *N Engl J Med* 1993, **328**:1–9.

Aortic regurgitation — J.R. Clague

Diagnosis

Symptoms
- Many patients are asymptomatic.

Dyspnoea and fatigue: due to left ventricular impairment and low cardiac output initially on exertion.

Symptoms of left ventricular failure: later.

Angina: less common than in aortic stenosis; usually indicates coronary artery disease.

Signs

Pulse
Large volume, rapid fall with low diastolic pressure: 'collapsing'.

Head nodding in time with pulse: de Musset's sign.

Visible pulsation in neck: Corrigan's sign.

Capillary pulsation in fingernails: Quincke's sign.

A booming sound heard over femorals: 'pistol-shot femorals'.

Systolic and diastolic murmur: produced by compression of femorals by stethoscope; Duroziez sign.

Heart
- Heart sounds are usually normal.

Forceful, displaced, 'heaving' apex: may be seen and felt.

Ejection click: in early systole with bicuspid valve.

Third heart sound: in early diastole with left ventricular failure.

High-frequency early diastolic murmur: maximal at left sternal edge in expiration.

Ejection systolic murmur: resulting from increased flow across valve.

Low-frequency mid-diastolic murmur (Austin–Flint): at apex, similar to murmur of mitral stenosis but without preceding opening snap.

Pulmonary hypertension, loud pulmonary component of second heart sound: in advanced cases.

Investigations

Chest radiography: usually normal in mild aortic regurgitation; possibly valvular calcification; cardiomegaly almost always in severe aortic regurgitation; possibly pulmonary venous congestion after left ventricular failure.

ECG: signs of left ventricular hypertrophy (increased QRS amplitude and ST/T wave changes in precordial leads) and left atrial hypertophy (wide P wave in lead II and biphasic P in lead V_1).

Echocardiography: for left ventricular size and function; valve may appear normal; fluttering on anterior leaflet of mitral valve and early closure of mitral valve in diastole indicate important aortic regurgitation; may also give useful information on state of aortic root.

Doppler ultrasonography: best method of detecting aortic regurgitation.

Cardiac catheterization: essential when coronary artery disease suspected (e.g. in patients >40 years) and when severity of aortic regurgitation doubted; injection of contrast into aortic root gives information on degree of regurgitation and state of aortic root (presence of dilatation, dissection, root abscesses).

MRI: for assessment of aortic root.

Complications

Cardiac failure: most important cause of disability and death.

Infective endocarditis: should be considered in patients with unexplained illness; may lead to sudden and catastrophic aortic regurgitation.

Arrhythmias: ventricular tachycardia, usually indicating left ventricular failure.

Differential diagnosis
Pulmonary regurgitation: usually accompanying signs of pulmonary hypertension; echo-Doppler examination should resolve the issue.

Patent ductus arteriosus: continuous murmur heard well to the left of sternum; again, echo-Doppler is definitive investigation.

Aetiology
- Causes include the following:

Rheumatic disorder in 30% of patients: e.g. coexistent mitral valve disease.

Aortic root dilatation in 20%: e.g. aortic dissection (frequently leads to aortic regurgitation, an indication for urgent surgery) or degeneration of aortic media (frequently idiopathic but may underlie more generalized conditions, e.g. Marfan syndrome, Ehler–Danlos syndrome, osteogenesis imperfecta).

Inflammations in 10%: e.g. rheumatoid arthritis, syphilis, ankylosing spondylitis, Reiter's syndrome.

Bicuspid valve in 15%: usually causes stenosis, can become regurgitant (bicuspid valves present in 1% of population).

Infective endocarditis in 20%: may occur on a bicuspid valve, leading to rupture of a valve cusp.

Epidemiology
- Aortic regurgitation is one of the most common valve lesions.

Treatment

Diet and lifestyle
- Competitive sport should be discouraged.

Pharmacological treatment

Antibiotic prophylaxis
- Prophylaxis is needed against infective endocarditis in asymptomatic patients with known aortic regurgitation; it is particularly important before dental procedures. See Endocarditis *for specific details*.

Vasodilatation
- Surgery is the main treatment, but angiotensin-converting enzyme inhibitors have a role in reducing systemic vascular resistance and decreasing aortic regurgitation.

Standard dosage	Captopril 6.25 mg test dose, then 25 mg twice daily.
Contraindications	Hypotension, severe left ventricular impairment, renal failure; extreme caution with coexistent aortic stenosis.
Main drug interactions	Increased hypotensive effect with beta blockers, diuretics, calcium antagonists.
Main side effects	Hypotension, renal failure.

Non-pharmacological treatment
- Surgery is the main form of treatment for aortic regurgitation.
- Aortic valve and root replacement is indicated for onset of symptoms, increased heart size, and change in ECG, all of which indicate onset of left ventricular dysfunction.

Treatment aims
To prevent or delay deterioration of left ventricular function.

Prognosis
- Prognosis depends mainly on the underlying condition.
- Rheumatic aortic regurgitation, if detected early, has an excellent prognosis.
- Acute aortic regurgitation due to a dissection or endocarditis is fatal unless treated promptly.
- Patients with an underlying collagen disorder, e.g. Marfan syndrome, have a poor prognosis.

Follow-up and management
- Patients with aortic regurgitation should be seen at regular intervals in a cardiology clinic; signs of deteriorating left ventricular function should be vigorously sought by follow-up echocardiography.
- Patients who have had valve replacement should also be seen regularly and monitored for signs of failure of the aortic valve prosthesis (particularly in patients with biological valves) and endocarditis.

Key references

Bonow RO: Management of chronic aortic regurgitation. *N Engl J Med* 1994, **331**:736–737.

Davies MJ: *Pathology of Cardiac Valves*. London: Butterworth, 1980.

Hall RJ: Aortic regurgitation: In *Diseases of the Heart*. Edited by Julian DG *et al*. London: Baillière Tindall, 1989, pp 731–750.

Thompson R: Aortic regurgitation–how do we judge optimal timing for surgery? *Aust N Z J Med* 1984, **14**:514–517.

Aortic stenosis — J.R. Clague

Diagnosis

Symptoms
- Many patients are asymptomatic.

Angina: in ~70% of adult patients.

Syncope: in ~25% of patients, during or immediately after exercise.

Dyspnoea: common presenting symptom; severe dyspnoea, paroxysmal nocturnal dyspnoea, and orthopnoea late manifestations indicating left ventricular dysfunction.

Signs

Pulse
- The pulse is normal in mild aortic stenosis (gradient <50 mmHg).

Slow rise, sometimes with 'notch' on upstroke ('anacrotic'): indicating severe aortic stenosis; with associated aortic regurgitation, double pulse may be felt ('bisferiens').

Heart
Undisplaced, 'thrusting' apex beat: thrill may be palpable at base of heart.

Delayed or absent aortic component in second heart sound: in severe aortic stenosis and calcified valves, respectively.

Added sounds: ejection click may be heard at apex; fourth heart sound may be heard in severe aortic stenosis; third sound implies impaired left ventricular function.

Murmurs: midsystolic, rough; best heard at base of heart in second right interspace but often heard anywhere over precordium, almost always radiating to neck in severe aortic stenosis, increased in expiration; may be very soft with poor left ventricular function and low cardiac output.

Investigations
ECG: usually shows left ventricular hypertrophy, possibly left axis deviation, later left atrial hypertrophy (negative P wave in V_1), conduction abnormalities due to calcification of conducting tissues (first-degree heart block, left bundle branch block).

Chest radiography: may show cardiac enlargement, post-stenotic dilatation of aorta, calcification of aortic valve (particularly in older patients).

Echocardiography: normal valve appearance excludes significant aortic stenosis in adults; also helps to define level of obstruction (i.e. valvar, supravalvar, subvalvar); left ventricular function can also be assessed; Doppler examination permits determination of peak gradient across the valve.

Cardiac catheterization: necessary if coronary artery disease suspected or diagnosis doubted; aortography useful in presence of concomitant aortic regurgitation; retrograde crossing of valve only indicated if echocardiography inadequate; gradient obtained using this method is peak-to-peak, 10–15 mmHg less than peak instantaneous gradient measured by Doppler examination.

Complications
Sudden death: in 10–20% of adults and 1% of children.

Cardiac failure: indicates poor prognosis unless valve replaced.

Arrhythmias and conduction abnormalities: ventricular arrhythmias more common than supraventricular arrhythmias; heart block may occur because of calcification of conducting tissues.

Systemic embolization: caused by deposits breaking off valve apparatus.

Infective endocarditis: should be considered in patients with aortic stenosis who present with unexplained illness.

Differential diagnosis

Aortic sclerosis: old age, normal pulse character, normal echocardiogram, no gradient.

Flow murmur (pregnancy, anaemia, thyrotoxicosis): large-volume pulse, normal echocardiogram, no gradient.

Mitral regurgitation: pansystolic murmur, no radiation to neck, mitral valve abnormality on echo-Doppler examination.

Hypertrophic cardiomyopathy: late systolic murmur, jerky pulse, echocardiogram showing left ventricular hypertrophy, asymmetric septal hypertrophy, systolic anterior motion of mitral valve.

Ventricular septal defect: pansystolic murmur at left sternal edge with thrill, jet detected on Doppler examination.

Aetiology

Congenital: bicuspid or unicuspid valve
- The disease is usually manifest in early childhood or adolescence.
- It may be associated with other congenital abnormalities (coarctation of aorta and patent ductus arteriosus).
- Subvalvar stenosis is more common in boys and accounts for 10% of congenital cases.
- Supravalvar aortic stenosis is rare, usually a component of Williams syndrome.

Acquired
- The disease can be calcific (calcified bicuspid or tricuspid aortic valves manifest in adults) or rheumatic (rarely isolated; usually accompanies rheumatic mitral valve disease).

Epidemiology
- Valvar aortic stenosis is the most common valve lesion in adults in industrialized countries.
- 70% of patients suffer from calcific stenosis (60% bicuspid, 10% tricuspid), 15% rheumatic, and 15% other forms.

Treatment

Diet and lifestyle
- Patients must avoid strenuous exercise and competitive sports.

Pharmacological treatment
- Drug treatment has no place in the treatment of aortic stenosis, but patients should be given antibiotic prophylaxis against infective endocarditis (*see* Endocarditis *for specific details*).

Non-pharmacological treatment

Surgery
- Surgery is mandatory for symptomatic patients.
- It should be considered in asymptomatic patients with severe aortic stenosis (peak-to-peak gradient >50 mmHg).
- Age alone is not a contraindication.
- Patients with severe aortic stenosis should have valve replacement early to avoid deterioration in left ventricular function.

Balloon valvuloplasty
- This is useful in infants (in whom the results of surgery are poor) and in children and young adults (in whom the valve apparatus is not calcified).
- It should only be considered in adults when surgery is contraindicated.

Treatment aims
To replace valve before left ventricular dysfunction occurs.

Prognosis
- Up to 20% of patients with severe congestive aortic stenosis die during childhood, mainly because of progressive heart failure.
- In adults, the 5-year survival rate is 40%.
- The prognosis after surgery depends on age and left ventricular function.

Follow-up and management
- Patients with mild to moderate aortic stenosis should be monitored for increasing severity.
- Patients who have had valve replacement should be monitored for failure of the valve prosthesis (particularly biological valves) and endocarditis.

Key references
Hall RJ: Aortic stenosis. In *Diseases of the Heart.* Edited by Julian DG *et al*. London: Baillière Tindall, 1989, pp 707–730.

Lombard JT, Seltzer A: Valvular aortic stenosis: clinical and haemodynamic profile of patients. *Ann Intern Med* 1987, **106**:292–298.

Selzer A: Changing aspects of the natural history of valvular aortic stenosis. *N Engl J Med* 1987, **317**:91–98.

Atrial septal defect — S.J.D. Brecker

Diagnosis

Symptoms

Ostium secundum defect
- Patients are often asymptomatic in early life.
- Children may have increased incidence of chest infections.
- Symptoms increase with age: >70% of adults are symptomatic by 40 years.

Palpitation: indicating atrial arrythmias.
Dyspnoea.
Productive cough: indicating recurrent chest infections.
Fatigue, ankle swelling: indicating congestive heart failure.
Symptoms of paradoxical emboli.

Ostium primum defect
- Patients will more probably develop symptoms and heart failure in childhood.

Failure to thrive.
Chest infections.
Poor development.

- In adults, in addition to the same symptoms as secundum defect, the following occur:

Syncope: indicating heart block.
Symptoms of infective endocarditis.

Signs

Ostium primum and secundum defects
Normal or small-volume pulse.
Normal or raised venous pressure: raised pressure with pulmonary hypertension and right ventricular disease.
Prominent right ventricular impulse.
Widely split second sound in inspiration and expiration (fixed).
Ejection systolic flow murmur in pulmonary area and mid-diastolic tricuspid flow murmur: increased right-sided flows, louder on inspiration.

Ostium primum defect only
Pansystolic murmur at apex: indicating mitral regurgitation (mitral valve abnormal).

Both
- The following signs of pulmonary hypertension may be manifest:

Right ventricular hypertrophy, palpable pulmonary closure, pulmonary ejection click, early diastolic murmur of pulmonary regurgitation.

Investigations

ECG: for ostium secundum defect, shows right axis deviation, right bundle branch block; for ostium primum defect, shows left axis deviation, right bundle branch block, prolonged PR interval.
Chest radiography: for secundum and primum defects, shows moderate cardiac enlargement, small aortic knuckle, large pulmonary artery, pulmonary plethora.
Two-dimensional echocardiography: identifies precise anatomy in most patients; contrast studies may reveal site of shunting.
Cardiac catheterization: often unnecessary in diagnosis but may be used to assess shunt with saturation samples taken from right and left heart, right heart pressures, and pulmonary vascular resistance.

Complications
Atrial arrhythmias: atrial fibrillation most common.
Pulmonary hypertension and development of right ventricular disease.
Eisenmenger syndrome with reversal of shunt.
Paradoxical embolus.
Infective endocarditis: in patients with ostium primum defect only.

Differential diagnosis

Uncomplicated ostium secundum defect
Mild pulmonary stenosis.

Atrial septal defect with pulmonary hypertension
Rheumatic mitral and tricuspid valve disease.
Primary pulmonary hypertension.
Cor pulmonale.

Aetiology
- The cause is unknown.

Epidemiology
- Atrial septal defect constitutes 7% of all congenital heart disease and 30% of congenital heart disease in adults.
- The female:male ratio is 2:1.

Types

Ostium secundum
Defect of fossa ovalis (most common; 70% of all defects).

Ostium primum
Defect in septum inferior to fossa ovalis; may occur in isolation or as atrial component of atrioventricular septal defect.

Sinus venosus
Defect at base of superior vena cava/upper part of interatrial septum; often associated with anomalous pulmonary venous drainage.

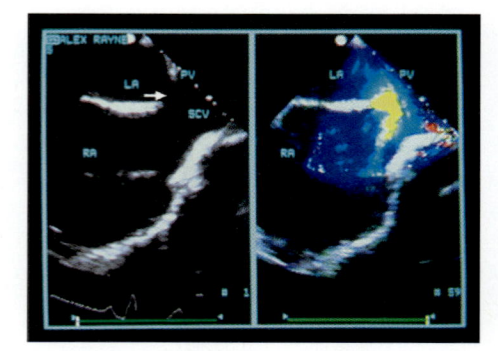

Sinus venosus atrial septal defect (arrow).

Treatment

Diet and lifestyle
- No special precautions are necessary.

Pharmacological treatment
- Drug treatment has a role only in the management of complications of the defect such as atrial fibrillation (digoxin), right ventricular disease (diuretics), and infective endocarditis of a primum defect (antibiotics).

Non-pharmacological treatment
- Treatment of the defect itself involves surgical closure or transcatheter delivery of an umbrella or clamshell device across the defect.

Ostium secundum defect
- Asymptomatic infants and children are usually followed, with closure advocated before the age of 10 years, if the pulmonary:systemic flow ratio is >1.5:1; the feasibility of device closure is determined on transthoracic and transoesophageal echocardiography.
- If the child is unsuitable for transcatheter closure, surgical placement of pericardial or dacron patch should be used.
- For adults, the debate continues on whether closure is worthwhile, but, if symptomatic with shunt >2:1, most experts advocate closure; transcatheter device closure may be feasible.
- Contraindications to closure are pulmonary vascular resistance >6 units and age >65 years with small shunt.

Ostium primum defect
- All patients with significant shunt, unless complicated by severe pulmonary vascular disease should have surgical closure, with repair of associated mitral valve abnormalities.

Treatment aims
To prevent late-onset pulmonary hypertension.
To avoid right ventricular disease.
To reduce or delay incidence of atrial arrhythmias.

Prognosis
- In patients with ostium secundum defect, mortality of repair in an uncomplicated case is <1%; in older patients with rise in pulmonary vascular resistance, mortality is higher.
- Most patients with unoperated ostium primum defect die by the age of 30 years; operative mortality varies with the complexity of the defect but is usually 5–10%.

Follow-up and management
- Patients must be observed for symptoms of atrial arrhythmias, developing pulmonary hypertension, and right ventricular disease.
- After repair of an ostium primum defect, heart block is possible.

Key references
Dexter L: Atrial septal defect. *Br Heart J* 1956, **18**:209–225.

Hamilton WT *et al.*: Atrial septal defect secundum: clinical profile with physiologic correlates. In *Adult Congenital Heart Disease*. Edited by Roberts WC. Philadelphia: FA Davis, 1987, pp 395–408.

O'Toole JD *et al.*: The mechanism of splitting of the second heart sound in atrial septal defect. *Circulation* 1977, **56**:1047–1053.

Perloff JK: Atrial septal defect. In *The Clinical Recognition of Congenital Heart Disease* edn 3. Edited by Perloff JK. Philadelphia: WB Saunders, 1987, pp 272–349.

Sutton MGS, Tajik AJ, McGoon DC: Atrial septal defect in patients aged 60 years or older: operative results and long-term postoperative follow-up. *Circulation* 1981, **64**:402–409.

Cardiac failure and dilated cardiomyopathy — A.J.S. Coats

Diagnosis

Symptoms
- Dilated cardiomyopathy starts as asymptomatic left ventricular dysfunction.
- Cardiac failure is defined as symptomatic left ventricular dysfunction.

Exertional fatigue, dyspnoea, ankle oedema: major symptoms.

Nocturia, urinary frequency, chest discomfort: less common symptoms.

Signs

Cardiac failure
- Cardiac failure can be free of objective signs.

Oedema, raised jugular venous pressure, lung crepitations: signs of fluid retention.

Cold clammy skin, low blood pressure: signs of impaired perfusion.

Displaced apex, right ventricular heave, third or fourth heart sound, functional mitral or tricuspid regurgitation, tachycardia: signs of ventricular dysfunction.

Underlying disorder
Valvular disease.

Atherosclerotic vascular disease.

Severe hypertension.

Severe anaemia or volume overload: e.g. arteriovenous shunt.

Pathological arrhythmia.

Evidence of generalized myopathy or poisoning.

Investigations

Chest radiography, echocardiography, cardiopulmonary exercise testing: to confirm diagnosis.

ECG: to look for underlying cause, e.g. ischaemia or infarction, left ventricular hypertrophy, arrhythmia, other causes of pathological Q-waves.

Echocardiography: to look for valvular disease; differentiates globally impaired left ventricle (e.g. dilated cardiomyopathy) from segmental dysfunction (e.g. ischaemic heart disease).

Blood tests: for rare causes, e.g. hypocalcaemic cardiomyopathy, thyroid heart disease, iron-storage diseases, anaemia, heavy metal poisons, amyloid (serum electrophoresis, rectal biopsy), sarcoid (serum angiotensin-converting enzyme, Kveim test).

Coronary angiography: occasionally, to identify ischaemic heart failure.

Ventricular biopsy: rarely, for specific myocarditis, especially viral.

Radionuclide ventriculography or echocardiography: for ejection fraction, to assess severity.

24-h Holter ECG monitoring: for ventricular arrhythmias.

Blood tests: for associated disease; renal, liver, and electrolyte disturbances common.

Complications

Atrial and ventricular brady- and tachyarrhythmias: especially atrial fibrillation and ventricular tachycardia.

Peripheral emboli, postural hypotension.

Renal failure.

Hepatic congestion and dysfunction.

Poor gastrointestinal absorption.

Muscle wasting, tissue abnormalities, oxidative enzyme depletion, early fatigue.

Pulmonary congestion, non-asthmatic bronchial constriction, respiratory muscle weakness.

Pulmonary hypertension and right ventricular failure: rare.

Differential diagnosis
Chronic lung disease.
Psychogenic dyspnoea.

Aetiology
- Causes include the following:
Ischaemic heart disease: in 40–70% of patients.
Hypertension: in 10–30%.
Idiopathic, alcoholic, puerperal, or familial dilated cardiomyopathy: in 10–20%.
Valvular heart disease: in 5–10%.
Post-viral myocarditis: possibly in 1–10%.
Rare underlying causes.

Epidemiology
- 1% of the general adult population suffers from cardiac failure or dilated cardiomyopathy.
- The incidence increases with age (>10% in people aged 80 years or more).

Treatment

Diet and lifestyle
- Patients should be encouraged to restrict sodium and alcohol intake and to maintain ideal weight.
- Patients with stable moderate cardiac failure should undertake exercise training; patients with unstable cardiac failure or intercurrent illness should rest.

Pharmacological treatment

Diuretics
- Patients with fluid retention should be given thiazides for mild disease, loop diuretics for moderate disease, or combinations of loop, thiazide, and potassium-sparing agents for severe cardiac failure; metolazone is particularly effective with loop diuretics.

Standard dosage	Depends on degree of fluid retention.
Contraindications	Renal failure, hypokalaemia (both relative).
Main drug interactions	Low potassium with digoxin.
Main side effects	Hypokalaemia, renal impairment.

Angiotensin-converting enzyme inhibitors
- These are used for symptomatic heart failure without contraindications and asymptomatic left ventricular dysfunction in some patients (e.g. after myocardial infarction).

Standard dosage	Higher doses, e.g. captopril 25 mg 3 times daily or enalapril 10 mg twice daily.
Contraindications	Worsening renal function, allergy, severe cough.
Main drug interactions	Hyperkalaemia with potassium-sparing agents.
Main side effects	Cough, renal failure.

Digoxin
- Digoxin is used to control ventricular response rate in atrial fibrillation; its role in sinus rhythm is controversial.

Standard dosage	Digoxin 0.0625–0.25 mg daily.
Contraindications	Renal failure.
Special points	Serum concentrations must be monitored.
Main drug interactions	Diuretic-induced low potassium.
Main side effects	Arrhythmias, nausea, visual disturbances.

Beta blockers and partial beta agonists
- These are indicated only for selected patients in specialist units.

Standard dosage	Slow-dose increments.
Contraindications	Worsening cardiac failure, heart block, asthma.
Main drug interactions	Other bradycardic agents (digoxin, some calcium antagonists).
Main side effects	Worsening cardiac failure, heart block.

Sympathomimetics and phosphodiesterase inhibitors
- Such agents are indicated only for acute short-term support, not for chronic oral administration.
- No beneficial effect has been found in ambulant patients.
- They interact with monoamine oxidase inhibitors.
- They can cause ventricular arrhythmias.

Antiarrhythmics
- With the exception of digoxin, antiarrythmics are advisable only in symptomatic life-threatening arrhythmias. Amiodarone is probably the best choice (implantable defibrillators are an expensive alternative).

Standard dosage	Amiodarone 100–200 mg daily.
Contraindications	Severe heart failure, heart block.
Main drug interactions	Digoxin, warfarin doses must be reduced.
Main side effects	Proarrhythmic effects, worsening heart failure, liver and lung toxicity, thyroid dysfunction.

Treatment aims
To alleviate symptoms.
To delay disease progression.
To reduce mortality.

Other treatments
Coronary bypass grafting: in selected patients with severe coronary disease.
Heart transplantation: for younger patients with severe left ventricular disease; organ supply remains inadequate for demand.
Myoplasty.

Prognosis
- Adverse prognostic features include the following:
Old age.
Low ejection fraction.
Poor exercise tolerance.
Ischaemic origin.
Ventricular arrhythmias.
Reduced heart rate variability.
High plasma noradrenaline concentration.
Low serum sodium concentration.
- The annual mortality is 50% in patients with severe heart failure and 10–20% in patients with mild to moderate heart failure.

Follow-up and management
- Life-long regular review is needed.

Key references
Cohn JN et al.: A comparison of enalapril with hydralazine-isosorbide dinitrate in the treatment of chronic congestive heart failure. *N Engl J Med* 1991, **325**:303–310.

CONSENSUS Trial Study Group: Effects of enalapril on mortality in severe congestive heart failure: results of the Co-operative North Scandinavian Enalapril Survival Study. *N Engl J Med* 1987, **316**:1429–1435.

Pfeffer MA et al.: Effect of captopril on mortality and morbidity in patients with left ventricular dysfunction after myocardial infarction. Results of the Survival and Ventricular Enlargement trial. *N Engl J Med* 1992, **327**:669–677.

SOLVD Investigators: Effect of enalapril on survival in patients with reduced left ventricular ejection fractions and congestive heart failure. *N Engl J Med* 1991, **325**:293–302.

Cardiopulmonary resuscitation — G. Wynne and N. Chronos

Basic life support

Definition
- The term 'basic life support' refers to maintaining an airway and supporting breathing and the circulation without equipment.
- This is a practical skill, and training must be sought.
- Health-care professionals should also have more complex skills, including the use of airway adjuncts, e.g. Guedel airway plus face-mask (with or without a non-return valve) or bag-mask ventilation and two-rescuer resuscitation.

Assessment

Approach
- Safety for the rescuer and the patient must be assessed.

Responsiveness
- The rescuer should gently shake the patient's shoulders and ask loudly 'Are you alright?'
- If the patient is unresponsive, the rescuer should call for help.
- The airway is opened by the combined manoeuvre of head tilt and chin lift; in most cases, this alone lifts the tongue from the back of the throat.
- If neck injury is likely, a chin lift or jaw thrust must be performed without moving the head or neck to open the airway.
- Any obvious obstruction should be removed from the mouth.
- Well fitting dentures should be left in place because these help to maintain a mouth seal during ventilation.

Breathing
- After opening the airway, the rescuer should look for chest movements, listen for breath sounds at the mouth, and feel for exhaled air with the cheek.
- These must be done for 5 s before deciding that breathing is absent.

Pulse
- The best pulse to feel in any emergency is the carotid.
- This should be palpated for 5 s to ensure that circulation is absent.

Action

For respiratory arrest
- If the patient is not breathing but a pulse is present, 10 breaths/min expired-air ventilation must be given.
- The pulse must be checked again after every 10 breaths, instituting full cardiopulmonary resuscitation if the pulse disappears.

For cardiorespiratory arrest
- If the patient is unconscious, not breathing, and the pulse is absent, ventilation and initiation of chest compression are needed at a rate of 2 breaths:15 compressions, with 80 compressions/min (single rescuer).
- Chances are remote that effective spontaneous cardiac action will be restored without other techniques of advanced life support (including defibrillation), so time should not be wasted by further checks for the presence of a pulse.
- If, however, the patient makes a movement or takes a spontaneous breath, the carotid pulse should be checked to establish whether the heart is beating, taking no more than 5 s, and breathing should be checked.
- Otherwise, resuscitation must not be interrupted.

Safety for the rescuer
- No evidence is available for the transmission of HIV or hepatitis B virus during mouth-to-mouth ventilation.
- Up to 70% of cardiac arrests occur in the home and involve people who are known to the rescuer.
- In hospital, if patients are suspected or known to have an infection, mouth-to-mouth ventilation should not be attempted; airway adjuncts should be available for use.

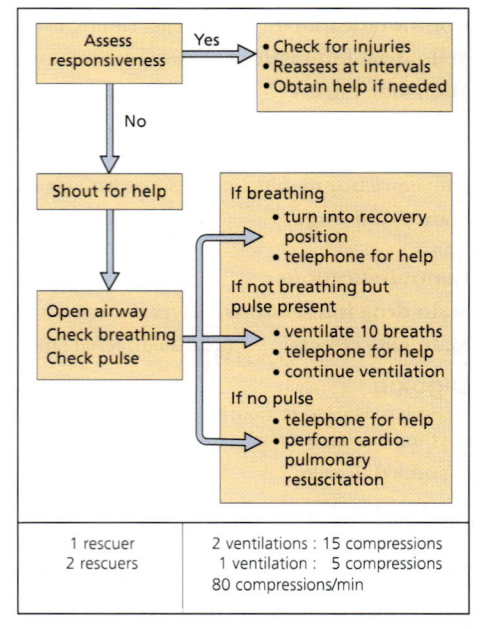

Basic life support flowchart:

Assess responsiveness
- Yes → Check for injuries; Reassess at intervals; Obtain help if needed
- No → Shout for help → Open airway, Check breathing, Check pulse
  - If breathing: turn into recovery position; telephone for help
  - If not breathing but pulse present: ventilate 10 breaths; telephone for help; continue ventilation
  - If no pulse: telephone for help; perform cardiopulmonary resuscitation

1 rescuer	2 ventilations : 15 compressions
2 rescuers	1 ventilation : 5 compressions
	80 compressions/min

Basic life support.

Advanced life support

Defibrillation

- Electrical defibrillation is the only effective method of terminating ventricular fibrillation, a lethal rhythm disturbance, and of restoring a perfusing cardiac rhythm.
- The success of electrical defibrillation depends on time and the metabolic state of the myocardium.
- The delay in the administration of defibrillating shocks should be minimal.
- If the first three shocks, at 200 J, 200 J, and 360 J, can be delivered quickly (within 30–45 s), the sequence should not be interrupted by basic life support.
- If the time to charge a manual defibrillator or to confirm that the rhythm is still ventricular fibrillation is likely to be unduly prolonged, one or two sequences of basic life support should be administered between shocks.
- The prospects of success decrease relatively rapidly over a few minutes after cardiac arrest.
- Basic life support is unlikely to improve the odds of successful defibrillation; its value is in maintaining some cerebral perfusion and in slowing myocardial deterioration.
- After repeating the loops 3 times, different paddle position, a different defibrillator, and other antiarrythmic drugs (e.g. amiodarone, lignocaine, bretylium tosylate) are still worth considering for refractory ventricular fibrillation.
- The position of the defibrillation paddles influences current flow through the myocardium; one electrode should be placed below the second intercostal space midclavicular line on the right and the other just outside the usual position of the cardiac apex (V_4–V_5).

Precordial thump

- The precordial thump is recommended for patients in ventricular fibrillation, pulseless ventricular tachycardia, or asystole.
- The application of a precordial thump takes only 2–3 s and should not cause a significant delay in the application of electric defibrillation; it should be used only when advanced life support is available.

Pharmacological treatment

Indications

For ventricular fibrillation and pulseless ventricular tachycardia: adrenaline.

For asystole: adrenaline, atropine.

For electromechanical dissociation: treatment of cause (e.g. hypovolaemia, tension pneumothorax, cardiac tamponade, pulmonary embolism, drug overdose or intoxication, hypothermia, electrolyte imbalance); consideration of routine pressor agents, calcium chloride, alkalizing agents, or high-dose adrenaline (one or more of these may be of value in some circumstances).

For prolonged resuscitation or according to blood gas analysis: sodium bicarbonate.

Specific drugs

Adrenaline 1 mg i.v. (10 ml 1:10 000 solution); should be followed by 10 sequences of 5 compressions:1 ventilation; high-dose adrenaline (5 mg) should be considered in asystole and electromechanical dissociation, although value unproven if no response after 3 cycles.

Atropine 3 mg.

Sodium bicarbonate 50 mmol (50 ml 8.4% solution).

Calcium chloride 1 g (10 ml 10% solution).

- A large peripheral or central vein should be the standard route, with rapid infusion.
- The endotracheal route should be used only if an i.v. line cannot be established, in which case, double or triple doses of adrenaline or atropine should be given through an endotracheal tube.

Treatment aims

To resuscitate the patient.
To enhance basic life support (adrenaline).

Prognosis

- Survival from cardiac arrest is greatest when the event is witnessed, when a bystander starts resuscitation, when the heart arrests in ventricular fibrillation, or when defibrillation is carried out at an early stage.

Follow-up and management

- After resuscitation, patients should be observed, monitored, and treated in an intensive care unit.
- Patients must be checked by assessing responsiveness, airway, breathing, circulation, and blood pressure; arterial blood gas and electrolyte measurements should be taken; chest radiography is advised.

Training

- Doctors need regular formal practical training in resuscitation.
- Advanced life support courses are being run under the direction of the Resuscitation Council (UK).

Further information:
ALS Coordinator, 9 Fitzroy Square, London W1P 5AH, tel 0171 388 5686.

Key references

ALS Working Party of the ERC: Guidelines for advanced life support. *Resuscitation* 1992, **24**:111–121.

BLS Working Party of the ERC: Guidelines for basic life support. *Resuscitation* 1992, **24**:103–110.

Bosseart L, Koster R: Defibrillation: methods and strategies. *Resuscitation* 1992, **24**:211–215.

Hapres SA, Robertson C: CPR drug delivery routes and systems. *Resuscitation* 1992, **24**:137–140.

O'Nunain S, Ruskin J: Cardiac arrest. *Lancet* 1993, **341**:1631–1647.

Robertson C: The precordial thump and cough techniques in advanced life support. *Resuscitation* 1992, **24**:133–135.

von Planta M, Chamberlain D: Drug treatment of arrhythmias during cardiopulmonary resuscitation. *Resuscitation* 1992, **24**:227–232.

Dyslipoproteinaemia A.F. Winder

Diagnosis

Symptoms
Myocardial infarction, angina, claudication, transient ischaemic attacks, cerebrovascular accident: indicating accelerated atheroma.

Pancreatitis, confusional states: rare, caused by chylomicronaemia.

- Adverse lipid profiles without symptoms are often revealed by well-person screening or through other risk associations, e.g. bad family history.

Signs
- Ectopic lipid deposits should be sought because they suggest the duration of lipidaemia (and thus the degree of risk) and alert to asymptomatic lipidaemia.

Corneal arcus: traces in 50% of UK adults by age of 50 years; heavy or early presence can reveal hypercholesterolaemia; differential arcus can reveal carotid stenosis.

Xanthomas of tendons: heels, knees, knuckles; indicating long-standing severe hypercholesterolaemia, almost always familial.

Xanthomas of soft tissues: elbows, eyelids, palmar creases, rarely elsewhere; typical of mixed lipidaemia and triglyceride excess.

Lipidaemia retinalis and eruptive xanthomas: indicating chylomicronaemia.

Corneal clouding: rare major disorder of high-density lipoprotein.

Carotid bruit, poor or absent peripheral pulses: vascular abnormalities.

Investigations
- The aim of investigations is to clarify the pattern of lipid abnormality and its cause.
- Lipid profiles can be disturbed and difficult to interpret for up to 3 months after myocardial infarction.

Lipid profile: for concentrations of cholesterol, triglycerides, and high-density lipoprotein cholesterol after overnight fasting; random sample adequate for cholesterol.

Secondary lipidaemia tests: for thyroid-stimulating hormone concentration, glucose tolerance, alcohol markers; other tests suggested by history or examination.

Second-level tests: apolipoprotein E typing for moderate mixed excess or palmar xanthomas; fibrinogen level, platelet function, lipoprotein (a) concentration also of interest.

Special procedures: for major hypertriglyceridaemia, measurement of apolipoprotein CII and lipoprotein lipase; for major high-density lipoprotein deficiency, measurement of lecithin cholesterol acyltransferase activity and apolipoprotein AI and DNA studies.

Family screening: to review suspected genetic problem, notably polygenic or familial hypercholesterolaemia.

- Other problems, notably blood pressure, cardiac status, cigarette smoking, and fibrinogen concentration, should be considered in the overall assessment of clinical risk and options for benefit.

Complications
Progressive atheromatous disease.

Graft or angioplasty restenosis.

Attacks of abdominal pain and pancreatitis.

Differential diagnosis
Other causes of premature vascular disease, pancreatitis, corneal clouding.

Aetiology

Genetic causes

Monogenic dominant: forms of heterozygous familial hypercholesterolaemia (rare homozygotes) and familial combined hypercholesterolaemia.

Recessive: most cases of familial dysbetalipoproteinaemia (type III).

Polygenic.

Secondary causes

Hypothyroidism in older hypercholesterolaemic women.

Alcoholism in executive men.

Diabetes or impaired glucose tolerance in older men or women with mixed lipidaemia.

Chronic renal or liver disease.

Etretinate sensitivity.

Unknown causes

Includes diet-dependent effects and possible genetic basis ('common hypercholesterolaemia').

Epidemiology

- UK cholesterol levels are high by world standards.
- High-density lipoprotein levels are higher and low-density lipoprotein levels lower in women than in men.
- High-density lipoprotein levels are not affected by age after puberty; low-density lipoprotein levels continue to rise in women and young men.
- Heterozygous familial hypercholesterolaemia is present in 0.2% of live births and 6% of patients <50 years admitted to coronary care units.
- Major apolipoprotein E variants are present in 1.7% of live births (type III lipidaemia), but only 1% of these have major pulmonary vascular or cardiovascular disease as adults; a secondary problem (e.g. alcohol) is usually needed to provoke clinical expression.

Treatment

Diet and lifestyle
- Reduction in total fat intake (with a greater proportion taken as unsaturates), weight loss, and more steady physical activity should be encouraged.
- Much ingenuity and interpersonal skill is needed to maintain compliance, and committed support by skilled dietitians is invaluable.
- Diet change can also sharpen responses to any subsequent lipid drug treatment.

Pharmacological treatment
- The cause of the abnormal lipid profile must be identified and treated.
- No single drug is universally appropriate; combinations are useful.

Priorities for lipid-lowering treatment in diet-resistant patients
Proposed by the British Hyperlipidaemia Association (1993).
1. Existing coronary heart disease or previous coronary artery bypass grafting, angioplasty, or cardiac transplantation.
2. Several risk factors or major genetic lipid disorder (e.g. familial hypercholesterolaemia).
3. Asymptomatic dyslipoproteinaemia in men or in postmenopausal women.

Resins
- Resins divert bile acids, lower cholesterol, and raise triglycerides; they are first-line treatment in children with familial hypercholesterolaemia.

Standard dosage	Resins 1–2 sachets twice daily (up to 4 sachets daily).
Contraindications	Biliary obstruction.
Special points	Compliance is better with newer formulations, e.g. Colestipol orange.
Main drug interactions	May reduce absorption of other medication (should be given before or well after).
Main side effects	Gastric irritation, constipation, wind.

Statins
- Statins are powerful cholesterol-lowering agents, alone or with resins.

Standard dosage	Statins 10–40 mg single daily dose, depending on product (e.g. fluvastatin, pravastatin, simvastatin).
Contraindications	Liver disease, pregnancy, breast feeding.
Special points	Not licensed for children.
Main drug interactions	Occasional severe myositis or rhabdomyolysis when used with cyclosporin or fibrates.
Main side effects	Rheumatic complaints, severe myositis alone or in combination treatment; reaction time may be delayed.

Fibrates
- Fibrates are used in patients with mixed lipidaemia or low high-density lipoprotein levels; they promote turnover of triglyceride lipoproteins and can generate high-density lipoproteins; some lower fibrinogens, and the level may affect choice.

Standard dosage	Depends on product, e.g. fenofibrate and cipro-fibrate (long half-lives) 100–200 mg single daily dose.
Contraindications	Severe renal or liver disease, pregnancy.
Special points	Some fibrates are licensed for children but rarely so used.
Main drug interactions	If used with statins, can affect prothrombin time on oral anticoagulants.
Main side effects	Changed bowel habit, rashes, myositis (rare).

Second-line drugs
- Probucol can cause xanthoma regression, but high-density lipoprotein concentrations are reduced.
- Fish oils or polyunsaturates (vegetable or marine) may be antithrombotic.
- Nicotinates can raise high-density lipoproteins and lower lipoprotein (a), but compliance is difficult.

Treatment aims
To improve overall lipid profile in patients with or at risk of coronary heart disease.

Prognosis
- Increase in high-density lipoprotein levels is associated with plaque regression.

Follow-up and management
- Dietary support must be reinforced, enthusiastic, and family-based.
- For failing lipid response, compliance and the prospect of a second lipid-related disorder (e.g. hypothyroidism, alcoholism) must be checked.
- Diet or medication changes must be given time to act (e.g. review after 4 months).

Key references
Barth JD, Arntzenius HC: Progression and regression of atherosclerosis, what roles for LDL cholesterol and HDL cholesterol. *Eur Heart J* 1991, **12**:952–957.

Betteridge DJ et al.: Management of hyperlipidaemia: guidelines of the British Hyperlipidaemia Association. *Postgrad Med J* 1993, **69**:359–369.

Brown BG et al.: Lipid-lowering and plaque regression: new insights into prevention of plaque disruption and clinical events in coronary disease. *Circulation* 1993, **87**:1781–1791.

Eisenmenger complex S.J.D. Brecker

Diagnosis

Definition

Eisenmenger complex
- Originally described by Eisenmenger, this is defined as pulmonary hypertension at systemic levels due to raised pulmonary vascular resistance, with reversed shunting (i.e. right to left) through a large ventricular septal defect.

Eisenmenger syndrome
- This extension of the term by Wood includes all defects associated with pulmonary hypertension at systemic levels and pulmonary vascular disease; this includes all shunts whether they are atrial, ventricular, or even at the aortopulmonary level.

Symptoms

Dyspnoea: related to degree of hypoxia; breathlessness least marked in an Eisenmenger patent ductus arteriosus because blue blood is shunted to lower body.

Angina of effort.

Exertional syncope: low cardiac output.

Haemoptysis: pulmonary infarction or capillary rupture.

Ankle swelling: right ventricular disease.

Palpitation: sinus tachycardia, atrial arrhythmias.

Signs

Central cyanosis.

Clubbing: with patent ductus arteriosus, toes clubbed and more cyanosed than hands.

Low-volume pulse, arrhythmias.

Raised venous pressure: with a dominant 'a' wave.

Prominent right ventricular impulse with palpable pulmonary second sound.

Right atrial fourth heart sound, pulmonary ejection click, loud pulmonary second sound.

Murmurs: not from defects; low flow across large defects, thus murmurs from effects of pulmonary hypertension; early diastolic murmur due to pulmonary regurgitation, pansystolic murmur of tricuspid regurgitation.

Second sound fixed and split with atrial septal defect, single with ventricular septal defect, normally split with patent ductus.

Ankle oedema: with right ventricular disease.

Investigations

ECG: shows P pulmonale (right atrial hypertrophy), right axis deviation, with tall R waves and inverted T waves in right precordial leads (right ventricular hypertrophy).

Chest radiography: shows large main pulmonary artery with narrowed 'pruned' peripheral vessels.

Two-dimensional echocardiography: shows anatomy of defect and effects of right ventricular disease (enlarged right ventricle compressing small left ventricle).

Cardiac catheterization: pulmonary pressures at systemic levels, with evidence of shunting on saturation samples.

Complications

Right ventricular failure.
Sudden death.
Polycythaemia.
Cerebral abscess.
Haemorrhage.
Paradoxical embolus.
Infective endocarditis.
Haemoptysis.
Hyperuricaemia.

Differential diagnosis

Fallot's tetralogy.
Transposition with pulmonary stenosis.
Primary pulmonary hypertension.
Secondary pulmonary hypertension: e.g. pulmonary vasculitis or pulmonary thromboembolic disease.
- Any of these may coexist with a patent foramen ovale and may confuse the significance of the defect.

Aetiology

- Associated defects include the following:
Ventricular septal defect.
Atrial septal defect.
Patent ductus arteriosus.
Aortopulmonary defect.
Double outlet right ventricle.
Truncus arteriosus.
Transposition of great vessels.

Epidemiology

- The incidence of congenital heart disease is ~10 in 1000 live births; only a few of these progress to the Eisenmenger syndrome.

Treatment

Diet and lifestyle
- Pregnancy carries significant mortality and should be avoided.
- Travel to high altitude is extremely poorly tolerated.
- Strenuous exertion and competitive sports must be avoided.
- Oxygen should be given during flights, and dehydration avoided.

Pharmacological treatment

Diuretics
- Standard diuretic treatment is appropriate for right ventricular disease, but care must be taken to avoid dehydration.

Digoxin
- Digoxin remains the mainstay for treatment of atrial fibrillation.

Standard dosage	Digoxin 0.0625–0.25 mg daily.
Contraindications	Renal failure.
Special points	Hypokalaemia must be avoided.
Main drug interactions	None.
Main side effects	Anorexia, nausea, vomiting, arrhythmias.

Antibiotics
- Antibiotics are indicated for invasive procedures and to treat infective endocarditis (see Endocarditis *for specific details*).

Anticoagulants
- Anticoagulants are indicated when thromboembolism is clinically evident (e.g. transient ischaemic attacks).

Standard dosage	Warfarin guided by INR.
Contraindications	Pregnancy, peptic ulcer, severe hypertension.
Main drug interactions	*See drug data sheet.*
Main side effects	Haemorrhage.

Other options
- Non-pharmacological methods of contraception are preferred, but the progesterone-only pill may be used.
- No effective pulmonary vasodilators can be recommended routinely; controlled trials on an individual patient basis may be appropriate.
- Haemoptysis should be treated as a medical emergency; specialist treatment at a cardiac centre is recommended.

Treatment aims
To improve symptoms and prolong survival.

Other treatments
- Surgical correction of the anatomical defect is not possible when pulmonary vascular resistance is raised.
- Heart–lung transplantation offers the best chance of survival in severely disabled patients, but they must be free from other disease, e.g. renal failure.
- Venesection should be done, with simultaneous fluid replacement, to avoid symptoms of polycythaemia.

Prognosis
- Death occurs most often in the fourth decade, with sudden death being the most common mechanism.
- Long-term survival after heart–lung transplantation is possible, but studies are in progress at present.

Follow-up and management
- Patients need careful follow-up.
- Attention must be paid to haematocrit and venesection in polycythaemic patients.
- Cardiological input to all aspects of the patient's medical care is essential (e.g. contraception and pregnancy, non-cardiac surgery, infections).

Key references
Graham TP Jr: The Eisenmenger syndrome. In *Adult Congenital Heart Disease*. Edited by Roberts WC. Philadelphia: FA Davis, 1987, pp 567–582.

Somerville J: Eisenmenger reaction (syndrome). In *Oxford Textbook of Medicine* edn 2. Edited by Weatherall DJ, Ledingham JGG, Warrell DA. Oxford: Oxford University Press, 1987, pp 13.256–13.258.

Wood P: The Eisenmenger syndrome, or pulmonary hypertension with reversed central shunt. *BMJ* 1958, **ii**:755–762.

Endocarditis J.A. Hall

Diagnosis

Definition
- Endocarditis is an infection (usually bacterial) of the lining of the heart (usually the valves); the hallmark is endocardial vegetations consisting of platelet or fibrin thrombi with bacteria and mononuclear cells.

Subacute endocarditis: low-virulence organisms on previously abnormal valves.
Acute endocarditis: high-virulence organisms on previously normal valves.
Culture-negative endocarditis: negative blood cultures may be due to previous partial treatment, infection by an unusual organism (e.g. chlamydiae, rickettsiae, *Brucella* spp., fungi), or noninfective endocarditis.
Noninfective endocarditis: Libman–Sacks endocarditis in SLE; noninfected vegetations occur (mitral more than aortic) with valvular stenosis or regurgitation.
Marantic endocarditis in terminal illnesses: sterile vegetations, rarely embolizing, often chance post-mortem finding.

Symptoms
Fever, malaise, anorexia, weight loss, rigors: nonspecific symptoms of inflammation.
Progressive heart failure: due to valve destruction (can be dramatic).
Stroke, pulseless limb, renal infarct, pulmonary infarct: due to embolization of vegetations.
Arthralgia, loin pain: due to immune-complex deposition.

Signs
Fever: unless patient is moribund or immunosuppressed.
Murmurs: except in right-sided endocarditis.
Pallor, purpura, petechiae, vasculitis, splinter haemorrhages, erythematous nodules in finger pulps, flat red spots on palms and soles, haemorrhagic retinal infarcts.
Rashes.
Heart failure.
Clubbing, café-au-lait pigmentation, splenomegaly: if disease is chronic.

Investigations
- Diagnosis depends on a high index of suspicion; no single test is 'diagnostic'.

Blood culture: at least three cultures needed to identify organism.
Full blood count: shows anaemia, raised leucocyte count, haemolysis with paraprosthetic leaks.
Urinalysis: shows microscopic haematuria, proteinuria.
Urea and creatinine analysis: concentrations raised with glomerulonephritis.
CRP, ESR, plasma viscosity analysis: raised as markers of inflammation.
ECG: may reveal conduction disturbances indicative of septal abscess formation (e.g. onset of left bundle branch block may presage heart block or sudden death).
Two-dimensional echocardiography: may reveal vegetations to support diagnosis (absence does not exclude diagnosis); can be used to assess valvular regurgitation or heart chamber size; may detect complications early (e.g. abscess formation).
Transoesophageal echocardiography: more sensitive than two-dimensional; indicated if diagnosis in doubt and in patients with prosthetic valves.
Serological tests: e.g. to diagnose infection by *Brucella* spp., chlamydiae, rickettsiae.

Complications
Valve destruction: acute regurgitation, pulmonary oedema, heart failure.
Embolism: leading to infarction; in any vascular bed.
Local extension of infection: purulent pericarditis, aortic root abscess (may cause sinus of valsalva fistula), myocardial abscess (conduction disturbance).
Septic emboli to vasa vasorum: may lead to mycotic aneurysms anywhere on vascular tree; most worrying in cerebral vessels, resulting in cerebral haemorrhage.
Distal infection (metastatic): due to septic emboli, e.g. brain abscess, cerebritis.
Candida endocarditis: may be manifest by fungal endophthalmitis.
Glomerulonephritis.

Differential diagnosis
Pyrexia of unknown origin, tuberculosis, staphylococcal septicaemia, paraneoplastic phenomenon (lymphoma, carcinoma).
Systemic vasculitis.
Chordal rupture, aortic dissection, left atrial myxoma.

Aetiology
- Damaged valves carry small, short-lived, sterile platelet or fibrin thrombi on their surfaces; these thrombi become infected during transient bacteraemia.
- Bacteraemia can result from dental manipulations (*Streptococcus viridans*), genitourinary instrumentation or surgery (*Escherichia coli*, *Strep. faecalis*), mucosal damage due to carcinoma of the colon (*Strep. bovis*), or insertion of intravenous lines or injections (*Staphylococcus aureus* or *epidermidis*).
- Alpha haemolytic streptococci (*Strep. viridans* group) account for 50% of patients.
- Other bacteria include *Strep. pyogenes*, *Haemophilus parainfluenzae*, *Neisseria*, *Pseudomonas*, and *Brucella* spp.
- Non-bacterial organisms include fungi (e.g. *Candida* spp., *Aspergillus* spp.), chlamydiae (e.g. *Chlamydia psittaci*), and ricketsiae (e.g. *Coxiella burnetti*).
- Groups at risk include the following: Patients with previously damaged endocardium (75% of cases: 25% rheumatic heart disease; 25% prosthetic heart valves; 15% bicuspid aortic valve, mitral valve prolapse; 10% congenital heart disease). Intravenous drug abusers. Patients with long-standing intravenous lines, e.g. for feeding, chemotherapy, or haemodynamic monitoring: recurrent bacteraemia, immunosuppression, and valve trauma caused by the line itself.

Epidemiology
- An average district general hospital admits one patient with endocarditis each month.
- An average GP sees one patient with endocarditis every 10 years.

Treatment

Diet and lifestyle
- No special precautions are necessary.

Pharmacological treatment
- The key is accurate, early diagnosis and close cooperation between cardiologist, microbiologist, and cardiac surgeon.
- Patients presenting with fever and suspected endocarditis do not need emergency antibiotic treatment (unless acutely unwell); a delay of 48–72 h allows efforts to make an accurate diagnosis.
- Positive blood cultures allow the initiation of antibiotic treatment based on probable sensitivities, while laboratory confirmation is awaited.
- If the blood culture is negative, appropriate serology for culture-negative organisms should be sent, while 'best-bet' antibiotics are given.
- Successful treatment should result in a fall in fever within 10 days and a fall in CRP within 2 weeks.

Standard dosage	*For Streptococcus viridans:* benzylpenicillin 8–24 mU i.v. daily as 6-hourly boluses or continuous infusion. *For Staphylococcus aureus:* flucloxacillin 8 g i.v. daily as 6-hourly boluses or continuous infusion. Each with aminoglycoside in synergistic doses (e.g. 60 mg i.v. twice daily), depending on renal function and blood concentrations. *For Strep. faecalis:* ampicillin and gentamicin. *For Staph. epidermidis:* vancomycin. *For fungi:* amphotericin B.
Contraindications	Penicillin allergy (vancomycin, teicoplanin, or fucidin with rifampicin can be used instead).
Special points	Adequacy of dosing can be checked by using patient's serum to inhibit or kill organisms *in vitro* (back titrations should be >1:8).
Main drug interactions	Warfarin dose needs may be altered. Risk of ototoxicity and nephrotoxicity with combined vancomycin and gentamicin, especially if renal function impaired, also when given with high-dose frusemide.
Main side effects	Anaphylaxis, rashes, fever (allergic reactions to initial treatment), oropharyngeal candidiasis and rarely neutropenia (benzylpenicillin), cholestatic jaundice (flucloxacillin, fucidin), hepatitis (flucloxacillin, rifampicin, amphotericin), ototoxicity (vancomycin, gentamicin).

Non-pharmacological treatment
- If the portal of entry was bad teeth, these should be removed.
- After the need for surgery has been identified, treatment must not be delayed.
- Surgery is indicated in the following situations:

Failure of medical treatment to control infective process (possible abscess formation), indicated by continuing fever >10 days, rising CRP concentration, worsening nephritis.

Indications of abscess formation, e.g. conduction abnormalities, cavity on echocardiography, or prosthetic valve dehiscence.

Haemodynamic deterioration, e.g. pulmonary oedema or increasing cardiomegaly.

Infection by organisms that are difficult to eradicate, e.g. *Staphylococcus aureus, Candida* spp., *Aspergillus* spp.

Infection on a prosthetic valve.

Emboli or large vegetations.

Treatment aims
To eradicate infection and prevent valve damage.

Prognosis
- Despite advances in diagnosis and treatment, mortality remains high at >20%; avoiding delay before diagnosis, isolation of an organism, use of high-dose antibiotics, and appropriate use of cardiac surgery should reduce this figure.
- Some patients have recurrent infection (<10%), and all are at risk of re-infection.

Follow-up and management
- Blood culture, blood count, CRP concentration, and echocardiograph should be checked 3–4 weeks after apparently successful antibiotic treatment has been stopped.
- Removal of the predisposing factor (e.g. ventricular septal defect, patent ductus arteriosus) should be considered.

Prevention
- Patients at risk should maintain good dental hygiene and receive antibiotic prophylaxis for potentially bacteraemic manoeuvres, e.g. tooth extraction, genitourinary surgery, instrumentation.
- This will, however, probably prevent only 10% of cases.

Key references
Larbalestier RI *et al.*: Acute bacterial endocarditis. Optimising surgical results. *Circulation* 1992, **86 (suppl)**:II68–II74.

Working Party of the British Society of Antimicrobial Chemotherapy: Antibiotic prophylaxis of infective endocarditis. *Lancet* 1990, **335**:88–89; 1992, **339**:1292–1293.

Heart block — S.J.D. Brecker

Diagnosis

Definition
- Heart block is a disturbance of conduction of the electrical impulse from atrium to ventricle.
- Failure of the sinus impulse to penetrate the atrium (sinoatrial block) and bundle branch block are not considered here.

First-degree atrioventricular block: delayed conduction of impulses from atrium to ventricle, with a prolonged PR interval, but all impulses are conducted.

Second-degree atrioventricular block: intermittent complete failure of conduction of atrial impulse to ventricle, with dropped (non-conducted) P waves on ECG.
Mobitz type I (Wenckebach): progressive lengthening of PR interval until conduction completely fails; atrioventricular conduction recovers after dropped beat, and sequence is repeated.
Mobitz type II: occasional or repetitive failure of conduction without previous lengthening of PR interval; may be every second (2:1) or third (3:1) beat or occasional random dropped P waves.

Third-degree (complete) atrioventricular block: complete failure of conduction of all atrial impulses to ventricles; escape rhythm is either narrow complex (if level of block is in atrioventricular node, escape pacemaker arises in His bundle) or broad complex (if block is infranodal).

Symptoms

First-degree and Mobitz type I
- Patients are usually asymptomatic but may progress to higher-grade atrioventricular block.

Mobitz type II and complete heart block
Syncope (Stokes–Adams attack): loss of consciousness is abrupt, without warning, and the patient appears pale; rare in Mobitz type II.
Presyncope and dizzy spells, fatigue, dyspnoea, sudden death.

Signs

First-degree
- No signs are manifest.

Mobitz type I
Irregular pulse with dropped beats.

Mobitz type II
Occasional dropped beats: irregular pulse.
2:1/3:1 block, etc.: bradycardia, oedema, raised venous pressure.

Complete heart block
Bradycardia, large-volume pulse, raised venous pressure with occasional cannon waves, variable intensity of first heart sound, peripheral oedema.

Investigations
Resting ECG: usually diagnostic.
24-h Holter monitoring: if heart block is intermittent.

Complications
Injury: from syncope.
'Heart failure': underlying ventricular function may be normal, but low cardiac output due to bradycardia may mimic ventricular disease.
Ventricular tachycardia and fibrillation: leading to sudden death, may complicate complete heart block.

Differential diagnosis
- ECG diagnosis is usually definitive; the only differential should be in aetiology.

Aetiology
- Causes include the following:

Idiopathic fibrosis: increasing frequency with age.
Ischaemic heart disease, particularly acute myocardial infarction.
Calcific aortic stenosis: involvement of ring close to atrioventricular node.
Drug toxicity: many antiarrhythmic agents, including digoxin.
Postoperative: especially aortic valve replacement.
Congenital complete heart block.
Complex congenital heart disease.
Infection: aortic valve endocarditis with root abscess, diphtheria, Lyme disease, rheumatic fever.
Multisystem disease: sarcoidosis, amyloidosis, ankylosing spondylitis, Reiter's syndrome, rheumatoid arthritis, scleroderma, SLE.
Muscular dystrophy, myotic dystrophy, Refsum's disease.

Epidemiology
- >200 000 permanent pacemakers are implanted world wide each year; most of these are for heart block.

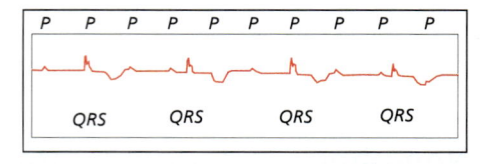

Rhythm strip of ECG for complete heart block showing complete dissociation between P waves and QRS complexes and slow ventricular escape rhythm of 32 beats/min.

Treatment

Diet and lifestyle
- Patients should lead a normal life after heart block has been treated.
- Permanent pacemaker implantation places certain restrictions on patients, e.g. avoidance of contact sports, which might damage the device or lead.

Pharmacological treatment
- Atropine (0.5–1 mg i.v. bolus) and isoprenaline (200 µg i.v. bolus or 0.5–10 µg/min infusion) may be used as temporary measures before temporary or permanent pacemaker implantation or when heart block needs treatment during resuscitation, although external temporary pacing should also be considered in such circumstances.

Non-pharmacological treatment
- Implantation of a permanent pacemaker to a patient with complete heart block is one of the most cost-effective interventions in modern medicine.

Indications for permanent pacemaker implantation
Second-degree Mobitz type II heart block.
Complete heart block.

Indications for temporary pacing
Symptomatic second-degree Mobitz type II and complete heart block, pending implantation of a permanent pacemaker.

Acute myocardial infarction: complete heart block, second-degree Mobitz type II, development of alternating bundle branch block, development of right bundle branch block with left axis deviation.

Treatment aims
To return patient to a full and active life.

Prognosis
- Implantation of a permanent pacemaker dramatically improves the prognosis of patients with complete heart block.

Follow-up and management
- Patients with first-degree or second-degree Mobitz type I heart block should be followed carefully to check for development of higher-grade atrioventricular block.
- Patients with a permanent pacemaker need regular follow-up in a pacemaker clinic to ensure continued normal function of the device.
- Permanent pacemakers must be changed every 7–10 years.

Key references
Rowlands DJ: Conduction disturbances. In *Understanding the Electrocardiogram: Rhythm Abnormalities*. Macclesfield: ICI, 1987, pp 483–507.

Hypertension — A.J.S. Coats

Diagnosis

Symptoms
- Patients are usually symptomless; hypertension is discovered at opportunistic or organized screening visits or detected after a hypertensive complication has intervened (myocardial infarction, cardiovascular accident, peripheral vascular disease, heart failure).
- Patients should be asked about symptoms of underlying causes of hypertension, e.g. flushing and palpitations with phaeochromocytoma, also other endocrine causes.

Headaches: occasionally.

Poor vision, shortness of breath, angina: rare.

Signs

Uncomplicated mild hypertension
- No signs other than raised blood pressure are manifest.

Moderate to severe hypertension
Displaced forceful apex beat, fourth heart sound, left atrial lift: signs of cardiac damage.
Silver wire arterioles, arteriovenous nipping, haemorrhages, exudates, papilloedema.

Hypertensive complications
Signs of heart failure, renal failure, peripheral vascular disease, strokes.

Underlying causes
Signs of Cushing's syndrome, renal artery stenosis, aortic coarctation, phaeochromocytoma, acromegaly.

Investigations

Blood pressure measurement: to confirm diagnosis; repeated over several visits or by ambulatory monitoring.
Chest radiography: for coarctation, e.g. rib-notching and double aortic shadow.
U&E analysis: to check for renal failure, low potassium in Conn's syndrome.
Urine microscopy: for haematuria, casts, proteinuria in nephritis.
24-h urinary catecholamines, metanephrines, vanillylmandelic acid analysis: for phaeochromocytoma.
Ultrasonography of kidneys: show small scarred kidneys of pyelonephritis or end-stage renovascular disease; obstructive nephropathy.
Nuclear renography or renal angiography: for renal artery stenosis.
Endocrine tests: for Cushing's syndrome, acromegaly, thyroid disease.
ECG or echocardiography: for left ventricular hypertrophy in patients with moderate to severe hypertension.
Microalbuminuria measurement: for kidney damage in patients with moderate to severe hypertension.

Complications
Atrial fibrillation, ischaemic heart disease, heart failure.
Peripheral vascular disease.
Nephrosclerosis, renovascular disease, renal failure.
Transient ischaemic attacks, cardiovascular accidents, encephalopathy.
Haemorrhage, infarction, papilloedema, blindness.

Differential diagnosis
'White-coat' hypertension.
Pseudohypertension.

Aetiology
- In most patients, no cause is found (essential hypertension).
- Underlying causes include the following.

Renal artery stenosis, nephritis, obstructive uropathy.
Coarctation.
Phaeochromocytoma, Cushing's syndrome, Conn's syndrome, acromegaly, thyroid disease.
Cyclosporin, steroids, NSAIDs.
Pre-eclampsia, occasional autonomic neuropathy.

Epidemiology
- The frequency of hypertension depends on diagnostic cut-off levels of blood pressure: 10–15% of the adult population have hypertension, increasing with age.
- Incidence and associations differ in non-white populations: e.g. with insulin resistance (Reaven's syndrome) in Asians, low-renin hypertension in Afro-Caribbeans

Treatment

Diet and lifestyle
- Patients should be encouraged to lose weight, increase physical exercise, reduce salt intake, moderate alcohol intake, stop smoking, and consider other risk factors, e.g. hyperlipidaemia.

Pharmacological treatment

ACE inhibitors
Standard dosage	Depends on choice of agent.
Contraindications	Angioedema, renal artery stenosis, pregnancy.
Main drug interactions	Hyperkalaemia, synergistic with potassium-sparing diuretics.
Main side effects	Cough, renal impairment, angioedema (rare).

Calcium antagonists
Standard dosage	Depends on choice of agent.
Contraindications	Heart failure (relative).
Special points	Useful in black patients.
Main drug interactions	Bradycardia with diltiazem or verapamil and beta blockers.
Main side effects	Oedema, flushing.

Beta blockers
Standard dosage	Depends on choice of agent.
Contraindications	Asthma, heart failure, heart block.
Special points	Less effective in elderly patients.
Main drug interactions	Bradycardia with diltiazem or verapamil.
Main side effects	Lethargy, fatigue, impotence.

Thiazide diuretics
Standard dosage	Low doses, depending on choice of agent.
Contraindications	Diabetes (relative).
Special points	Particularly beneficial in elderly patients.
Main drug interactions	Other diuretics.
Main side effects	Hypokalaemia, glucose intolerance.

Alpha blockers
Standard dosage	Depends on choice of agent.
Contraindications	Known hypersensitivity.
Special points	First-dose hypotension and tolerance may occur.
Main drug interactions	Few specific interactions.
Main side effects	Flushing, occasionally lupus-like syndrome.

Combination therapy
- Logical and synergistic combinations should be chosen, such as thiazides and ACE inhibitors; fixed-dose combinations are a disadvantage.

Treatment aims
To reduce blood pressure to <140/90 mmHg and to improve other cardiovascular risk factors.

Prognosis
- Prognosis is excellent if blood pressure is controlled (almost always possible).

Follow-up and management
- Follow-up must be for life.

Key references

Collins R et al.: Blood pressure, stroke, and coronary heart disease: part II. Short-term reductions in blood pressure: overview of randomised drug trials in their epidemiologic context. Lancet 1990, **335**:827–838.

Dahlöf B et al.: Morbidity and mortality in the Swedish Trial in Old Patients with Hypertension (STOP-Hypertension). Lancet 1991, **338**:1281–1285.

MRC Working Party: Medical Research Council trial of treatment in older adults: principal results. BMJ 1992, **304**:405–412.

SHEP Co-operative Research Group: Prevention of stroke by antihypertensive drug treatment in older persons with isolated systolic hypertension. JAMA 1991, **265**:3255–3264.

Sever P et al.: Management guidelines in essential hypertension: report of the second working party of the British Hypertension Society. BMJ 1993, **306**:983–987.

Hypertrophic cardiomyopathy
W.J. McKenna and A. Anastasakis

Diagnosis

Symptoms
- Patients may be asymptomatic.

Severe cardiac failure: in infants.
Premature unexpected death: may be presenting symptom in children or young adults.
Dyspnoea on exertion: in ~50% of patients.
Chest pain: in ~50%; may be exertional or occur at rest.
Syncope: in 15–25%.
Dizziness, palpitations.

Signs
- In patients without outflow tract gradient, abnormalities may be subtle.

Rapid upstroke arterial pulse: best felt in carotid area.
Forceful left ventricular impulse: best appreciated on full held expiration in left lateral position.
Ejection systolic murmur: best heard at left sternal border; radiating towards aortic and mitral areas but not into neck.
Palpable atrial beat: reflecting forceful atrial systolic contraction.

Investigations
Two-dimensional echocardiography: important for assessing left ventricle structure and function, gradients, valvular regurgitation, and atrial dimensions.
ECG: may be normal in <5% of patients or show abnormalities reflecting left ventricular hypertrophy, atrial fibrillation, left axis deviation, right bundle branch block, and myocardial disarray (e.g. ST- and T-wave changes, intraventricular conduction defects, abnormal Q waves); bizarre or abnormal findings in young patients should raise suspicion of hypertrophic cardiomyopathy, especially if a family member also affected.
Chest radiography: may be normal or show evidence of left or right atrial or left ventricular enlargement.
Treadmill exercise test with maximum oxygen ventilatory capacity: simple and non-invasive; provides useful functional information; maximum oxygen ventilatory capacity often moderately reduced; one-third of patients have abnormal blood pressure response, with drops of 25–150 mmHg from peak systolic recordings (probably of prognostic significance); ST segment changes of >2 mm documented in 25%, associated with symptoms of angina.
48-h Holter monitoring: arrhythmias common during ECG monitoring; established atrial fibrillation in ~10% of patients, paroxysmal supraventricular arrhythmias in 30%, non-sustained ventricular tachycardia in 25%; ventricular tachycardia invariably asymptomatic during Holter monitoring, but most useful marker of risk of sudden death in adults; sustained supraventricular arrhythmias often symptomatic and predispose to thromboembolic complications.
Thallium scintigraphy: fixed and reversible perfusion defects common, useful in assessment of ischaemia, particularly when resting ECG grossly abnormal and exercise changes uninterpretable.
Cardiac catheterization and left ventriculography: invasive evaluation not needed for diagnosis, but coronary arteriography often necessary in older patients with angina to exclude coronary artery disease; endomyocardial biopsy possibly necessary to exclude specific heart muscle disorder (amyloid, sarcoid) but has no other role in diagnosis because of patchy nature of myofibre disarray.

Complications
Atrial fibrillation.
Systemic embolism.
Infective endocarditis.
Sudden death.

Differential diagnosis
Aortic valve disease.
Systemic hypertension.

Aetiology
- Hypertrophic cardiomyopathy is an autosomal dominant heart muscle disorder.
- Mutations in the gene encoding contractile proteins cause disease in 50–60% of patients.

Pathology
Macroscopic: hypertrophied myocardium; thickened anterior leaflet of mitral valve; contact lesion upper anterior septum.
Histological: interstitial fibrosis; myofibre disorganization and whorling; myocyte hypertrophy.

Pathophysiology
Systolic: hyperdynamic contraction; left ventricular outflow tract gradient (30%; associated mitral regurgitation).
Diastolic: impaired relaxation; impaired filling; decreased compliance.

Epidemiology
- The male:female ratio is equal, although the disease tends to affect younger men and older women.
- In children and adolescents, myocardial hypertrophy often occurs during growth spurts; a negative diagnosis made before adolescent growth has been completed must be tempered by the proviso of subsequent reassessment.
- Myocardial hypertrophy does not progress after adolescent growth is completed.
- The annual mortality from sudden death is 2.5% in adults and at least 6% in children and young adults.
- First-degree relatives of affected patients have a 50% chance of carrying the disease gene; they should be investigated by ECG and two-dimensional echocardiography.

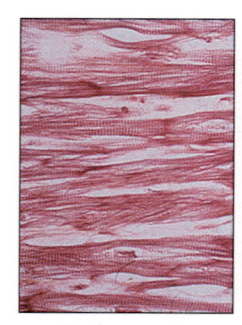

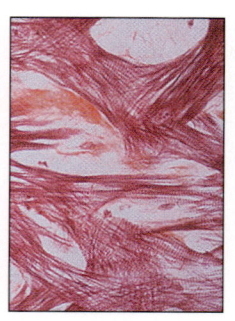

Myofibrillar stain from a normal person (left) and showing myocardial disarray (right).

Treatment

Diet and lifestyle
- Competitive exercise is not recommended, especially in high-risk patients.

Pharmacological treatment

Beta blockers
- Beta blockers may reduce symptoms and increase exercise capacity but they do not reduce the incidence of ventricular arrhythmia or risk of sudden death.

Standard dosage	Propranolol 80–320 mg daily. Atenolol 50 mg daily.
Contraindications	Conduction disease.
Main drug interactions	Other drugs that suppress impulse formation.
Main side effects	Other unwanted adrenergic blocking effects.

Calcium antagonists
- Calcium antagonism can improve haemodynamics and relieve symptoms but gives no reduction in risk of sudden death.

Standard dosage	Verapamil 120–480 mg daily.
Contraindications	Outflow-tract gradient.
Special points	Verapamil fails to abolish ventricular arrhythmia.
Main drug interactions	Digoxin.
Main side effects	High-grade conduction block, negative inotropic effect.

Antiarrhythmics
- Antiarrhythmics are effective in short-term and long-term control of supraventricular and ventricular arrhythmias and can improve survival in adults with nonsustained ventricular tachycardia (low dose).

Standard dosage	Amiodarone 100–200 mg daily.
Contraindications	Hyperthyroidism.
Special points	Plasma concentration should be maintained <1.5 mg/L.
Main drug interactions	Anticoagulants, digoxin.
Main side effects	Photosensitivity, sleep disturbance.

Other options
Anticoagulation: important in patients with paroxysmal or established atrial fibrillation.

Endocarditis prophylaxis: for patients with obstruction and valvular regurgitation (*see* Endocarditis *for details*).

Treatment aims
To improve symptoms.
To prevent complications.
To prevent sudden death.

Other treatments

Surgical myectomy
- In patients with left ventricle outflow tract obstruction, this provides symptomatic and haemodynamic improvement.
- Perioperative mortality is high, at 5–10%.

Dual-chamber permanent pacing
- Recently proposed for treatment of obstructions, this provides a reduction in outflow gradient and improvement in symptoms.
- Further assessment is needed.

Cardiac transplantation
- Transplantation is limited to patients who develop severe systolic impairment.

Prognosis
- Non-sustained ventricular tachycardia is the best marker of high risk in adults.
- Other patients at high risk are children and adolescents who have had recurrent syncope and patients with two or more siblings with hypertrophic cardiomyopathy who have died suddenly.

Follow-up and management
- Patients must be monitored for disease progression and risk of complications.

Key references

McKenna WJ: Hypertrophic cardiomyopathy. In *Diseases of the Heart*. Edited by Julian DG *et al*. London: Baillières Tindall, 1989, pp 933–950.

McKenna WJ: The cardiomyopathies and heart disease in general medicine. In *Oxford Textbook of Medicine* edn 3. Edited by Weatherall D, Ledingham JGG, Warrell DA. Oxford: Oxford University Press, 1995.

Mitral regurgitation — M. Norell

Diagnosis

Symptoms
- Symptoms are often mild or absent.

Dyspnoea: due to pulmonary congestion.
Fatigue: due to low cardiac output.
Palpitation: due to atrial fibrillation.
Fluid retention: in late-stage disease.

Signs
Irregular pulse: if patient is in atrial fibrillation.
Low-amplitude pulse pressure.
Raised venous pressure.
Parasternal heave: right ventricular hypertrophy and systolic left atrial expansion.
Laterally displaced and hyperdynamic apical impulse.
Pansystolic murmur.
Third heart sound.
Loud pulmonary second sound: if patient has pulmonary hypertension.

Investigations
ECG: shows broad bifid P wave (P mitrale), atrial fibrillation.
Chest radiography: shows pulmonary congestion, left atrial enlargement, cardiac enlargement, pulmonary artery enlargement (if severe and long-standing).
Echocardiography and Doppler ultrasonography: large left atrium, large left ventricle, increased fractional shortening, regurgitant jet (Doppler), leaflet prolapse (floppy valve or flail leaflet).
Transoesophogeal echocardiography: may give better visualization of valve apparatus.
Cardiac catheterization: large 'V' wave in wedge trace, angiographic evidence of mitral regurgitation.

Complications
Systemic embolism.
Pulmonary hypertension, right heart failure.
Endocarditis.

Differential diagnosis
Floppy mitral valve: late systolic murmur and midsystolic click.
Hypertrophic cardiomyopathy: ECG and echocardiographic evidence of left ventricular hypertrophy.

Aetiology
- Causes include the following:

Rheumatic disease.
Floppy mitral valve.
Chordal rupture.
Papillary muscle dysfunction or rupture.
'Functional' disorder, i.e. secondary to dilated, poorly contracting left ventricle.

- Floppy valve and chordal rupture are associated with connective tissue abnormalities, papillary muscle dysfunction and rupture with coronary artery disease.

Epidemiology
- The increasing availability of echocardiography may result in more patients with mitral regurgitation being found.

Treatment

Diet and lifestyle
- Patients should avoid being overweight, stop smoking, and maintain normal activities, if possible.

Pharmacological treatment

Digoxin
- If the patient is in atrial fibrillation, digoxin is indicated for control of ventricular rate (less easy than with mitral stenosis).

Standard dosage	Digoxin 0.5 mg loading dose, repeated after 8 h; maintenance dose usually 0.25 mg daily.
Contraindications	Caution in patients who are elderly, relatively small, or renally impaired (reduced dosage).
Main drug interactions	Diuretic-induced hypokalaemia enhances effect of digoxin.
Main side effects	Nausea, vomiting, diarrhoea, yellow discoloration to vision (xanthopsia), bradycardia.

Diuretics
- Diuretics are indicated to relieve pulmonary congestion.

Standard dosage	Frusemide 20–80 mg daily with potassium supplements or potassium-sparing agent (particularly if patient is also taking digoxin).
Contraindications	None.
Special points	May precipitate attacks of gout in susceptible patients and may interfere with diabetic control.
Main drug interactions	Digoxin.
Main side effects	Hypokalaemia, dehydration.

Vasodilators
- Vasodilatation is used to reduce regurgitant factor by reducing afterload unless systemic blood pressure is low.

Standard dosage	Angiotensin-converting enzyme (ACE) inhibitors, e.g. enalapril 5–20 mg twice daily or captopril 12.5–50 mg 3 times daily. Calcium antagonists, e.g. nifedipine 5–20 mg 3 times daily. Hydralazine 12.5–50 mg 3 times daily. Initially given at night to avoid immediate hypotensive effects.
Contraindications	Hypotension.
Special points	*ACE inhibitors*: treatment best started in hospital if patient taking large dose of diuretic or other vasodilator at same time.
Main drug interactions	*ACE inhibitors*: potassium-sparing diuretics or supplements.
Main side effects	*ACE inhibitors*: hypotension, renal dysfunction, dysgeusia (taste dysfunction), rashes, dry unproductive cough. *Calcium antagonists*: flushing, headache, fluid retention. *Hydralazine*: hypotension, headache, lupus-like syndrome (rare).

Anticoagulants
- Anticoagulants are indicated to reduce the risk of systemic embolism in patients with moderate to severe mitral regurgitation, atrial fibrillation, and dilated left atrium.

Standard dosage	Warfarin 10 mg daily for 3 days; maintenance dose depends on regular checks of INR.
Contraindications	Bleeding tendency.
Main drug interactions	Any drug that displaces warfarin from protein-binding sites or increases liver enzyme activity may cause alteration in the INR and thus necessitate dose adjustment.
Main side effects	Increased bleeding tendency.

Treatment aims
To achieve normal functional capacity.

Other treatments
Surgical mitral valve repair or replacement.

Prognosis
- Prognosis is good unless pulmonary artery pressures have been chronically high.

Follow-up and management
- Drug treatment needs regular review to ensure that it has not become inadequate.

Key references
Kay, GL *et al.*: Probability of valve repair for pure mitral regurgitation. *J Thorac Cardiovasc Surg* 1994, **108**:871–879.

Mitral stenosis — M. Norell

Diagnosis

Symptoms
Fatigue: insidious onset; due to low cardiac output.
Dyspnoea, orthopnoea: due to pulmonary congestion.
Palpitation: due to atrial fibrillation.

Signs
Irregular pulse: in atrial fibrillation.
Loud (palpable) first heart sound.
Opening snap: if valve is mobile.
Mitral diastolic murmur: long if severe.
Raised venous pressure.
Parasternal heave: right ventricular hypertrophy.
Loud pulmonary second sound.

Investigations
ECG: shows broad bifid P wave (P mitrale), usually atrial fibrillation if disease advanced.
Chest radiography: shows left atrial enlargement, pulmonary congestion, prominent pulmonary arteries (in pulmonary hypertensive patients).
Echocardiography and Doppler ultrasonography: show thickened mitral valve with reduced movement, large left atrium, reduced left ventricular filling rate, reduced mitral valve area.
Cardiac catheterization: shows raised right heart pressures and an end-diastolic gradient from pulmonary artery wedge pressure (or left atrium if transeptal puncture done) to left ventricle.

Complications
Systemic embolism: from left atrium.
Pulmonary hypertension, right heart failure.
Endocarditis: unusual.

Differential diagnosis
Left atrial myxoma: physical signs may be identical (echocardiography confirms diagnosis).

Aetiology
- Causes include the following:
Rheumatic disease.
Congenital abnormality (rare).

Epidemiology
- The occurrence of mitral stenosis is decreasing in developed countries as a result of the declining incidence of rheumatic fever.

Treatment

Diet and lifestyle
- Patients should avoid being overweight, give up smoking, and maintain normal activities, if possible.

Pharmacological treatment

Digoxin
- If the patient is in atrial fibrillation, digoxin is indicated for control of ventricular rate.

Standard dosage	Digoxin 0.5 mg loading dose, repeated after 8 h; maintenance dose usually 0.25 mg daily, adjusted according to serum digoxin concentration.
Contraindications	Caution in patients who are elderly, relatively small, or renally impaired (reduced dosage).
Main drug interactions	Diuretic-induced hypokalaemia enhances effect of digoxin.
Main side effects	Nausea, vomiting, diarrhoea, yellow discoloration to vision (xanthopsia), bradycardia.

Diuretics
- Diuretics are indicated for dyspnoea or fluid retention.

Standard dosage	Frusemide 20–80 mg daily with potassium supplements or potassium-sparing agent (particularly if patient is also taking digoxin).
Contraindications	None.
Special points	May precipitate attacks of gout in susceptible patients and may interfere with diabetic control.
Main drug interactions	Digoxin.
Main side effects	Hypokalaemia, dehydration.

Anticoagulants
- Anticoagulants are mandatory if the degree of stenosis is high, even if the patient is still in sinus rhythm.

Standard dosage	Warfarin 10 mg daily for 3 days; maintenance dose depends on regular checks of INR.
Contraindications	Bleeding tendency.
Main drug interactions	Any drug that displaces warfarin from protein-binding sites or increases liver enzyme activity may cause alteration in INR and thus necessitate dose adjustment.
Main side effects	Increased bleeding tendency.

Treatment aims
To achieve normal exercise capability and normal functional capacity.

Other treatments
Balloon valvuloplasty if valve is mobile and not heavily calcified.
Surgical valvotomy or replacement.

Prognosis
- The prognosis is good unless pulmonary hypertension is chronic.

Follow-up and management
- Restenosis may occur after valvotomy or valvuloplasty.
- Drug treatment may become inadequate and indicate intervention eventually.
- Patients should have prophylactic treatment against endocarditis (see Endocarditis for details).

Key references
Inoue K: Percutaneous trans-venous mitral commissurotomy using the Inoue Balloon. *Eur Heart J* 1991, **12**:B99–108.

Myocardial infarction
S.R.M. Holmberg

Diagnosis

Symptoms
Chest pain: typically precordial, often with radiation to left or right arm, throat, lower jaw, epigastrium, or back; usually severe; crushing or vice-like; pain often described as indigestion-like, may be relieved by belching.

Breathlessness: common, often without cardiac failure.

Malaise, nausea, vomiting, syncope, apprehension.

Signs
- Few cardiovascular signs may be apparent on acute presentation.

Malaise, pallor, sweating, restlessness.

Pyrexia: usually developing the day after infarction.

Unexpectedly slow or rapid pulse.

Raised jugular venous pressure: only with significant right ventricular damage.

Third or fourth heart sounds, dyskinetic apical impulse: indicating significant myocardial dysfunction.

Chest crackles: may indicate left ventricular failure.

New murmurs or pericardial rub: may be heard in patients with complications.

Investigations
12-lead ECG: often sufficient to establish diagnosis; adjunctive tests may be necessary for confirmation if infarction is minor or if ECG shows pre-existing abnormalities, e.g. previous infarction, conduction abnormalities (especially left bundle branch block).

Chest radiography: to check for pulmonary congestion.

Cardiac enzymes evaluation: creatine kinase, aspartate transaminase, and lactate dehydrogenase rise characteristically after myocardial infarction; creatine kinase MB cardiospecific isoenzyme may be helpful with skeletal muscle damage.

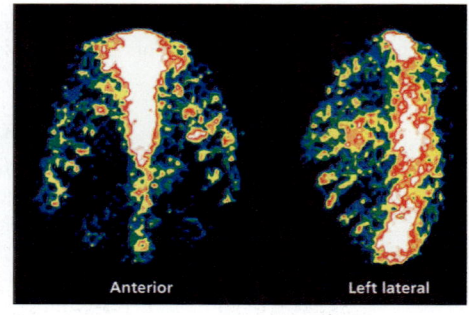

Abnormal uptake of pyrophosphate in the heart indicating recent myocardial infarction.

Echocardiography: to assess wall motion abnormalities, ventricular septal defect, regurgitation, and mural thrombus.

Scintigraphy: ^{99m}Tc pyrophosphate scan may detect myocardial infarction 4 h to 7 days after onset.

Complications
Left ventricular failure.
Cardiogenic shock.
Bradyarrhythmias.
Tachyarrhythmias.
Cardiac rupture.
Pericarditis.
Acute ventricular septal defect.
Acute mitral regurgitation.
Systemic emboli.
Aneurysm formation.

Differential diagnosis
Angina without infarction.
Pericarditis.
Oesophageal or gastrointestinal pain.
Aortic dissection.
Pulmonary embolus.
Musculoskeletal or nonspecific chest pain.

Aetiology
Causes
Thrombotic occlusion of a coronary artery, related to rupture of an atherosclerotic plaque and subsequent intraluminal haemorrhage.

Risk factors
Increasing age.
Family history.
Hypertension.
Diabetes mellitus.
Lack of exercise.
Male gender.
Smoking.
Hyperlipidaemia.
Thrombotic tendency (fibrinogen).
Obesity.

Epidemiology
- 10–17 in 1000 men aged 40–69 years sustain myocardial infarction in the UK.
- In the UK, ~160 000 deaths annually are related to coronary heart disease.

Treatment

Diet and lifestyle
- Patients must give up smoking, reduce weight, and take up regular exercise.

Pharmacological treatment

Immediate treatment
Analgesia: i.v. diamorphine with antiemetic.
Oxygen.
Aspirin: 300 mg orally initially, then maintenance dose 75 mg daily.
Nitrates: particularly in patients with continuing ischaemia.
Beta blockade: atenolol i.v. and then orally, except in patients with left ventricular failure, pulse rate <70/min, or blood pressure <100 mmHg.

Thrombolytic treatment
- Treatment should be given as soon as possible, unless contraindicated.
- It is indicated for all suitable patients within 12 h of onset of symptoms.
- Maximum benefit is with large myocardial infarction and early administration (especially <4 h).
- The value is proven for patients with acute myocardial infarction and ST elevation or bundle branch block; no definite benefit has been shown in patients with ST depression or normal ECG.
- rt-PA may be more effective than streptokinase but is much more expensive; it should be used in patients for whom streptokinase is unsuitable and may be considered for patients with large anterior myocardial infarction or hypotension.

Standard dosage	Streptokinase, 1.5 MU over 1 h. rt-PA, 15 mg bolus, then 50 mg in 30 min, then 40 mg in 60 min, followed by i.v. heparin.
Contraindications	Possible aortic dissection, active peptic ulceration, recent surgery, haemorrhagic diathesis, possible pregnancy, sub-arachnoid haemorrhage, cardiovascular accident with residual defect, recent transient ischaemic attack, unconscious patient, severe hypertension, systemic thrombus (e.g. aortic aneurysm, left atrial clot), prolonged or traumatic resuscitation, recent central venous or arterial puncture. Few contraindications are absolute.
Special points	Streptokinase should be avoided in patients with known allergy or who have been treated between 5 days and 1 year previously.
Main drug interactions	None of importance.
Main side effects.	Haemorrhage (treated by tranexamic acid 1 g slow i.v. injection and fresh frozen plasma to restore clotting factor).

Follow-up treatment
- Secondary prevention is needed for patients at high risk from recurrent cardiac events, including those with late ischaemic pain or arrhythmias, a history of angina or hypertension, or significant left ventricular dysfunction.

Beta blockers: e.g. timolol 10 mg twice daily (drug of choice); alternatively, verapamil 360 mg daily or warfarin.

Angiotensin-converting enzyme (ACE) inhibitors: e.g. captopril titrated to maximum tolerated dose, if possible 50 mg 3 times daily (12.5 mg 3 times daily by hospital discharge); indicated for all patients with left ventricular ejection fractions <40%.

Treatment aims
To relieve pain and other symptoms.
To salvage threatened myocardium.
To prevent and treat complications.

Other treatments
Early coronary angiography: possibly for patients with continuing pain or arrhythmias.

Prognosis
- In-hospital mortality after acute myocardial infarction is ~10%; subsequent mortality is higher than for age-matched control populations.
- Mortality is falling because of therapeutic advances and changes in the natural history.
- Poor prognosis is indicated by advanced age, severe left ventricular dysfunction, and multivessel coronary disease.
- Coronary artery bypass grafting may improve prognosis in some high-risk groups.

Follow-up and management
- Risk factors, e.g. hyperlipidaemia, hypertension, or diabetes, should be controlled.
- Exercise testing is needed to check for residual ischaemia, followed by coronary angiography if the test is positive.

Key references
DAVIT-II: Effect of verapamil on mortality and major events after acute myocardial infarction. *Am J Cardiol* 1990, **66**:779–785.
GUSTO Investigators: An international randomized trial comparing four thrombolytic strategies for acute myocardial infarction. *N Engl J Med* 1993, **329**:673–682.
Pfeffer MA *et al.*: Effect of captopril on mortality and morbidity in patients with left ventricular dysfunction after myocardial infarction. *N Engl J Med* 1992, **327**:669–677.

Pericarditis and tamponade — A.H. Gershlick

Diagnosis

Symptoms

Pericarditis
Mild to severe precordial pain: on inspiration or worse on inspiration; may radiate to neck and shoulders; worse on coughing, swallowing, or sneezing; improved by leaning forward.

Dyspnoea, nausea.

Tamponade
Precordial discomfort: occasionally, due to large effusions.

Cough, hoarseness, tachypnoea, dysphagia: due to pressure.

Malaise, cyanosis, dyspnoea, sweating, anxiety, hypotension: rapidly developing.

Signs

Pericarditis
Fever.

Pericardial, often pleuropericardial, coarse rub: best heard at left sternal edge with patient leaning forward; may come and go over a few hours, may decrease with development of effusion.

Initially normal venous pressure.

Tamponade
Tachycardia: nearly always present.

Low blood and pulse pressures.

Pulsus paradoxus: pulse may disappear on inspiration; may occur in asthma.

Raised venous pressure: with prominent 'y' descent and no 'x' descent; may increase on inspiration.

Investigations
- For any pericardial disease, the underlying cause must always be sought.

Pericarditis
Full blood count, ESR and U&E measurement.

Antistreptolysin O titre, antineutrophil factor, rheumatoid factor analysis.

Cardiac enzyme tests: enzymes may be normal or increase, but creatinine phosphokinase MB probably is not significantly increased unless accompanying myocarditis.

Paired viral antibody screening: increase in neutralizing antibodies (up to 4 times) within 3–4 weeks of onset.

Mantoux test.

ECG: changes throughout all leads; raised ST segment, inverted T waves only in some patients, pericardial effusion (low-voltage QRS and T wave in large effusions), electrical alternans (caused by heart swinging about).

Chest radiography: normal unless pericardial fluid >250 ml; cardiac contour may be globular, with no congestion in lungs.

Tamponade
Echocardiography: essential in any patient in whom pericardial fluid is suspected (e.g. cardiomegaly on chest radiography with hypotension); right ventricular collapse characteristic of tamponade.

Complications
Relapsing or constrictive pericarditis, pericardial effusion and tamponade: complications of pericarditis.

Hypotension, renal failure: complications of tamponade.

Differential diagnosis

Pericarditis
Extension of infarct after infarction.
Myocardial infarction, unstable angina, ulcer dyspepsia, acute aortic dissection, spontaneous pneumothorax, pleurisy.

Tamponade
Cardiomyopathy or constrictive pericarditis.

Aetiology

Causes of pericarditis
Viral: may be associated with pleurisy.
Immune or collagen diseases: SLE, scleroderma.
Rheumatic fever, rheumatoid arthritis.
Myocardial infarction or cardiac surgery.
Metabolic: uraemia, myxoedema.
AIDS, opportunistic infections (e.g. tuberculosis).
Association with neoplasia, particularly lymphomas, leukaemia, carcinoma of bronchus or breast.

Causes of tamponade
Any of the above, but particularly the following:
Carcinoma of bronchus or breast.
Uraemia.
Cardiac surgery.
Viral infection (in young patients).

Epidemiology
- The incidence at post-mortem examination is 2–6%.
- The clinical incidence is <1 in 100 hospital admissions.
- More men than women are affected.
- The disorder may recur after treatment but is usually a one-off event, depending on the cause.

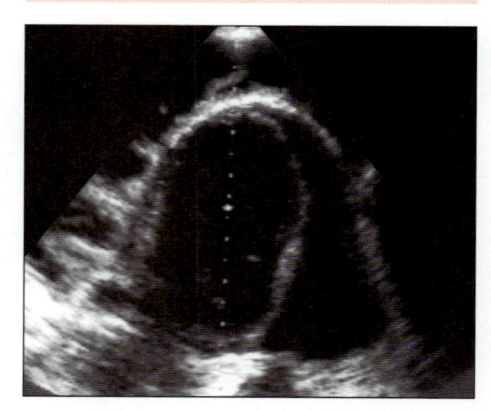

Pericardial space containing fluid (top centre); bright pericardium (mid centre); left ventricle (lower centre); fibrinous strands in pericardial fluid (lower left).

Treatment

Diet and lifestyle
- No special dietary precautions are necessary.
- Overactivity is contraindicated until the symptoms have resolved.

Pharmacological treatment
- Drugs are indicated for pericarditis.
- Aspirin usually settles both pain and fever; indomethacin is particularly useful in preventing recurrence; a short course of steroids may be needed.
- Specific treatment is needed for any related condition.

Standard dosage	Aspirin 300–600 mg every 3–4 h.
	Indomethacin 50–200 mg in divided doses (adults).
	Prednisolone 30 mg for 2–3 weeks, then reduced depending on symptoms.
Contraindications	*Aspirin:* peptic ulceration, hypersensitivity.
	Indomethacin: peptic ulceration.
	Prednisolone: osteoporosis, history of gastrointestinal symptoms, tuberculosis, pregnancy.
	Caution in renal or hepatic impairment.
Main drug interactions	*All:* warfarin.
	Indomethacin: aspirin, steroids.
	Prednisolone: aspirin.
Main side effects	*Aspirin:* dyspepsia.
	Indomethacin: gastrointestinal problems, including bleeding.
	Prednisolone: hypertension, peripheral oedema, potassium loss, hyperglycaemia.

Non-pharmacological treatment
- For tamponade, pericardial aspiration may be life-saving with large effusions.
- As much fluid as possible should be drained; blood-stained effusions usually signify malignancy, but all samples should be sent for cytology and bacteriology.
- Recurrent effusions may need balloon pericardotomy or surgical drainage.
- Chemotherapy can be started if malignant disease has been confirmed.

Treatment aims
To prevent adverse haemodynamic changes of tamponade.
To treat underlying condition.

Prognosis
- Prognosis depends on the underlying condition: it is good for pericarditis but poor for malignant pericardial effusion.
- Patients with pericarditis usually recover completely in 1–2 weeks.

Follow-up and management
- Regular echocardiographic follow-up is necessary for pericardial effusions.

Key references
Fowler NO: Cardiac tamponade. A clinical or an echocardiographic diagnosis. *Circulation* 1993, **87**:1738–1741.

Friman G, Fohlman J: The epidemiology of viral heart disease. *Scand J Inf Dis* 1993, **88**:7–10.

Spodick DH: Pericarditis in systemic diseases. *Cardiol Clin* 1990, **8**:709–716.

Pulmonary embolism
K. Priestley and S.P. Hanley

Diagnosis

Symptoms
Pleuritic chest pain, dyspnoea, haemoptysis: indicating acute minor pulmonary embolism.

Acute-onset dyspnoea, syncope, central chest pain: indicating acute massive pulmonary embolism.

Gradual-onset dyspnoea, pleuritic chest pain, decreasing exercise tolerance: indicating subacute massive pulmonary embolism.

Increasing dyspnoea, effort syncope: indicating chronic pulmonary embolism.

Signs
- Pulmonary embolism is manifest in several ways, depending on the extent of pulmonary vascular obstruction, the time during which the obstruction accumulates, and the presence or absence of pre-existing heart or lung disease.

Shortness of breath, pleural rub, signs associated with pleural effusion: indicating pulmonary infarction.

Tachypnoea or hyperventilation, reduced cardiac output, right heart failure: indicating massive pulmonary embolism.

Pulmonary hypertension: indicating chronic pulmonary embolism.

Investigations
- The diagnosis of pulmonary embolism needs a high index of clinical suspicion, combined with the results of investigations that may confirm or refute these suspicions.

Pulmonary angiography: allows definitive diagnosis but is invasive and needs specialized facilities; emboli seen as filling defects within contrast-filled pulmonary arteries.

Chest radiography: helps to exclude other conditions; may show vascular markings or large pulmonary artery shadow in massive embolism; may also show linear basal atelectasis in pulmonary infarction; but this is a nonspecific sign.

ECG: the classic S_1, Q_3, T_3 pattern is nonspecific and unusual.

Ventilation perfusion scanning: easily performed, low-risk procedure; normal scan virtually excludes pulmonary embolus; nondiagnostic scans need investigation for presence of peripheral venous thrombosis to support diagnosis of pulmonary embolism (if negative, untreated patient has <3% chance of subsequent pulmonary embolism) or pulmonary angiography; high-probability scan usually diagnostic, with 98% specificity, 91% positive predictive value (74% in patients with previous pulmonary embolism), but low sensitivity (41%); investigation must not be delayed because 14% of high-probability scans and 45% of indeterminate scans become normal by day 7 of treatment.

Echocardiography: primarily useful in differential diagnosis of dyspnoea; thrombus seen within right heart or proximal pulmonary artery and high index of clinical suspicion may be considered diagnostic.

Doppler ultrasonography, phlebography, impedance phlethysmography: indirect investigations for proximal leg vein thrombosis; if positive, they may provide a useful alternative to pulmonary angiography in patients with suspected minor pulmonary embolism but indeterminate lung scan.

Complications
Death.

Pulmonary infarction, infection, cavitation, or hypertension.

Differential diagnosis
- Pulmonary embolism has a wide differential diagnosis and hence its reputation as 'The Great Masquerader'.

Acute minor pulmonary embolism
Pneumonia.

Acute massive pulmonary embolism
Septicaemia.
Myocardial infarction.
Hypovolaemia.
Pericardial tamponade.

Subacute massive pulmonary embolism
Pulmonary oedema
Pneumonia
Hyperventilation.

Chronic pulmonary embolism
Primary pulmonary hypertension.

Aetiology
- >90% of pulmonary emboli originate as deep venous thrombosis of the lower extremities.
- Common causes include the following:
Surgery within past 1 month.
Medical illness (e.g. myocardial infarction or stroke).
Immobility, cancer, obesity, or oral contraception.
Pregnancy or oestrogen therapy.
Indwelling central venous lines.
Hypercoagulable states, which may be acquired (e.g. lupus anticoagulant, anticardiolipin antibodies) or inherited (e.g. antithrombin III deficiency, protein C deficiency).

Epidemiology
- In England and Wales, ~1600 deaths due to pulmonary embolism are registered each year, although the annual death rate is estimated to be 20 000.
- Deaths are more common in women and increase with age.
- At necropsy, pulmonary embolism has been found in 9–26% of all patients; it was suspected before death in only ~16%.

Treatment

Diet and lifestyle
- Patients should avoid periods of sustained immobility, e.g. during longhaul flights.

Pharmacological treatment

Anticoagulant treatment: heparin
- Heparin is used for acute treatment of haemodynamically stable patients; it prevents further fibrin deposition and thrombus extension.
- Treatment must be commenced immediately if clinical suspicion is high.

Standard dosage	Heparin bolus 5000–8000 units followed by i.v. infusion to maintain activated partial thromboplastin time at 1.5–2.5 times control.
Contraindications	Active bleeding, recent cerebral haemorrhage or brain, eye, or spinal-cord surgery, malignant hypertension.
Special points	High-dose s.c. heparin reduces need for i.v. infusion and increases patient mobility.
Main drug interactions	Oral anticoagulants or drugs that interfere with platelet function, e.g. aspirin or dextran solutions.
Main side effects	Bleeding, heparin-induced thrombocytopenia.

Anticoagulant treatment: warfarin
- Warfarin has no role in immediate treatment but prevents recurrence; it impairs coagulation, thus reducing thrombus formation.

Standard dosage	Warfarin 10 mg daily for 2 days (average-sized adult); maintenance dose adjusted to obtain INR 2.0–3.0
Contraindications	As for heparin; avoided in pregnancy.
Special points	Should be started at same time as heparin treatment.
Main drug interactions	Many drugs may enhance or reduce the activity of warfarin; drug data sheets should be consulted.
Main side effects	Bleeding.

Thrombolytic treatment
- This is indicated for haemodynamically compromised patients with proven pulmonary embolism (i.e. high clinical suspicion and high-probability lung scan or pulmonary artery thrombus seen on echocardiography or angiography).
- Treatment promotes the dissolution of recently formed thrombus. It produces a more rapid resolution of emboli and improvement in cardiopulmonary status than heparin therapy alone does. No reduction in mortality, however, has been shown.

Standard dosage	Streptokinase 250 000 units for 30 min followed by 100 000 units/h for 24 h. Urokinase 4400 units/kg for 10 min followed by 4400 units/kg/h for 12–24 h. rt-PA 100 mg by continuous infusion for 2 h.
Contraindications	Active bleeding, recent cerebrovascular accident, recent trauma, major surgery, or organ biopsy.
Special points	Local administration is no more effective and is not safer than peripheral administration, which is simpler. All thrombolytic agents appear equally effective. Should be followed by heparin treatment.
Main drug interactions	None.
Main side effects	Bleeding (the risk of major haemorrhage is twice that with heparin), allergic reactions to streptokinase.

Prophylactic treatment
- Most deaths from pulmonary emboli are sudden or occur in patients in whom the diagnosis was not suspected; therefore a significant reduction in mortality is only achieved by adequate prevention.
- Physical measures: early mobilization, pneumatic calf compression, and graduated compression stockings.
- Drugs: conventional heparin 5000 units s.c. every 8–12 h, low molecular weight heparin 3500–5000 units once daily depending on type used, or low-dose warfarin.

Treatment aims
To reduce morbidity of acute episode.
To prevent recurrence of pulmonary embolism or chronic pulmonary hypertension.

Other treatments
Inferior vena cava filters: used when anticoagulation is contraindicated or fails.
Pulmonary embolectomy.

Prognosis
- One-third of acute or subacute pulmonary emboli result in sudden death or are undiagnosed during life.
- Patients with untreated clinically apparent pulmonary emboli have a 30% mortality from recurrent emboli; this is reduced to 8% with effective treatment.
- Survivors of the acute or subacute episode usually have no clinical sequelae.
- Chronic pulmonary embolism carries a grave prognosis and pharmacological treatment is generally ineffective; elective thromboendarterectomy may produce long-term improvement in some patients.
- Patients who have had pulmonary emboli are at increased risk of further thromboembolic episodes when exposed to situations in which thrombosis might occur.

Follow-up and management
- Oral anticoagulant treatment and monitoring are continued for at least 3–6 months but may be continued indefinitely if underlying risk factors cannot be controlled.

Key references
Becker DM, Philbrick JT, Selby JB: Inferior vena cava filters indications, safety, effectiveness. *Arch Intern Med* 1992, **152**:1985–1994.

Goldhaber SZ, Morpurgo M, WHO/ISFC Task Force on Pulmonary Embolism: Diagnosis, treatment, and prevention of pulmonary embolism. *JAMA* 1992, **268**:1727–1733.

PIOPED Investigators: Value of the ventilation/perfusion scan in acute pulmonary embolism. *JAMA* 1990, **263**:2753–2759.

Stein PD et al.: Complications and validity of pulmonary angiography in acute pulmonary embolism. *Circulation* 1992, **85**:462–468.

Restrictive cardiomyopathy and constrictive pericarditis
I.A. Simpson

Diagnosis

Symptoms
Dyspnoea.
Fatigue.
Ankle or abdominal swelling.

Signs

Restrictive cardiomyopathy
Raised jugular venous pressure.
Inspiratory increase in jugular venous pressure: Kussmaul's sign.
Palpable apex beat.
Mild or moderate cardiomegaly.
Third or fourth heart sounds.
Peripheral oedema.
Ascites.

Constrictive pericarditis
Raised jugular venous pressure, with rapid diastolic 'y' descent.
Kussmaul's sign.
Diffuse or impalpable apex beat.
Intercostal indrawing of apex in systole: Broadbent's sign.
Early diastolic pericardial 'knock'.
Widened splitting of second heart sound.

Investigations
- The two conditions overlap considerably, and separating them on clinical findings and investigations may be impossible; thoracotomy may be needed to exclude or confirm the diagnosis.

Chest radiography: *restrictive cardiomyopathy*, shows mild or moderate cardiomegaly; *constrictive pericarditis*, shows normal heart size and pericardial calcification.

ECG: *restrictive cardiomyopathy*, shows T-wave changes or bundle branch block, and atrial arrhythmias; *constrictive pericarditis*, shows nonspecific T-wave flattening and atrial fibrillation; *both*, shows low voltage complexes.

Echocardiography: *restrictive cardiomyopathy*, shows myocardial thickening and characteristic 'ground-glass' appearance (in amyloid); *constrictive pericarditis*, shows normal myocardial thickness and thickened pericardium; *both*, shows normal ventricular dimensions with enlarged atria and good systolic and poor diastolic function.

CT: *restrictive cardiomyopathy*, shows myocardial thickening and normal pericardium; *constrictive pericarditis*, shows normal myocardial thickness and pericardial calcification.

Cardiac catheterization: *restrictive cardiomyopathy*, shows left ventricular filling pressure exceeding right ventricular filling pressure and pulmonary artery systolic pressure often >45 mmHg, with myocardial biopsy possibly diagnostic; *constrictive pericarditis*, shows identical left and right ventricular filling pressures and pulmonary artery systolic pressure usually <45 mmHg, with normal myocardial biopsy; *both*, shows rapid 'y' descent in atrial pressure and early dip in diastolic pressure, with pressure rise to plateau in mid or late diastole.

Complications
Symptomatic hypotension.
Atrial and ventricular arrhythmias.
Progressive 'heart failure': in constrictive pericarditis, the 'heart' itself is not failing, but the resulting clinical features are similar to restrictive cardiomyopathy.
Hepatic failure: resulting from chronic hepatic venous congestion.
Nephrotic syndrome.
Conduction abnormalities: in restrictive cardiomyopathy.

Differential diagnosis
Biventricular heart failure: myocardial infarction, myocardial ischaemia, dilated cardiomyopathy.
Myocardial thickening: hypertension, aortic stenosis, hypertrophic cardiomyopathy.
Cardiac tamponade.
Nephrotic syndrome (other causes).

Aetiology

Causes of restrictive cardiomyopathy
Amyloidosis.
Glycogen storage disorders.
Haemochromatosis.
Endomyocardial fibrosis.
Eosinophilia.
Neoplastic infiltration.
Collagen vascular disorders.
Pseudoxanthoma elasticum.
Myocardial fibrosis of any origin.

Causes of constrictive pericarditis
- Most causes are unknown.

Tuberculosis (<15% of patients).
Chronic renal failure.
Connective tissue disorders.
Neoplastic infiltration.
Irradiation (often years earlier).
Post-purulent pericarditis.
Haemopericardium after surgery (rare).

Epidemiology
- Both conditions are rare.
- All age groups are affected.
- Glycogen storage disorders are incompatible with progression to adult life.

Treatment

Diet and lifestyle
- Patients' daily activities are restricted by fatigue, breathlessness, and fluid retention.

Pharmacological treatment

Restrictive cardiomyopathy
- Specific measures are generally unsatisfactory.
- Amyloid has no known pharmacological treatment.
- Patients with haemochromatosis should be given iron-chelating agents, e.g. desferrioxamine.
- Corticosteroids are only effective during the acute myocardial phase of eosinophilia.

Constrictive pericarditis
- The only satisfactory treatment is surgical.
- Patients with tuberculous pericarditis should be pretreated by antituberculous therapy; if the diagnosis is confirmed after pericardial resection, full antituberculous therapy should be continued for 6–12 months after resection. *See* Tuberculosis, extrapulmonary *for details*.

Non-pharmacological treatment

Restrictive cardiomyopathy
Permanent pacing for conduction abnormalities in amyloid.

Bimonthly venesection often for 2–3 years to reduce iron storage in haemochromatosis.

Endocardial resection after fibrosis is established in eosinophilia.

Transplantation occasionally.

Constrictive pericarditis
Complete surgical resection of the pericardium (myocardial inflammation or fibrosis may delay symptomatic response).

Treatment aims
To relieve symptoms.
To remove underlying causes.

Prognosis
- Prognosis is good after resection for constrictive pericarditis.
- Restrictive cardiomyopathy has poor prognosis.

Follow-up and management
- Management is purely palliative.

Key references
Maisch B: Pericardial diseases, with a focus on etiology, pathogenesis, pathophysiology new diagnostic imaging methods, and treatment. *Curr Opin Cardiol* 1994, **9**:379–388.

Spyrou N, Foale R: Restrictive cardiomyoptahies. *Curr Opin Cardiol* 1994, **9**:344–348.

Ward D: Pericardial and myocardial disease. *Practitioner* 1993, **237**:929–932.

Shock, acute hypotensive   A. Pitkin and D. Smith

Diagnosis

Symptoms
- Symptoms of hypotensive shock are nonspecific; they include the following:

Restlessness.
Confusion or stupor.
Breathlessness.
Chest pain.
- Symptoms of the underlying cause may predominate.

Signs
Hypotension: a useful definition is systolic blood pressure <90 mmHg.
Oliguria: <30 ml/h.
Cyanosis.
Confusion.
Peripheral vasoconstriction or vasodilatation: may indicate high or low systemic vascular resistance, respectively.
Tachycardia and third heart sound.

Investigations

Initial investigations
Full blood count, haematocrit, U&E, and creatinine analysis.
Cardiac enzyme analysis: if myocardial injury suspected.
Blood culture: if any infective process known or suspected.
Arterial blood gas analysis: to assess hypoxaemia and acidosis.
ECG and chest radiography: mandatory.

Circulatory assessment
- This should ideally be done in an intensive care unit.

Central venous cannulation: to measure central venous pressure.
Arterial cannulation: sphygmomanometry may be unreliable in shock.
Pulmonary artery catheterization: for pulmonary artery pressure, pulmonary capillary wedge pressure, and thermodilution cardiac output.
Echocardiography: for left ventricular function or if valve lesion, ventricular septal defect, or tamponade suspected.

Complications
Myocardial ischaemia or infarction.
Acute renal failure.
Ischaemic stroke.
Hepatic dysfunction.
Paralytic ileus.
Lactic acidosis: an indicator of severe tissue hypoxia.

Differential diagnosis
Not applicable.

Aetiology

Central venous pressure < −3 cm H_2O*
Indicates hypovolaemia.
Warm peripheries (low systemic vascular resistance): vasodilatation due to septicaemia or drug overdose.
Cool peripheries (high systemic resistance): normal haemoglobin or hamatocrit indicates haemorrhage; high haemoglobin indicates salt and water loss, e.g. from peritonitis, pancreatitis, diabetic ketoacidosis, burns, polyuric phase of acute tubular necrosis.

Central venous pressure > +1 cm H_2O*
Indicates 'pump failure'.
Tension pneumothorax.
Pulmonary embolism.
Impaired myocardial contractility due to acute myocardial infarction or ischaemia, sepsis, acidaemia, electrolyte disturbance, negatively inotropic agents (e.g. beta antagonists, antiarrhythmic agents).
Arrhythmia.
Cardiac tamponade.
Ruptured interventricular septum.
Acute mitral or aortic valve regurgitation.
Aortic stenosis.

*Measured from the sternal angle.

Epidemiology
Not applicable.

Septicaemia and hypotensive shock
- The circulatory hallmark of sepsis is an unpredictable derangement of regional blood flow. Inappropriate vasodilatation of muscle and skin arterioles may coexist with profound vasoconstriction of the renal and splanchnic vascular beds.
- The hypotension has many causes: a fall in systemic vascular resistance to <25% of normal, depression of myocardial contractility by hypoxaemia and acidaemia, dilatation of venous capacitance vessels resulting in low central venous pressure, and disruption of capillary function causing leakage of intravascular fluid and plasma proteins into alveoli, gastrointestinal tract, peritoneal cavity, and other tissues.
- The combination of myocardial impairment and damage to alveolar capillary basement membranes means that attempts to restore the blood pressure by rapid intravenous infusion of fluid will probably result in pulmonary oedema.

Treatment

Diet and lifestyle
Not applicable.

Pharmacological treatment
- Whenever possible, the underlying cause should be treated.
- Immediate measures include the following:

Provision of oxygen: hypoxaemia contributes to lactic acid production.
Treatment of arrhythmias: cardioversion preferable to negatively inotropic anti-arrhythmic drugs.
Plasma expander administration, if central venous pressure < −3 cm H_2O.
Correction of any electrolyte disturbance.
Broad-spectrum antibiotic treatment, if sepsis suspected.
Inotropic support for hypotension without hypovolaemia, as follows:

For oliguria
- Dopamine is the first choice in oliguria; it enhances renal blood flow at a low dose, inotropic and vasoconstrictor at doses >5 µg/kg/min ($beta_1$, alpha agonism). It must be administered centrally.

Standard dosage	Dopamine 3–5 µg/kg/min.
Contraindications	Phaeochromocytoma.
Main drug interactions	Monoamine oxidase inhibitors.
Main side effects	Vomiting, tachycardia, angina, headache.

After myocardial infarction
- Dobutamine is the first choice after myocardial infarction; it is predominantly a $beta_1$ agonist; it improves myocardial oxygen supply:demand ratio and causes peripheral vasodilatation (hence its use if the systemic vascular resistance is high).

Standard dosage	Dobutamine 5–20 µg/kg/min.
Contraindications	Outflow tract obstruction, proarrhythmic tendencies.
Main drug interactions	Hypotension with other vasodilators.
Main side effects	Tachycardia, local phlebitis, hypokalaemia.

For severe hypotension
- Adrenaline is the most positively inotropic catecholamine; it acts as a beta agonist at low dose, and an alpha agonist at doses >10 µg/min and causes peripheral vasoconstriction (hence its use if systemic vascular resistance is low).

Standard dosage	Adrenaline 2–40 µg/min.
Contraindications	Hypertension, tachyarrhythmias.
Main drug interactions	Inhalational anaesthetics, tricyclic antidepressants.
Main side effects	Tachycardia, arrhythmias.

For bradycardia, atrioventricular block, and right heart failure
- Isoprenaline is used in bradycardia, atrioventricular block, and right heart failure; it causes pulmonary and systemic vasodilatation; it worsens myocardial supply:demand ratio and ventilation/perfusion mismatch.

Standard dosage	Isoprenaline 1–10 µg/min.
Contraindications	Cardiac ischaemia, hyperthyroidism.
Main drug interactions	Inhalational anaesthetics, tricyclic antidepressants.
Main side effects	Atrial and ventricular tachyarrhythmias.

If systemic vascular resistance is profoundly low
- Noradrenaline is used if the systemic vascular resistance is profoundly low; its alpha agonism causes vasoconstriction; a rise in blood pressure occurs at the expense of a fall in cardiac output.

Standard dosage	Noradrenaline 1–10 µg/min.
Contraindications	Myocardial dysfunction.
Main drug interactions	Tricyclic antidepressants.
Main side effects	Digit necrosis, myocardial ischaemia.

Treatment aims
To increase cardiac output, blood pressure, and tissue oxygen delivery to a level that avoids the detrimental end-organ effects of anaerobic metabolism and lactic acid production.

Other treatments

Mechanical ventilation
- This allows effective correction of hypoxaemia and eliminates the work of breathing (most useful in acute left ventricular failure).

Intra-aortic balloon pump
- This is a temporary measure (24–48 h) while spontaneous improvement or definitive treatment (e.g. valve or ventricular septal defect repair) is awaited.
- It is useful in cardiac surgery and refractory unstable angina.
- Complications, in 20% of patients, include leg ischaemia, aortic dissection, haemolysis, thrombocytopenia, infection.

Surgery
- Surgery is indicated early in rupture of interventricular septum or papillary muscle, aortic dissection, and subacute myocardial rupture causing tamponade.

Prognosis
- The main determinant of outcome is the underlying disorder: for example, hypotension due to diabetic ketoacidosis in a young person has a favourable prognosis, whereas cardiogenic shock resulting from acute anterior myocardial infarction has a mortality of 80–90%.

Follow-up and management
- No follow-up is needed.

Key references
Barnard MJ, Linter SPK: Acute circulatory support. *BMJ* 1993, **307**:35–41.

Bradley RD: Intensive care. In *Oxford Textbook of Medicine*. Edited by Weatherall DJ, Ledingham JGG, Warrell DA. Oxford: Oxford University Press, 1993, pp 14.1–14.21.

Tachycardia, supraventricular — C.J. Garratt

Diagnosis

Definition
- Supraventricular tachycardias include the following:

Sinus tachycardia.

Atrial fibrillation.

Atrial flutter.

Atrial tachycardia.

Atrioventricular re-entrant tachycardia.

Atrioventricular nodal re-entrant tachycardia.

- Atrioventricular re-entrant and nodal re-entrant tachycardias, the two common supraventricular tachycardias arising from the atrioventricular junction, are discussed here.

Symptoms
Palpitation: paroxysms of regular palpitation at 140–240 beats/min, with sudden onset and offset.

Syncope: palpitation may be associated with syncope or presyncope at onset of attack, when blood pressure is probably at its lowest.

Chest pain: unusual but may occur during attacks, particularly in presence of ischaemic heart disease.

Paroxysmal attacks: occasionally precipitated by postural changes or may be associated with particular times in menstrual cycle.

Signs
Fast, regular pulse.

Signs of left ventricular failure: unusual unless structural heart disease is coexistent.

- Atrioventricular dissociation is not evident (no cannon waves in neck).
- Blood pressure is usually well maintained after the first few seconds of an attack.

Investigations
ECG: regular rhythm present, usually with narrow QRS complexes; occasionally, pre-existing or rate-related bundle branch block leads to broad QRS complexes.

Chest radiography: usually normal unless structural heart disease coexistent.

Electrophysiology: indicated if catheter ablation contemplated or for risk assessment in symptomatic patients with Wolff–Parkinson–White syndrome.

Complications
Left ventricular failure: caused by coexistent structural heart disease; supraventricular tachycardia may cause ventricular failure in the absence of pre-existing structural heart disease only if tachycardia is incessant and has continued uninterrupted for many months or years.

Differential diagnosis
Atrial tachycardia or atrial flutter.

Ventricular tachycardia: if atrioventricular re-entrant tachycardia is conducted with bundle branch block.

- When the history is being taken, establishing the presence or absence of structural heart disease, e.g. cardiomyopathy or previous myocardial infarction, is important. A history or known diagnosis of either of these conditions makes a diagnosis of ventricular tachycardia much more probable than atrioventricular re-entrant or nodal re-entrant tachycardia. If the QRS complex is broad and has a pattern unlike that of classic left or right bundle branch block, then diagnosis is probably ventricular tachycardia.

Aetiology
Atrioventricular re-entrant tachycardia
- The structural substrate is a congenital abnormality of the conducting system of the heart, whereby an extra electrical connection exists between the atria and the ventricles.
- Tachycardia arises when an electrical impulse passes from the atrium to the ventricle through the normal atrioventricular node but returns to the atria by the accessory pathway.

Atrioventricular nodal re-entrant tachycardia
- Patients have two functionally separate pathways within or close to the atrioventricular node.
- Tachycardia arises in a similar way to that arising in patients with atrioventricular re-entrant tachycardia.

Epidemiology
- These arrhythmias occur frequently and form most of the tachycardias in patients with structurally normal hearts.
- Men are more likely to have atrioventricular re-entrant tachycardia, and women atrioventricular nodal re-entrant tachycardia.
- Paroxysms of palpitation may start in infancy but more usually in teenage years or twenties.

Tachycardia, supraventricular

C.J. Garratt

Treatment

Diet and lifestyle
- If the tachycardias are initiated by atrial premature beats, abstinence from caffeine may help.
- Otherwise, no special precautions are necessary.

Pharmacological treatment

Acute treatment

Standard dosage	Adenosine i.v. bolus dose followed by saline flush, starting at 3 mg, with a second dose of 6 mg if tachycardia does not terminate after 60 s; a further dose of 12 mg is given if tachycardia does not terminate after another 60 s. Verapamil 5 mg i.v slowly (30 s); if tachycardia has not terminated after 5 min, a second 5 mg dose may be given, if hypotension has not occurred.
Contraindications	*Adenosine:* asthma. *Verapamil:* poor ventricular function.
Special points	*Adenosine:* although 12 mg is maximum adult dose recommended in product licence, bolus doses of 18 mg may occasionally be need to terminate tachycardia; may exacerbate bronchoconstriction. *Verapamil:* negatively inotropic and should not be given to patients with known abnormal ventricular function or with signs of cardiomegaly on chest radiography; best not given to patients with a broad complex tachycardia because it may cause cardiovascular collapse if erroneously given to patients with ventricular tachycardia; i.v. verapamil should not be given to patient taking oral beta blockers be-cause sinus arrest or dramatic hypotension may occur.
Main drug interactions	*Adenosine:* increased effect with dipyridamole; decreased effect with theophylline.
Main side effects	*Adenosine:* flushing and chest tightness (transient).

Prophylaxis
- Beta blockade (e.g. atenolol 50–100 mg) is often effective in this role, particularly if the attacks are exercise-induced.
- Digoxin 0.125 mg and verapamil 120 mg 3 times daily may be effective but are contraindicated in the presence of a delta wave because they may increase the ventricular rate if atrial fibrillation complicates the Wolff–Parkinson–White syndrome.

Treatment aims
To terminate an acute paroxysm of tachycardia.
To suppress tachycardia.
To cure tachycardia.

Other treatments

Vagal manoeuvres
- Deep breathing or the Valsalva manoeuvre (best done with patient lying down), with straining for at least 15 s, should terminate tachycardia a few seconds after strain release.

Radiofrequency catheter ablation
- This is the treatment of choice for patients with recurrent symptomatic junctional tachycardias that do not respond to prophylactic drug treatment.

Prognosis
- Prognosis is generally excellent, and life expectancy does not differ from that of the normal population.
- Symptomatic patients with the Wolff–Parkinson–White pattern on the ECG during sinus rhythm have a small risk of sudden death, associated with the development of atrial fibrillation.

Follow-up and management
- Oral aspirin is advisable for 6 weeks after catheter ablation because the damaged endothelium may provide a focus for thrombus formation.
- Patients should be assessed for recurrence of symptoms or re-emergence of the Wolff–Parkinson–White pattern on the ECG.

Key references
Bennett DH: Cardiac Arrhythmias. Oxford: Butterworth Heinemann, 1993.

Camm AJ, Garratt CJ: Drug therapy: adenosine and supraventricular tachycardia. *N Engl J Med* 1991, **325**:1621–1629.

Nathan AW: Cardiac arrhythmias. In *Essentials of Cardiology*. Edited by Timmis AD, Nathan AW. Oxford: Blackwell, 1993.

Tachycardia, ventricular
D.E. Ward

Diagnosis

Symptoms
- Symptoms are not always manifest.

Palpitations.

Sudden shortness of breath.

Dizzy spell.

Blackouts.

Cardiac arrest.

Sudden death.

Signs
- Signs are not always manifest.

Tachycardia: 100–300 beats/min.

Hypotension and associated signs.

Cannon waves in jugular venous pressure, variable blood pressure, variation in intensity of first heart sound: signs of atrioventricular dissociation.

Investigations

12-lead ECG: initially, to confirm diagnosis, after treatment, for comparison of sinus rhythm; reveals tachycardia with QRS complexes 140 ms duration, evidence of atrio-ventricular dissociation (independent P waves, fusion beats, capture beats, second-degree ventriculo-atrial block), marked left or right axis deviation during tachycardia, absence of RS complexes in chest leads during tachycardia.

Adenosine test: initially, to distinguish from junctional or atrial tachycardia; if patient presents with stable tachycardia and if 12-lead ECG cannot be interpreted as showing ventricular tachycardia, incremental boluses of adenosine 0.05–0.20 mg/kg i.v. should be given, which terminates almost all junctional tachycardias, slows most atrial tachycardias, but affects almost no ventricular tachycardia except those arising in the right ventricular outflow tract.

Cardiac enzymes analysis: after treatment, if history suggests infarction.

Exercise test: under supervision of arrhythmia specialist to look for coronary disease, to provoke arrhythmia, and to assess drug efficacy.

24-h ambulatory ECG recording: to quantify frequency of ventricular arrhythmia and associated arrhythmias (e.g. ventricular premature beat).

Echocardiography: to assess left and right ventricular function.

Left ventricular and coronary angiography.

Complications

Cardiac arrest.

Sudden death.

Cardiogenic shock.

Pulmonary oedema.

Differential diagnosis
Supraventricular tachycardia: either atrial or junctional, with either right or left bundle branch block.
- All wide-complex tachycardias should be considered ventricular in origin until proved otherwise.

Aetiology
- Causes include the following:

Acute ischaemia: coronary obstruction by thrombus.

Large scar old infarction: previous surgery, dysplasias.

Microscopic scar infiltration: fibrosis.

No clinical disease: e.g. right ventricular outflow tachycardia, right ventricular dysplasia.

Functional disease: 'fascicular' tachycardia.

Tumours, malformations, other causes (rare).

Epidemiology
- 2–10% of patients suffering a myocardial infarction have a sustained ventricular tachycardia or cardiac arrest within 12 months.

Tachycardia, ventricular
D.E. Ward

Treatment

Diet and lifestyle
- Patients should avoid strenuous exercise and eat a normal diet unless they have evidence of coronary disease.

Pharmacological treatment
- The underlying disease process (e.g. coronary artery disease) or associated cardiogenic fluid retention must be treated.

Emergency
Cardiopulmonary resuscitation if necessary.

Lignocaine 50 mg i.v. in stable patients.

Direct-current cardioversion in unstable patients (synchronized) or if drug treatment fails.

- A succession of drugs is unwise, especially in patients with coronary disease and impaired ventricular function.
- Verapamil must not be given: it may cause profound collapse and even death.

Long-term
- Drug treatment should be supervised by a cardiologist with a special interest in arrhythmias.
- All antiarrhythmic drugs have arrhythmogenic properties, especially when used in combination with other antiarrhythmic drugs.
- Whether long-term drug treatment improves prognosis is not known.

Standard dosage	Disopyramide 250 mg slow release twice daily; alternatively procainamide or quinidine.
	Flecainide 100 mg twice daily; alternatively encainide or propafenone.
	Sotalol 80 mg twice daily; alternatively amiodarone.
Contraindications	*Disopyramide:* very poor left ventricular function.
	Flecainide: previous myocardial infarction; caution in patients with coronary disease.
	Sotalol: as for beta blockers generally.
Special points	*Flecainide:* increases pacing threshold.
	Sotalol: prolongs action potential duration (unlike other beta blockers).
	Amiodarone: high incidence of toxic effects, long elimination half-life; should be considered as a last-resort drug.
Main drug interactions	*Disopyramide:* antihistamines, antiepileptics.
	Flecainide: antidepressant, fluoxetine, antimalarial agents.
	Sotalol: as for beta blockers generally.
Main side effects	*Disopyramide:* vagolytic effects (dry mouth, slow stream).
	Flecainide: dizziness, arrhythmias.
	Sotalol: as for beta blockers generally.

Treatment aims
To suppress recurrence of tachycardia (drug treatment).

To terminate recurrence of tachycardia (device treatment).

To destroy the arrhythmia 'substrate', possibly offering a cure (ablation).

To correct mechanical heart disease and refractory arrhythmias (transplantation).

Other treatments
- Alternative long-term treatments include the following:

Implantation of automatic defibrillator device to terminate tachycardia: this also treats ventricular tachycardia by rapid pacing.

Ablation of localized focus or circuit causing tachycardia: radiofrequency energy and low-energy direct current are most popular sources; success rate <50%.

Electrophysiologically guided surgery.

Transplantation in selected patients with severe ventricular impairment.

Prognosis
- Prognosis depends on the underlying disease process and presentation.
- 1-year mortality in patients resuscitated from cardiac arrest occurring out of hospital is up to 50%.
- Long-term prognosis is excellent for ventricular tachycardia associated with a normal heart.

Follow-up and management
- Patients should be referred to a centre specializing in ventricular tachycardia to allow the correct choice of treatments to be selected.
- Long-term drug treatment can be assessed by ambulatory monitoring (in patients with frequent ventricular premature contractions) or electrophysiological studies (in patients with inducible tachycardia).
- Ventricular tachycardia is not a curable disease and needs long-term follow-up.

Key references
O'Nunain S, Ruskin J: Cardiac arrest. *Lancet* 1993, **341**:1641–1647.

Shenasa M *et al.*: Ventricular tachycardia. *Lancet* 1993, **341**:1512–1518.

Wolff–Parkinson–White syndrome
J. Morgan

Diagnosis

Definition
- Myocardial activation from atrial to ventricular myocardium occurs over an accessory connection (accessory to the normal His Purkinje system).
- If conduction occurs in sinus rhythm, pre-excitation is apparent on the ECG.
- The substrate for atrioventricular re-entry tachycardia is present; conduction in tachycardia from ventricle to atrium over the accessory connection is orthodromic (90%) or from atrium to ventricle is antidromic.

Symptoms
- Most patients who are found to have the Wolff–Parkinson–White syndrome are asymptomatic; the only feature is the presence of pre-excitation on the surface ECG.

Palpitation: most common symptom; caused by re-entry tachycardia (sudden onset and termination, regular, rapid – often >200 beats/min); may also be caused by paroxysmal atrial fibrillation (in ~5% of patients).
Chest pain: during tachycardia; pain or discomfort similar to angina; rarely indicates coronary artery disease.
Impaired consciousness: dizziness or faintness common; syncope less frequent (5%) and usually follows vasodilatation occurring as a secondary response to tachycardia.
Polyuria: accompanying sustained episodes of tachycardia.

Signs
- In sinus rhythm, no clinical signs indicate the presence of the condition; during tachycardia, clinical signs associated with the impaired circulation and abnormal cardiac action may be found, principally the following:

Rapid pulse.
Hypotension.
Alteration in the venous pulse wave form.

Investigations
Pre-excitation ECG: pre-excitation is the QRS configuration generated by fusion of ventricular activation wave fronts from normal His Purkinje system and accessory atrioventricular connection; myocardium activated through accessory connection gives rise to delta wave (slurred initial QRS); precise delta wave pattern depends on location of accessory connection on atrioventricular ring, and QRS configuration may be subtly or dramatically changed from normal; pre-excitation ceases with temporary cessation of anterograde conduction through accessory connection, or pre-excitation changes may vary depending on balance of activation between normal conduction system and accessory connection, (both influenced by autonomic tone); PR interval shortening results from myocardial activation through the accessory connection which lacks decremental conduction properties.
ECG during tachycardia: usually (90%) narrow complex tachycardia; retrograde atrial activation may be seen as P waves of altered configuration inscribed in ST segments; rate-related bundle branch block (aberrancy) or antidromic tachycardia results in broad QRS complex tachycardia.
Ambulatory monitoring: paroxysms of tachycardia may be seen on 24-h or 48-h monitoring; usually too infrequent for capture of tachycardia to be probable; self-activated recording devices (cardiac memo/wrist recorder) with transtelephonic transmission to a recording centre may be more useful.
Electrophysiological study: cardiac extrastimulation techniques and recording of endocardial ECG allows diagnosis and characterization of the condition in almost all cases; complex studies rarely done for diagnosis alone but used as prelude to radiofrequency catheter ablation of accessory connection; single wire study determines ventricular response rate through accessory connection conduction during atrial fibrillation to assess risk of malignant arrhythmias secondary to rapid ventricular activation; this is an imprecise means of assessing the risk of sudden death.
Exercise stress testing: no role in defining connection conduction properties.

Complications
Atrial fibrillation.
Sudden cardiac death: rare.

Differential diagnosis
Atrioventricular nodal re-entry tachycardia: tachycardia due to dual atrioventricular node physiology allowing re-entry within the atrioventricular node; other types of supraventricular tachycardia (e.g. atrial flutter, fibrillation, ectopic atrial tachycardia, Mahaim re-entry).
Ventricular tachycardia: broad QRS complexes (due to antidromic tachycardia or aberrant conduction) may be misdiagnosed as tachycardia arising from a ventricular focus; algorithms are available to aid ECG differentiation.

Aetiology
- Wolff–Parkinson–White syndrome is not inherited.
- During early cardiac development, direct physical continuity exists between ventricular and atrial myocardium; in growth of atrioventricular sulcus, tissue at a later stage in cardiac development interrupts this, but defects may persist into neonatal and subsequently adult life.
- Term infants have frequently been found to have these connections, but they are presumed to be nonfunctional in most.
- Accessory connections appear microscopically to be normal myocardial muscle bundles bridging atrial and ventricular myocardium; they may have subepicardial or subendocardial locations; they are multiple in ~10% of patients with the condition.
- Ebstein's anomaly is associated with their presence, and multiple pathways are more common in these patients.

Epidemiology
- Early studies have suggested that ECG evidence of pre-excitation can be found in 0.3% of the population; probably only a few of such patients are symptomatic, but the evidence is conflicting.
- Depending on the nature of the population studies, documentation of tachycardia has varied from 5% to 90% of patients.

Treatment

Diet and lifestyle
- In patients with frequent symptoms, lifestyle is restricted by the occurrence of palpitations (often apparently related to stress or exertion) or by the side effects of drug treatment.

Pharmacological treatment
- Drugs are now considered second-line treatment for the Wolff–Parkinson–White syndrome.
- Asymptomatic patients need no drug treatment unless their occupation demands removal of all risk of tachycardia (e.g. airline pilots, certain military, police, and fire-brigade personnel).
- Symptomatic patients who need treatment but who do not wish to have radio-frequency catheter ablation can be given antiarrhythmic drugs; these exert their effect by altering atrioventricular nodal conduction or accessory connection conduction, or both, so that re-entry tachycardia will less probably be sustained.
- Drugs that slow atrioventricular nodal conduction but enhance accessory pathway conduction (e.g. digoxin) should not be used in isolation.
- Antiarrhythmic drugs often have unacceptable side effects, and some have been shown to have dangerous proarrhythmic effects.
- Drugs must be taken continuously, and not on an ad-hoc basis, to give optimal control of symptoms; even then, abolition of symptoms is rare.
- Adenosine can be used as an i.v. bolus to abort an episode of atrioventricular re-entry tachycardia.

Non-pharmacological treatment

Catheter ablation
- Catheter ablation is technically demanding but is associated with very low mortality and morbidity in skilled hands.
- Apposition of an ablation electrode to the endocardial location nearest the accessory connection results in cessation of accessory connection conduction on delivery of radiofrequency energy through the electrode.
- This is a low-voltage, high-frequency energy source, which results in heating of the electrode tip, in turn producing a small endocardial lesion (5–7 mm) that extends into the myocardium.
- Primary success is >90%.
- Failure to achieve complete abolition of accessory connection conduction leads to a small recurrence rate after apparently successful procedures.
- Radiofrequency catheter ablation is the treatment of choice because it is curative; other energy sources are available but are associated with various disadvantages.

Surgery
- Although curative, surgical division of accessory connections needs major cardiac surgery and so is associated with higher morbidity and mortality than catheter ablation.
- It should be reserved for patients in whom catheter ablation has been a repeated failure.

Treatment aims
To abolish accessory connection conduction and therefore risk of tachycardia and palpitation.
To remove risk of sudden cardiac death.
To assess risk in asymptomatic patients.

Prognosis
- The prognosis is probably that of the normal population after successful catheter ablation.
- Lesions induced by radiofrequency catheter ablation have not been associated with impairment of ventricular function or arrhythmogenic complications except in infant hearts, when lesions may grow with heart size.
- Untreated asymptomatic Wolff–Parkinson–White syndrome carries a good prognosis; the risk of sudden death in asymptomatic patients is probably very small.

Follow-up and management
- Recurrence of pre-excitation may occur early after a primarily successful catheter ablation (within 6 weeks) in as many as 10% of patients; occasionally, recurrence is not accompanied by symptom recurrence because of modification of the connection conduction properties.
- Late recurrence after successful catheter ablation (>3 months) is rare; patients usually experience short-lived episodes of palpitation or rhythm irregularity for some months after successful ablations, which may relate to a learning effect through which individuals have become sensitized to any short-lived change in heart rhythm (e.g. ectopic activity) because, before treatment, these heralded onset of tachycardia; these symptoms resolve with time and reassurance.
- After surgical treatment, standard follow-up is needed.
- Follow-up of patients treated by anti-arrhythmic drugs is determined by their symptoms and drug side effects.

Key references
Jackman WM et al.: Catheter ablation of accessory atrioventricular pathways (Wolff–Parkinson–White syndrome) by radiofrequency current. *N Engl J Med* 1991, **324**:1605–1611.

Index

A

ablation, radiofrequency catheter
  for supraventricular tachycardia 45
  for Wolff–Parkinson–White syndrome 49

abscess
  aortic root 22
  cerebral 20, 22
  myocardial 22

ACE inhibitors *see* angiotensin-converting enzyme inhibitors

acidosis, lactic 42

adenosine
  for supraventricular tachycardia 45
  for Wolff–Parkinson–White syndrome 49

adrenaline
  for asystole 17
  for electromechanical dissociation 17
  for pulseless ventricular tachycardia 17
  for severe hypotension 43
  for ventricular fibrillation 17

alkalizing agents for electromechanical dissociation 17

alpha blockers for hypertension 27

aminoglycoside for endocarditis 23

amiodarone
  for cardiac failure and dilated cardiomyopathy 15
  for hypertrophic cardiomyopathy 29
  for ventricular tachycardia 47

amlodipine for angina
  pectoris 3
  unstable 5

amphotericin B for endocarditis 23

ampicillin for endocarditis 23

analgesics for myocardial infarction 35

aneurysm 34
  mycotic 22
  thoracic aortic 6

angina 4, 10, 18, 20, 34
  pectoris 2
  preinfarction *see* unstable angina
  stable *see* angina pectoris
  unstable 2, 4, 36

angiography
  coronary 35
    percutaneous transluminal, for unstable angina 5

angioplasty, percutaneous transluminal coronary, for angina pectoris 3

angiotensin-converting enzyme inhibitors
  for aortic dissection 7
  for aortic regurgitation 9
  for cardiac failure and dilated cardiomyopathy 15

angiotensin-converting enzyme inhibitors *cont.*
  for hypertension 27
  for myocardial infarction 35

angor pectoris *see* angina pectoris

antiarrhythmics
  for cardiac failure and dilated cardiomyopathy 15
  for hypertrophic cardiomyopathy 29
  for Wolff–Parkinson–White syndrome 49

antibiotics
  broad-spectrum for sepsis in acute hypotensive shock 43
  for endocarditis 23
    in aortic regurgitation 9
    in aortic stenosis 11
    in atrial septal defect 13
    in Eisenmenger complex 21

anticoagulants
  for Eisenmenger complex 21
  for hypertrophic cardiomyopathy 29
  for mitral regurgitation 31
  for mitral stenosis 33
  for pulmonary embolism 39
  for unstable angina 5

antiemetics for myocardial infarction 35

antiplatelet agents for angina
  pectoris 3
  unstable 5

antituberculous therapy for tuberculous pericarditis 41

aortic
  dissection 2, 4, 6, 22, 34, 36
  incompetence *see* aortic regurgitation
  regurgitation 6, 8, 10
  root abscess 22
  rupture 6
  sclerosis 10
  stenosis 2, 10, 40
  valve
    disease 28
    incompetence *see* aortic regurgitation
    insufficiency *see* aortic regurgitation
    regurgitation *see* aortic regurgitation
    stenosis *see* aortic stenosis

arrhythmia 2, 8
  atrial 12, 20, 40
  supraventricular 10
  ventricular 10, 40

aspiration, pericardial, for tamponade 37

aspirin
  for angina
    pectoris 3
    unstable 5
  for myocardial infarction 35
  for pericarditis 37

asystole 17

atenolol
  for hypertrophic cardiomyopathy 29
  for myocardial infarction 35
  for supraventricular tachycardia 45

atheroma 18

atrial
  arrhythmia 12, 20, 40
  bradyarrhythmia 14
  fibrillation 12, 14, 26, 28, 30, 32, 44, 48
  flutter 44, 48
  myxoma 22, 32
  septal defect 12, 20
  tachyarrhythmia 14
  tachycardia 44, 48

atrioventricular
  block 24 *see also* heart block
  dissociation 46
  excitation, anomalous *see* Wolff–Parkinson–White syndrome
  nodal re-entrant tachycardia 44, 48
  re-entrant tachycardia 44, 48

atropine
  for asystole 17
  for heart block 25

auricular *see* atrial

auriculoventricular dissociation *see* heart block

Austin–Flint murmur 8

B

balloon
  pump, intra-aortic, for acute hypotensive shock 43
  valvuloplasty for aortic stenosis 11

benzylpenicillin for endocarditis 23

beta blockers
  for angina
    pectoris 3
    unstable 5
  for aortic dissection 7
  for cardiomyopathy
    dilated 15
    hypertrophic 29
  for hypertension 27
  for myocardial infarction 35
  for supraventricular tachycardia 45

blood pressure
  high *see* hypertension
  low *see* hypotension

bradyarrhythmia 34 *see also* bradycardia
  atrial 14
  ventricular 14

bradycardia 22 *see also* bradyarrhythmia

Broadbent's sign 40

bundle branch block 44, 46

Index

C

calcium
 antagonists
  for angina
   pectoris 3
   unstable 5
  for aortic dissection 7
  for hypertension 27
  for hypertrophic cardiomyopathy 29
  for mitral regurgitation 31
 chloride for electromechanical dissociation 17

captopril
 for aortic regurgitation 9
 for cardiac failure and dilated cardiomyopathy 15
 for mitral regurgitation 31
 for myocardial infarction 35

cardiac *see also* heart
 arrest 46
 damage 26
 failure 8, 10, 14, 28
 output, low 8, 10, 20, 30, 32, 38
 rupture 34
 tamponade 6, 36, 40

cardiogenic shock 34, 46

cardiomyopathy 36, 44
 congestive *see* dilated cardiomyopathy
 dilated 14, 40
 hypertrophic 2, 10, 28, 30, 40
 restrictive 40

cardiopulmonary resuscitation 16
 for ventricular tachycardia 47

cardiorespiratory arrest 16

cardiovascular accidents 26

cardioversion
 for acute hypotensive shock 43
 for ventricular tachycardia 47

cerebral *see also* brain
 abscess 20, 22
 arterial attack *see* transient ischaemic attack
 haemorrhage 22
 ischaemia, transient *see* transient ischaemic attack
 vasospasm *see* transient ischaemic attack

cerebritis 22

cerebrovascular accident *see* stroke

cervical spondylosis 2

chest
 discomfort 2
 infections, recurrent 12
 pain 28, 34
  musculoskeletal 6
  pleuritic 38

chordal rupture 22

chylomicronaemia 18

ciprofibrate for dyslipoproteinaemia 19

claudication 18

coarse rub
 pericardial 36
 pleuropericardial 36

colestipol for dyslipoproteinaemia 19

conduction abnormalities 10, 40

cor pulmonale 12

coronary
 angiography 35
  percutaneous transluminal, for unstable angina 5
 angioplasty, percutaneous transluminal, for angina pectoris 3
 artery
  bypass grafting
   for angina 3, 5
   for cardiac failure and dilated cardiomyopathy 15
  disease 8

Corrigan's sign 8

corticosteroids
 for pericarditis 37
 for restrictive cardiomyopathy 41

CPR *see* cardiopulmonary resuscitation

D

Da Costa's syndrome 2

defibrillation for ventricular fibrillation 17

de Musset's sign 8

desferrioxamine for restrictive cardiomyopathy 41

diabetes 2

diamorphine for myocardial infarction 35

digoxin
 for atrial septal defect 13
 for cardiac failure and dilated cardiomyopathy 15
 for Eisenmenger complex 21
 for mitral regurgitation 31
 for mitral stenosis 33
 for supraventricular tachycardia 45

diltiazem for angina
 pectoris 3
 unstable 5

dipyridamole for unstable angina 5

disopyramide for ventricular tachycardia 47

diuretics
 for atrial septal defect 13
 for cardiac failure and dilated cardiomyopathy 15

diuretics *cont.*
 for Eisenmenger complex 21
 for mitral regurgitation 31
 for mitral stenosis 33

dobutamine for acute hypotensive shock after myocardial infarction 43

dopamine for oliguria 43

ductus arteriosus, patent 8, 20

Duroziez sign 8

dyslipoproteinaemia 18

dysrhythmia *see* arrhythmia

E

effusion
 pericardial 36
 pleural 38

Eisenmenger
 complex 20
 syndrome 12, 20

electromechanical dissociation 17

embolism 22
 pulmonary 4, 6, 38
 systemic 10, 28, 30, 32

embolization of vegetations 22

embolus
 paradoxical 12, 20
 peripheral 14
 pulmonary 34
 septic 22
 systemic 34

enalapril
 for cardiac failure and dilated cardiomyopathy 15
 for mitral regurgitation 31

encainide for ventricular tachycardia 47

encephalopathy 26

endocardial vegetations 22

endocarditis 22, 30, 32
 acute 22
 Candida 22
 culture-negative 22
 infective 8, 10, 12, 20, 28
 Libman–Sacks 22
 marantic 22
 noninfective 22
 subacute 22

endophthalmitis 22

epinephrine *see* adrenaline

erythrocytosis *see* polycythaemia

excitation, anomalous atrioventricular *see* Wolff–Parkinson–White syndrome

Index

F

Fallot's tetralogy 20
fenofibrate for dyslipoproteinaemia 19
fibrates for dyslipoproteinaemia 19
fibrillation
    atrial 12, 14, 26, 28, 30, 32, 44, 48
    ventricular 4, 17, 24
fish oils for dyslipoproteinaemia 19
flecainide for ventricular tachycardia 47
flucloxacillin for endocarditis 23
fluvastatin for dyslipoproteinaemia 19
foramen ovale, patent 20
frusemide
    for mitral stenosis 33
    for mitral regurgitation 31
fucidin for endocarditis 23
furosemide see frusemide

G

gentamicin for endocarditis 23
glomerulonephritis 22
glyceryl trinitrate for angina pectoris 3

H

haemorrhage, cerebral 22
heart see also cardiac
    block 10, 12, 24
    disease, ischaemic 26, 44
    failure 24, 26
        biventricular 40
        congestive 12
        progressive 22, 40
        right 30, 32, 38
    Pick's disease of the see constrictive pericarditis
    transplantation
        for cardiac failure 15
        for cardiomyopathy
            dilated 15
            hypertrophic 29
            restrictive 41
heart–lung transplantation for Eisenmenger complex 21
heparin
    for myocardial infarction 35
    for pulmonary oedema 39
    for unstable angina 5
hepatic
    congestion 14
    dysfunction 14, 42
    failure 40

hydralazine for mitral regurgitation 31
hypercholesterolaemia 18
hyperlipidaemia 2 see also lipidaemia
hypertension 2, 6, 26, 40
    pulmonary 8, 12, 14, 20, 30, 32, 38
    systemic 28
    'white-coat' 26
hypertrophic cardiomyopathy 2, 10, 28, 30, 40
hypertrophy, right ventricular 30
hyperventilation 38
hypotension 6, 36, 48
    postural 14
    symptomatic 40
hypotensive shock, acute 42
hypovolaemia 38
hypoxia 20
    tissue 42

I

indomethacin for pericarditis 37
infarction
    myocardial 2, 4, 6, 18, 34, 36, 38, 40, 42, 44
    pulmonary 20, 22, 38
    renal 6, 22
infection
    pulmonary 38
    recurrent chest 12
intra-aortic balloon pump for acute hypotensive shock 43
iron-chelating agents for haemochromatosis 41
ischaemia
    limb 6
    myocardial 6, 40, 42
    transient cerebral see transient ischaemic attack
ischaemic
    attack, transient 18, 26
    heart disease 26, 44
    stroke 42
isoprenaline
    for acute hypotensive shock 43
    for heart block 25
isoproterenol see isoprenaline
isosorbide for unstable angina 5

K

kidney see renal
Kussmaul's sign 40

L

lactic acidosis 42
lidocaine see lignocaine
life support
    advanced 17
    basic 16
lignocaine for ventricular tachycardia 47
lipidaemia 18
lipoprotein
    (a) 18
    high-density 18
    lipase 18
liver see hepatic
loop diuretics for cardiac failure and dilated cardiomyopathy 15

M

mechanical ventilation for acute hypotensive shock 43
metolazone for cardiac failure and dilated cardiomyopathy 15
mitral
    regurgitation 10, 12, 30, 34
    stenosis 32
    valve, floppy 30
Mobitz
    type I block 24
    type II block 24
mouth-to-mouth resuscitation see cardiopulmonary resuscitation
myectomy for hypertrophic cardiomyopathy 29
myocardial
    abscess 22
    damage 2
    infarction 2, 4, 6, 18, 34, 36, 38, 40, 42, 44
    ischaemia 6, 40, 42
    thickening 40
myxoma, atrial 22, 32

N

nephrosclerosis 26
nephrotic syndrome 40
nicotinates for dyslipoproteinaemia 19
nifedipine for mitral regurgitation 31
nitrates
    for angina
        pectoris 3
        unstable 5
    for myocardial infarction 35

Index

nitroglycerine for unstable angina 5
noradrenaline for acute hypotensive shock 43
norepinephrine *see* noradrenaline

O

oedema
  peripheral 40
  pulmonary 22, 38, 46
oesophageal spasm 2
oesophagitis, reflux 2
ophthalmia *see* endophthalmitis
ostium
  primum defect 12
  secundum defect 12
oxygen
  for acute hypotensive shock 43
  for myocardial infarction 35

P

pacing
  permanent
    for heart block 22
    for restrictive cardiomyopathy 41
    dual-chamber, for hypertrophic cardiomyopathy 29
  temporary, for heart block 22
partial beta agonists for cardiac failure and dilated cardiomyopathy 15
pericardial
  aspiration for tamponade 37
  coarse rub 36
  effusion 36
  tamponade 36, 38
pericarditis 2, 4, 6, 22, 34, 36
  constrictive 36, 40
  relapsing 36
phosphodiesterase inhibitors for cardiac failure and dilated cardiomyopathy 15
Pick's disease of the heart *see* constrictive pericarditis
plasma expanders for acute hypotensive shock 43
pleural effusion 38
pleurisy 36
pneumonia 38
pneumothorax, spontaneous 36
polyunsaturates for dyslipoproteinaemia 19
potassium-sparing diuretics
  for cardiac failure and dilated cardiomyopathy 15
  for mitral regurgitation 31
  for mitral stenosis 33
pravastatin for dyslipoproteinaemia 19
precordial
  discomfort 36
  pain 36
  thump
    for asystole 17
    for pulseless ventricular tachycardia 17
    for ventricular fibrillation 17
prednisolone for pericarditis 37
pressor agents for electromechanical dissociation 17
probucol for dyslipoproteinaemia 19
procainamide for ventricular tachycardia 47
propafenone for venricular tachycardia 47
propranolol for hypertrophic cardiomyopathy 29
pseudohypertension 26
pulmonary
  cavitation 38
  congestion 30, 32
  embolism 4, 6, 38
  embolus 34
  hypertension 8, 12, 14, 20, 30, 32, 38
  incompetence *see* pulmonary regurgitation
  infarction 20, 22, 38
  infection 38
  oedema 22, 38, 46
  regurgitation 8, 20
  stenosis 12, 20
  thromboembolic disease 20
  valve
    incompetence *see* pulmonary regurgitation
    insufficiency *see* pulmonary regurgitation
    stenosis *see* pulmonary stenosis
  vasculitis 20
pulsus paradoxus 36
pyrexia of unknown origin 22

Q

Quincke's sign 8
quinidine for ventricular tachycardia 47

R

radiofrequency catheter ablation
  for supraventricular tachycardia 45
  for Wolff–Parkinson–White syndrome 49
regurgitation
  aortic 6, 8, 10
  mitral 10, 12, 30, 34
  pulmonary 8, 20
  tricuspid 20
  valvular 22
renal
  failure 14, 26, 36
    acute 42
  infarction 6, 22
  insufficiency *see* renal failure
renovascular disease 26
resins for dyslipoproteinaemia 19
respiratory arrest 16
restrictive cardiomyopathy 40
resuscitation, cardiopulmonary 16
  for ventricular tachycardia 47
revascularization for unstable angina 5
rheumatic valve disease 12
rifampicin for endocarditis 23
rt-PA
  for myocardial infarction 35
  for pulmonary oedema 39
rupture
  aortic 6
  cardiac 34
  chordal 22

S

sclerosis, aortic 10
septal defect
  atrial 12, 20
  ventricular 10, 20, 34
septicaemia 38, 42
  staphylococcal 22
shock
  acute hypotensive 42
  cardiogenic 34, 46
simvastatin for dyslipoproteinaemia 19
sinus
  tachycardia 20, 44
  venosus atrial septal defect 12
sodium
  bicarbonate for prolonged resuscitation 17
  nitroprusside for aortic dissection 7
sotalol for ventricular tachycardia 47
spondylosis, cervical 2
statins for dyslipoproteinaemia 19
stenocardia *see* angina pectoris
stenosis
  aortic 2, 10, 40
  carotid 18
  mitral 32
  pulmonary 12, 20

Index

valvular 22
steroids *see* corticosteroids
Stokes–Adams attack 24
streptokinase
    for myocardial infarction 35
    for pulmonary oedema 39
stroke 6, 20, 26
    ischaemic 42
supraventricular
    arrhythmia 10
    tachycardia 44, 46, 48
sympathomimetics for cardiac failure and dilated cardiomyopathy 15
syncope 24
    effort 38
    exertional 20

T

tachyarrhythmia 34
    atrial 14
    ventricular 14
tachycardia
    atrial 44
        ectopic 48
    atrioventricular
        nodal re-entrant 44, 48
        re-entrant 44, 48
    sinus 20, 44
    supraventricular 44, 46, 48
    ventricular 4, 8, 14, 24, 44, 46, 48
        pulseless 17
tamponade 36
    cardiac 6, 40
    pericardial 36, 38
teicoplanin for endocarditis 23
thiazide diuretics
    for cardiac failure and dilated cardiomyopathy 15
    for hypertension 27
thrombolytic treatment
    for myocardial infarction 35
    for pulmonary embolism 39
timolol for myocardial infarction 35
transient
    cerebral ischaemia *see* transient ischaemic attack
    ischaemic attack 18, 26
transplantation
    heart
        for cardiac failure 15
        for cardiomyopathy
            dilated 15
            hypertrophic 29
            restrictive 41
heart–lung for Eisenmenger complex 21
tuberculosis 22

U

urokinase for pulmonary oedema 39

V

vagal manoeuvres for supraventricular tachycardia 45
valsalva manoeuvre for supraventricular tachycardia 45
valve
    aortic
        disease 28
        incompetence *see* aortic regurgitation
        insufficiency *see* aortic regurgitation
        regurgitation *see* aortic regurgitation
        stenosis *see* aortic stenosis
    destruction 22
    disease, rheumatic 12
    floppy mitral 30
    pulmonary
        incompetence *see* pulmonary regurgitation
        insufficiency *see* pulmonary regurgitation
        stenosis *see* pulmonary stenosis
valvular
    regurgitation 22
    stenosis 22
valvuloplasty, balloon, for aortic stenosis 11
vancomycin for endocarditis 23
vascular
    abnormality 18
    disease, peripheral 26
vasculitis
    pulmonary 20
    systemic 22
vasodilators
    for aortic dissection 9
    for mitral regurgitation 31
vasospasm, cerebral *see* transient ischaemic attack
vegetations, endocardial 22
venesection
    for Eisenmenger complex 21
    for restrictive cardiomyopathy 41
ventilation, mechanical, for acute hypotensive shock 43
ventricular
    arrhythmia 10, 40
    bradyarrhythmia 14
    disease, right 12, 20
    dysfunction, left 10, 14
    failure
        left 8, 34, 44
        right 14, 20
    fibrillation 4, 17, 24
ventricular *cont.*
    hypertrophy, right 30
    impairment 8
    septal defect 10, 20, 34
    tachyarrhythmia 14
    tachycardia 4, 8, 14, 24, 44, 46, 48
        pulseless 17
verapamil
    for hypertrophic cardiomyopathy 29
    for myocardial infarction 35
    for angina pectoris 3
    for tachycardia, supraventricular 45

W

warfarin
    for Eisenmenger complex 21
    for mitral regurgitation 31
    for mitral stenosis 33
    for myocardial infarction 35
    for pulmonary oedema 39
Wolff–Parkinson–White syndrome 44, 48

X

xanthoma 18

CURRENT DIAGNOSIS & TREATMENT

in

Dermatology

Edited by
Malcolm Rustin

Series editors
Roy Pounder
Mark Hamilton

A QUICK Reference for the Clinician

Contributors

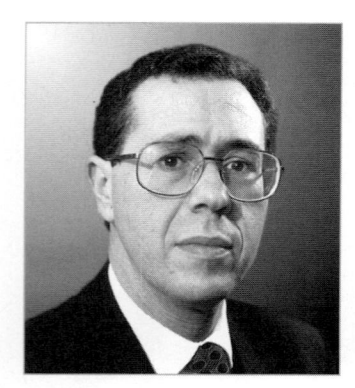

EDITOR

M RUSTIN

Dr Malcolm Rustin is a Consultant Dermatologist at the Royal Free Hospital, London. He runs a dedicated clinic for patients with atopic eczema and has a research interest in developing new treatments for this disease and investigating its immunological abnormalities.

REFEREES

Dr C Bunker
Consultant Dermatologist
Westminster and Chelsea Hospital
London, UK

Dr John SC English
Department of Dermatology
North Staffordshire Hospital Centre
Stoke-on-Trent, UK

AUTHORS

ACNE
Dr Nicholas Simpson
Department of Dermatology
Royal Victoria Infirmary
Newcastle upon Tyne, UK

ALOPECIA
Dr David de Berker
Department of Dermatology
Royal Victoria Infirmary
Newcastle upon Tyne, UK

BULLOUS DISORDERS
Dr Sara H Wakelin
Department of Dermatology
John Radcliffe Hospital
Oxford, UK

Dr Fenella Wojnarowska
Department of Dermatology
Slade Hospital
Oxford, UK

ECZEMA
Dr Jane M McGregor
Department of Dermatology
Royal Free Hospital
London, UK

Dr Malcolm Rustin
Department of Dermatology
Royal Free Hospital
London, UK

FUNGAL NAIL INFECTIONS
Dr David T Roberts
Department of Dermatology
Southern General Hospital
Glasgow, UK

PSORIASIS
Dr Claire Fuller
St John's Institute of Dermatology
Guy's and St Thomas's Hospitals
London, UK

Dr Jonathan Barker
St John's Institute of Dermatology
Guy's and St Thomas's Hospitals
London, UK

URTICARIA
Dr Richard Barlow
St John's Institute of Dermatology
Guy's and St Thomas's Hospitals
London, UK

Professor MW Greaves
St John's Institute of Dermatology
Guy's and St Thomas's Hospitals
London, UK

VASCULITIS, SKIN MANIFESTATIONS
Dr Nick Levell
Department of Dermatology
University College Hospital
London, UK

Dr Tony Bewley
Department of Dermatology
Middlesex Hospital
London, UK

Dr Pauline M Dowd
Department of Dermatology
Middlesex Hospital
London, UK

VIRAL WARTS
Dr E Claire Benton
Consultant Dermatologist
Royal Infirmary
Edinburgh, UK

Contents

2 Acne

4 Alopecia
  alopecia areata
  fungal infections
  lichenoid alopecia
  traumatic alopecia

6 Bullous disorders
  dermatitis herpetiformis
  epidermolysis bullosa
  pemphigoid
  pemphigoid gestationis
  pemphigus

8 Eczema

10 Fungal nail infections

12 Psoriasis
  flexural psoriasis
  guttate psoriasis
  nail psoriasis
  palmoplantar psoriasis
  scalp psoriasis

14 Urticaria
  acute urticaria
  angioedema
  chronic urticaria
  urticarial vasculitis

16 Vasculitis, skin manifestations

18 Viral warts
  anogenital warts (condyloma acuminata, condyloma plana)
  cutaneous warts ('butcher's', common, deep plantar, facial, mosaic, palmar/plantar, plane)

20 Index

Acne — N. Simpson

Diagnosis

Symptoms
Dissatisfaction with appearance.
Localized pain: from inflammatory cysts and nodules.

Signs
- Distribution is confined to the face and upper trunk predominantly, but occasionally the upper arms are involved in more severe cases.

Non-inflamed lesions: open and closed comedones.

Inflamed lesions: inflammatory papules, pustules, nodules, and cysts.

Seborrhoea.

Scars.

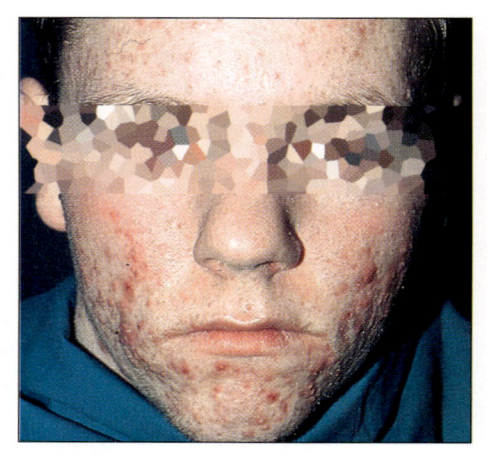

Moderate to severe facial acne.

Investigations
- Acne is a clinical diagnosis.

Cutaneous microbiology: may identify resistant strains of *Propionobacterium acnes*.

Complications
Scarring: from resolution of inflamed lesions, type of scarring depending on original lesion: superficial lesions may lead to 'ice-pick' scars; nodules and deep cysts may leave atrophic wedge-shaped scars; keloid scars may occur after lesions on upper chest and back.

Differential diagnosis
Rosacea: facial flushing and no comedones.
Perioral dermatitis: clustering of inflammatory papules around mouth and on cheeks, without comedones and often with clear unaffected zone around vermilion border of lips.
Steroid acne: many inflammatory lesions on face and trunk but with no comedones, cysts, or nodules.

Aetiology
- Causes include the following:
Increased sebum production.
Blockage of the pilosebaceous outflow tract, which may be due to comedogenic substances produced by *Propionobacterium acnes* or abnormal linoleic acid metabolism within the epidermal cells lining the duct.

Epidemiology
- 85% of teenage boys and 75% of teenage girls have acne of some degree.
- More severe grades of acne occur in the late teens and early twenties in 1–5% of the population.

Treatment

Diet and lifestyle
- Diet has little effect on acne, despite folklore about chips and chocolate consumption.
- Kitchens and hot humid environments aggravate acne.
- Greasy cosmetics should be avoided.

Pharmacological treatment
- Treatment plans should be discussed with the patient to encourage compliance.

For mild acne: topical treatment
Standard dosage	Benzoyl peroxide 2.5–10% once daily. Azelaic acid 20% twice daily. Tretinoin 0.25–0.1% in various bases once daily. Isotretinoin gel 0.05% once or twice daily.
Contraindications	None.
Special points	Compliance can be increased by advising patient to reduce frequency of application if necessary.
Main drug interactions	None.
Main side effects	Irritation, desquamation.

For mild acne: topical antibiotics
Standard dosage	Clindamycin 1% solution and lotion twice daily. Erythromycin 2% lotion and 4% lotion, with 1.2% zinc acetate twice daily. Tetracycline 4% lotion twice daily.
Contraindications	Systemic antibiotic treatment.
Main drug interactions	None.
Main side effects	Some local irritation and mild scaliness.

For moderate acne: oral antibiotics
Standard dosage	Tetracycline 1 g daily. Erythromycin 1 g daily, minocycline 100 mg daily, or doxycycline 100 mg daily. Treatment should last at least 3–6 months.
Contraindications	*Tetracycline:* mid and last trimester of pregnancy, breast feeding, age <12 years, SLE. *Erythromycin, minocycline, doxycycline:* caution in hepatic or renal impairment.
Special points	*Tetracycline:* headaches and visual disturbance may indicate benign intracranial hypertension.
Main drug interactions	May affect oral contraceptive pill.
Main side effects	*Tetracycline:* nausea, vomiting, photosensitivity (unusual, but treatment should be stopped). *Erythromycin, minocycline, doxycycline:* abdominal discomfort (common), nausea and vomiting (less common, may be avoided by dividing dose).

For moderate or severe acne
Standard dosage	Isotretinoin daily for 16–24 weeks under specialist supervision.
Contraindications	Pregnancy; caution in pre-existing renal or hepatic disease or abnormal fasting lipids.
Special points	May be prescribed only through hospital pharmacy. Blood donation should cease during course and for 1 month afterwards.
Main drug interactions	Preparations containing high doses of vitamin A.
Main side effects	Chapping of exposed skin of face, neck, and hands, with marked cheilitis, dry nasal and conjunctival mucosae, with mild epistaxis and conjunctivitis, fetal malformation.

Treatment aims
To reduce inflammatory lesions.
To reduce sebum production (antiandrogen and oral isotretinoin).
To prevent scarring.

Other treatments
Abrasive therapies: aluminium oxide 38–52% or polyethylene granules 2%; unpopular with patients because of irritation.
Sulphur: various concentrations in various bases; smell often leads to poor compliance.
Salicylic acid: various concentrations; causes peeling and irritation.
Intradermal collagen injections for correction of atrophic scars: expensive and benefit may be temporary because the collagen is remodelled.

Prognosis
- Prognosis is excellent in most groups.
- Persistent minor acne may be a problem for women in mid to late 20s.

Follow-up and management
- Follow-up is always necessary because of the slow rate of response to first-line agents.
- All courses should last at least 3 months before change of treatment is contemplated.
- Referral for hospital treatment with isotretinoin should be preferred to continued changing of oral antibiotics.

Key references
Healey E, Simpson N. Acne vulgaris. *BMJ* 1994, 308:381–383
Simpson NB: *Acne and the Mature Woman.* London: Science Press, 1992.

Alopecia   D. de Berker

Diagnosis

Symptoms and signs
- Alopecia is a physical sign and not a clinical diagnosis.
- It is a feature of many processes, some normal (e.g. male-pattern baldness) and others pathological, such as these described here.
- It is primarily seen on the scalp but may affect any hair-bearing part of the body.

Alopecia areata
Localized or generalized hair loss: resulting in completely bald or diffusely thinned areas.

Evident follicular orifices.

Exclamation-mark hairs.

Depigmented hairs: may grow before return of normal hair.

Pitted or roughened nails.

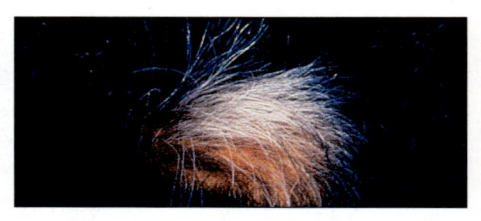

Alopecia areata, with deficient melanin in area of regrowth.

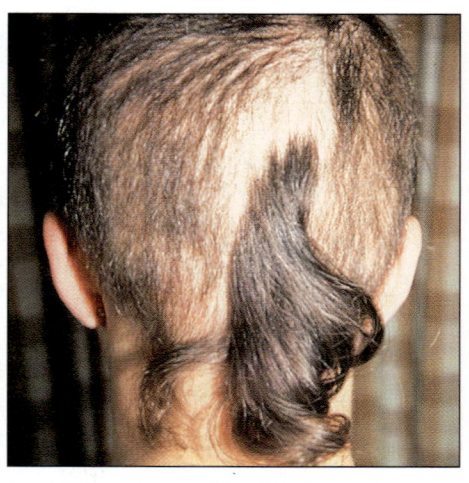

Traumatic alopecia
Signs of trauma: from cosmetic processes or self-injury (trichotillomania).

Lichenoid alopecia
- Lichen planus and discoid lupus erythematosus produce a lichenoid histological process in the scalp; they may be detected by the following:

Characteristic rash or mucosal changes.

Scalp changes: scarring, atrophy, perifollicular erythema with scale.

- Potential for scarring makes diagnosis and management a dermatological emergency.

Fungal infection
Kerion.

Tinea capitis.

Spared pony tail growth in trichotillomania.

Investigations

Alopecia areata
Autoimmune profile: in adults to screen for associated thyroid disease and pernicious anaemia.

Traumatic alopecia
Hair microscopy: may reveal chemical or heat trauma, with features of weathering (poor cuticle, brush ends, trichorrhexis nodes).

Scalp histology: can help to distinguish from alopecia areata, with distortion of hairs within a follicle, empty follicles, and interfollicular haemorrhage.

Lichenoid alopecia
Scalp histology: may reveal lymphocytic dermal infiltrate focusing on follicles being destroyed and on vessels in discoid lupus; early discoid lupus may reveal deposits of IgG and complement on immunofluorescence.

Antinuclear factor analysis: in discoid lupus in case of overlap with SLE.

Fungal infections
Fungal scrapings: for mycology.

Wood's light examination: glows green for *Microsporum* or *Trychophyton* spp.

Complications
- These conditions are not complicated by anything other than local persistence.

Squamous cell carcinoma: in discoid lupus lesions (rare).

Differential diagnosis

Alopecia areata
Trichotillomania, pseudopelade, iron deficiency, telogen effluvium, thyroid dysfunction.

Traumatic alopecia
Alopecia areata, androgenic alopecia, thyroid dysfunction, iron deficiency.

Lichenoid alopecia
Sarcoid, necrobiosis lipoidica, pseudopelade.

Fungal infection
Folliculitis decalvans, erosive pustular dermatosis, bacterial folliculitis.

Aetiology

Alopecia areata
- Alopecia areata is part of an autoimmune diathesis.
- It may be associated with thyroid disease, pernicious anaemia, and vitiligo.

Traumatic alopecia
- Traction and heat processes of coiffure damage the hair shaft and root.

Lichenoid alopecia
- This is a form of autoimmunity, resulting in keratinocyte death, with lymphocytic infiltration and hair follicle destruction.

Epidemiology

Alopecia areata
- Up to 80% of patients present between the ages of 20 and 40 years.
- 10% of sufferers are atopic; they have a 75% chance of progressing to alopecia totalis.

Traumatic alopecia
- Peak presentation is between the ages of 11 and 17 years, with few patients >40 years; patients are predominantly female.

Lichenoid alopecia
- The female:male ratio is 2:1 in discoid lupus erythematosus.
- More women than men suffer from lichen planus, usually presenting between the ages of 30 and 60 years.

Fungal infection
- *Microsporum* spp. infection is associated with animal contact and occurs most often in childhood.

Treatment

Diet and lifestyle
- Arresting self-mutilating behaviour, by direct advice or psychiatric help, is important in traumatic alopecia.

Pharmacological treatment

Alopecia areata
- Alopecia areata may resolve with no treatment or may fail to resolve with maximum treatment.
- Topical or locally injected steroids may be used; short systemic courses have poor evidence of sustained benefit and a risk of dependence, with consequent long-term sequelae.
- Other treatments include contact sensitization with diphencyprone and irritant treatment with dithranol.

Standard dosage	Clobetasol propionate 0.05% cream or ointment <10 g weekly, massaged into affected area twice daily. Triamcinolone acetonide up to 3 ml (10 mg/ml), delivered by Dermojet to the treatment area, every 1–2 weeks for 6–12 weeks or 2 ml (2.5–10 mg/ml) intradermally every 4–6 weeks.
Contraindications	Local infection, pregnancy, infants.
Special points	A potent steroid: use over a large area results in systemic absorption. Topical steroids should be used for 4–8 weeks to assess response and possible side effects; treatment may be stopped (if ineffective) or reduced (if effective) at this point. The risk of focal atrophy is greater with injected steroids.
Main drug interactions	None.
Main side effects	Local steroid atrophy, steroid folliculitis, systemic steroid absorption.

Traumatic alopecia
- Hairstyles involving traction and heat processes must be avoided. Some hair loss and weathering may be reversible after taking this advice.
- Hair conditioners may help slightly in combination with reducing frequency of hair washing to 2–3 times weekly.
- Trichotillomania has no pharmacological treatment unless it is part of psychiatric therapy.

Lichenoid alopecia
- Potent topical (clobetasol propionate 0.05%) or intralesional steroids may be used as for alopecia areata.
- Systemic steroids have a clearer justification in lichenoid alopecia than in alopecia areata because, if the disease is not arrested rapidly, it results in areas of permanent hair loss.
- After the condition is under control, alternative treatment should be substituted, e.g. antimalarials and sun block for discoid lupus.

Standard dosage	Prednisolone 5–30 mg in the morning.
Contraindications	Pregnancy, diabetes mellitus, hypertension, obesity, tuberculosis, systemic infection.
Main drug interactions	Anticonvulsants, antihypertensives, rifampicin.
Main side effects	Weight gain, sodium and fluid retention, hypertension, diabetes mellitus, adrenal suppression, osteoporosis.

Treatment aims
To arrest and reverse pathological hair loss. To help patient come to terms with irreversible changes.

Other treatments
Multiple micrografts to give a new, feathered hairline.
Expansion of existing hair-bearing scalp with fluid chambers.
Wigs.

Prognosis

Alopecia areata
- If onset is in childhood, family or personal history of atopy and involvement of the hairline or complete baldness are bad prognostic factors. In older patients, although 50% may recover in <1 year, the chances of relapse are > 80%.

Traumatic alopecia
- Cosmetically induced changes may be partly reversible with cessation of the cause. Trichotillomania resolves in most children and adolescents. Adults with tonsure-type changes have poor prognosis.

Lichenoid alopecia
- Treatment may allow considerable regrowth if scarring is minimal. The condition may burn out over several years. Some patients have relentlessly active disease despite aggressive treatment and suffer considerable permanent hair loss.

Follow-up and management
- Hospital follow-up is not necessary for mild alopecia areata.
- Patients should be followed to assess the efficacy of treatment and the need for continuation.
- When potent treatment is commenced or scarring is a risk, hospital follow-up should be arranged until the condition has resolved or is stable.

Key references
Rook A, Dawber RPR (eds). *Diseases of the Hair and Scalp.* Oxford: Blackwell Scientific Publications, 1991.

MacDonald-Hull S, Cunliffe W: Successful treatment of alopecia areata using the contact allergen diphencyprone. *Br J Dermatol* 1991, **124**:212–213.

Bullous disorders
S.H. Wakelin and F. Wojnarowska

Diagnosis

Symptoms

General
Chronic blistering of skin: primary feature in this heterogeneous group of disorders.

Inherited or mechanobullous
Trauma-induced blistering: present at birth (epidermolysis bullosa).

Acquired or immunobullous
Spontaneous blistering rash: onset in adults and elderly patients (pemphigoid).
Itch: characteristically severe in dermatitis herpetiformis and pemphigoid gestationis.
Painful ulcers: 50% of patients with pemphigus present with oral ulceration.
Erosions of mucous membranes.

Signs

Blisters: large and tense on erythematous bases (pemphigoid); flaccid and easily ruptured, leaving raw areas and crusts (pemphigus); possibly not identifiable.
Scarring: feature of cicatricial pemphigoid and dystrophic epidermolysis bullosa.
Characteristic patterns of lesions: e.g. elbows and buttocks in dermatitis herpetiformis.

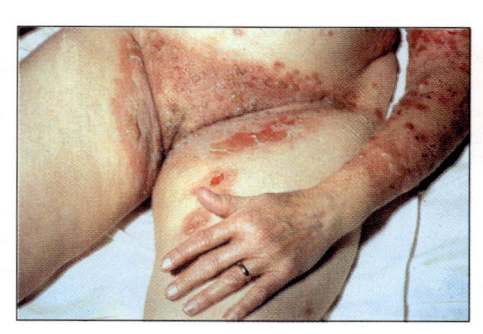

Bullous pemphigoid.

Investigations

Histology of fresh blister (<48 h): to define level of cleavage
Direct immunofluorescence of perilesional or uninvolved skin: to detect tissue-bound immunoglobulins and complement, e.g. IgA at dermal papillae in dermatitis herpetiformis, IgG and C3 at dermoepidermal junction in pemphigoid, interepidermal IgG in pemphigus.
Indirect immunofluorescence of serum: to identify circulating immunoglobulin against skin; pemphigus antibody titre correlates with disease activity.
Cytology: can provide immediate diagnosis in pemphigus (Tzank test) and herpes infections (balloon cells).
Fetal skin biopsy: for prenatal diagnosis.

Complications

Secondary infection.
Disturbed fluid and electrolyte balance: in untreated pemphigus.

Pemphigus Blister = flaccid and easily ruptured.
Pemphigoid Blister = large and tense on erythematous base.

Differential diagnosis

Infections: e.g. varicella zoster, bullous impetigo.
Insect bites: may cause giant bullae on legs.
Burns or friction.
Drug eruptions: e.g. frusemide.
Porphyria cutanea tarda.
Pompholyx eczema.

Aetiology

- Causes include the following:

Mechanobullous
Absent or abnormal structural components of skin: keratin in epidermolysis bullosa simplex, nicein in junctional epidermolysis bullosa, collagen VII in dystrophic epidermolysis bullosa.

Immunobullous
- The initiating cause is poorly understood.
Genetic influence: HLA association.
Pathogenic autoantibodies.
Drugs (rare): e.g. penicillamine-induced pemphigus.

Epidemiology

- All forms of bullous disorders are rare.
- ~1 in 5000 people are affected.
- Pemphigoid is much more common than pemphigus.

Treatment

Diet and lifestyle
- Dietary measures are only of proven value in dermatitis herpetiformis, when a gluten-free diet may be curative, but drug dosage cannot be decreased for at least 6 months.
- Protection against trauma and wound care are the mainstay of treatment for epidermolysis bullosa.

Pharmacological treatment
- For immunobullous disorders, moderate to potent topical steroids may control limited disease; a topical antimicrobial agent is often co-administered.
- Systemic treatment options include prednisolone, azathioprine (as a steroid-sparing drug), dapsone (for dermatitis herpetiformis, linear IgA disease, and, rarely, other diseases), and sulphonamides (when dapsone not tolerated).
- Other drugs include methotrexate, cyclophosphamide, and tetracyclines.
- Treatment should be given under specialist supervision.

Standard dosage	Dose depends on agent, disease, and severity.
Contraindications	*Prednisolone:* systemic infection. *Azathioprine:* pregnancy. *Dapsone:* porphyria; caution in patients with glucose-6-phosphate dehydrogenase deficiency.
Special points	*Prednisolone:* high doses must be avoided in elderly patients. *Azathioprine:* full blood count and liver function must be checked regularly. *Dapsone:* causes dose-related haemolysis.
Main drug interactions	*Azathioprine:* allopurinol enhances effect and toxicity. *Dapsone:* probenecid.
Main side effects	*Prednisolone:* weight gain, hypertension, diabetes. *Azathioprine:* bone-marrow toxicity, hepatotoxicity. *Dapsone:* anaemia, methaemoglobinaemia, hepatotoxicity, agranulocytosis, motor neuropathy. *Sulphonamides:* skin rashes, nausea, agranulocytosis, hepatitis.

Treatment aims
To relieve pain and heal wounds (in epidermolysis bullosa).
To suppress disease activity with lowest possible dose of drug (in inflammatory bullous disorders).
To treat secondary infection.

Prognosis
- Most patients have chronic disease, with spontaneous remission.
- In patients with epidermolysis bullosa simplex, blistering may decrease in adult life.
- Pemphigoid gestationis almost always recurs in subsequent pregnancies and may also occur if the patient takes an oral contraceptive.
- Pemphigus carries a mortality of <10%.
- The risk of death in bullous pemphigoid increases with the age of the patient at onset because of side effects of treatment and general debilitation of severe illness; average duration is ~3 years.

Follow-up and management
- Long-term follow-up by a specialist is advised for all but the mildest disorders.
- Genetic counselling for inherited bullous disorders is advised.

Key references
Crosby DL *et al.*: Bullous diseases. Introduction. *Dermatol Clin* 1993, **11**:373–378.

Guillaum JC *et al.*: Controlled trial of azathioprine and plasma exchange in addition to prednisolone in the treatment of bullous pempigoid. *Arch Dermatol* 1993, **129**:49–53.

Oliver GF *et al.*: Treatment of lichen planus. *Drugs* 1993, **45**:56–65.

Rabinowitz LG *et al.*: Inflammatory bullous diseases in children. *Dermatol Clin* 1993, **11**:419–427.

Roujeau JC, Stern RS: Severe adverse cutaneous reactions to drugs. *N Engl J Med* 1994, **331**:1272–1285.

Eczema
J.M. McGregor and M.H.A. Rustin

Diagnosis

Symptoms
Itching.
Soreness, dryness, vesiculation and occasionally blistering of skin.

Signs

Major
Erythema.
Scaling.
Papulovesicles or blisters.

Minor
Excoriation.
Increased skin markings or lichenification.
Horizontal ridging of nails or 'shiny' nails.

Investigations
- History and examination are often sufficient for diagnosis.
- Although serological abnormalities may be identified, laboratory investigations are not diagnostic; they may be helpful in excluding an underlying systemic disease or in establishing a differential diagnosis.

Full blood count: to exclude thrombocytopenia (Wiskott–Aldrich syndrome), anaemia (dermatitis herpetiformis or pellagra), or lymphoma.

U&E analysis, liver function tests: patients with severe or erythrodermic eczema become dehydrated, lose albumin through skin and gut, and may have nonspecific abnormal liver enzymes.

HIV test: should be considered in patients with persistent seborrhoeic dermatitis.

Prick testing: rarely helpful in diagnosis or management of eczema.

Patch and photopatch testing: useful in establishing potential allergic contact component in development of eczema (e.g. rubber, nickel, topical corticosteroids).

Skin biopsy: for histology (possibly with immunofluorescence) if diagnosis in doubt (dermatitis herpetiformis, chronic superficial scaly dermatitis, mycosis fungoides, drug eruptions).

Skin scraping: microscopy for fungal hyphae and scabies, mycological culture (tinea corporis/capitis may mimic eczema).

Skin and nose swab: for microscopy and culture; coagulase-positive *Staphylococcus aureus* may colonize eczematous skin and contribute to the disease process; treatment by systemic antibiotics may speed resolution.

Complications
Secondary infection: by *Staphylococcus aureus* (may be severe in atopic dermatitis) or herpes simplex virus (Kaposi's varicelliform eruption, may be life-threatening in children with atopic dermatitis).

Erythroderma: hospital admission needed for bed-rest and careful monitoring of vital signs and electrolytes.

Differential diagnosis
Wiskott–Aldrich syndrome: bruising, recurrent infections (in children).
Zinc deficiency: perioral or perianal involvement.
Leiners disease: failure to thrive.
Netherton's syndrome: abnormal hair.
Drug eruptions.
Malignancy: e.g. leukaemia or lymphoma.
Malnutrition: pellagra (photosensitive).
Dermatitis herpetiformis.
Mycosis fungoides.
Chronic superficial scaly dermatoses.
Skin infections: tinea corporis/capitis, Scabies.

Aetiology
- The cause of eczema is poorly understood, but many factors are currently considered to play a role, including the following:

Genetic family history of atopy (allergic rhinitis, eczema, and asthma): in >70% of patients with atopic dermatitis.
Environmental challenges (immunologically mediated): including house dust mite (atopic eczema), irritant contact (e.g. bleaches, detergents), allergic contact (e.g. rubber, nickel).
Stress.

Epidemiology
- Up to 20% of the population may develop eczema at some time in their lives.
- ~15% of infants are affected by atopic dermatitis.
- Eczema accounts for ~20% of all dermatological consultations with general practitioners.
- The male:female ratio is equal.

Classification

Exogenous
Irritant contact.
Allergic contact.
Photoallergic contact.
Phototoxic.

Endogenous
Atopic.
Asteatotic.
Discoid.
Lichenified.
Varicose.
Seborrhoeic.
Erythrodermic.
Pompholyx.

Treatment

Diet and lifestyle
- Dairy-product-free diets have been helpful in some children with atopic eczema; no evidence indicates that diet influences other forms of eczema.
- Breast feeding may decrease the incidence or severity of atopic eczema in predisposed children if the mother avoids eggs and dairy products; soya or other non-allergen milks may be substituted for cow's milk later on.
- Natural fibres should be worn next to the skin; extremes of temperature should be avoided; fingernails should be filed daily to reduce damage caused by scratching; gortex mattress covers may reduce exposure to dust mite allergen.
- Patients, particularly children, should be encouraged to participate fully in sports and other activities; a positive and encouraging atmosphere within the family can help reduce anxiety caused by eczema.

Pharmacological treatment

Topical treatment
- Creams are recommended for exudative eczema and ointments for dry and lichenified eczema.

Emollients: various preparations available ranging from light aqueous cream to greasy white soft paraffin or emulsifying ointment; these can be used as soap substitutes; emollient bath additives containing oat (Aveeno), liquid paraffin (Oilatum), and soya (Balneum) to be used daily.

Steroids: strength depends on severity of eczema and site of involvement (supervised by physician, not patient).
Mild: 1% hydrocortisone for face and body (infants), facial eczema (adults).
Moderately potent: 0.05% clobetasone butyrate for face (adults for 1–2 weeks), trunk, and limbs.
Potent: 0.1% betamethasone valerate, 0.05% fluocinonide for moderate to severe eczema on trunk and limbs (adults), palmoplantar eczema.
Very potent: 0.05% clobetasol propionate for severe eczema on trunk and limbs (adults for short periods), palmoplantar eczema (penetration may be increased by occlusion).
Side effects include skin atrophy and bruising, systemic absorption (particularly in children).

Systemic treatment
- Systemic treatment is indicated for eczema complicated by infection or unresponsive to topical treatment alone.

Antibiotics: erythromycin or flucloxacillin; secondary infection probable after sudden deterioration in eczema; 2–3 week courses may be needed.
Antivirals: oral acyclovir 5-day course mandatory in atopic patients with herpes simplex infection; prophylaxis in atopic children with recurrent herpes simplex infection.
Antihistamines: sedative antihistamines used to allay pruritis; recent evidence also suggests that cetirizine is beneficial.
- Systemic treatment for severe eczema involves immunosuppression by oral prednisolone (causes hypertension, diabetes, skin atrophy, osteoporosis), azathioprine (causes bone-marrow suppression), or cyclosporin (causes hypertension, hirsutism, gynaecomastia, reduced renal function).
- Traditional Chinese herbal therapy is currently under trial; side effects have not yet been established, but hepatotoxicity has been reported.

Other treatments
Evening primrose oil (Epogam): useful in some patients, particularly with prominent pruritis; expensive and benefit unproven.
Phototherapy: ultraviolet B, narrow-band ultraviolet B, psoralen and ultraviolet A (PUVA) effective in some patients; time-consuming, inconvenient for patient.

Treatment aims
To reduce itch.
To clear eczema.
To prevent relapse.
To treat superinfection.

Prognosis
- 50% of patients with atopic dermatitis are clear of eczema at 5 years and 90% at puberty; 10% have persistent disease.
- The prognosis for patients with irritant or allergic dermatitis is good if the relevant agent is identified and effective avoidance measures are taken.
- Endogenous eczema is usually a chronic, relapsing condition.

Follow-up and management
- Most patients are treated by topical preparations and are followed until their eczema is stable.
- Patients on systemic treatment need long-term follow-up in order to monitor potential side effects and to maintain a good quality of life with minimum possible immunosuppression.

Key references
Bos JD, Kapsenberg ML, Sillevis Smith JH: Pathogenesis of atopic eczema. *Lancet* 1994, **343**:1338–1341.

Przybilla B, Eberlein-König B, Rueff F: Practical management of atopic eczema. *Lancet* 1994, **343**:1342–1346.

Roujeau JC, Stern RS: Severe adverse cutaneous reactions to drugs. *N Engl J Med* 1994, **331**:1272–1285.

Fungal nail infection
D.T. Roberts

Diagnosis

Symptoms and signs
- In its early stages, the disease is usually asymptomatic.

Cosmetic disability: particularly in fingernails.

Hyperkeratosis: in toenails.

Mechanical problems: caused by pressure from footwear.

Discoloration of nail: grey-green or black discoloration often associated with specific types of fungi; green-black discoloration caused by secondary *Pseudomonas* infection; black or partly black discoloration of nail should always be referred for specialist opinion (unless recent trauma evident) in order not to miss a subungual melanoma.

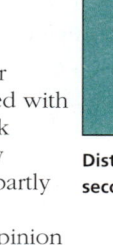

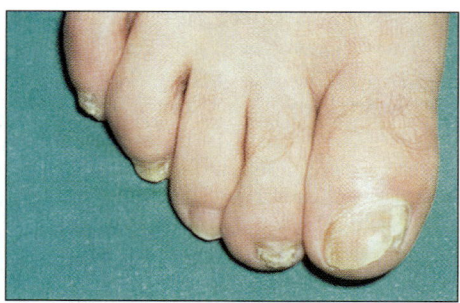

Disruption of nail plate.

Distal and lateral subungual onychomycosis secondary to dermatophyte infection.

Investigations
Microscopy: nail clippings should be sent for microscopic examination to a laboratory with expertise in mycological diagnosis.

Nail fragment culture: if specific organism cannot be identified on microscopy, nail fragments should be cultured on Sabouraud's agar and incubated for up to 3 weeks at 28–30°C; 30% of microscopy-positive nails do not yield fungal growth in culture because fungi found in distal nail clippings are often not viable; specimens must be obtained from more proximal part of infection (not always possible).

Complications
Spread of infection to other nails: toenail infection can spread to fingernails.

Infection of the skin adjacent to infected nails.

Secondary sensitization rash elsewhere: acute blistering of palms and soles (cheiropodopompholyx) or widespread allergic dermatitis reaction.

Differential diagnosis
Toenails
Psoriasis, onychogryphosis, congenital pachyonychia, sarcoidosis.

Fingernails
Psoriasis, lichen planus, alopecia areata, bacterial infection, transverse leukonychia.

Aetiology
- 90% of toenail infection and >50% of fingernail infection is caused by dermatophyte fungi, usually *Trichophyton rubrum*, followed by *Tricophyton mentagrophytes*, and, much more rarely, *Epidermophyton floccosum*.
- Candidal yeasts, usually *C. albicans*, closely followed by *C. parapsilosis*, may be manifest as proximal disease in fingernails.
- The saprophytic mould *Scopulariopsis brevicaulis* causes toenail disease in previously damaged nails; *Hendersonula toroloidea*, a tropical-plant pathogen, typically produces a black nail dystrophy and is usually seen in immigrants.

Epidemiology
- Dermatophyte infection starts in the toe clefts and is contracted in communal bathing places; ~15% of the population have toe-cleft infection (athlete's foot).
- A recent population-based survey has shown the prevalence of dermatophyte nail infection to be ~2.7%.

Classification
Distal and lateral subungual onychomycosis
Affects distal end and side of nail; most common type of fungal nail dystrophy seen in dermatophyte and some secondary mould infections.

Superficial white onychomycosis
Relatively rare; usually caused by *Trichophyton mentagrophytes*.

Proximal subungual onychomycosis
Arises in proximal part of nail; often secondary to chronic paronychia caused by *Candida* spp.

Total dystrophic onychomycosis
All of the nail plate destroyed; may be end result of any of the above.

Treatment

Diet and lifestyle
- Prophylaxis of fungal foot infection using antifungal powder or plastic oversocks in communal bathing places helps to prevent the establishment of nail infection (dermatophyte fungi, endemic on the floors of communal bathing places, are protected within small pieces of keratin and are therefore relatively immune to destruction by disinfectant).

Pharmacological treatment
- Fungal nail infection should be considered a medical rather than a surgical disease.
- Modern drugs, notably terbinafine, provide cure rates of >80% in both finger and toenail infection.
- Although the duration of treatment is relatively short, the nail takes some time after the end of treatment to grow out normally; this should be explained to the patient.

Topical treatment
- Treatment should not be initiated before infection is confirmed.

Amorolfine 5% nail lacquer: a broad-spectrum antimycotic, active against various types of fungi; useful in early distal disease only; works better on fingernails than on toenails because fingernails grow faster.

Tioconazole 28% (Trosyl): a broad-spectrum antifungal agent; probably not as effective as amorolfine in dermatophyte nail infection; probably significantly beneficial only in early distal disease.

Systemic treatment
- For established nail infection, systemic treatment produces higher cure rates than topical treatment.
- Long-term systemic treatment should not be used as a trial to confirm diagnosis.

Standard dosage	Griseofulvin 1 g daily for 6–9 months in fingernail infection, 12–18 months in toenail infection. Terbinafine 250 mg daily for 6 weeks in fingernail infection, 3 months in toenail infection.
Contraindications	*Griseofulvin:* porphyria, severe liver disease, SLE, pregnancy, lactation. *Terbinafine:* hypersensitivity, pregnancy, lactation.
Special points	*Griseofulvin:* weakly fungistatic antifungal agent; cure rates in toenail infection are disappointing (~30%); fingernails respond better (60–70% cure rates). *Terbinafine:* allylamine and a potent fungicidal agent against dermatophytes; not as active against yeasts.
Main drug interactions	*Griseofulvin:* coumerin anticoagulants, phenobarbitone; decreases efficacy of birth control pill. *Terbinafine:* rifampicin, cimetidine.
Main side effects	*Griseofulvin:* photosensitivity, nausea, headache, rashes. *Terbinafine:* delay in gastric emptying, taste disturbance, rash.

- Oral ketoconazole is licensed only for fingernail infections that have failed to respond to other antifungal agents. A few fatal cases of hepatotoxicity have occurred with this drug; its use in nail infection is no longer recommended.

Treatment aims
To eradicate the infection.
To allow growth of healthy nails.

Other treatments
- Surgical or chemical removal is indicated only when rapid alleviation of troublesome symptoms is necessary (unusual).
- Nails can be simply avulsed, and regrowth covered with a systemic antifungal agent.
- Nail removal alone almost inevitably leads to reinfection.

Prognosis
- The advent of terbinafine has significantly improved the prognosis of fungal nail infection; the cure rates in dermatophyte infection are much higher than with griseofulvin.
- In elderly patients with peripheral vascular disease, nail growth is often slow or nonexistent; the appearance of the nail does not improve, even though the antifungal drug may eradicate the offending organism.

Follow-up and management
- Elderly patients should be reviewed after 6 months to ensure that the nail is growing adequately; if it is not, then nail removal is the only alternative in symptomatic disease.

Key references
Goodfield MJD, Andrew L, Evans EGV: Short term treatment of dermatophyte onychomycosis with terbinafine. *BMJ* 1992, **304**:1151–1154.

Williams HC: The epidemiology of onychomycosis in Britain. *Br J Dermatol* 1993, **129**:101–109.

Psoriasis
L.C. Fuller and J.N.W.N. Barker

Diagnosis

Symptoms
- Usually no symptoms are manifest.

Itching.

Painful, tender skin: occasionally.

Signs
Symmetrical, well demarcated erythematous plaques: with thick adherent, silvery scale, often affecting extensor aspects, e.g. elbows, knees, scalp, sacrum; may occur at sites of trauma, e.g. surgical scars (Koebner phenomenon); signs of chronic plaque.

Pitting, onycholysis, subungual hyperkeratosis, salmon patches: signs of nail psoriasis.

Multiple 1–2 cm diameter lesions scattered over trunk and limbs: sudden onset, usually in adolescents; signs of guttate psoriasis.

Shiny, well demarcated plaques: signs of flexural psoriasis.

Erythematous plaques studded with multiple sterile pustules: signs of palmoplantar psoriasis.

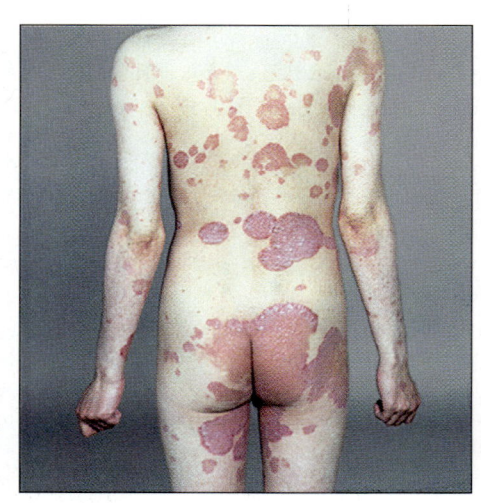

Chronic plaque psoriasis.

Investigations
- Most patients do not need any investigations.

Skin biopsy: to detect psoriasiform papillomatosis, acanthosis, hyperkeratosis, and parakeratosis, with intra-epidermal collections of neutrophils (microabscesses of Munro), capillary dilatation and elongation, and lymphocytic infiltrate.

Throat swab: to exclude streptococcal carriage, which may precipitate guttate psoriasis.

Nail clippings analysis: to exclude onychomycosis as cause of dystrophic nails.

Skin swabs: to exclude candidiasis or bacterial intertrigo as cause of flexural eruption.

Radiography of joints: for associated arthritis.

Blood cultures: for erythrodermic psoriasis and generalized pustular psoriasis, to exclude secondary infection.

Antistreptolysin O titre: for guttate psoriasis.

Complications
Sheets of sterile pustules associated with fever and malaise: with generalized pustular psoriasis; high mortality.

Generalized exfoliative dermatitis: involving 80% of skin surface; with erythroderma; high mortality.

Distal arthropathy, rheumatoid-type, seronegative, oligoarthritis, ankylosing spondylitis, arthritis mutilans: with psoriatic arthropathy.

Differential diagnosis
Plaque
Hypertrophic lichen planus, drug eruption, eczema.

Scalp psoriasis
Seborrhoeic dermatitis.

Guttate psoriasis
Pityriasis rosea or lichenoides chronica.

Flexural psoriasis
Candidal or bacterial intertrigo, seborrhoeic dermatitis.

Palmoplantar psoriasis
Cheiropomphylyx, Reiter's disease.

Nail psoriasis
Onychomycosis.

Aetiology
Causes
Genetics: positive family history in 35% of patients, 70% concordance in monozygotic twins, association with HLA CW6 (20-fold increased risk).

Immunology: many features indicating cell-mediated immune mechanisms in lesional skin; multiple mediators of inflammation detected in lesional skin but no evidence for circulating immune abnormality.

Epidermal kinetics: 20-fold increase in involved psoriatic keratinocyte turnover.

Vascular: increased blood flow in neighbouring, clinically unaffected skin.

Precipitating factors
Trauma: Koebner phenomenon.

Infection: streptococcal sore throat (guttate psoriasis).

Drugs: beta blockers, lithium, antimalarials; oral corticosteroid withdrawal.

Psychological stress: difficult to assess but often reported.

Sunlight: 10% aggravated, 90% improved.

Heavy drinking: alcohol probably does not directly exacerbate psoriasis but may reduce therapeutic compliance.

Smoking: particular association with palmoplantar pustular psoriasis.

Epidemiology
- 2% of people in industrialized countries are affected.
- The male:female ratio is equal.
- Peak onset is at about 20 years, with a second, smaller peak in the 60s.

Treatment

Diet and lifestyle
- No special precautions are necessary.

Pharmacological treatment
- Patients should be referred to a consultant in the case of diagnostic difficulty, need for patient counselling or education (including initial demonstration of topical treatment), failure of topical treatment used appropriately for 3 months, need for increasing amounts or potency of topical corticosteroids, need for systemic drugs, or generalized pustular or erythrodermic psoriasis (emergency referral).

Topical treatment
Coal tar: safe and effective in plaque psoriasis; messy to apply (limiting compliance).

Dithranol (in Lassar's paste or Dithrocream): effective topical agent; treatment started at low concentration, e.g. 0.1%, built up by doubling concentrations, titrating against clinical response compared with irritation; application must be closely supervised; main side effects include staining of the skin and clothes and burning.

Steroids: effective and cosmetically acceptable; long-term use needs close supervision.

Vitamin D3 analogues: calcipotriol safe and effective in mild to moderate psoriasis; may be irritant but does not stain.

Phototherapy: ultraviolet B useful for chronic plaque and guttate psoriasis; alone or with other treatments.

Systemic therapy
- Treatment should be given under specialist supervision.
- Methotrexate is used in widespread plaque, acute generalized pustular and erythrodermic psoriasis, and psoriatic arthropathy as short-term or maintenance treatment.
- Retinoids are effective particularly in acral or generalized pustular psoriasis.
- Cyclosporin is effective for severe refractory psoriasis and psoriatic arthropathy.
- Long-term photochemotherapy (oral or topical psoralens with ultraviolet A) is complicated by increased risk of cutaneous squamous-cell carcinoma.

Standard dosage	Methotrexate single weekly oral dose titrated against response, always commencing with low dose. Acitretin 25–50 mg daily.
Contraindications	*Methotrexate:* hepatic disease, alcohol abuse, malignancy. *Retinoids:* hepatic and renal damage. *Cyclosporin:* renal disease, uncontrolled hypertension, infection, malignancy.
Special points	*Methotrexate:* conception must be avoided in both men and women. *Retinoids:* pregnancy must be avoided during treatment and for up to 2 years afterwards. *Cyclosporin:* sudden withdrawal may lead to relapse within a few weeks but not to the severe rebound seen with systemic steroids; monitoring should include blood pressure, serum creatinine, and glomerular filtration rate.
Main drug interactions	*Methotrexate:* alcohol, salicylates, NSAIDs, co-trimoxazole, probenecid, phenytoin, retinoids, pyrimethamine, frusemide. *Retinoids:* reduce effect of warfarin. *Cyclosporin:* NSAIDs may potentiate nephrotoxicity.
Main side effects	*Methotrexate:* hepatic fibrosis (liver biopsy every 1.5 g cumulative dose), acute bone-marrow suppression. *Retinoids:* raised serum lipids, liver enzymes (abnormalities return to normal on cessation of treatment), spinal changes after prolonged treatment (diffuse idiopathic skeletal hyperostosis). *Cyclosporin:* dose-related hypertension and nephrotoxicity (plasma creatinine should be monitored at baseline and then monthly).

Treatment aims
To clear existing psoriasis by 80% (systemic regimens).

Prognosis
- Psoriasis is a chronic disease; sufferers tend to relapse and remit over many years.
- Severity and occurrence of complications are highly variable.

Follow-up and management
- All patients on systemic regimens must be followed up regularly by a dermatologist.
- Regular clinical review is needed if the patient is using topical steroids.

Patient support
- The noninfectious, non-malignant nature of psoriasis and the need for long-term treatment to control rather than to eradicate the disease must be explained to the patient.
- The patient should be referred to support groups, e.g. the Psoriasis Association.

Key references
Barker JNWN: Pathophysiology of psoriasis. *Lancet* 1991, **338**:227–230.

Menne T, Larsen K: Psoriasis treatment with vitamin D derivatives. *Semin Dermatol* 1992, **11 (suppl 4)**:5–10.

Mihatsch MJ, Welbb K: Consensus conference on cyclosporin A for psoriasis. *Br J Dermatol* 1992, **126**:621–623.

RCP/BAD Working Party: Guidelines for management of patients with psoriasis. *BMJ* 1991, **303**:829–835.

Theeuwes M, Leder R: Hereditary insights into psoriasis. *Eur J Dermatol* 1993, **3**:335–341.

Urticaria   R.J. Barlow and M.W. Greaves

Diagnosis

Symptoms
Itching and swelling of skin.
Arthralgia: in severe urticaria.
Angioedema: in ~50% of patients.

Signs
Erythematous skin swellings (wheals): may have pale centres and blanch on pressure; individual lesions may coalesce into giant wheals or annular and serpiginous forms; wheals usually resolve without trace after a few hours.

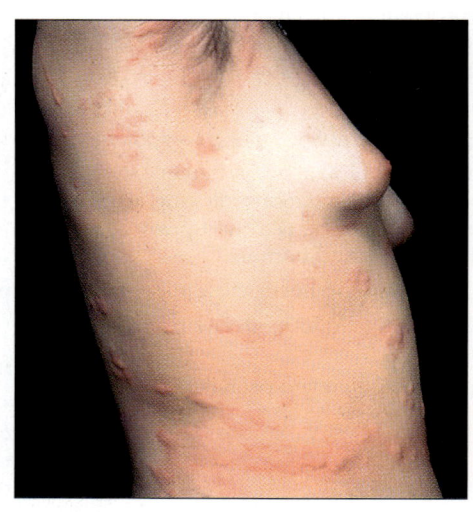

Scattered urticarial wheals on the trunk.

Investigations

Acute urticaria (<6 weeks)
- A detailed history and examination are important, particularly in relation to food and drug ingestion.

Confirmatory skin prick tests: only indicated if suspected food or drug consistently induces wheals within several hours of ingestion.

Radioallergosorbent testing (RAST): for IgE, may be helpful in suspected penicillin allergy.

Chronic urticaria (>6 weeks)
- Extensive investigations are not cost-effective unless indicated clinically or by an abnormal differential leucocyte count or ESR.

Challenge tests: for physical urticarias if indicated.

Complications

Acquired angioedema: characterized by local swellings of subcutaneous or submucous tissue, usually without itching or erythema.

Physical urticarias: with chronic idiopathic urticaria; physical urticarias are distinct syndromes elicited by mechanical stimuli (dermographism, delayed pressure, vibration-induced), temperature change (cholinergic, contact heat, cold), light (solar), and water (aquagenic).

Differential diagnosis
Urticarial vasculitis.
Erythema marginatum rheumaticum.

Aetiology
- Urticaria may be exacerbated by alcohol and NSAIDs, especially aspirin.

Acute urticaria
- Causes include the following:
Idiopathic.
Non-immunologically determined intolerance to drugs and foodstuffs.
True IgE-mediated allergic reactions (<5% of patients).

Chronic urticaria
- No cause is identified in most patients.
- Rarely, previously unrecognised intolerance to food (including dyes and preservatives), chronic low-grade infection, or parasite infestation may be involved.
- Thyroid auto-antibodies have been reported in 12% of patients.
- Chronic idiopathic urticaria frequently runs a relapsing course and may itself be an autoimmune disorder in some patients in whom histamine-releasing IgG autoantibodies have been shown.

Epidemiology
- 10–15% of the general population experience an urticarial eruption at some stage.
- A slight female predominance is seen.
- The incidence is highest in the third and fourth decades.

Treatment

Diet and lifestyle
- Known triggering agents, e.g. alcohol, aspirin, foodstuff, if identified, must be avoided.
- Death is a risk in patients with cold urticaria on immersion in cold water.

Pharmacological treatment
- In the absence of an identifiable cause, treatment should be supportive and symptomatic until the urticaria resolves spontaneously.

H_1 receptor antagonists
- The minimally sedating H_1 blockers terfenadine, cetirizine, loratidine, and astemizole have fewer anticholinergic side effects than older antihistamines and are as potent in relieving itching and whealing.
- Ketotifen 2–6 mg daily is also a mast cell membrane stabilizing drug and calcium antagonist; doxepin 25–100 mg 3 times daily is also an antidepressant and may occasionally be justified.

Standard dosage	Chlorpheniramine maleate 4 mg every 4–6 h. Promethazine hydrochloride 10–20 mg every 8–12 h or up to 50 mg at night. Hydroxyzine hydrochloride 25 mg every 6–8 h. Terfenadine 60 mg twice daily; cetirizine 10 mg twice daily; loratidine 10 mg once daily; astemizole 10 mg once daily.
Contraindications	Porphyrias.
Special points	*Chlorpheniramine maleate:* understood to be safe in pregnancy and the porphyrias.
Main drug interactions	Potentiate the effects of alcohol. *Terfenadine:* with concurrent erythromycin or ketoconazole, can cause ventricular arrythmias.
Main side effects	Drowsiness (night-time administration), antimuscarinic effects; ventricular arrythmias have been reported after excessive dosage of astemizole or terfenadine.

Systemic corticosteroids
- High doses may be needed, resulting in serious adverse effects. They should be avoided except in acute, severe exacerbations.

For angioedema associated with urticaria
Ephedrine 2% intraoral spray in 100 ml aqueous solution containing 1 g chlorbutol and 1 g sodium chloride: for mild involvement of mouth and throat.

Maintenance of airway and intravascular fluid volume, adrenaline 1:1000 (1 mg/ml; 0.5–1 ml subcut), chlorpheniramine maleate 10–20 mg i.v. (maximum, 40 mg in 24 h), hydrocortisone sodium succinate 100–300 mg i.v.: for severe angioedema.

Treatment aims
To relieve itching and reduce whealing.

Prognosis
- Acute urticaria resolves within 6 weeks.
- Most cases or chronic urticaria resolve within 2 years, but up to 20% of patients experience episodes for >20 years.

Follow-up and management
- Follow-up is needed to monitor the efficacy and complications of treatment.

Urticarial vasculitis
- This rare syndrome is manifest clinically with urticaria but shows vasculitis on histological examination (needed to confirm diagnosis).
- Compared with other forms of chronic urticaria, wheals are more likely to be painful or burning, to persist for >24 h, and to resolve with bruising.
- Usually no response to antihistamines is seen.

Key references
Greaves MW: Urticaria: new molecular insights and treatments. The Parkes Weber Lecture 1991. *J R Coll Physicians Lond* 1992, **26**:199–203.

Huston DP, Bressler RB: Urticaria and angio-oedema. *Clin Allergy* 1992, **76**:805–840.

Lawlor F: Urticaria. *J Eur Acad Dermatol Venereol* 1993, **2**:35–43.

Vasculitis, skin manifestations
N.J. Levell, A.P. Bewley, and P.M. Dowd

Diagnosis

Symptoms
Crops of painful purple areas on skin.
Symptoms of the predisposing disease.

Signs
Painful, palpable purpura: the thee 'P's.
Crops of **purple nodules** usually in dependent areas.
Lesions: tender; do not blanch; haemorrhagic blisters; black, necrotic, ulcerating in severe disease.
Finger pulp 2–3 mm lesions: indicating connective tissue disease, particularly rheumatoid arthritis.
Nail-bed linear lesions: indicating trauma, connective tissue disease, or systemic infection.
Net-like pattern (livedo reticularis): indicating connective tissue disease, cryoglobulinaemia, antiphospholipid syndrome, or polyarteritis nodosa.
Subcutaneous nodules along arteries: indicating polyarteritis nodosa.

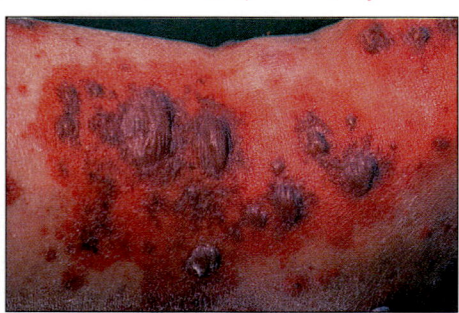

Cutaneous vasculitis on the legs, showing red/purple palpable painful lesions, some of which have overlying haemorrhagic blisters.

Investigations
Urinalysis, urine microscopy, serum creatinine measurement: to identify renal involvement.
Blood culture, culture of possible sites of infection: to identify infective cause.
Measurement of rheumatoid factor, antinuclear antibodies, antineutrophil cytoplasmic antibodies, anticardiolipin antibodies: to identify connective tissue disorders.
Cryoglobulin measurement: collected after fasting and taken to laboratory at 37°C.
Skin biopsy: not indicated if clinical picture is typical, because histology often shows nonspecific leucocytoclastic vasculitis, but may help in patients with drug-induced, infective, or inflammatory vasculitis; may also be helpful in identifying infiltrating inflammatory cells, type and size of blood vessels involved, and whether granulomatous changes are present.

Complications
Ulceration: particularly on lower limbs; may follow skin biopsy.
Secondary infection.
Renal involvement: in 30–60% of patients.
Joint, gastrointestinal tract, CNS, or lung involvement.

Differential diagnosis
Purpura.
Thrombocytopenia.
Platelet dysfunction.
Corticosteroid treatment.
Old age.
Scurvy.
Trauma.
Non-accidental injury in children.
Haemangioma.
Kaposi's sarcoma.
Bacillary angiomatosis.

Aetiology
- Causes include the following:

Environmental factors
Gravitational stasis.
Cold exposure.

Infection
Acute: meningococcal meningitis (1–3 weeks after throat infection), gonorrhoea.
Chronic: urinary infections, dental abscess, leprosy, hepatitis B and C.

Drugs
Antibiotics: e.g. sulphonamides.
Warfarin (rarely causes haemorrhagic skin infarction).

Inflammation
Immune complexes: e.g. connective tissue disorders.
Cryoglobulins: e.g. in malignancy.
Autoantibodies: e.g. antineutrophil cytoplasmic antibody in Wegener's granulomatosis (may be secondary phenomenon).

Epidemiology
- Vasculitis is a common condition.
- The male:female ratio is equal.
- It can affect people at any age.

Treatment

Diet and lifestyle
- Patients must avoid cold, gravitational effects (with bed-rest during acute episodes), and tight garments.

Pharmacological treatment
- Drugs that are probable causes of vasculitis should be discontinued.
- Precipitating infections should be treated by antibiotics.

Prednisolone
- Prednisolone may be ineffective, and side effects limit use to patients with severe progressive systemic disease.

Standard dosage	Prednisolone 60–80 mg daily initially.
Contraindications	Untreated infection; caution in pregnancy because causes neonatal adrenal suppression.
Main drug interactions	Antihypertensives, antidiabetics, diuretics, antiepileptics.
Main side effects	Diabetes, osteoporosis, mental disturbance, peptic ulceration, infections, suppressed growth in children, proximal myopathy, cataracts, hypertension, acute adrenal insufficiency.

Dapsone
- Dapsone is often effective against chronic vasculitis, although this is not mentioned on the drug data sheet.

Standard dosage	Dapsone 50–100 mg daily.
Contraindications	Porphyrias, severe anaemia, glucose 6-phosphate dehydrogenase.
Special points	Folate supplements needed in pregnancy (causes neonatal haemolysis and methaemoglobinaemia). Regular blood checks necessary.
Main drug interactions	Probenecid.
Main side effects	Agranulocytosis, haemolytic anaemia, headaches, nausea, neuropathy, exfoliative dermatitis, hepatitis.

Indomethacin
- Indomethacin is sometimes effective in urticarial vasculitis, although this is not mentioned on the drug data sheet.

Standard dosage	Indomethacin 50–150 mg daily.
Contraindications	Active peptic ulceration; caution in renal impairment, epilepsy, parkinsonism, salicylate hypersensitivity.
Special points	Excreted in breast milk.
Main drug interactions	Warfarin, angiotensin-converting enzyme inhibitors, haloperidol, digoxin, diuretics, lithium, probenecid.
Main side effects	Gastrointestinal discomfort, nausea, ulceration and bleeding, asthma, tinnitus, headache, vertigo, drowsiness, convulsions, fluid retention, renal failure, hypertension, corneal deposits, thrombocytopenia, angioedema.

Treatment aims
To alleviate discomfort.
To prevent skin ulceration.
To detect systemic involvement early.

Other treatments
- Plasmapheresis: has been used to remove immune complexes in patients with SLE; no evidence of benefit has been shown in controlled studies.

Prognosis
- Individual episodes may clear after 3–6 weeks.
- Relapse and chronic disease are common.
- Patients with infective or drug-induced vasculitis usually recover fully on removal of the cause, although chronic vasculitis or, rarely, fatal systemic necrotizing vasculitis occur.
- The prognosis of inflammatory vasculitis depends on the cause: up to 25% of patients with renal involvement develop chronic renal problems in Henoch–Schönlein purpura.

Follow-up and management
- Renal involvement must be detected by weekly urinalysis and microscopy during an episode and serum creatinine and blood pressure measurement every 2 weeks.
- Cutaneous complications must be treated.
- Patients must be monitored for side effects of treatment.

Key references
D'Cruz D, Hughes D: Systemic vasculitis. *BMJ* 1992, **304**:269–270.
Jorizzo K: Classification of vasculitis. *J Invest Dermatol* 1993, **100**:106S–110S.
Scott DGI et al.: Vasculitis. In *Oxford Textbook of Rheumatology*. Edited by Maddison PJ et al. Oxford: Oxford Medical Publications, 1993, pp 842–884.

Viral warts — E.C. Benton

Diagnosis

Symptoms
- Many viral warts are asymptomatic but unsightly.

Pain: especially from deep plantar warts.

Signs

Cutaneous warts

Well demarcated papule, compressed keratin edge, central tow-like substance containing thrombosed capillaries: deep plantar warts.

Flesh-coloured hyperkeratotic papules: often on dorsum of hands or knees or at other sites of trauma: common warts.

Fleshy base, hyperkeratotic, papilliferous surface: facial warts.

Small punctate lesions, central depression, thrombosed capillaries: endophytic palmar/plantar warts.

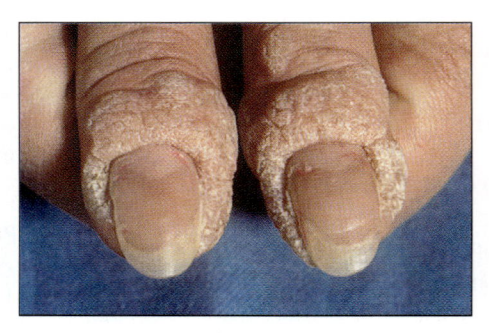

Proliferative friable warts: 'Butchers' warts' in meat handlers or fishmongers.

Superficial saucer-shaped warts: in mosaic pattern on sole of foot, periungal area, or knuckles: mosaic warts.

2–5 mm flat-topped papules: usually on sites exposed to light: plane warts.

Periungual viral warts.

Anogenital warts

Soft fleshy cauliflower-like papules with friable surface: condyloma acuminata; occurring anywhere on anogenital skin or mucosa.

Areas of aceto-white staining on genital mucosa after application of 3% acetic acid solution: condyloma plana (aceto-white staining may also occur with other disorders).

Investigations

Cutaneous warts

Histology: if diagnosis uncertain.

Anogenital warts

Screening for other sexually transmitted diseases: all sexual contacts should be examined.

Cervical cytology: for women and contacts of infected men.

Cytobrush smear: of anal canal for homosexual men with perianal warts.

Biopsy: may be necessary to detect dysplasia associated with human papilloma virus infection.

Complications

Increased risk of genital tract dysplasia: in patients with anogenital warts, especially if immunosuppressed.

Differential diagnosis

Cutaneous warts
Molluscum contagiosum.
Fibroepithelial skin tag.
Seborrhoeic wart.
Cellular naevus.
Punctate palmar/plantar keratoses.
Actinic keratosis.
Squamous cell cancer.

Anogenital warts
Molluscum contagiosum.
Condylomata lata of syphilis.

Aetiology

Cause

Human papilloma virus infection involving cutaneous and mucocutaneous sites; classified by different cleavage patterns of viral DNA, (>60 types identified). Virus occurs in clinical, subclinical, or latent forms; no viral particles are shed in latent form, but this form could act as reservoir for the virus in relapsing infections.

Spread

Skin warts: direct or indirect passage of infected skin scales, enhanced by breaks in or maceration of skin surface or increased exposure, e.g. in communal showers or swimming pools.

Anogenital warts: usually by sexual contact; inoculation of cutaneous human papilloma virus types may occur; neonates may acquire virus from maternal genital tract.

Epidemiology

- The prevalence of viral warts is 7–13% of the population.
- Skin warts occur most often in patients aged 12–16 years.
- Anogenital warts occur most often in young sexually active adults.

Treatment

Diet and lifestyle
- No special precautions are necessary.
- Patients with genital warts should use condoms.

Pharmacological treatment
- The choice of treatment depends on the extent of the warts, symptoms, and response to previous treatment.
- Scarring treatments should be avoided, if possible.

For cutaneous warts
- Topical treatment suitable for application by patient is indicated.

Standard dosage	Salicylic acid as paint, gel, ointment or impregnated plasters; concentration varies from 10 to 50%. Glutaraldehyde 10%. Formalin 1.5% gel or 20% in Unguentum Merck for mosaic warts.
Contraindications	Facial or anogenital warts; caution in diabetes or peripheral vascular disease.
Main drug interactions	None.
Main side effects	Skin irritation.

- Second-line treatment consists of cryotherapy with liquid nitrogen or carbon dioxide snow; this is a first-line treatment for facial warts.
- Third-line treatments in hospital clinics only include monochloracetic acid for plantar warts, intralesional bleomycin (on a named-patient basis), and systemic or intralesional interferon for recalcitrant warts.

For anogenital warts

Standard dosage	Podophyllin 15–25% applied once weekly. Podophyllotoxin 0.5%.
Contraindications	Pregnancy.
Special points	Extensive application must be avoided because of risk of systemic absorption and toxicity.
Main drug interactions	None.
Main side effects	Skin irritation.

- Other treatments include cryotherapy, electrocautery, scissor excision, and carbon dioxide laser.
- Topical 5-fluorouracil is an alternative for vaginal warts.

Treatment aims
To clear clinical disease without scarring and with minimum of adverse effects.

Prognosis
- In many patients, warts resolve spontaneously, leaving no scarring.
- Depression of cell-mediated immunity predisposes to persistent infection.
- Up to 70% of cutaneous warts resolve spontaneously in 2 years.

Follow-up and management
- Regular cervical cytology is needed for women with anogenital warts.
- Ideally, colposcopy should be done especially if the cervical cytology is abnormal.

Key references
Bunney MH, Benton EC, Cubie HA: *Viral Warts–Biology and Treatment* edn 2. Oxford: Oxford University Press, 1992.

Dawber R, Colver GB, Jackson M (eds): *Cutaneous Cyrosurgery.* London: Martin Dunitz, 1992.

Jablonska S, Orth G (eds): *Clinics in Dermatology: Warts/Human Papillomavirus* vols 3/4. Philadelphia: JB Lippincott, 1985.

Index

A

acitretin for psoriasis 13
acne 2
acyclovir for eczema 9
adrenaline for angioedema associated with urticaria 15
alopecia
    androgenic 4
    areata 4, 10
    lichenoid 4
    traumatic 4
aluminium oxide for acne 3
amorolfine for fungal nail infection 11
angiitis *see* vasculitis
angioedema 14
angiomatosis, bacillary 16
antibiotics *see also* antimicrobials
    for acne 3
    for eczema 9
    for skin manifestations of vasculitis 17
antifungal agents for fungal nail infection 11
antihistamines
    for eczema 9
    for urticaria 15
antimalarials for discoid lupus erythematosus 5
antimicrobials *see also* antibiotics
    for bullous disorders 7
antimycotic agents for fungal nail infection 11
antivirals for eczema 9
aqueous cream for eczema 9
arthritis
    mutilans 12
    rheumatoid 16
arthropathy
    distal 12
    psoriatic 12
astemizole for urticaria 15
Aveeno for eczema 9
azathioprine
    for bullous disorders 7
    for eczema 9
azelaic acid for acne 3

B

baldness *see* alopecia
Balneum for eczema 9
benzoyl peroxide for acne 3
betamethasone for eczema 9
bites, insect 6
bleomycin for cutaneous warts 19
blistering 6, 8
    haemorrhagic 16
    rash, spontaneous 6
    trauma-induced 6
bulla *see* blistering
bullous
    disorders 6
    impetigo 6
burns 6

C

calcipotriol for psoriasis 13
carbon dioxide
    laser treatment for anogenital warts 19
    snow for cutaneous warts 19
carcinoma, squamous-cell 4, 18
cetirizine
    for eczema 9
    for urticaria 15
cheiropodopompholyx 10
cheiropompholyx 12
chlorpheniramine for urticaria 15
clindamycin for acne 3
clobetasol propionate
    for alopecia areata 5
    for eczema 9
clobetasone for eczema 9
coal tar for psoriasis 13
collagen injection, intradermal, for acne 3
comedones 2
condyloma
    acuminata 18
    plana 18
condylomata lata of syphilis 18
corticosteroids
    for alopecia areata 5
    for bullous disorders 7
    for eczema 9
    for psoriasis 13
    for urticaria 15
cryoglobulinaemia 16
cryotherapy for cutaneous warts 19
cyclophosphamide for bullous disorders 7
cyclosporin A 338
    for eczema 9
    for psoriasis 13
cysts, inflammatory 2

D

dapsone
    for bullous disorders 7
    for skin manifestations of vasculitis 17
dermatitis
    allergic 10
    atopic 8
    eczematous *see* eczema
    exfoliative 12 *see also* erythroderma
    herpetiformis 6, 8
    medicamentosa *see* drug eruption
    perioral 2
    seborrhoeic 12
dermatosis, pustular
    chronic superficial scaly 8
    erosive 4
    subcutaneous *see* bullous disorders
diphencyprone for alopecia areata 5
dithranol
    for alopecia areata 5
    for psoriasis 13
doxepin for urticaria 15
doxycycline for acne 3
drug eruption 6, 8, 12

E

eczema 8, 12
    allergic contact 8
    asteototic 8
    atopic 8
    discoid 8
    endogenous 8
    erythrodermic 8
    exogenous 8
    exudative 9
    irritant contact 8
    lichenified 8
    palmoplantar 9
    photoallergic contact 8
    phototoxic 8
    pompholyx 6, 8
    seborrhoeic 8
    varicose 8
effluvium, telogen 4
electrocautery for anogenital warts 19
emollients for eczema 9
ephedrine for angioedema associated with urticaria 15
epidermolysis bullosa 6
Epogam for eczema 9
erythema 8
    marginatum rheumaticum 14
erythroderma 8, 12

Index

erythromycin
  for acne 3
  for eczema 9
evening primrose oil for eczema 9

F

flucloxacillin for eczema 9
fluocinonide for eczema 9
fluorouracil for anogenital warts 19
folate supplements for vasculitis 17
folliculitis 4
formalin for cutaneous warts 19
frusemide eruptions 6

G

genital tract dysplasia 18
glutaraldehyde for cutaneous warts 19
griseofulvin for fungal nail infection 11

H

H_1 blockers for urticaria 15
haemangioma 16
hair loss *see* alopecia
herbal therapy, Chinese, for eczema 9
hydrocortisone
  for angioedema associated with urticaria 15
  for eczema 9
hydroxyzine for urticaria 15
hyperkeratosis 10
  palmaris et plantaris *see* keratosis punctate palmarplantar
  subungual 12

I

impetigo
  bullous 6
  contagiosa *see* bullous impetigo
indomethacin for urticarial vasculitis 17
infection 6
  bacterial 10
  fungal 4
    nail 10
  Pseudomonas 10
  secondary
    by herpes simplex 8
    by *Staphylococcus aureus* 8
  skin, by tinea corporis/capitis 8
  systemic 16

varicella–zoster 6
insect bites 6
interferon for cutaneous warts 19
intertrigo
  bacterial 12
  candidal 12
iron deficiency 4
isotretinoin for acne 3
itching 6, 8, 12, 14

K

Kaposi's
  sarcoma 16
  varicelliform eruption 8
keratoma *see* keratosis
keratosis
  actinic 18
  palmaris et plantaris *see* keratosis punctate palmarplantar
  palmarplantar *see* keratosis punctate palmarplantar
  punctate palmarplantar 18
kerion 4
ketotifen for urticaria 15

L

lesion 6, 12, 16
  nail-bed linear 16
leukonychia, transverse 10
lichen
  planus 4, 10
    hypertrophic 12
  ruber planus *see* lichen planus
lichenification 8
livedo reticularis 16
loratidine for urticaria 15
lupus erythematosus, discoid 4

M

malnutrition 8
Marie–Streumpell disease *see* spondylitis, ankylosing
melanoma, subungual 10
methotrexate
  for bullous disorders 7
  for psoriasis 13
micrografts for alopecia 5
minocycline for acne 3
molluscum contagiosum 18

monochloracetic acid for plantar warts 19
mucous membranes, erosion of 6
mycosis fungoides 8

N

naevus, cellular 18
nail
  discoloration 10
  infection, fungal 10
  plate disruption 10
  psoriasis 12
  removal, surgical or chemical 11
  ridging 8
  'shiny' 8
necrobiosis lipoidica 4
nitrogen, liquid, for cutaneous warts 19
nodules
  inflammatory 2
  subcutaneous 16

O

oat for eczema 9
oil
  evening primrose for eczema 9
  mineral *see* paraffin
Oilatum for eczema 9
oligoarthritis 12
onchogryphosis 10
onycholysis 12
onychomycosis 10, 12
  distal and lateral subungual 10
  proximal subungual 10
  superficial white 10
  total dystrophic 10

P

pachonychia 10
papules
  hyperkeratotic 18
  inflammatory 2
papulovesicles 8
paraffin for eczema 9
pellagra 8
pemphigoid 6
  gestationis 6
pemphigus 6
photochemotherapy for psoriasis 13
photoradiation therapy *see* phototherapy
phototherapy

Index

for eczema 9
for psoriasis 13
pitting 12
pityriasis
lichenoides chronica 12
rosea 12
plaque 12
erythematous 12
psoriasis, chronic 12
platelet dysfunction 16
podophyllin for anogenital warts 19
podophyllotoxin for anogenital warts 19
polyarteritis nodosa 16
polyethylene granules for acne 3
porphyria cutanea tarda 6
prednisolone
for bullous disorders 7
for eczema 9
for lichenoid alopecia 5
for skin manifestations of vasculitis 17
promethazine for urticaria 15
pruritus *see* itching
pseudopelade 4 *see also* alopecia
psoralen and ultraviolet A
for eczema 9
for psoriasis 13
psoriasis 10, 12
chronic plaque 12
flexural 12
guttate 12
nail 12
palmoplantar 12
pustular 12
scalp 12
purpura 16
painful, palpable 16
pustules 12
inflammatory 2
PUVA *see* psoralen with ultraviolet A

R

Reiter's disease 12
retinoids for psoriasis 13
rosacea 2

S

salicylic acid
for acne 3
for cutaneous warts 19
salmon patches 12

sarcoid 4
sarcoidosis 10
sarcoma, Kaposi's 16
scarring 2
'ice-pick' 2
keloid 2
Schaumann's disease *see* sarcoidosis
scurvy 16
seborrhoea 2
skin
disease
vesicular *see* bullous disorders
vesiculobullous *see* bullous disorders
infection by tinea corporis/capitis 8
manifestations of vasculitis 16
tag, fibroepithelial 18
Sneddon–Wilkinson disease *see* bullous disorders
soya for eczema 9
spondylarthritis *see* spondylitis, ankylosing
spondylitis
ankylosing 12
rheumatoid *see* spondylitis, ankylosing
steroids *see* corticosteroids
sulphonamides for bullous disorders 7
sulphur for acne 3
sun block for discoid lupus erythematosus 5

T

telogen effluvium 4
terbinafine for fungal nail infection 11
terfenadine for urticaria 15
tetracycline
for acne 3
for bullous disorders 7
thrombocytopenia 16
thyroid dysfunction 4
tinea
capitis 4, 8
corporis 8
unguium *see* onychomycosis
tioconazole for fungal nail infection 11
trauma 16
tretinoin for acne 3
triamcinolone acetonide for alopecia areata 5
trichotillomania 4

U

ulceration 16
painful 6
ultraviolet B
for eczema 9
for psoriasis 13
urticaria 14
aquagenic 14
cholinergic 14
cold 14
contact heat 14
delayed-pressure 14
physical 14
solar 14
vibration-induced 14

V

varicelliform eruption, Kaposi's 8
vasculitis
skin manifestations 16
urticarial 14
vesicular skin diseases *see* bullous disorders
vesiculation 8 *see also* blistering
vesiculobullous skin diseases *see* bullous disorders
vitamin D3 analogues for psoriasis 13

W

warts
anogenital 18
'Butchers' 18
common 18
cutaneous 18
deep plantar 18
endophytic palmar/plantar 18
facial 18
mosaic 18
plane 18
seborrhoeic 18
viral 18
wheals 14
wigs for alopecia 5
Wiskott–Aldrich syndrome 8

Z

zinc
acetate with erythromycin for acne 3
deficiency 8

CURRENT DIAGNOSIS & TREATMENT

in

Endocrinology & metabolic disorders

Edited by
John Wass

Series editors
Roy Pounder
Mark Hamilton

A QUICK Reference for the Clinician

Contributors

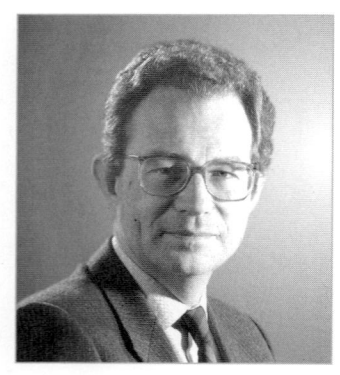

EDITOR

Professor JAH Wass

Professor John Wass runs the Endocrine Unit at the Radcliffe Infirmary and Nuffield Orthopaedic Centre, Oxford. He edited Clinical Endocrinology from 1991 to 1994. He is Linacre Fellow at the Royal College of Physicians, London. His main research interests are acromegaly, the treatment of pituitary tumours, and growth factors in general.

ENDOCRINOLOGY AND METABOLIC DISORDERS

Dr Pierre Bouloux
Reader in Endocrinology
Royal Free Hospital
London, UK

Dr David Hadden
Metabolic Unit
Royal Victoria Hospital
Belfast, UK

AUTHORS

ACROMEGALY
Dr Richard Sheaves
Department of Endocrinology
St Bartholomew's Hospital
London, UK

ADDISON'S DISEASE
Dr Shern L Chew
Department of Endocrinology
St Bartholomew's Hospital
London, UK

CUSHING'S SYNDROME
Dr Trevor A Howlett
Department of Endocrinology
Leicester Royal Infirmary
Leicester, UK

DIABETES INSIPIDUS
Professor PH Baylis
Department of Medicine
Royal Victoria Infirmary
Newcastle upon Tyne, UK

DIABETES MELLITUS, INSULIN-DEPENDENT
Dr Paul L Drury
Auckland Diabetes Centre
Diabetes Education and Advisory Service
Auckland, New Zealand

DIABETES MELLITUS, NON-INSULIN-DEPENDENT
Dr Paul L Drury
Auckland Diabetes Centre
Diabetes Education and Advisory Service
Auckland, New Zealand

DIABETIC MANAGEMENT IN CHILDREN
Dr Clara Lowy
Endocrine and Diabetes Unit
St Thomas's Hospital
London, UK

DIABETIC MANAGEMENT IN PREGNANCY
Dr David JB Thomas
Department of Medicine
Mt Vernon Hospital
Northwood, Middlesex, UK

DIABETIC MANAGEMENT IN SURGERY
Dr David JB Thomas
Department of Medicine
Mt Vernon Hospital
Northwood, Middlesex, UK

FEMALE HYPERGONADOTROPHIC HYPERGONADISM
Dr Robert Fox
Department of Obstetrics and Gynaecology
St Michael's Hospital
Bristol, UK

Dr David J Cahill
Department of Obstetrics and Gynaecology
St Michael's Hospital
Bristol, UK

FEMALE HYPOGONADOTROPHIC HYPERGONADISM
Dr Robert Fox
University Department of Obstetrics and Gynaecology
St Michael's Hospital
Bristol, UK

Dr David J Cahill
Department of Obstetrics and Gynaecology
St Michael's Hospital
Bristol, UK

GROWTH ABNORMALITIES, SHORT STATURE
Professor Charles GD Brook
Department of Medicine
University College Hospital
London, UK

GROWTH ABNORMALITIES, TALL STATURE
Professor Charles GD Brook
Department of Medicine
University College Hospital
London, UK

HYPERCALCAEMIA
Dr David Heath
Division of Medicine
Queen Elizabeth Hospital
Birmingham, UK

HYPERGLYCAEMIC EMERGENCIES
Dr Sally Marshall
Department of Medicine
School of Clinical Medical Studies
The Medical School
Newcastle upon Tyne, UK

HYPERPROLACTINAEMIA
Dr Peter J Trainer
Division of Endocrinology
Oregon Health Sciences University
Portland, Oregon, USA

HYPERTHYROIDISM
Dr Jayne A Franklyn
Department of Medicine
Queen Elizabeth Hospital
Birmingham, UK

HYPOCALCAEMIA
Dr David Heath
Division of Medicine
Queen Elizabeth Hospital
Birmingham, UK

HYPOGLYCAEMIA
Dr Stephanie A Amiel
Department of Endocrinology
Guy's Hospital
London, UK

HYPOPITUITARISM
Dr Paul Jenkins
Department of Endocrinology
St Bartholomew's Hospital
London, UK

HYPOTHYROIDISM
Dr Jayne A Franklyn
Department of Medicine
Queen Elizabeth Hospital
Birmingham, UK

OBESITY
Professor J Garrow
Department of Human Nutrition
St Bartholomew's Hospital
London, UK

PHAEOCHROMOCYTOMA
Dr Paul M Stewart
Department of Medicine
Queen Elizabeth Hospital
Birmingham, UK

POLYCYSTIC OVARIAN DISEASE
Dr Robert Fox
University Department of Obstetrics and Gynaecology
St Michael's Hospital
Bristol, UK

Dr David J Cahill
Department of Obstetrics and Gynaecology
St Michael's Hospital
Bristol, UK

PUBERTAL ABNORMALITIES
Dr Martin O Savage
Reader in Paediatric Endocrinology
St Bartholomew's Hospital
London, UK

SYNDROME OF INAPPROPRIATE ANTIDIURESIS
Professor PH Baylis
Department of Medicine
Royal Victoria Infirmary
Newcastle upon Tyne, UK

TESTICULAR DISORDERS
Professor David Anderson
Honorary Visiting Professor of Medicine and Endocrinology
University of Manchester
Manchester, UK

THYROID CARCINOMA
Professor Michael C Sheppard
Department of Medicine
University of Birmingham
Birmingham, UK

Contents

- 2 Acromegaly
- 4 Addison's disease
- 6 Cushing's syndrome
- 8 Diabetes insipidus
- 10 Diabetes mellitus, insulin-dependent
- 12 Diabetes mellitus, non-insulin-dependent
- 14 Diabetic management in children
- 16 Diabetic management in pregnancy
- 18 Diabetic management in surgery
- 20 Female hypergonadotrophic hypogonadism
- 22 Female hypogonadotrophic hypogonadism
- 24 Growth abnormalities, short stature
- 26 Growth abnormalities, tall stature
- 28 Hypercalcaemia
- 30 Hyperglycaemic emergencies
  - hyperglycaemia
  - ketoacidosis
- 32 Hyperprolactinaemia
  - hyperprolactinaemia
  - macroadenoma
- 34 Hyperthyroidism
- 36 Hypocalcaemia
- 38 Hypoglycaemia
- 40 Hypopituitarism
  - growth hormone deficiency
  - pituitary–adrenal axis deficiency
  - pituitary–gonadal axis deficiency
  - posterior pituitary deficiency
  - thyroid deficiency
- 42 Hypothyroidism
  - congenital hypothyroidism
  - iodine-deficient hypothyroidism
- 44 Obesity
- 46 Phaeochromocytoma
- 48 Polycystic ovarian disease
- 50 Pubertal abnormalities
  - delayed puberty
  - precocious puberty
  - pseudoprecocious puberty
- 52 Syndrome of inappropriate antidiuresis
- 54 Testicular disorders
  - adult male infertility
  - androgen deficiency
  - delayed puberty and hypogonadism
  - gynaecomastia
  - male congenital adrenal hyperplasia
  - male pseudohermaphroditism
  - 5α-reductase deficiency
- 56 Thyroid carcinoma
- 58 Index

Acromegaly
R. Sheaves

Diagnosis

Symptoms

General
Coarsening of facial features, enlargement of hands and feet.
Headache.
Sweating.
Musculoskeletal abnormalities: associated with joint degeneration.
Neuropathy: particularly carpal tunnel syndrome.
Sleep apnoea: due to nasopharyngeal soft-tissue hypertrophy.

Local effects of pituitary tumour
Visual deterioration: due to chiasmal compression.
Hypopituitarism: hypothyroidism, gonadotrophin deficiency, adrenal insufficiency.
Hyperprolactinaemia: impaired libido, impotence, amenorrhoea, galactorrhoea.

Signs

General
Large hands and feet with soft tissue overgrowth.
Coarse features and frontal bossing.
Prognathism and dental separation.
Hypertension: in 30% of patients.
Carpal tunnel syndrome: in 40%.
Multinodular goitre: in 10%.
Gigantism and eunuchoid features: if disease was manifest during childhood.

Local effects of pituitary tumour
Decreased visual acuity.
Visual field defects.
Optic atrophy.
Hypopituitarism: loss of body hair, hypothyroidism.
Hyperprolactinaemia: galactorrhoea.

Investigations
Tests of growth hormone secretion: diagnosis can be established by failure of growth hormone suppression to undetectable concentrations (<1 mU/L) during oral glucose tolerance test; may also show impaired glucose tolerance (in 40% of patients) or diabetes mellitus (in 20%); confirmed by raised level of insulin-like growth factor 1.
Pituitary function tests: thyroid function; pituitary–gonadal axis (luteinizing hormone, follicle-stimulating hormone, oestradiol, testosterone); 09.00 h cortisol (dynamic testing with insulin tolerance test may be indicated); serum prolactin (raised in 30%).
Lateral skull radiography: shows thickened skull, enlarged frontal sinuses, abnormal pituitary fossa.
MRI or CT of pituitary fossa.
Visual field test: Goldman perimetry.

Complications
Coronary artery disease and cardiac failure: high prevalence of hypertension and diabetes mellitus are significant risk factors.
Respiratory disease: small airway function abnormal; additional extrathoracic upper airway obstruction (macroglossia, goitre, nasopharyngeal soft-tissue hypertrophy); mortality significantly increased.
Arthropathies: frequent; contribute significantly to overall morbidity.
Hypercalciuria: in 50% of patients.
Hypercalcaemia: in 5% of patients.
Renal stones: occasionally.
Colorectal polyps: increased incidence, although association between acromegaly and colonic malignancy inferred but so far unproved.

Differential diagnosis
- The facial appearance and enlargement of the hands and feet is characteristic for acromegaly.
Pseudoacromegaly (severe hypothyroidism).

Aetiology
- Causes include the following:
Pituitary growth hormone producing adenoma in 99% of patients.
Occasionally, excess secretion of growth hormone-releasing hormone from neuro-endocrine tumours (gut, pancreas, lung) or from hypothalamic ganglioneuromas.
- An association has been found with multiple endocrine neoplasia type 1 syndrome.

Epidemiology
- The annual incidence is 2.8–4.0 in one million.
- The prevalence is 40–60 in one million.
- Up to 200 new patients are afflicted with acromegaly annually in the UK.

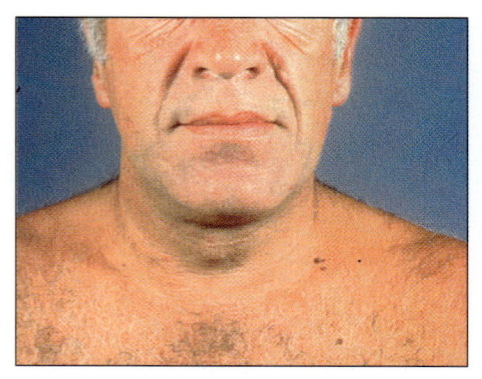

Typical coarse features of acromegaly.

Treatment

Diet and lifestyle
- Unless the patient suffers from diabetes mellitus or hyperlipidaemia, no special dietary precautions are necessary.
- Measures to reduce known vascular risk factors (stopping smoking, controlling hypertension and diabetes, and normalizing lipids) are paramount from the outset.

Pharmacological treatment
- Octreotide may be used when growth hormone concentrations remain >5 mU/L after surgery or in elderly patients as first-line treatment.
- Bromocriptine reduces growth hormone concentrations in some patients.

Standard dosage	Octreotide 100 µg s.c. 3 times daily. Bromocriptine 1.25 mg at night initially, increasing to 20–30 mg daily over a period of weeks.
Contraindications	*Octreotide*: pregnancy and breast-feeding. *Bromocriptine*: psychotic disorders, porphyria.
Special points	*Octreotide*: growth hormone may be further suppressed in some cases by a dose of 200 µg 3 times daily; little gain from further dose increases. *Bromocriptine*: if effective, treatment costs much reduced.
Main drug interactions	*Octreotide*: may alter insulin and hypoglycaemic drug needs in patients with diabetes mellitus. *Bromocriptine*: dopamine antagonists (e.g. metoclopramide) interfere with action.
Main side effects	*Octreotide*: local transient discomfort at injection site, which can be minimized by warming the solution before administration; colicky abdominal pain, diarrhoea, nausea, bloating, flatulence, which usually resolve during first 2–3 weeks of treatment; gallstones, gastritis (long-term). *Bromocriptine*: nausea, vomiting, headache, nasal congestion, postural hypotension, digital vasospasm, constipation.

Non-pharmacological treatment

Trans-sphenoidal surgery
- This is the treatment of choice.
- Cure rates of 40–90% have been achieved.
- The probability of success is influenced by preoperative growth hormone concentrations, tumour size, and invasion.

Pituitary radiotherapy
- Radiotherapy is indicated for patients declining or unfit for surgery or for those not adequately treated by surgery.
- The greatest decrease in growth hormone concentration occurs during the first 2 years.
- Continued decrease in growth hormone concentration is seen for many years.
- Increasing development of hypopituitarism is seen.

Treatment aims
To relieve symptoms.
To reduce growth hormone concentrations to <5 mU/L.
To treat local effects of pituitary tumour.
To maintain normal pituitary function.

Prognosis
- Patients with long-standing acromegaly have twice the mortality of the general population.
- Reduction of the serum growth hormone concentration to <5 mU/L is associated with mortality similar to that of the general population.

Follow-up and management
- Patients with acromegaly need lifelong follow-up to assess the response to treatment and to determine the function of the normal pituitary gland.

Key references
Acromegaly Therapy Consensus Development Panel: Benefits versus risks of medical treatment for acromegaly. *Am J Med* 1994, **97**:468-473.

Bates AS et al.: An audit of outcome of treatment in acromegaly. *QJM* 1993, **86**:293–299.

Ezzat S, Melmed S: Are patients with acromegaly at increased risk for neoplasia? *J Clin Endocrinol Metab* 1991, **72**:245–249.

Wass JAH (ed): *Treating acromegaly, 100 Years On*: Society for Endocrinology, 1994.

Addison's disease — S.L. Chew

Diagnosis

Symptoms
- Onset is usually insidious.

Dizziness and syncope.

Weakness, fatigue, weight loss: common.

Gastrointestinal symptoms: in ~50% of patients.

Pigmentation, persistent tan after holiday, increase in normal skin pigmentation: common.

Mental changes.

Symmetrical musculoskeletal pain: in 10%.

Acute back pain: in anticoagulated patients; rare.

Signs
Postural hypotension.

Hypotension: usually systolic blood pressure <110 mmHg.

Generalized pigmentation: common; extensor and exposed skin should be checked.

Buccal pigmentation: usually manifest with generalized pigmentation.

Scar pigmentation: only scars inflicted after onset of Addison's disease.

Signs of organ-specific autoimmune disease: e.g. vitiligo, thyroid signs.

Hyponatraemia: inability to excrete water due to raised antidiuretic hormone concentration (common).

Hyperkalaemia: usually mild (normal in 40% of patients).

Hypercalcaemia: in 10% of patients.

Hypoglycaemia: sometimes seen in children or undernourished patients.

Investigations
Chest radiography: to check for tuberculosis.

Blood count and film: eosinophilia, macrocytosis with coexistent vitamin B_{12} deficiency, normocytic anaemia after volume replacement.

Serum cortisol measurement: concentration usually <200 nmol/L; may be 200–500 nmol/L during stress; >500 nmol/L makes diagnosis improbable.

Plasma adrenocorticotrophic hormone measurement: concentration usually >80 ng/L (sample must be centrifuged and frozen immediately).

Plasma renin activity and aldosterone measurement: high renin, low aldosterone concentrations.

Short Synacthen test: tetracosactrin 250 μg i.m.; cortisol measured at 0, 30, and 60 min (normal rise >500 nmol/L, with increment of 200 nmol/L); does not distinguish primary from secondary adrenal failure.

Long Synacthen test: tetracosactrin depot 1 mg i.m; cortisol measured at 0, 30, 60, 90, and 120 min and at 4, 6, 8, 12, and 24 h (in secondary adrenal failure, cortisol rises at 24 h; in Addison's disease, no rise occurs).

- The 0, 30, and 60 min values of both Synacthen tests are usually very similar.

Complications
Death: if diagnosis missed, if patient not given extra steroids in stress situations, or if replacement steroids not taken; hydrocortisone must be given before thyroxine when hypothyroidism and Addison's disease coexist (Schmidt's syndrome).

Associated autoimmune endocrine failure: vitamin B_{12} deficiency, hypothyroidism, hypoparathyroidism.

Differential diagnosis
Secondary adrenal insufficiency: low adrenocorticotrophic hormone, cortisol response to long Synachten test at 24 h.

Other causes of pigmentation: e.g. haemochromatosis.

Aetiology
- Causes include the following:

Autoimmune adrenalitis: cortex atrophy only, with anti-adrenal antibodies (>80%).

Tuberculosis: whole-gland involvement, calcification on radiography or CT (less common now).

- Rare causes include the following (80–90% of both adrenals must be affected):

Adrenal haemorrhage: usually in anticoagulated or septicaemic patients.

Adrenoleukodystrophy.

Amyloidosis.

Congenital adrenal hyperplasia.

Drugs: e.g. ketoconazole.

Familial glucocorticoid deficiency: adrenocorticotrophic hormone receptor mutation.

Glucocorticosteroid receptor defects.

Haemochromatosis.

HIV-related adrenalitis.

Metastases.

Sarcoidosis.

Epidemiology
- The prevalence of Addison's disease is 6 in 100 000 in North East Thames Region.
- The female:male ratio is 2:1.

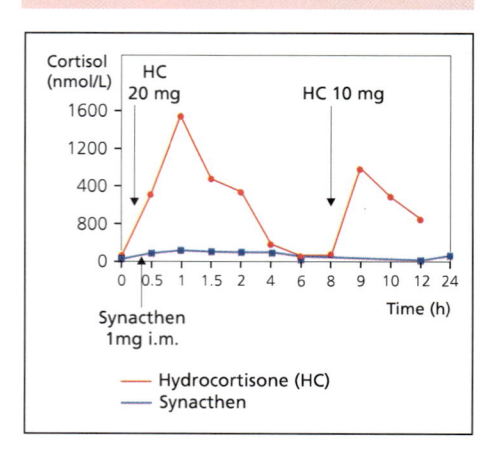

Poor response of serum cortisol to depot synacthen, with cortisol profile of hydrocortisone on a separate day.

Treatment

Diet and lifestyle

- Patients should always carry a steroid-warning card, Medicalert bracelet, and 'emergency pack' (hydrocortisone 100 mg ampule with saline solution, green needle, and 2 ml syringe).
- Patients and partners should be taught how to give an i.m. injection in case of vomiting or coma.
- Patients should be educated about the need for extra hydrocortisone in case of illness or physical stress (surgery).
- Patients should have 24-h direct access to a specialist endocrine centre.

Pharmacological treatment

For acutely ill or hypotensive patients

- If the diagnosis is suspected, action must be taken immediately.

Hydrocortisone 100 mg i.v. bolus.

Saline infusion 1 L initially in 4–6 h.

20% glucose i.v. bolus to correct hypoglycaemia.

- Inotropic agents are useless.

Continued treatment

Standard dosage	Hydrocortisone 100 mg i.m. every 6 h until clinical improvement; patients in intensive care units or on anticoagulants can be treated by 100 mg in 50 ml saline solution at 2 mg/h i.v. infusion.
Contraindications	None.
Special points	When conscious and taking fluids orally, most patients can be converted to oral hydrocortisone. Prednisolone and dexamethasone sometimes used instead.
Main drug interactions	None.
Main side effects	Short-term treatment at these doses rarely has side effects, but diabetes mellitus and psychosis must be considered.

Treatment aims

To alleviate symptoms and restore circulating mineralosteroid and corticosteroids to physiological levels.

Prognosis

- Patients have a normal life expectancy if adequately treated.
- Adrenal function is rarely recovered.

Follow-up and management

- Cortisol concentrations must be monitored during the day; ideally, the peak concentration should be 800–1000 nmol/L, with concentration before the evening dose at least 100 nmol/L.
- Plasma renin activity may be monitored 2 h after fludrocortisone dose.
- Long-term management includes referral to a specialist endocrine unit, hydrocortisone 20 mg orally on waking and 10 mg in the evening before 19.00 h (dose and frequency vary), and fludrocortisone 0.1–0.2 mg daily.

Key references

De Bellis A et al.: Remission of subclinical adrenocortical failure in subjects with adrenal autoantibodies. *J Clin Endocrinol Metab* 1993, **76**:1002–1007.

Oelkers W, Diederich S, Bahr V: Diagnosis and therapy surveillance in Addison's disease: rapid adrenocorticotrophin (ACTH) test and measurement of plasma ACTH, renin activity, and aldosterone. *J Clin Endocrinol Metab* 1992, **75**:259–264.

Ur E et al. Mania in association with hydrocortisone replacement for Addison's disease. *Postgrad Med J* 1992, **68**:41–43.

Werbel SS, Ober, KP: Acute adrenal insufficiency. *Endocrinol Metab Clin North Am* 1993, **22**:303–328.

Cushing's syndrome — T.A. Howlett

Diagnosis

Symptoms
Weight gain: face, chest, and abdomen more than arms and legs.
Hirsutism, acne.
Thin skin, easy bruising, stretch marks.
Muscle weakness and aching.
Menstrual disturbance, impotence, loss of libido.
Back pain, loss of height, pain from other osteoporosis-related fractures.
Depression, anxiety, psychiatric disturbance.
Thirst, polyuria, nocturia: sometimes associated with diabetes mellitus.

Signs
Centripetal obesity: may be simply a relative change in fat distribution; many patients with Cushing's syndrome are overweight rather than obese; morbid obesity rare.
'Moon face', hirsutism, facial plethora.
Thin skin relative to age, easy bruising, pigmentation, acne, red abdominal striae (not just stretch marks, which are common in obese patients and after pregnancy).
Proximal myopathy: e.g. difficulty rising from squat without assistance.
Hypertension: incidental finding or with symptoms of cardiovascular complications.
Kyphosis, loss of height.
Lower-limb oedema: common.
Androgenic hair loss: occasionally.

Investigations
- All tests may give false-positive and false-negative results, so only the simple screening tests should be done by nonspecialists.

Simple screening tests for Cushing's syndrome
24-h urinary free cortisol measurement: raised concentration in Cushing's syndrome; a simple test when diagnosis is clinically unlikely but must be excluded.
Low-dose (2 mg) dexamethasone suppression test: normal suppression of serum cortisol is to <50 nmol/L; patients with Cushing's syndrome fail to suppress.

Confirmatory investigations for diagnosis of Cushing's syndrome
Midnight serum cortisol measurement: normal sleeping midnight serum cortisol <100 nmol/L; normal circadian rhythm lost in Cushing's syndrome.
Insulin stress test: loss of normal cortisol stress response in Cushing's syndrome; not a standard test and should only be done in specialist unit.

Differential diagnosis of the cause of proven Cushing's syndrome
Plasma adrenocorticotrophic hormone (ACTH) measurement: undetectable concentration confirms adrenal Cushing's syndrome; values >400 ng/L suggest ectopic tumour.
Plasma potassium measurement: low concentration in most patients with ectopic ACTH.
CT or MRI of adrenals: shows adrenal tumours or macronodular hyperplasia.
MRI or CT of pituitary gland: may show corticotroph adenoma, but false-positives and false-negatives common.
High-dose (8 mg) dexamethasone suppression test: pituitary Cushing's disease usually shows partial suppression; adrenal tumours and ectopic ACTH do not.
Corticotrophin-releasing hormone test: pituitary Cushing's disease frequently shows exaggerated response; other causes do not.
Petrosal sinus sampling catheterization: confirms pituitary ACTH secretion with near certainty.

Complications
Diabetes, infections, osteoporosis, thromboembolism, ischaemic heart disease, cerebrovascular disease, peripheral vascular disease.

Differential diagnosis
Simple obesity.
Polycystic ovarian syndrome.
- Few patients with obesity, hirsutism, bruising, stretch marks, hypertension, or diabetes have Cushing's syndrome.

Aetiology

Adrenocorticotrophic hormone (ACTH)-dependent Cushing's syndrome
- Pituitary Cushing's disease (70% of patients) is usually due to a (basophil) corticotroph microadenoma, but macroadenoma, corticotroph hyperplasia, and normal tissue structure are found.
- Ectopic ACTH secretion (10%) is usually due to bronchial or thymic carcinoid tumour.
- Ectopic corticotrophin-releasing hormone secretion is rare.

Adrenal Cushing's syndrome
- Causes include adrenal adenoma (10%), adrenal carcinoma (10%), and macronodular adrenal hyperplasia (rare).

Iatrogenic Cushing's syndrome
- The most common cause of the clinical syndrome, this is due to steroid or ACTH treatment.

Epidemiology
- Spontaneous Cushing's syndrome is rare.
- Cushing's syndrome and adrenal adenomas occur more often in women.

Ectopic adrenocorticotrophic hormone (ACTH) syndrome

Occult ectopic ACTH syndrome
- This is usually seen when a neuroendocrine tumour (mostly carcinoid, of bronchial or thymic origin) secretes large amounts of ACTH and mimics a pituitary adenoma.
- The tumour may be only a few millimetres in diameter and only discovered after intensive imaging; diagnosis may prove difficult with conventional tests.

Overt ectopic ACTH secretion
- Many malignant tumours secrete ACTH, most often bronchial small-cell carcinoma; usually the tumour is clinically obvious.
- Patients are rarely cushingoid; they may have no endocrine symptoms or may exhibit pigmentation, myopathy, weight loss, and debility, associated with high cortisol and ACTH concentrations and profound hypokalaemic alkalosis.

Treatment

Diet and lifestyle
- Patients must avoid the risk of fractures or skin abrasions.
- Patients should avoid high salt intake when hypertension is present.

Pharmacological treatment
- Medical treatment for Cushing's syndrome is effective in improving the clinical syndrome but is a short-term measure to prepare the patient for surgery, while awaiting the long-term benefit of other treatment, or in patients with inoperable tumours.
- Drugs include metyrapone, ketoconazole, aminoglutethamide, and op'DDD (mitotane); all have significant problems and should be used only under specialist supervision.

Non-pharmacological treatment

For Cushing's disease
Trans-sphenoidal surgery: treatment of choice for proven pituitary disease, with selective adenomectomy if possible; successful surgery usually results in temporary adrenal insufficiency (due to suppression of normal axis).

Alternatives for surgical failures: pituitary irradiation, bilateral adrenalectomy.

For ectopic adrenocorticotrophic hormone syndrome
Surgical excision: treatment of choice if technically possible and if tumour secreting hormone can be localized.

Radiotherapy or chemotherapy: for some ectopic tumours.

Alternatives if tumour cannot be localized or removed: longer-term medical treatment, bilateral adrenalectomy.

For adrenal tumours
Excision of adrenal adenomas: usually complete, with cure of clinical syndrome and temporary adrenal insufficiency due to suppression of normal axis.

Excision of adrenal carcinomas: sometimes complete, although these carcinomas are often inoperable and usually recur (in which case, medical treatment is essential).

Treatment aims
To restore a normally functioning hypothalamo–pituitary axis, without damage to other endocrine axes.

Prognosis
- Young patients with mild Cushing's disease cured by trans-sphenoidal surgery without recurrence should have normal life expectancy.
- Patients with adrenal carcinoma usually suffer recurrence and death within months.
- Before effective treatment was available, 50% of patients with Cushing's syndrome died within 5 years of diagnosis.
- The overall 'cure' rate for trans-sphenoidal surgery is usually 75–80% but can be as low as 50% (depending on the criteria used to define cure).
- Bilateral adrenalectomy is 100% effective, but patients suffer from life-long hypoadrenalism and are at risk of Nelson's syndrome.
- For adrenal adenomas, surgical excision cures most patients.

Follow-up and management
- Follow-up must be life-long because of the risk of recurrence and morbidity.
- Management depends on the individual patient and should be done by specialists.

Key references
Burke CW *et al.*: Transsphenoidal surgery for Cushing's disease: does what is removed determine endocrine outcome? *Clin Endocrinol* 1990, **33**:525–537.

Howlett TA, Rees LH, Besser GM: Cushing's syndrome. *Clin Endocrinol Metab* 1985, **14**:911–945.

Oldfield EH *et al.*: Petrosal sinus sampling with and without corticotrophin-releasing hormone for the differential diagnosis of Cushing's syndrome. *N Engl J Med* 1991, **325**:897–905.

Trainer PJ, Grossman A: The diagnosis and differential diagnosis of Cushing's syndrome. *Clin Endocrinol* 1991, **34**:317–330.

Diabetes insipidus — P.H. Baylis

Diagnosis

Symptoms
Polyuria, nocturia, excessive thirst (polydipsia).
Enuresis, sleep disturbances, difficulties at school: in children.
- Patients with mild disorder may be asymptomatic.
- During pregnancy, cranial diabetes insipidus symptoms may worsen because of the placental enzyme, vasopressinase.

Signs
- Cranial diabetes insipidus has few signs if patients drink enough.

Urine output 3–20 L/24 h.

Hypernatraemic dehydration: due to loss of thirst sensation and resulting lack of water intake.

Investigations
Blood glucose and serum sodium, potassium, urea, creatinine, and calcium measurement: to confirm diagnosis of cranial diabetes insipidus, to identify patients needing specific tests, to exclude other causes of polyuria.

Fluid deprivation test: cheap and easy to perform but often gives equivocal results; fluid intake during night before test; all fluids withdrawn for up to 8 h (supervision essential); patient weighed hourly (test must be stopped if weight loss >5% of initial body weight); measurement of urine volume and urine and blood osmolality every 1–2 h for 12–16 h; administration of desmopressin 2 µg i.m.

Infusion of 5% hypertonic saline solution: 2 h infusion, with measurements of plasma osmolality and vasopressin; provides definitive diagnosis of cranial diabetes insipidus and quick to perform but is expensive and needs facility to measure plasma vasopressin.

Therapeutic trial of desmopressin: 1–2 week trial with close supervision of body weight, urine volume and osmolality, and plasma osmolality differentiates the three major causes of diabetes insipidus (cranial, nephrogenic, primary polydipsia).

MRI: to identify cause of cranial diabetes insipidus, shows loss of hyperintense signal in neurohypophysis and presence of tumour.

Serum angiotensin-converting enzyme measurement: to detect sarcoid.

Complications
Bladder distension, hydroureter, hydronephrosis: with bladder outflow obstruction.
Secondary nephrogenic diabetes insipidus: due to renal interstitial solute washout.
Hypernatraemic dehydration: if fluid intake inadequate.

Differential diagnosis
Nephrogenic diabetes insipidus.
Primary polydipsia.
Excessive fluid intake (e.g. due to psychogenic polydipsia).
Diabetes mellitus.

Aetiology
- Diabetes insipidus is caused by inadequate quantities of osmoregulated vasopressin due to the following:

Familial causes
Dominant inheritance; gene deletions or substitutions.
Diabetes insipidus, diabetes mellitus, optic atrophy, nerve deafness (DIDMOAD).

Acquired causes
Idiopathic: possible infundibular hypophysitis.
Trauma: neurosurgery, head injury.
Tumours: craniopharyngioma, dysgerminoma, metastases.
Granulomas: sarcoidosis, histiocytosis.
Infection: meningitis, encephalitis.
Vascular disorders: Sheehan's syndrome, sickle cell disease.

Epidemiology
- Diabetes insipidus is a rare condition.
- The estimated prevalence is ~1 in 50 000.
- The male:female ratio is 3:2.

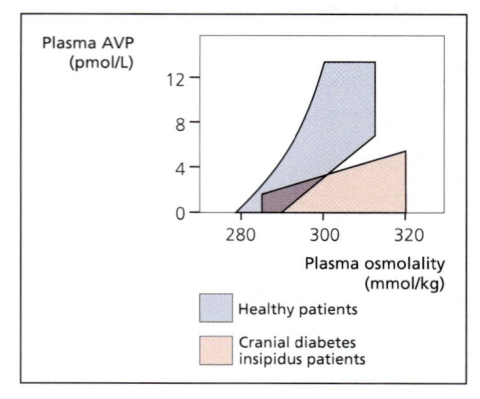

Responses of plasma osmolality and arginine vasopressin (AVP) to hypertonic saline infusion in healthy patients and those with cranial diabetes insipidus, who have subnormal AVP responses.

Treatment

Diet and lifestyle
- Patients must drink sufficient fluid to quench thirst in order to maintain water balance.

Pharmacological treatment

DDAVP (desmopressin)
- DDAVP is a synthetic vasopressin analogue with minimal pressor activity and some resistance to degradation *in vivo*; it is the drug of choice.

Standard dosage	DDAVP 100–600 µg orally in divided doses daily; 5–40 µg intranasally daily, divided doses as spray or delivery by rhinyle; or 0.5–4 µg i.m. or i.v. daily.
Contraindications	Rare hypersensitivity to drug vehicle; caution in renal disease.
Special points	Excessive fluid intake must be avoided. Intranasal preparations less well absorbed when patients have colds or chronic rhinitis. Administration technique must be checked with patients using the rhinyle.
Main drug interactions	None known.
Main side effects	Hyponatraemia (caused by persistent antidiuresis due to DDAVP with continued inappropriate fluid intake).

Lysin vasopressin
- This is a vasopressin of the pig family, synthetically prepared; it has pressor activity and short action.

Standard dosage	Lypressin 2.5–10 units intranasally 3–7 times daily.
Contraindications	Renal disease, hypertension, cardiovascular disease.
Special points	Excessive fluid intake must be avoided.
Main drug interactions	None known.
Main side effects	Pallor, nausea, renal colic, abdominal colic, abdominal cramps, constriction of coronary arteries.

Pitressin
- This synthetically produced natural human hormone (arginine vasopressin) is not recommended for treatment of cranial diabetes insipidus because of its pressor activity and very short action.

Other options
- Specific treatment of the cause of cranial diabetes insipidus may relieve symptoms, e.g. steroids for sarcoidosis (rare).
- Less effective oral preparations include chorpropamide 250–500 mg daily, (hypoglycaemia a major side effect) and carbamazepine 200–600 mg daily.

Treatment aims
To reduce urine volume to 1–2 L/24 h.
To relieve thirst.
To avoid hyponatraemia.

Prognosis
- Prognosis is excellent for treated patients.
- Patients with cranial diabetes insipidus rarely manage without replacement therapy unless the underlying disease is treated successfully.

Follow-up and management
- Care must be taken to avoid hyponatraemia due to overtreatment with vasopressin analogues.
- Withdrawal of desmopressin once a week for 1 day is recommended, with monthly measurement of serum sodium or plasma osmolality to ensure normal sodium concentrations.
- When administering analogues with pressor activity (lypressin), blood pressure should be checked 3-monthly.

Key references
Baylis PH: Vasopressin: physiology and disorders of hormone secretion. *Med Internat* 1993, **21**:189–196.

Kovacs L, Robertson G: Disorders of water balance – hyponatraemia and hypernatraemia. *Baillières Clin Endocrinol Metab* 1992, **6**:107–127.

Diabetes mellitus, insulin-dependent
P.L. Drury

Diagnosis

Symptoms
- Symptoms are usually of short duration (days to weeks), often longer in older patients.

Polyuria.

Polydipsia.

Weight loss.

Lethargy.

Diabetic ketoacidosis or coma: if disease undetected or ignored; symptoms more severe, followed by progressive loss of consciousness, with vomiting, abdominal pain, air hunger.

Signs
- Initially no symptoms are manifest.

Mild dehydration, weight loss, ketones on breath.

Shock, severe dehydration, Kussmaul respiration, reduced level of consciousness: later signs.

Investigations
Laboratory blood glucose measurement: essential for diagnosis; glucose strips, even with meters, not sufficient.

Urinalysis: shows glycosuria and ketonuria.

Arterial blood gas measurement: shows metabolic acidosis.

Electrolyte analysis: wide variation, may show marked hyperkalaemia and dehydration.

Complications
- Complications are rare before 5–10 years duration of diabetes.

Diabetic retinopathy: background affects >75% by 30 years, only affects vision if near macula; proliferative affects fewer but threatens vision by vitreous haemorrhage/fibrosis; treated by laser; most common cause of new adult blindness <65 years.

Diabetic nephropathy: affects up to 40% after 30 years, but rate probably now falling; proteinuria is hallmark, with progressive renal impairment; can be slowed by vigorous antihypertensive treatment; end-stage failure can be treated by continuous ambulatory peritoneal dialysis or transplantation.

Diabetic neuropathy: many forms, most common being symmetrical sensory polyneuropathy leading to loss of temperature, vibration, and pain sense, hence easy progression to foot ulceration; also several painful forms.

Large-vessel disease (coronary, cerebrovascular, peripheral): also much more common, especially when patient has nephropathy; possibly more diffuse than non-diabetic large-vessel disease, but otherwise generally similar.

- Other problems include skin disorders, especially necrobiosis, joint disorders, mononeuropathies, and cataracts.

- Intensive treatment and good glycaemic control reduce the subsequent incidence of retinopathy, nephropathy, and neuropathy, but at the expense of more frequent hypoglycaemia.

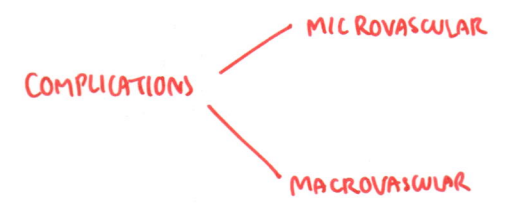

Differential diagnosis
- Diagnosis is not usually a problem, after diabetes mellitus has been considered; possible errors include the following:

Drug overdose and other causes of coma.

Pancreatitis or acute abdomen when abdominal pain is prominent.

Anorexia, thyrotoxicosis, malignancy when weight loss is severe.

- Deciding whether the patient is insulin-dependent can be difficult if the diagnosis is made early; in case of doubt, short-term insulin treatment should be given.

Aetiology
- Insulin-dependent diabetes mellitus is associated with HLA DR3 and DR4.
- The process occurs via an autoimmune mechanism with antibodies against pancreatic islet-cells, which show insulitis and are progressively destroyed.
- The triggering environmental agent is not known.

Epidemiology
- Insulin-dependent diabetes mellitus can occur at any age, but onset is frequently in juveniles (hence the alternative term 'juvenile-onset diabetes mellitus').
- It occurs most often in people of white race, especially in those furthest from the equator (Scandinavia, southern New Zealand); other races differ in genetic susceptibility (e.g. West Indians have similar acute diabetes, but often not truly insulin-dependent or ketosis-prone).
- It affects ~3 in 1000 of the UK population.
- It is increasing in incidence throughout Europe, possibly also occurring earlier.

[Handwritten annotation: COMPLICATIONS → MICROVASCULAR / MACROVASCULAR]

P.L. Drury | **Diabetes mellitus, insulin-dependent**

Treatment

Diet and lifestyle
- Dietetic advice is essential; the diet should be high in unrefined carbohydrate, low in simple sugars, with high fibre and low fat, spread throughout the day, ideally as three meals and three snacks, including one before bedtime.
- Normal activity is advised, except for a few career and driving limitations.

Pharmacological treatment
- After insulin dependency has been established, exogenous insulin is needed.

Types of insulin
- Mainly human biosynthetic insulins are used; pork and beef insulins are still available in some preparations.

Short-acting (soluble/clear): Actrapid, Velosulin, Humulin S.
Intermediate-acting (isophane/cloudy): Protophane, Insulatard, Humulin I.
Longer-acting (zinc-based/cloudy): Monotard, Ultratard, Humulin Zn.
Ready-mixed (soluble isophane, cloudy): e.g. Mixtard 30/70, Humulin M3.

Types of regimen
Once-daily: suited only for elderly, frail patients and those unable to self-inject.
Twice-daily: minimum for all normal patients, including variable dose self-mixing.
Added bedtime dose: mixture in morning, short-acting before supper, intermediate-acting before bedtime; flexible regimen, especially for patients troubled by overnight hypoglycaemia.
Basal-bolus: long-acting overnight, short-acting boluses before meals.

Practical issues
Sites of injection: abdomen, leg or buttock, arm (s.c.)
Timing: usually 30 min before meal.
Exercise needs: extra food or reduced insulin dose.
Insulin infusion (variable rate): best method for ketoacidosis, for unstable diabetes, and during surgery.

Hypoglycaemia
- This is the major unwanted effect of insulin treatment and the predominant concern of many patients.
- It is more common with long duration of diabetes, 'tight control', and previous severe hypoglycaemia.
- It mostly occurs between 10.00 and 13.00 h and overnight.
- Symptoms include sweating, shaking, hunger, palpitation, lack of concentration, confusion, and restlessness, later fits and coma.
- Hypoglycaemia should be treated by oral glucose or food, i.v. glucose, or i.m. glucagon.

See Hypoglycaemia for details.

Treatment aims
To restore normal well-being.
To achieve optimal glycaemic control without significant hypoglycaemia.
To provide patient education and self-care.
To prevent complications.

Prognosis
- The prognosis is excellent and improving in the short and medium terms, provided that the diagnosis is made and patient and carers are competent; ketoacidosis and hypoglycaemia are rare causes of death.
- Longer-term prognosis largely depends on long-term glycaemic control and compliance with screening and treatment.
- Major causes of death are end-stage renal failure and coronary artery disease.
- Major causes of morbidity include proliferative retinopathy leading to blindness, coronary artery disease and peripheral vascular disease, and neuropathy leading to foot ulceration, claudication, or gangrene.

Follow-up and management
- Long-term follow-up is essential for continued education, checks on control, haemoglobin A_{1c} and finger-print sugar levels preprandially and screening for complications (especially eye and foot examination, proteinuria).
- Potentially fertile women should have good control before conception.
- Full patient and family education by specialist nurses and dietitians is essential.
- Most patients should test their own blood glucose and learn to adjust insulin.

Patient support
British Diabetic Association, 10 Queen Anne St, London W1M 0BD; tel 0171 323 1531.

Key references
Day JL: *The Diabetes Handbook: Insulin-Dependent Diabetes*. London: Thorsons/British Diabetic Association, 1992.
Diabetes Control and Complications Trial Research Group: The effect of intensive treatment of diabetes on the development and progression of long-term complications in insulin dependent diabetes. *N Engl J Med* 1993, **329**:977–986.
Tattersall RB, Gale EAM (eds): *Diabetes. Clinical Management*. Edinburgh: Churchill Livingstone, 1990.

Diabetes mellitus, non-insulin-dependent — P.L. Drury

Diagnosis

Symptoms
- ~50% of patients are symptomatic, 50% found on routine or accidental screening.
- Common symptoms, often manifest over many months or years, include the following:

Polyuria, polydipsia.

Pruritus vulvae or balanitis.

Weight loss, tiredness, blurred vision.

Hyperglycaemic non-ketotic coma, with severe dehydration or hyperosmolality: rare manifestation.

Signs
- Generally, no signs are manifest.
- Patients may present with the following:

Obesity.

Foot ulceration or infection.

Diabetic retinopathy.

Signs of secondary causes of diabetes: e.g. acromegaly, Cushing's disease, thyrotoxicosis.

Investigations
Blood glucose measurement: random capillary/venous blood glucose concentration >11 mmol/L in symptomatic patient is diagnostic; two values >11 mmol/L needed in asymptomatic patients.

Glucose tolerance test: needed when diagnosis in doubt (75 g glucose).

Measurement of haemoglobin A_{1c}: raised concentration.

Measurement of iron and total iron-binding capacity: to rule out haemochromatosis.

Measurement of thyroxine and thyroid-stimulating hormone: to rule out thyrotoxicosis.

- Glycosuria alone and blood strip readings are never diagnostic.

Complications
- Complications are often present at the time of diagnosis (after years of hyperglycaemia).

Diabetic retinopathy: may be present at diagnosis, only affects vision if near macula; macular oedema frequent with major reduction of visual acuity; proliferative affects fewer but threatens vision by vitreous haemorrhage/fibrosis; both treated by laser.

Diabetic nephropathy: less common than in insulin-dependent diabetes mellitus, except in non-white races; proteinuria is marker for high cardiovascular risk, but not necessarily progressive renal impairment; can be slowed by vigorous antihypertensive treatment; end-stage failure can be treated by continuous ambulatory peritoneal dialysis or transplantation.

Diabetic neuropathy: many forms, most common being symmetrical sensory polyneuropathy leading to loss of temperature, vibration, and pain sense, hence easy progression to foot ulceration.

Large-vessel disease (coronary, cerebrovascular, peripheral): much more common especially when patient has nephropathy; possibly more diffuse than non-diabetic large-vessel disease, but otherwise generally similar; these, especially coronary artery disease, are major causes of premature death.

Differential diagnosis
- Diagnosis is not usually a problem, after diabetes mellitus has been thought of; possible errors include the following:

Urinary tract infection.

Prostatic hyperplasia.

Vaginal prolapse.

Aetiology
- The cause of non-insulin-dependent diabetes mellitus is unknown; the disorder may be part of a constellation with hypertension and hyperlipidaemia (Reaven's syndrome, syndrome X).
- Patients may have a mixture of 'relative' insulin deficiency and insulin resistance, contributions of the two varying widely between individuals.
- Very rarely, patients have insulin receptor abnormalities.
- A strong familial component is evident, but the disorder is not directly inherited.
- A marked link with obesity is seen.

Epidemiology
- The prevalence varies widely between races, some populations having a prevalence of >50% by the age of 50 years.
- The UK prevalence is 1–2%, rising rapidly with age.
- The disease is six times more common in Asians, about twice as common in Afro-Carribeans.
- It is probably becoming more common in the developed world.

Treatment

Diet and lifestyle
- The diet should be high in unrefined carbohydrate, low in simple sugars, with high fibre and low fat, spread throughout the day.
- Patients should aim to reduce excess body weight.
- Patients should engage in physical exercise and resume full activities; minimal limitations for those on some drugs include not driving goods vehicles, buses, etc.

Pharmacological treatment
- Diet alone should be used initially unless the patient is losing too much weight or is seriously symptomatic, in which case diet should be supplemented by pharmacological treatment.

Sulphonylureas
- These increase insulin response to glucose and tend to cause weight gain.

Standard dosage	Glibenclamide 1.25–15 mg orally daily. Gliclazide 40–320 mg orally daily. Glipizide 2.5–20 mg orally daily.
Contraindications	Breast-feeding, porphyria, pregnancy; caution in elderly patients and those with renal or hepatic failure (glibenclamide contraindicated).
Special points	Used only in conjunction with a diet.
Main drug interactions	Few of major clinical relevance (*see drug data sheet*).
Main side effects	Hypoglycaemia is common; otherwise occasional rashes, jaundice, headache.

Biguanide
- Metformin reduces hepatic gluconeogenesis and probably decreases carbohydrate absorption.

Standard dosage	Metformin 1–2.5 g daily in divided doses.
Contraindications	Hepatic or renal impairment, heart failure, pregnancy.
Special points	Does not cause hypoglycaemia; may rarely cause lactic acidosis.
Main drug interactions	Alcohol-dependence may predispose to lactic acidosis.
Main side effects	Flatulence, anorexia, diarrhoea, sometimes transient.

Insulin
- Insulin is indicated for symptomatic or uncontrolled diabetes mellitus despite maximal oral agents, in addition to diet.
- Usually, it is needed only once or twice daily; a longer-acting formulation may be used to control basal hyperglycaemia.

See Diabetes mellitus, insulin-dependent *for details*.

Other options
Guar gum 5 g 3 times daily: slows absorption of food; poorly tolerated.

Acarbose 50 mg 3 times daily (alpha-glucosidase inhibitor): decreases rate of glucose absorption, thereby reducing postprandial glycaemia; recent introduction.

Treatment aims
To restore normal well-being.
To achieve optimal glycaemic control without significant hypoglycaemia.
To provide patient education and self-care.
To prevent complications.

Prognosis
- Mortality is increased as a result of excess cardiovascular disease, myocardial infarction, stroke, and peripheral vascular disease.
- Morbidity is due to the same causes and also to retinopathy, renal disease, and foot ulceration.
- Oral hypoglycaemics have not been proved to reduce mortality or morbidity.

Follow-up and management
- Patients need long-term follow-up for treatment aims and screening for development of complications.
- Glycosylated haemoglobin is an objective marker of glycaemic control.

Patient support
British Diabetic Association, 10 Queen Anne St, London W1M 0BD; tel 0171 323 1531.

Key references
Day JF: *The Diabetes Handbook: Non Insulin-Dependent Diabetes.* London: Thorsons, British Diabetic Association, 1992.
Tattersall RB, Gale EAM (eds): *Diabetes: Clinical Management.* Edinburgh: Churchill Livingstone, 1990.

Diabetic management in children — C. Lowy

Diagnosis

Symptoms
- Children may not admit to any symptoms until very late.

Thirst: including unusual forms, e.g. drinking bath water.

Polyuria: bed wetting.

Weight loss.

Decreased appetite.

Vomiting: possibly with abdominal pain.

Confusion: without coma.

Signs

Uncomplicated
Misery, irritability.
Dehydration.

Complicated
Semi-coma.
Deep but rapid respiration: Kussmaul respiration.
Hypotension.
Infection: in ear, throat, lung, urinary tract.

Investigations
- The urine must always be tested for glucose in a sick child with some of the above symptoms or signs, even if atypical.

Urinalysis: urine should contain 2% glucose, maximum ketones read on text strip, should be cultured to exclude infection.

Blood glucose and plasma sodium, potassium, bicarbonate, and urea measurement: glucose >20 mmol/L, sodium usually within normal range, potassium low, normal, or high (value governs i.v. replacement), bicarbonate low.

Blood pH, oxygen, carbon dioxide, acid–base status analysis: arterial pH <7.3, oxygen normal, carbon dioxide low.

Blood culture: to identify septicaemia and responsible organism.

Chest radiography: to identify consolidation due to pneumonia.

Complications

Hypovolaemia, circulatory failure, cardiac arrest.

Disequilibrium, with cerebral oedema: caused by over-rapid reversal of high hyperglycaemia or electrolyte imbalance.

Hypokalaemia or hyperkalaemia: due to inappropriate i.v. potassium replacement.

Hypoglycaemia: due to insulin treatment.

Retinopathy, nephropathy and associated hypertension, neuropathy: long-term complications unusual in childhood.

Differential diagnosis

Newly diagnosed child
Any condition manifest by nausea and vomiting.
Any condition manifest by polyuria.
Any condition manifest by coma.

Previously diagnosed child
Uncontrolled diabetes mellitus due to intercurrent infection.
Coma due to hypoglycaemia.

Aetiology
- Causes include the following:

Failure of insulin production and secretion due to lymphocytic infiltration and destruction of beta cells of the islets of langerhans of the pancreas.

Particular HLA phenotypes (HLA DQ8 and DQ2) and circulating compliment-fixing antibodies to islet tissue and antibodies to insulin itself.

Epidemiology
- ~1–2 in 1000 children in Europe have diabetes mellitus, with higher incidences reported from northern European countries.

Treatment

Diet and lifestyle

- Refined carbohydrates must be avoided.
- Diet must be well balanced, with 50% carbohydrates (100 g plus 10 g for each year of childhood life), no high-saturated fats, vegetable oils used for cooking, and high-fibre food (whole-wheat bread, baked beans).
- Meals should be regular, with snacks between main meals and at bedtime.
- No restrictions should be placed on children, but bouts of physical exercise may require additional carbohydrate intake. Hypoglycaemia is particularly dangerous during activities in which children are exposed to cold because their thermal regulation fails and hypothermia may occur; this is a major problem, especially in small children. Glucose in the form of Dextrosol or Lucozade must be carried by a child or an accompanying adult. Parents should be taught to give glucagon, given when a hypoglycaemic child cannot take oral glucose.

Pharmacological treatment

- Oral agents have no place in the management of childhood-onset insulin-dependent diabetes mellitus.
- Insulin is injected before meals, usually twice daily before breakfast and the evening meal, using a mixture of short- and intermediate-acting insulins.
- In small children, this may present a problem because of their sleep patterns. The evening injection can be divided so that the soluble insulin is given before the evening meal and intermediate-acting insulin later in the evening; this can be given while the child is asleep.
- Insulin-containing pens have been produced containing both short- and intermediate-acting insulin.
- Regimens can be altered so that insulin is injected before each meal and intermediate-acting insulin at bedtime, the latter to provide sufficient insulin during the resting period.

Standard dosage	Insulin 0.5–1 unit/kg daily, adjusted according to blood glucose concentration.
Contraindications	Very rare hypersensitivity (usually due to preservatives in insulin preparation).
Special points	Home blood glucose monitoring essential if hyper- and hypoglycaemia is to be avoided.
Main drug interactions	High-dose beta agonists cause severe insulin resistance.
Main side effects	Hyper- or hypoglycaemia due to inappropriate dosing.

- Insulin can also be given by continuous infusions (subcutaneous or implanted intraperitoneal) using pumps.

Treatment aims

To return child to health.
To achieve glycaemic control.

Prognosis

- Childhood-onset diabetes mellitus is associated with significant complications.
- Life expectancy is reduced by one-third, although this is rapidly improving.

Follow-up and management

- Regular attendance at a combined paediatric and diabetic clinic is vital to monitor growth, provide advice on diet as child gets older, monitor long-term glycaemic control, and check for complications.
- Management at presentation requires the following:

With hyperglycaemia and ketonuria but no vomiting, outpatient management (fluids not needed).
Frequent visits to specialist diabetic unit or frequent visits of staff of the centre to the child's home.
Adjustment of dose of insulin on the basis of blood glucose values.
Two or more s.c. insulin injections and change in diet.
With vomiting, hospital admission for i.v. rehydration, insulin treatment, and identification of immediate cause of diabetic ketoacidosis.
Depending on age, education of child about the diabetic process and basic physiology of glucose homeostasis by a skilled member of the diabetic team, usually a specialist nurse.
Education of parents about their child's disease and its control (treatment of hyperglycaemia, hypoglycaemia, alteration of diet for physical activities, holidays).
Counselling to enable parents to come to terms with their child's life-long disability.

Key references

Diabetes Control and Complication Trial Group: The effect of intensive treatment of diabetes on the development and progression of longterm complications in insulin dependent diabetes. *N Engl J Med* 1993, **329**:977–986.

Kostraba JN et al.: Increasing trend of outpatient management of children with newly diagnosed IDDM. *Diabetes Care* 1992, **15**:95–100.

Sonksen P, Fox C, Judd S: *Diabetes at your Fingertips* vol 7. 1991, pp 166–179.

Diabetic management in pregnancy
D.J.B Thomas

Diagnosis

Symptoms and signs
- Diabetes may already be present or may be manifest for the first time in pregnancy; some patients remain insulin-dependent after pregnancy, whereas, in others, the diabetes disappears after pregnancy (gestational diabetes mellitus).
- Patients present with the usual symptoms and signs of pregnancy and possibly of diabetes mellitus; women with gestational diabetes mellitus, however, are usually asymptomatic, the diabetes being detected by screening (most effective at 28 weeks).

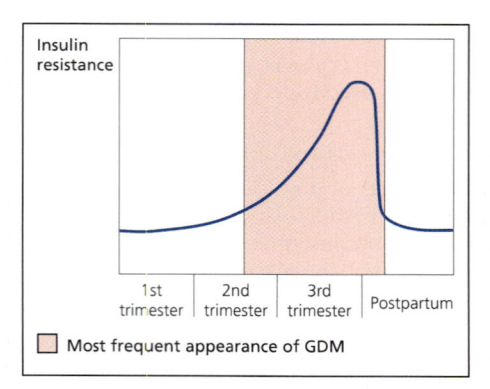

Increase of insulin resistance and the appearance of gestational diabetes mellitus (GDM).

Investigations
- All women suspected of having gestational diabetes mellitus should be screened.
- If fasting blood glucose is >5 mmol/L or random blood glucose is >7 mmol/L, a glucose tolerance test should be considered.
- All pregnant women should be screened at 28 weeks; high-risk women should have a fasting blood sugar assessment 3-weekly.

Blood glucose measurement: 2–6 times daily; targets are 3–5 mmol/L before meals, <9 mmol/L after meals.

U&E and creatinine analysis, full blood count: to assess renal function and anaemia.

Urinalysis: for protein, microalbumin; possibly 24-h for measurement of protein and creatinine clearance; haemoglobin A_{1c} should be kept in normal range.

Ultrasonography: at 17–19 weeks for fetal size and to check for malformations; possibly serial ultrasonography of biparietal diameter and abdominal circumference.

Fetal lung maturity measurement: to predict respiratory distress syndrome; lecithin:sphingomyelin ratio may be spuriously high in diabetic patients; low phosphatidyl choline or glycerol concentrations may be better predictors.

- When discrepancies are found between blood monitoring results and haemoglobin A_{1c}, the technique must be checked (meter device more reliable), results checked for falsification, and haemoglobinopathy, splenectomy, and gross anaemia considered.

Complications

Maternal
Worsening retinopathy, nephropathy.
Increased pre-eclamptic toxaemia.
Hydramnios.
Ketosis, hyperglycaemia.
Death.

Fetal
Respiratory distress, jaundice, macrosomia.
Hypoglycaemia.
Hypocalcaemia.
Polycythaemia.
Microcephaly, sacral agenesis.
Congenital malformations.
Congenital heart disease.

Differential diagnosis
Not applicable.

Aetiology

Causes of gestational diabetes (increased insulin resistance)
Increased concentrations of progesterone, cortisol, prolactin, and human placental lactogen, which also influence post-receptor metabolism.
Poorly understood immunological processes, which increase insulin need two- to threefold during pregnancy.

Risk factors for gestational diabetes mellitus
Previous gestational diabetes.
First-degree relative with diabetes.
Fasting glycosuria.
Previous unexplained fetal death.
Previous 'large for dates' baby.
Previous malformed baby.
Maternal obesity.
Hydramnios, macrosomia.

Epidemiology
- Diabetes mellitus occurs in 1–2% of the UK population.
- Gestational diabetes mellitus develops in 1–2% of pregnancies, depending on the diagnostic criteria.

Pregnancy counselling
- Diabetic women must be advised of the following:
- The risk of death is slightly higher than in non-diabetic women.
- Complications, e.g. retinopathy, nephropathy, and heart disease, may worsen in pregnancy.
- Caesarean section is more probable.
- Numerous antenatal visits and close supervision will be needed.
- Home blood glucose monitoring will be needed several times daily.
- Two or more insulin injections will be needed daily.
- Diet must be adhered to, and smoking and drinking must be stopped.
- The baby will be at increased risk of death, malformations, and serious neonatal complications.
- Risks are, however, minimized by close supervision and cooperation.

Treatment

Diet and lifestyle
- Known diabetic patients should already have consulted a dietitian; those with gestational diabetes must be referred.
- Patients must ensure that 50% of energy intake is carbohydrate and that their diet contains adequate calcium and vitamins.
- Iron and folate supplements are needed.
- Patients should aim to achieve the normal weight gain in pregnancy (average, 10 kg) by appropriate food intake; energy intake should be restricted to 6300–7560 kJ (1500–1800 kcal) daily in some overweight pregnant women.

Pharmacological treatment

During pregnancy
- All patients on oral agents should be transferred to insulin, usually given 2–4 times daily, occasionally more often; a mixture of short- and intermediate-acting insulin can be used depending on patient needs, or a late dose of intermediate-acting insulin before bed and short-acting insulin before meals.
- Two-thirds of patients with gestational diabetes mellitus may be treated by dietary advice; the remaining one-third need insulin, which can be given as a mixture of short- and intermediate-acting insulin twice daily, with possible supplement of short-acting insulin before lunch.
- Insulin needs increase during pregnancy; >100 units may be required; the need falls late in third trimester, dramatically after labour.

During labour and delivery
- 1–4 units of insulin are needed hourly.
- Blood glucose must be maintained at near-normal concentrations (monitoring needed at least hourly).
- In prolonged labour or in high-risk patients, an independent energy source, e.g. 10% dextrose 100 ml i.v. hourly is needed.
- Insulin can be delivered separately by a syringe driver (short-acting insulin 50 units in 50 ml normal saline solution).
- Beta agonists used for premature labour may cause insulin resistance.
- General anaesthesia and caesarean section increase insulin needs.
- After delivery, insulin needs fall dramatically.
- Patients with gestational diabetes mellitus do not need further insulin treatment but may need medical review.

Treatment aims
To maintain preprandial blood glucose at 3.5–5 mmol/L, postprandial blood glucose <9 mmol/L, and haemoglobin A_{1c} in normal range.
To achieve a mature fetus, born after 38 weeks by vaginal delivery, with no neonatal complications.

Prognosis
- Retinopathy and nephropathy can deteriorate during pregnancy but can be minimized by good metabolic control and supervision.
- Perinatal mortality is still increased in diabetic pregnancies; half of the increase is associated with poor control.
- Maternal mortality is slightly higher than in non-diabetic patients.

Follow-up and management

Initial assessment
- Patients are best seen in joint clinic with a diabetologist and an obstetrician.
- Patients should be screened for diabetic complications; visual acuity, fundal examination with dilated pupils, and assessment of renal function are important.
- Blood pressure must be monitored regularly.

Subsequent assessment
- Follow-up should be every 1–4 weeks, depending on the patient's need.
- Patients should be encouraged to change their insulin regimen to attain good metabolic control.

Key references

Dornhorst A: Implications of gestational diabetes for the health of the mother. *Br J Obstet Gynaecol* 1994, **101**:286–290.

Hellmuth E, Damm P, Molsted-Pedersen L: Congenital malformations in offspring of diabetic women treated with oral hypoglycaemic agents during pregnancy. *Diabetic Med* 1994, **11**:471–474.

Lowy C: Pregnancy and diabetes mellitus. In *Textbook of Diabetes*. Edited by Pickup J, Williams G. Oxford: Blackwell Scientific Publications, 1991, pp 835–850.

Nelson Piercy C, Gale EAM: Do we know how to screen for gestational diabetes? Current practice in one regional health authority. *Diabetic Med* 1994, **11**:493–498.

Diabetic management in surgery — D.J.B. Thomas

Diagnosis

Symptoms
- Well controlled diabetic patients having an operation have no symptoms.

Thirst and polyuria: indicating poor control in patients with any type of diabetes.

Nausea and abdominal pain: indicating very poor control in insulin-dependent patients.

Signs
Tachycardia, ketosis, dehydration, hypotension: signs of poor diabetic control in insulin-dependent patients; these will most probably develop after the operation if preoperative control of diabetes was poor.

Investigations

For elective surgery
Blood glucose profile: 2 days before patient has a major operation; haemoglobin A_{1c} should be within 10% of normal range.

- Other investigations are the same as for non-diabetic patients.

For emergency surgery
Blood glucose measurement: to assess hyperglycaemia.

U&E analysis: to assess renal function and electrolyte balance.

Blood gas analysis: to assess acid–base balance.

Complications
Cardiovascular problems: particularly myocardial infarction; the main perioperative causes of death in diabetic patients.

Infection and poor wound healing: in poorly controlled diabetic patients.

Differential diagnosis
- Acute surgical abdominal disorders can be confused with severely decompensated diabetes in insulin-dependent patients: a medical opinion is essential.

Aetiology
- The stress response to surgery and anaesthesia is characterized by hyperglycaemia, suppression of insulin release, and insulin resistance.
- This is due to increases in cortisol, catecholamines, and other counterregulatory hormones.
- The stress response is greater with major surgery.

Epidemiology
- 50% of diabetic patients have operations at some point in their lives.
- Patients with macrovascular disease will probably have several operations.

Treatment

Diet and lifestyle
- Major operations are often followed by a period of relative or absolute starvation: adequate energy intake and insulin must be supplied to diabetic patients because insulin depletion leads to severe catabolic disorders.
- Breakfast and oral agents are omitted if the operation is in the morning.
- If the operation is minor, eating and oral agents can soon be restarted.

Pharmacological treatment
- Patients with 'brittle' diabetes may need a glucose insulin infusion for 24 h before surgery.
- Regional anaesthesia does not produce the same degree of stress response as general anaesthesia.
- Infections should be treated aggressively by intravenous antibiotics.

For non-insulin-dependent diabetes: preoperative
- Metformin, which may cause lactic acidosis, and chlorpropamide, because its long action may lead to hypoglycaemia, should be avoided.
- Patients should be given shorter-acting sulphonylureas instead, e.g. glibenclamide 1.25–15 mg daily or gliclazide 40–360 mg daily.
- Blood glucose concentration must be monitored.
- The main side effect is hypoglycaemia.

For non-insulin-dependent diabetes: perioperative
- Intravenous solutions containing glucose should be avoided unless hypoglycaemia is a risk.
- If the operation is major, treatment should be the same as for insulin-dependent diabetes until the stress response of surgery is finished.

For insulin-dependent diabetes: preoperative
- Preoperative admission for stabilization may be needed to achieve a blood glucose concentration of 6–10 mmol/L.
- If control is good, the insulin regimen need not be changed until the day of surgery; if control is poor before a meal, short-acting insulin achieves rapid metabolic control.
- Blood glucose concentration must be monitored.
- The main side effect is hypoglycaemia.

For insulin-dependent diabetes: perioperative
Short-acting insulin 50 units in 50 ml normal saline solution with a syringe driver; 500 ml 10% dextrose with 10 mmol potassium chloride through a separate infusion pump infused 5-hourly.
- Blood glucose concentration must be maintained at 6–10 mmol/L; 1–4 units of insulin may be needed hourly via a syringe driver.

Alternatively, glucose–potassium–insulin infusion: 10% dextrose 500 ml with potassium chloride 10 mmol and short-acting insulin 15 units infused as a mixture 5-hourly.
- Premixed insulins are unsuitable when insulin need changes rapidly.
- If blood glucose is >11 mmol/L, 20 units insulin should be added; if blood glucose is <6 mmol/L, 10 units should be added; other parameters should not be changed.
- The insulin infusion must be continued until the patient's first meal, when s.c. insulin should be started immediately; insulin needs will probably be higher than usual.

Treatment aims
To maintain blood glucose at 6–10 mmol/L during the operation.

Prognosis
- Mortality should be similar to that in non-diabetic patients.

Follow-up and management
- Blood glucose should be monitored 3–4 times daily before the operation.
- During and early after an operation, blood glucose should be monitored at least hourly.
- Urea and electrolytes should be measured daily, and any deficiencies replaced.

Timing of surgery
- Routine surgery should be postponed in newly diagnosed diabetic patients until good control is attained.
- Acute surgical conditions may lead to ketoacidosis; if possible, surgery should be delayed until metabolic control is achieved.
- Surgery should be done in the morning if possible.

Special situations

Cardiac surgery
- Hypothermic bypass surgery with pump priming and inotropic drugs leads to marked insulin resistance and much higher insulin needs.
- The rapidly changing insulin need makes a separate infusion line for insulin essential.

Pregnancy
- Control of diabetes during caesarean section is critical for mother and fetus.

Key references
Clark JDA, Currie J, Hartog M: Management of diabetes in surgery: a survey of current practice by anaesthetists. *Diabetic Med* 1992, **9**:271–274.

Gill GV: Surgery and diabetes mellitus. In *Textbook of Diabetes* vol 2. Edited by Pickup J, Williams G. Oxford: Blackwell Scientific Publications, 1991, pp 820–825.

Sawyer RG, Pruett TL: Wound infections. *Surg Clin North Am* 1994, **74**:523–524.

Smith EA, Kilpatrick ES: Intra-operative blood glucose measurements. *Anaesthesia* 1994, **49**:129–132.

Female hypergonadotrophic hypogonadism
R. Fox and D. Cahill

Diagnosis

Symptoms
Primary or secondary amenorrhoea: erratic menstruation or oligomenorrhoea in earliest phases.

Delayed puberty.

Infertility.

Hot flushes, vaginal dryness and dyspareunia, thin skin, and scalp hair loss: symptoms of oestrogen deficiency.

Signs
- Few signs are manifest, particularly shortly after onset of amenorrhoea.

Incomplete pubertal maturation: indicating primary amenorrhoea.

Atrophic vaginal mucosa.

Features of Turner's syndrome: short stature, webbed neck.

Investigations

For the disorder
Serum follicle-stimulating hormone (FSH) measurement: persistently raised concentration (>25 IU/L); in women with possible incipient ovarian failure (erratic cycles and moderately raised serum FSH [10–25 IU/L]), care must be taken to ensure sampling was not done during a pre-ovulatory gonadotrophin surge (risk of false-positive results).

Progestogen challenge test: negative, indicating oestrogen deficiency; determination of oestrogen state (of the endometrium) helps to screen for other causes of raised FSH concentration; no value for measuring oestradiol.

For the underlying cause
Autoimmune profile: including anti-ovarian antibodies.

Chromosome analysis: to check for aneuploidy (45XO, 47XXX, 46XY).

Laparoscopy: if streak ovaries seen, possibility of conception is ruled out; if ovaries 'normal', biopsy unhelpful; conception has been recorded in women with no follicles at histology.

For assessment of bone state
Radiography for bone age: if delayed in girls with primary amenorrhoea, ultralow-dose oestrogen should be used to achieve maximum height (ethinyloestradiol 2 µg daily).

Bone densiometry: no clinical value.

Complications
Infertility: almost all women affected are sterile.

Unwanted pregnancy: fertility returns unexpectedly in a small proportion of women.

Osteoporosis or atraumatic fractures: resulting from oestrogen deficiency.

Cardiovascular disease: effect of oestrogen deficiency on lipid state.

Gonadal neoplasia: in women with gonadal dysgenesis and 46XY karyotype.

Differential diagnosis
- Gonadotrophin-secreting pituitary adenomas are rare; the distinguishing feature is oestrogenization.

Spurious elevation of follicle-stimulating hormone.

Resistant ovary syndrome.

Aetiology
- Causes include the following:

Gonadal dysgenesis: e.g. Turner's syndrome, pure gonadal dysgenesis.

Autoimmune: anti-ovarian antibodies.

Infection: mumps.

Irradiation or chemotherapy.

Extensive ovarian surgery: for endometriosis or recurrent cysts.

Idiopathic premature menopause.

Resistant ovary syndrome.

Treated galactosaemia.

17α-hydroxylase deficiency.

Epidemiology
- The lifetime risk (before 40 years) is 0.6%.
- ~5% of cases of anovulation, 10% of amenorrhoea, and 2% of oligomenorrhoea are due to hypergonadotrophic hypogonadism.

Treatment

Diet and lifestyle
- Advice about increasing dietary calcium and the risk of atraumatic fractures should be given to women with long-standing untreated amenorrhoea.
- Women not wishing to conceive should be warned of the small risk of conception.

Pharmacological treatment
- Sex-steroid therapy alleviates symptoms of oestrogen deficiency and prevents osteoporosis and cardiovascular disease.
- Oestrogen is the active agent; progestogens are used to prevent endometrial neoplasia.
- Standard hormone replacement preparations are not contraceptive; women who wish to avoid the small risk of conception should use low-dose combined oral contraceptive (ethinyloestradiol 20 µg, desogestrel 150 µg).

Standard dosage	Depends on patient's needs.
Contraindications	Undiagnosed abnormal menstruation.
Special points	*Transdermal oestradiol patches:* poor absorption in young women because of thick skin. *Subcutaneous oestradiol implants:* long duration of oestradiol release (up to 36 months); should be avoided in women who may request ovum donation. *Progestogens:* third-generation agent should be used to avoid deleterious effect on lipids.
Main drug interactions	Anticonvulsants, warfarin.
Main side effects	*Oestrogen:* nausea (avoided by slow introduction). *Progestogen:* premenstrual symptoms.

Treatment aims
To avoid general health risks.
To achieve conception.

Other treatments

Laparoscopic gonadectomy
- If gonads are found on laparoscopy of the internal genitalia, they should be removed laparascopically.
- If streak gonads only are found, no further action is needed.
- If gonads are not evident, the inguinal canal should be explored.

For infertility
- Hypergonadotrophic hypogonadism represents end-organ failure for which the chances of resumption of ovulation (spontaneous or induced) are small and difficult to predict.
- Several methods of inducing ovulation have been described, but, for most women, in-vitro fertilization with donated oocytes offers the only realistic chance of a pregnancy.
- Fostering, adoption, and surrogacy can also be considered.

Prognosis
- The results from one trial of oestrogen and human menopausal gonadotrophin treatment in 91 women with hypergonadotrophic amenorrhoea are as follows:
34 patients ovulated.
19 conceptions.
10 miscarriages (53% of conceptions).
1 stillbirth.
8 viable births.

Follow-up and management
- Yearly review is necessary to ensure compliance with hormone replacement therapy.

Key references
Check JH *et al.*: Ovulation induction and pregnancies in 100 consecutive women with hypergonadotrophic amenorrhoea. *Fertil Steril* 1990, **53**:811–817.

Davies MC *et al.*: Bone mineral loss in young women with amenorrhoea. *BMJ* 1990, **301**:790–793.

Rebar RW *et al.*: Clinical features of young women with hypergonadotrophic amenorrhoea. *Fertil Steril* 1990, **53**:804–810.

Female hypogonadotrophic hypogonadism
R. Fox and D. Cahill

Diagnosis

Symptoms
Primary or secondary amenorrhoea: oligomenorrhoea less often.
Delayed puberty: short stature.
Infertility.
Headaches and visual disturbance: indicating pituitary tumours.
Vaginal dryness, thin skin, and scalp hair loss: symptoms of oestrogen deficiency.
Eating disorders and weight-loss: often hidden from family and carers.

Signs
- Usually few signs are manifest, particularly shortly after onset of amenorrhoea.

Incomplete pubertal maturation: indicating primary amenorrhoea.
Low body-mass index: <19 kg/m² in eating disorders.
Galactorrhoea: in hyperprolactinaemia.
Anosmia: Kallmann syndrome.
Visual impairment: indicating pituitary tumours.
Atrophic vaginal mucosa.

Investigations

For the disorder
Serum follicle-stimulating hormone measurement: concentration not raised (<10 IU/L).
Progestogen challenge test: medroxyprogesterone acetate 5 mg daily for 5 days, followed by assessment of menstrual response for 7 days; bleeding indicates oestrogenization, no bleeding indicates oestrogen deficiency.
Ovarian ultrasonography: small inactive or multifollicular ovaries; occasionally, by coincidence, polycystic ovaries are found (pre-existing polycystic ovarian disease overridden by hypothalamo-pituitary failure).

For the underlying cause
Serum prolactin measurement: concentration persistently >1000 mU/L indicates hyperprolactinaemia.
Thyroid function tests: primary hypothyroidism is a cause of hyperprolactinaemia.
MRI: to define suspected hypothalamic or pituitary tumour.

For complications
Thyroid stimulating hormone measurement: to screen for panhypopituitarism.
Full pituitary testing: if low thyroid stimulating hormone, history of pituitary surgery or radiotherapy, or suspicion of pituitary or hypothalamic tumour.
Radiography for bone age: if delayed in girls with primary amenorrhoea, low-dose oestrogen hormone replacement therapy may be used to try to achieve maximum height potential (ethinyloestradiol 2 µg daily).
Bone densiometry: no clinical value.

Complications
Anovulatory infertility.
Unwanted pregnancy: resumption of ovulation common in hypothalamic disorders.
Osteoporosis, cardiovascular disease: long-term health risks resulting from oestrogen deficiency.
Compression of optic chiasma: rare.
Panhypopituitarism: rare.

Differential diagnosis
Uterine malformation (cryptomenorrhoea) or atresia.
Aschermann syndrome (uterine synechiae).

Aetiology
- Causes include the following:

Hypothalamic
Weight loss, psychological stress, exercise.
Tumours (craniopharyngioma).
Kallmann syndrome (anosmia/isolated gonadotrophin-releasing hormone deficiency).
Hyperprolactinaemia: anovulation mediated through hypothalamus.
Idiopathic hypothalamic dysfunction.

Pituitary
Prolactin-secreting macroadenomas.
Nonfunctioning pituitary tumours.
Surgery and radiotherapy.
Sheehan's syndrome (postpartum infarction).
Granulomas.

Hyperprolactinaemia
Pregnancy and lactation.
Drugs.
Primary hypothyroidism.
Hypothalamic disease.
Pressure on or section of pituitary stalk.
Prolactin-secreting pituitary adenomas.
See Hyperprolactinaemia for further details.

Epidemiology
- ~40% of cases of anovulation, 55% of amenorrhoea, and 6% of oligomenorrhoea are due to hypogonadotrophic hypogonadism.

Treatment

Diet and lifestyle
- Weight gain (supervised by dietitians and psychologists) is the most appropriate treatment for amenorrhoea associated with weight loss; ovulation may be restored.
- Vitamin D and calcium supplementation are needed in patients with anorexia.
- Advice about the risk of atraumatic fractures should be given to women with long-standing untreated amenorrhoea.

Pharmacological treatment

For hormone replacement (not hyperprolactinaemia)
- Sex-steroid therapy alleviates symptoms of oestrogen deficiency and prevents osteoporosis and cardiovascular disease.
- Oestrogen is the active agent; progestogens are used to prevent endometrial neoplasia.
- Standard hormone replacement preparations are not contraceptive; women who wish to avoid the small risk of conception should use low-dose combined oral contraceptive (ethinyloestradiol 20 µg, desogestrel 150 µg).

Standard dosage	Depends on patient's needs.
Contraindications	Undiagnosed abnormal menstruation.
Special points	*Transdermal oestradiol patches:* poor absorption in young women because of thick skin. *Subcutaneous oestradiol implants:* long duration of oestradiol release (up to 36 months); should be avoided in women who may request ovulation induction. *Progestogens:* third-generation agent should be used to avoid deleterious effect on lipids.
Main drug interactions	Anticonvulsants, warfarin.
Main side effects	*Oestrogen:* nausea (avoided by slow introduction). *Progestogen:* premenstrual symptoms.

For infertility (not hyperprolactinaemia)
- Serious causes (e.g. anorexia nervosa) must be treated first.
- Pregnancy must be ruled out before treatment is initiated.

For hypothalamic dysfunction: anti-oestrogen, pulsatile luteinizing-hormone releasing hormone, exogenous gonadotrophins are tried in turn.

For pituitary causes: exogenous gonadotrophins.

See Polycystic ovarian disease *for further details.*

For hyperprolactinaemia
Associated with primary hypothyroidism: thyroxine.

Associated with prolactinergic drugs: possible removal of drugs.

Associated with prolactinoma: dopamine agonists to reduce tumour size and restore ovulation; surgery and radiotherapy needed rarely for some macroadenomas.

If fertility not required: standard hormone replacement treatment, with low-dose dopamine agonist to prevent tumour expansion.

If fertility required: dopamine agonist to induce ovulation; alternatively, pulsatile luteinizing-hormone releasing hormone or exogenous gonadotrophin.

See Hyperprolactinaemia *for further details.*

Treatment aims
To alleviate underlying causes.
To prevent long-term health risks.
To achieve pregnancy.

Prognosis
- Eating disorders are difficult to control, and patients frequently relapse; sudden death is a risk, perhaps due to arrhythmias.
- Normal conception rates can be achieved for most of the common causes.
- The outcome of pregnancy is poor for underweight women.

Follow-up and management
- Most prolactinomas are <5 mm within 8 weeks of the start of dopamine agonist treatment.
- Prolactin concentration must be measured 6-monthly.
- Previously large prolactinomas may re-expand in pregnancy; visual fields must be checked.

Key references
Abraham S *et al.*: Should ovulation be induced in women recovering from an eating disorder or who are compulsive exercisers? *Fertil Steril* 1990, **53**:566–568.

Gulekli B *et al.*: Effect of treatment on established osteoporosis in young women with amenorrhoea. *Clin Endocrin* 1994, **41**:275–281.

Patton G *et al.*: The course of anorexia nervosa. *BMJ* 1989, **299**:139–140.

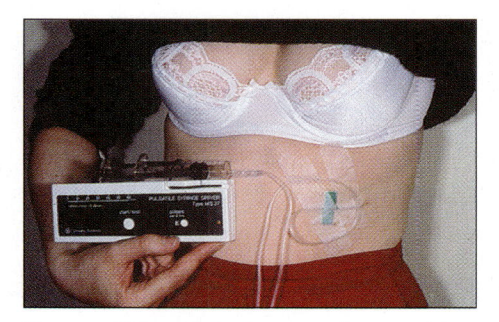

Woman with hypothalamic amenorrhoea receiving pulsatile luteinizing-hormone releasing hormone subcutaneously from battery-driven pump.

Growth abnormalities, short stature — C.G.D. Brook

Diagnosis

Symptoms
- Patients present with short stature at all ages.

Height less than the third height centile or short for family.

Delayed puberty: in patients short for a reason.

Signs
- Signs are not always manifest.
- Features of hypothyroidism with goitre may be seen.

Disproportionate growth: e.g. short legs.

Dysmorphic features: e.g. in Turner's syndrome, intrauterine growth retardation.

Investigations

Anthropometry: height of child should be recorded on two occasions separated by at least 3 months to calculate annual growth rate; assessments of nutrition (weight, skinfold thickness) helpful; Tanner stages of puberty must be elicited; heights of parents should be measured; short person growing at normal rate for age and stage of puberty may need explanation of how shortness arose (e.g. low birth weight).

Radiography: to assess skeletal maturity (bone age) as guide to long-term outlook; skeletal survey needed for disproportionate short stature and for children with height prediction small for family, who may have occult skeletal dysplasia.

Haematology: to identify anaemia (vitamin B_{12}, folate, ferritin malabsorption).

ESR measurement: to exclude inflammatory disease.

Chemical pathology: U&E analysis, measurement of calcium to exclude metabolic disease; measurement of thyroxine, gonadotrophins, and prolactin in short children of pubertal age showing no or few signs of puberty; measurement of growth hormone secretion for short children growing slowly for otherwise unexplained reasons.

Karyotyping: XO in Turner's syndrome.

Complications
Premature fusion of epiphyses: through injudicious treatment.

Differential diagnosis
Not applicable.

Aetiology
- All disease in childhood causes a decrease in growth velocity that ultimately becomes manifest as short stature.
- The following may play a role:

Nutritional disorders: in infants.

Diminished growth hormone secretion: in the absence of physical signs in children.

Functional or organic failure of the hypothalamo–pituitary–gonadal axis: at 14 years.

Endocrine condition: in short, fat patients with low growth velocity.

Disease in any body system: in thin patients.

Epidemiology
- Boys with delayed puberty (and its consequent short stature) outnumber girls by 20 to 1.
- Most other conditions have a roughly equal sex distribution.

C.G.D. Brook — Growth abnormalities, short stature

Treatment

Diet and lifestyle
- In infants, adequate nutrition must be promoted, including correction of malabsorption.

Pharmacological treatment
- In childhood, growth hormone is appropriately prescribed to correct insufficiency; at puberty, sex steroids are appropriate first-line treatment.
- Long-term alleviation of short stature is only achievable when an abnormal growth velocity can be corrected; the height of a normal child cannot be increased.

Growth hormone: depends on pretreatment growth rate, condition being treated, and response required; hypopituitary children need 15 units/m² s.c. weekly as daily divided injections; 20 units/m² weekly needed to increase normal pretreatment rate; 30–40 units/m² weekly for children with abnormal skeletons (e.g. in Turner's syndrome).

Thyroxine: 100 μg/m² orally as single daily dose.

Ethinyloestradiol: initially 2 μg daily, increased to 5, 10, 15, 20, and 30 μg daily at 6 monthly intervals; progestogen added when dose of 15 μg achieved or if breakthrough bleeding occurs earlier; contraindicated if family history of thrombotic disorder.

Testosterone: initially 50 mg testosterone esters at 4-weekly intervals, increased to 100 mg every 4 weeks after 6 months; increased to 3-weekly intervals over a further 6 months and then to 2-weekly intervals; causes accelerated fusion of epiphyses.

Treatment aims
To redress abnormal growth.

Prognosis
- The prognosis is not good in patients who are well developed at puberty.
- Treatment of disease promotes catch-up growth, but ultimate stature is determined by the deficit at presentation (height for bone age).
- Pre-existing deficits (low birth weight) or those caused by delay in diagnosis cannot be corrected.

Follow-up and management
- 6-monthly anthropometry is needed to record effects on growth and to readjust doses for increase in size.

Key references
Brook CGD: *A Guide to the Practice of Paediatric Endocrinology.* Cambridge: Cambridge University Press, 1993.

Brook CGD (ed.): *Clinical Paediatric Endocrinology* edn 3. Oxford: Blackwell Scientific Publications, 1995.

Growth abnormalities, tall stature — C.G.D. Brook

Diagnosis

Symptoms
- Symptoms are usually minimal.

Clumsiness or accident-proneness: e.g. because furniture is too small.

Aggression: patients stronger than their peers.

Behaviour disorder: patients trying to show that they are not as old as they seem.

Symptoms of hyperthyroidism: rarely.

Signs
- Tall children usually look normal.

Dysmorphic features.

Signs of early puberty or thyrotoxicosis.

Isolated signs of virilization: pubic hair, acne, cliteromegaly; probably due to adrenal androgen secretion, the cause of which should be investigated.

Joint hypermobility, arachnodactyly, iridonodesis, high arch palate: signs of Marfan syndrome.

Investigations
- Tall stature associated with precocious puberty must be fully investigated in boys; girls with no neurological signs and consonance of pubertal signs with pelvic ultrasonographic findings do not need invasive procedures.

Anthropometry: height of child and both parents should be measured; Tanner stages of puberty should be recorded; measurement of sitting height to determine leg length more helpful than measurement of span.

Radiography: assessment of skeletal maturity enables height prediction; radiographic appearance of iliac apophyses helps to asses potential for spinal growth; skull radiography (at least) for pituitary fossa.

Special tests: measurement of thyroxine and thyroid-stimulating hormone may reveal thyrotoxicosis; low basal concentration of growth hormone excludes gigantism, but proof of this diagnosis requires demonstration of measurable concentrations of growth hormone throughout 24 h, which leads to raised concentration of insulin-like growth factor 1.

Complications
Scoliosis.

Lens dislocation.

Cardiovascular problems.

Osteoarthritis.

Differential diagnosis
Not applicable.

Aetiology
- Causes include the following:

Normal growth rate and appearance
Tall parents.
Obesity of infantile onset.
Marfan, Klinefelter, or Sotos syndrome.

Excessive growth rate
Early puberty.
Androgen secretion (congenital adrenal hyperplasia, adrenal neoplasm, adrenarche).
Thyrotoxicosis.
Growth hormone excess.

Epidemiology
- 1% of the population is tall.

Treatment

Diet and lifestyle
- No special precautions are necessary.

Pharmacological treatment
- Treatment of children for limitation of tall adult stature after puberty has begun is probably a waste of time because insufficient time for manoeuvre is available; tall children should be referred before the age of 8 years.
- Precocious puberty and adrenal, thyroid, and pituitary conditions need appropriate treatment.
- Patients with Klinefelter syndrome and inadequate puberty need androgens to prevent gynaecomastia.
- If excessive height in adulthood is predicted, height can be lost by (early) induction of puberty at a height 30 cm less than that desired.
- If the age at which puberty induction would be needed to limit final stature is extremely low (i.e. the patient is and will be extremely tall), growth hormone secretion can be reduced using somatostatin analogues.

Ethinyloestradiol: initially 2 µg daily, increased to 5, 10, 15, 20, and 30 µg daily at 6 monthly intervals; progestogen added when dose of 15 µg achieved or if breakthrough bleeding occurs earlier; contraindicated if family history of thrombotic disorder.

Testosterone: initially 50 mg testosterone esters at 4-weekly intervals, increased to 100 mg every 4 weeks after 6 months; increased to 3-weekly intervals over a further 6 months and then to 2-weekly intervals; causes accelerated fusion of epiphyses.

Treatment aims
To reduce adult stature.

Prognosis
- The prognosis depends on the diagnosis.

Follow-up and management
- Children with Marfan syndrome need ophthalmological and cardiac opinions.

Key references
Brook CGD (ed): *Clinical Paediatric Endocrinology* edn. 3. Oxford: Blackwell Scientific Publications, 1995.

Hypercalcaemia — D.A. Heath

Diagnosis

Symptoms
- Hypercalcaemia causes either no symptoms or nonspecific symptoms, e.g. the following:

Tiredness and lethargy.

Nausea and vomiting.

Constipation.

Polydipsia and polyuria.

Muscle weakness.

Impaired mental function and occasional loss of consciousness: in severe cases.

Signs
- Specific signs of hypercalcaemia are rare.

Corneal and soft-tissue calcification.

Signs of dehydration: caused by moderate to severe hypercalcaemia.

Investigations
Serum calcium measurement: total serum calcium influenced by serum protein concentration, especially albumin.

Parathyroid hormone measurement: high concentration indicates probable hyperparathyroidism.

Tests for anaemia, liver function tests, alkaline phosphatase and ESR measurement: malignancy more probable if concentrations are abnormal or raised.

Chest and skeletal radiography: indicated if malignancy probable.

- Specific investigations of other causes of hypercalcaemia are indicated when the more common causes have been excluded.

Complications
Dehydration: common and, unless corrected, causes worsening of hypercalcaemia.

Kidney stones: may complicate hyperparathyroidism.

Bone pain: common in malignancy, rare in hyperparathyroidism.

Pancreatitis: rare complication of chronic hypercalcaemia.

Differential diagnosis
Not applicable.

Aetiology
- 97% of cases of hypercalcaemia in general medical practice are due either to primary hyperparathyroidism or to malignancy, which is usually disseminated.
- Other causes include the following:

Severe thyrotoxicosis.

Vitamin D overdose.

Calcium treatment to bind phosphate in chronic renal failure.

Sarcoidosis.

Familial benign or hypocalciuric hypercalcaemia.

Diuretic phase of acute renal failure.

Milk-alkali syndrome.

Epidemiology
- Primary hyperparathyroidism increases markedly after middle age and is three times more common in women than in men.
- Hyperparathyroidism may be a feature of multiple endocrine neoplasia type I or II.
- Many malignancies can be complicated by hypercalcaemia.
- Sarcoidosis is complicated by hypercalcaemia in <1% of patients.

Treatment

Diet and lifestyle
- A low-calcium diet is of no value in treating hypercalcaemia, although high calcium intake exacerbates the disorder.
- Patients with hyperparathyroidism treated conservatively should be advised to maintain an adequate fluid intake, especially when they are unwell.

Pharmacological treatment

For hyperparathyroidism
- The only effective treatment of primary hyperparathyroidism is surgical.

For malignancy
- Intravenous rehydration is mandatory.
- The bisphosphonate drugs are the initial treatment of choice for severe hypercalcaemia.

Standard dosage	*For severe hypercalcaemia:* clodronate 300 mg, palmidronate 30 mg, or etidronate 7.5 mg/kg slow i.v. infusion daily for 3–5 days. Clodronate 800 mg orally twice daily after serum calcium has fallen. *For mild hypercalcaemia:* clodronate 800 mg orally twice daily.
Contraindications	Caution in renal failure.
Special points	Serum calcium falls to or towards normal within 3–5 days. Oral bisphosphonates must be taken on an empty stomach.
Main drug interactions	Absorption of oral drug reduced by antacids, iron, and calcium.
Main side effects	Gastrointestinal upset.

For sarcoidosis
- Hypercalcaemia responds rapidly to steroids.

Standard dosage	Prednisolone 20 mg daily, reduced to lowest dose that controls hypercalcaemia.
Contraindications	Systemic infections; caution in peptic ulceration or diabetes.
Main drug interactions	None.
Main side effects	Cushingoid appearance (with maintained high doses), dyspepsia.

Non-pharmacological treatment

For hyperparathyroidism
- Surgery should be reserved for all younger patients and those with complications of the disease (e.g. renal stones).
- Elderly asymptomatic patients can be followed conservatively.
- Surgery must be done by an experienced parathyroid surgeon.
- After successful surgery, serum calcium is usually normal within 24 h.
- Transient hypocalcaemia may occur; rarely, permanent hypoparathyroidism may follow.

For malignancy
- Surgical cure is rare because the disease is usually disseminated.

Treatment aims

Hyperparathyroidism
To cure disease by surgery.
To monitor asymptomatic patients.

Malignancy
To alleviate symptoms.

Prognosis

Hyperparathyroidism
- Effective surgical treatment of hyperparathyroidism is associated with a normal life expectancy.
- After a patient has been cured, a recurrence of hypercalcaemia is unusual, except when hyperplastic glands are present.
- In hypercalcaemia of malignancy, unless curative chemotherapy can be offered, the prognosis is poor, most patients dying within 6 months.

Malignancy
- Hypercalcaemia frequently recurs unless the malignancy is well controlled.

Follow-up and management
- Follow-up of the malignant disease is essential, to check for recurrence of hypercalcaemia if the malignancy has not been cured.

Key references

Bilizikian JP: Management of hypercalcaemia. *J Clin Endocrinol Metab* 1993, **77**:1445–1449.

Heath DA: The treatment of hypercalcaemia of malignancy. *Clin Endocrinol* 1991, **34**:155–157.

Larsson K et al. The risk of hip fractures in patients with primary hyperparathyroidism: a population based cohort study with a follow-up of 19 years. *J Int Med* 1993, **234**:585–593.

Various: Proceedings of the NIH Consensus Development Conference on diagnosis and management of asymptomatic primary hyperparathyroidism. Bethesda, Maryland, October 29–31, 1990. *J Bone Miner Res* 1991, **6** (suppl 2):81–166.

Hyperglycaemic emergencies — S.M. Marshall

Diagnosis

Symptoms

Hyperglycaemia
Polyuria, thirst, polydipsia.
Weight loss.
Tiredness, lassitude, general malaise.
Decreasing level of consciousness.

Ketoacidosis
Nausea, vomiting, abdominal pain.
Dyspnoea.

Precipitating cause
Symptoms of infection, myocardial infarction, or other illness.

Signs

General
Dehydration: particularly marked in hyperosmolar coma.
Hypotension.
Variable level of consciousness.
Signs of precipitating cause.

Ketoacidosis
Kussmaul's respiration, ketones on breath.
Peripheral vasodilatation, warm skin, tachycardia, generalized abdominal tenderness.

Investigations

To establish diagnosis
Capillary blood glucose analysis.
Urinalysis: for glucose, ketones.

To confirm diagnosis
Laboratory blood glucose analysis.
Serum sodium, potassium, bicarbonate, and creatinine measurement.
Measurement of arterial or capillary pH, partial oxygen and carbon dioxide pressure, and base excess: if serum bicarbonate <20 mmol/L or ketonuria; shows acidosis, high oxygen pressure, low carbon dioxide pressure.

To identify precipitating cause
Chest radiography: may show infection or pulmonary oedema.
ECG: may show acute myocardial infarction or signs of electrolyte disturbance.
Blood, urine, and throat cultures.
Abdominal ultrasonography or paracentesis: to exclude acute abdominal disease if abdominal signs do not resolve quickly.

Complications

Cardiac arrest.
Thromboembolism: particularly if patient is hyperosmolar.
Inhalation pneumonia.
Renal failure.
Rhabdomyolysis: rare.

Differential diagnosis

Ketotic
Hyperventilation, chest infection, lactic acidosis.
Acute abdominal disease.

Non-ketotic
Hypercalcaemia.
Cerebrovascular disease.
Thyrotoxicosis.

Aetiology

- Causes include the following:
Diabetes (initial presentation).
Other physical stress, precipitating rise in counter-regulatory hormones and relative deficiency of insulin (e.g. infection, myocardial infarction, stroke).
Omission of insulin.

Epidemiology

- The incidence is not declining, despite advances in diabetes education.
- 3–8 episodes occur in 1000 diabetic patients each year.

Treatment

Diet and lifestyle
- No special precautions are necessary.

Pharmacological treatment
- Rehydration and correction of electrolyte imbalance must begin immediately.
- A central venous pressure measurement may be a useful guide to fluid replacement in elderly patients or those with cardiac disease.
- If the patient is comatose, a nasogastric tube should be passed.
- Urinary catheterization may be needed to allow accurate monitoring of urinary output.

Rehydration
1 L 0.154 mmol/L isotonic saline solution in first hour to restore circulating volume, raise blood pressure, and open renal circulation; then 1 L in 2 h, 1 L in 4 h, 1 L in 6 h, 1 L 8-hourly thereafter as needed.
- The infusion rates should be adjusted as clinically indicated.
- 0.077 mmol/L saline solution or 5% dextrose in water should be used if serum sodium is >155 mmol/L.
- Colloid solution can be given if the patient remains hypotensive.

Insulin
By continuous i.v. infusion: *if ketotic*: 6 units/h by pump; *if non-ketotic*: 3–4 units/h.
By intermittent intramuscular injection: *if ketotic*: 20 units initially, then 10 units/h; *if non-ketotic*: 10 units initially, then 6 units/h.
- Treatment is continued until blood glucose is <14 mmol/L; then the dose of insulin should be halved, and i.v. infusion of 10% dextrose commenced at 80 ml/h.
- Patients should be told not to stop insulin treatment if intercurrent illness supervenes associated with anorexia or vomiting; insulin needs increase in these circumstances.

Potassium
- The total body deficit of potassium is ~1000 mmol.
- Infusion should be started when serum potassium is <5.5 mmol/L.
- Potassium chloride 20–80 mmol /h, well diluted in rehydration fluid, should be given.
- Treatment should be monitored by serum potassium measurement and ECG.

Sodium bicarbonate
- This is indicated only if the pH is <6.9.
- Sodium bicarbonate 100 ml 8.4% in 30 min, with 20 mmol potassium chloride, should be given.
- The pH should be checked after 30 min, and treatment should be repeated if necessary until the pH is >6.9.

Other options
Anticoagulation: low-dose s.c. heparin for all; full-dose i.v. heparin if serum osmolality >360 mOsmol/L.
Antibiotics: broad spectrum if any suspicion of infection.
- Replacement of other electrolytes (magnesium, phosphate) is rarely indicated.

Complications of treatment
- Most complications are avoidable with meticulous care and attention to detail.

Hypo- or hyperkalaemia.
Hypoglycaemia.
Fluid overload, especially in elderly patients.
Cerebral oedema.
Adult respiratory distress syndrome.

Treatment aims
To save the patient's life.
To rehydrate the patient.
To restore acid-base and electrolyte balance to normal.
To achieve euglycaemia in 24–48 h.

Prognosis
- Mortality remains at 5–15% in diabetic ketoacidosis and 30–50% in hyperosmolar coma, even in experienced units.
- In elderly patients, the cause of death is often the underlying precipitating disorder rather than the metabolic upset.

Follow-up and management

Response to treatment
- Response should be monitored at the bedside (pulse, blood pressure, respiratory rate every 30–60 min, capillary glucose hourly) and in the laboratory (glucose, sodium, potassium, bicarbonate, creatinine, pH on admission and at 2, 5, and 12 h of treatment, or more often if clinically indicated).

Later management
- Patients should be given fluids or a light diet when able to eat, but i.v. or i.m. insulin should be continued.
- When patients can tolerate oral intake, they should be transferred to s.c. insulin: quick-acting before each of the three main meals and intermediate-acting before bed.
- A 30-min overlap must be allowed before i.v. insulin is discontinued, to allow time for s.c. absorption.

Follow-up
- The events leading to admission should be reviewed in an effort to educate the patient and prevent further admissions; all patients should be taught 'sick-day' rules, including advice on seeking professional help early.
- Patients presenting in hyperosmolar coma may not need long-term insulin, but continuing it for a few weeks is probably safer, before stopping under close supervision.

Key references
Berger W, Keller U: Treatment of diabetic ketoacidosis and non-ketotic hyperosmolar coma. *Clin Endocrinol Metab* 1991, **6**:1–22.

Marshall SM: Hyperglycaemic emergencies. *Care of the Critically Ill*, 1993, **9**:220–223.

Walker M, Marshall SM, Alberti KGMM: Clinical aspects of diabetic ketoacidosis. *Diabetes Metab Rev* 1989, **5**:651–663.

Hyperprolactinaemia — P.J. Trainer

Diagnosis

Symptoms
- Symptoms can be subdivided into those directly related to hyperprolactinaemia and those due to the mass effect of a pituitary macroadenoma.

Hyperprolactinaemia
Galactorrhoea.
Amenorrhoea, oligomenorrhoea: in women.
Impotence: in men.
Infertility.
Reduced libido.

Macroadenoma
Headache: frontal.
Visual field defect: bitemporal hemianopia.
Diplopia.
Convulsions: temporal-lobe epilepsy due to local extension of tumour.
Cerebrovascular accident.

Signs

Macroadenoma
Hypopituitarism.
Optic atrophy: if tumour compressing optic nerve.
Loss of secondary sexual characteristics, postural hypotension, hypothyroidism, delayed or arrested puberty: signs of hypopituitarism.

Investigations
Detailed drug history.
Serum prolactin measurement: thyroid-releasing hormone and other dynamic stimulation tests are of no value.
Thyroid function tests: hypothyroidism is a cause of raised serum prolactin.
Gonadotrophin and gonadal steroids measurement: to diagnose polycystic ovary syndrome, a cause of hyperprolactinaemia.
Skull radiography, pituitary MRI or CT: to identify tumour.

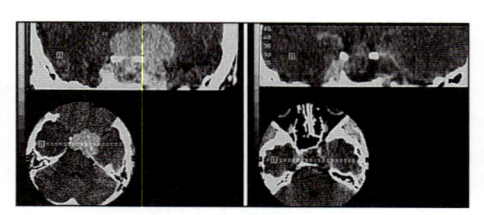

Axial and coronal view of large prolactinoma (left). Repeat scan (right) showing virtual disappearance of tumour on treatment by bromocriptine.

Complications

Hyperprolactinaemia
Infertility, impotence.
Osteoporosis.
Polycystic ovarian disease: in 25% of patients with a prolactinoma.

Macroadenoma
Hydrocephalus.
Blindness.
Hypopituitarism.
Cranial nerve palsy.

Differential diagnosis
Prolactinoma.
Pseudoprolactinoma (prolactin usually <3000 mU/L).
Hypothyroidism.
Medication (prolactin usually <3000 mU/L): substituted benzamides (metoclopropamide, sulpiride), phenothiazines, butyrophenones, reserpine, methyldopa.
Stress: e.g. venepuncture, epilepsy.
Polycystic ovarian disease (prolactin usually <1000 mU/L): hyperprolactinaemia can be secondary to polycystic ovarian disease; alternatively, polycystic ovarian disease occurs in 25% of patients with a prolactinoma.
Possible breast stimulation.

Aetiology
- Prolactinomas are monoclonal tumours that secrete prolactin.
- Pseudoprolactinomas are tumours of any type that interrupt the tonic inhibition, by hypothalamic dopamine, of prolactin secretion, i.e. the prolactin is secreted from the healthy pituitary.
- Oestrogens are not causative but can encourage prolactinoma growth, particularly the combined oral contraceptive pill and pregnancy.

Epidemiology
- Prolactinomas occur much more often in women than in men.

Treatment

Diet and lifestyle

- Oestrogens, e.g. the combined oral contraceptive, are contraindicated unless taken with dopamine agonists.
- Pregnancy and breast feeding can encourage tumour growth and must be undertaken with caution.

Pharmacological treatment

Standard dosage	Bromocriptine 1.25 mg initially, in the middle of a snack last thing at night; dose must be titrated against serum prolactin, median being 7.5 mg; ultimately, once-daily dose in the middle of a meal.
Contraindications	Toxaemia of pregnancy, sensitivity to ergot alkaloid, history of psychosis.
Special points	A depot preparation of bromocriptine is available and is rapidly effective in relieving pressure symptoms, e.g. visual loss.
	Other dopamine agonists in cases of bromocriptine intolerance or resistance are cabergoline, pergolide, lisuride, quinagolide (non-ergot), and terguride.
Main drug interactions	None.
Main side effects	Gastrointestinal disturbance, particularly nausea, postural hypotension, first-dose hypotension (effect negated by drugs that raise prolactin concentration).

Treatment aims
To normalize serum prolactin concentration.
To retain normal pituitary function.

Other treatments
Trans-sphenoidal microadenectomy: for dopamine agonist intolerance or resistance, infertility, pseudoprolactinoma.
Pituitary radiotherapy: for failed trans-sphenoidal hypophysectomy, macroprolactinoma (possibly before pregnancy to avoid expansion during pregnancy), dopamine agonist intolerance or resistance.

Prognosis
- 15–20% of microprolactinomas resolve during long-term dopamine agonist treatment.
- 40% of patients with macroadenomas have normal serum prolactinomas after trans-sphenoidal hypophysectomy.

Follow-up and management
- Patients must be maintained on the minimum dose of bromocriptine necessary to normalize serum prolactin concentrations.
- Bromocriptine must be stopped every 2 years, and serum prolactin concentrations must be checked.
- Long-term follow-up is necessary.

Key references
Cunnah D, Besser GM: Management of prolactinomas. *Clin Endocrinol* 1991, **34**:231–235.

Faglia G: Should dopamine agonist treatment for prolactinomas be life-long? *Clin Endocrinol* 1991, **34**:173–174.

Hyperthyroidism — J.A. Franklyn

Diagnosis

Symptoms
Weight loss, fatigue, sweating, heat intolerance, neck swelling.

Palpitations, shortness of breath.

Tremor, weakness, nervousness.

Increased frequency of bowel movements.

Staring, gritty eyes, swelling around eyes.

- Classic symptoms and signs may be absent in elderly patients.

Signs
Sinus tachycardia, atrial fibrillation, cardiac failure.

Fine tremor, proximal myopathy.

Goitre: diffuse, with or without bruit, nodular, solitary nodule.

Lid retraction, lid lag, periorbital puffiness, cheimosis, proptosis, corneal ulceration, ophthalmoplegia.

Pretibial myxoedema, palmar erythema, acropachy (finger clubbing).

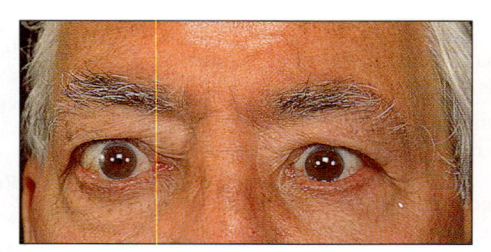

Periorbital oedema, mild lid retraction and cheimosis in a patient with Graves' ophthalmopathy.

Investigations
Serum thyroid hormone measurement: total or free thyroxine (T_4) to indicate severity of hyperthyroidism; total or free triiodothyronine (T_3) to indicate severity and diagnose T_3 toxicosis if T_4 normal but thyroid-stimulating hormone (TSH) low.

Serum TSH measurement: undetectable in hyperthyroidism; normal value excludes primary hyperthyroidism (use of a sensitive assay obviates need for thyrotrophin-releasing hormone testing); in pituitary-driven hyperthyroidism (rare), TSH is detectable.

Autoantibody tests: antithyroid peroxidase and antithyroglobulin antibodies often positive in Graves' disease; anti-TSH receptor antibodies often positive in Graves' disease but not measured routinely.

Radioisotope scanning and uptake measurements: not routinely indicated; ^{99m}Tc scintigraphy distinguishes Graves' disease from toxic nodular goitre; increased uptake of ^{131}I confirms hyperthyroidism; uptake low in thyroiditis.

Complications
Cardiac disease: especially atrial fibrillation and congestive cardiac failure (more common in elderly patients).

Reduced bone density and increased risk of osteoporotic fractures.

Graves' ophthalmopathy: may be progressive and occasionally sight-threatening because of corneal ulceration or optic nerve compression.

Differential diagnosis
Psychiatric disorders: e.g. anxiety.

Anaemia.

Malignancy.

Phaeochromocytoma.

Alcohol withdrawal.

Excess caffeine intake.

Aetiology
Common causes (95% of patients)
Graves' disease.
Autoimmune cause associated with antibodies to thyroid-stimulating hormone (TSH) receptor on thyroid cell.
Toxic nodular goitre: multinodular, single toxic adenoma.
Thyroiditis: subacute, silent, postpartum.

Uncommon causes
Exogenous iodide: kelp ingestion, amiodarone, radiographic contrast agents.
Factitious: ingestion of thyroid hormones.
Inappropriate secretion of TSH by pituitary: TSH-secreting tumour, thyroid hormone resistance syndromes.
Neonatal hyperthyroidism: baby born to mother with history of Graves' disease.

Epidemiology
- The prevalence of hyperthyroidism is ~20 in 1000 females and ~2 in 1000 males.
- Toxic nodular goitre is part of a spectrum of endemic or sporadic goitre, often found in patients with a long history of goitre; the peak incidence is at ~60 years.

Treatment

Diet and lifestyle
- Increased iodine intake may precipitate hyperthyroidism in patients with euthyroid goitre.
- Cigarette smoking significantly increases the risk of ophthalmopathy in Graves' disease.

Pharmacological treatment

Thionamides
- Thionamides are first-line treatment in patients <40 years with Graves' hyperthyroidism; they are short-term treatment in older patients and those with relapsed hyperthyroidism before radioiodine treatment.
- They produce biochemical improvement and symptomatic relief within 2 months in most patients; a full course of 18 months is important to allow remission of disease.

Standard dosage	Carbimazole 30 mg single daily dose at diagnosis, reduced to maintenance dose of 5–10 mg. Propylthiouracil 100 mg 3 times daily at diagnosis, reduced to maintenance dose of 50 mg 1–2 times daily.
Contraindications	Thionamide-induced agranulocytosis or other serious side effects.
Main drug interactions	No major interactions.
Main side effects	Agranulocytosis (rare; patients must be warned to stop treatment and seek an urgent blood test if they develop a sore throat or other infection), hepatitis, cholestatic jaundice and lupus-like syndromes (rare but serious), skin rashes and arthralgia (common but not serious).

Beta adrenergic blockers
- Beta-andergenic blockers are recommended for patients with moderate or severe symptoms until serum thyroid hormones have returned to normal; often they are the only treatment needed for thyroiditis.
- They provide quick symptomatic relief of tremor and palpitations that resemble sympathetic overactivity.

Standard dosage	Nadolol 80 mg once daily. Propranolol 20–80 mg 3 times daily (higher dose may be needed because of increased first-pass metabolism). Atenolol 50–100 mg daily.
Contraindications	Asthma, obstructive airways disease; caution in heart failure, even if induced by hyperthyroidism.
Main drug interactions	*See drug data sheets.*
Main side effects	*See drug data sheets.*

Radioiodine
- Radioiodine treatment must be done under specialist supervision.
- It is increasingly used as first-line treatment in patients with the first episode of hyperthyroidism; it is the treatment of choice in patients aged >40 years at presentation and in those with relapse after drug treatment or surgery.

Standard dosage	Radioiodine single dose initially; second dose after 6 months if hyperthyroidism not cured (one-third of patients); larger initial doses for elderly patients or those with severe disease to produce rapid effect and induce hypothyroidism.
Contraindications	Pregnancy (must be avoided for 6 months after treatment), breast feeding, hyperthyroidism secondary to thyroiditis; caution in patients with active ophthalmopathy.
Special points	Thionamides should be withdrawn at least 4 days before and avoided for 4 days after treatment. Can exacerbate hyperthyroidism and rarely induce 'thyroid storm'.
Main drug interactions	None.
Main side effects	Hypothyroidism (within 25 years of treatment), may be intended outcome if larger dose of radioiodine used for thyroid ablation and thyroxine replacement.

Treatment aims
To relieve symptoms.
To restore thyroxine and triiodothyronine values to normal range.
To obtain long-term euthyroidism.

Other treatments
Partial thyroidectomy: for Graves' disease in patients with large goitre and relapse after thionamide treatment or with large toxic nodular goitre.
- Patients must be rendered euthyroid before surgery by thionamide or beta blocker with potassium iodide.

Prognosis
- Only 30% of patients with Graves' hyperthyroidism remain euthyroid in the long term after a course of thionamide; 15% become hypothyroid even without treatment.
- Medium-dosed radioiodine treatment and partial thyroidectomy are each associated with a 50% risk of permanent hypothyroidism; larger doses ablate the thyroid.

Follow-up and management
- Serum thyroxine and thyroid-stimulating hormone concentration should be monitored every 4–6 weeks in patients on high-dose thionamides and every 3 months in those on maintenance doses.
- Thyroid function should be checked annually (continuing risk of hypothyroidism).

Management of hyperthyroidism in pregnancy
- Thionamides are the most appropriate agents; prophylthiouracil is preferred (crosses placenta less than carbimazole, excreted less in breast milk).
- Dosage must be adjusted to maintain serum thyroxine at the upper end of normal range (these drugs cause fetal goitre and hypothyroidism in high dose).
- Low doses are needed in Graves' hyperthyroidism (usually remits in pregnancy).
- Relapse is frequent after delivery.

Key references
Franklyn JA: The management of hyperthyroidism. *N Engl J Med* 1994, **330**:1731–1738.
Reinwein D *et al.*: A prospective randomised trial of antithyroid drug dose in Graves' disease therapy. *J Clin Endocrinol Metab* 1993, **76**:1516–1521.

Hypocalcaemia — D.A. Heath

Diagnosis

Symptoms
Paraesthesia: especially around face, hands, and feet.
Tetany: causing painful cramps culminating in hands going into tetanic spasm position.
Epilepsy.
Bone pain: common in vitamin D deficiency.

Signs
- Mild hypocalcaemia may be asymptomatic; signs are due to neuromuscular irritability.

Twitching of local facial muscles: after tapping over facial nerve in front of and below ear; Chvostek's sign (positive in some normal people, rarely in those with hypokalaemia).
Development of tetanic spasm: Trousseau's sign; after inflation of a sphygmomanometer cuff on arm (a painful procedure and not recommended).
Proximal myopathy: common in vitamin D deficiency.
Obesity, 'moon' face, shortened metacarpals and metatarsals: signs of pseudohypoparathyroidism.

Investigations
Serum calcium measurement: low concentration.
Serum phosphorus measurement: low concentration in vitamin D deficiency, high in hypoparathyroidism, pseudohypoparathyroidism, and renal failure.
Serum creatinine measurement: raised concentration in renal failure.
Serum alkaline phosphatase measurement: often raised concentration in vitamin D deficiency.
Serum magnesium measurement: low concentration can cause hypocalcaemia.
Serum parathyroid hormone measurement: raised concentration in vitamin D deficiency, pseudohypoparathyroidism, and renal failure.
Radiography: of wrists and knees in suspected rickets, chest and pelvis in suspected osteomalacia.

Complications
Epilepsy.
Cataracts and basal ganglia calcification: in longstanding hypocalcaemia.

Differential diagnosis
Previous neck surgery.
Hypomagnesaemia, especially if patient is an alcoholic, has extensive small-bowel disease or resection, or is on aminoglycoside drugs or cisplatinum.

Aetiology
- Causes include the following:

Low plasma proteins (not true hypocalcaemia).
Acute or chronic renal failure.
Vitamin D deficiency.
Hypoparathyroidism: rarely idiopathic, usually after neck surgery.
Pseudohypoparathyroidism.
Hypomagnesaemia.
Severe acute pancreatitis.
Malabsorption.

Epidemiology
- Vitamin D deficiency is more common in Asians who are vegetarians.
- It is manifest most often at times of increased requirements (i.e. neonates, growth spurt, and pregnancy).

Treatment

Diet and lifestyle

- Patients should have an adequate calcium intake (800–1000 mg daily).
- Low-dose vitamin D supplementation should be considered if exposure to sunlight is inadequate.

Pharmacological treatment

For acute symptomatic hypocalcaemia

Standard dosage	10% calcium gluconate 10 ml i.v. slowly, followed by 50–100 ml i.v. in 1 L saline solution over 24 h at a rate to relieve symptoms.
Contraindications	None.
Main drug interactions	None.
Main side effects	Tissue necrosis (if extravasation outside vein).

For hypoparathyroidism

Standard dosage	Calcitriol or alfacalcidol 0.5–1.0 µg orally daily.
Contraindications	None.
Special points	Regular serum calcium monitoring.
Main drug interactions	None.
Main side effects	Hypercalcaemia.

For vitamin D deficiency

Standard dosage	Calciferol 500–1000 units orally daily.
Contraindications	None.
Main drug interactions	None.
Main side effects	None at this dose range.

For renal failure

Standard dosage	Calcitriol or alfacalcidol 0.5–1.0 µg orally daily.
Contraindications	None.
Special points	Hyperphosphataemia should be controlled.
Main drug interactions	None.
Main side effects	Hypercalcaemia.

For hypomagnesaemic hypocalcaemia

- Patients with severe, symptomatic hypomagnesaemia are best treated initially by an intravenous preparation: magnesium sulphate 5–10 mg 50% solution in 1 L 5% dextrose over 3–4 h.
- Daily infusions may be needed until serum magnesium is maintained within the normal range.
- If magnesium losses continue (e.g. short bowel syndrome), this can be treated by intermittent infusions or oral therapy. Various oral preparations are available, all of which may cause gastrointestinal problems.

Treatment aims
To correct hypocalcaemia.

Prognosis
- Hypoparathyroidism usually needs life-long treatment.
- For vitamin D deficiency, treatment is needed throughout the period of increased vitamin D requirement.

Follow-up and management
- All patients on high doses of vitamin D need regular serum calcium measurements to prevent the occurrence of hypercalcaemia.

Key references
Tohme JF, Bilezilcian JP: Hypocalcaemic emergencies. *Endocrinol Metab Clin North Am* 1993, **22**:363–375.

Hypoglycaemia   S.A. Amiel

Diagnosis

Symptoms
Sweating, shaking, anxiety, feeling hot, nausea, palpitations, tingling lips: due to sympathetic and adrenergic response to low blood glucose concentration (autonomic).
Dizziness, tiredness, confusion, difficulty speaking, inability to concentrate, headache: due to impaired cerebral cortical function resulting from low blood glucose level.
Hunger, weakness, blurred vision.
Headache, malaise, confusion: post-hypoglycaemic.

- Patients with recurrent hypoglycaemic attacks often present with symptoms of decreased cognitive function or conscious level for which they have no subjective awareness.

Signs
Pallor, diaphoresis, tremor, tachycardia or occasionally bradycardia, increased pulse pressure, dilated pupils: autonomic.
Altered behaviour, irrational speech or behaviour, slurred speech, irritability, decreased level of consciousness, seizure, coma: neuroglycopenic.
Transient focal neurological defects: post-hypoglycaemic.

Investigations

For all cases
Blood glucose measurement: confirmed by laboratory measurement, although treatment may be started after bedside capillary blood glucose strip testing; concentration in men ≤2.8 mmol/L, in women ≤2.2 mmol/L, in treated diabetic patients ≤3.5 mmol/L.

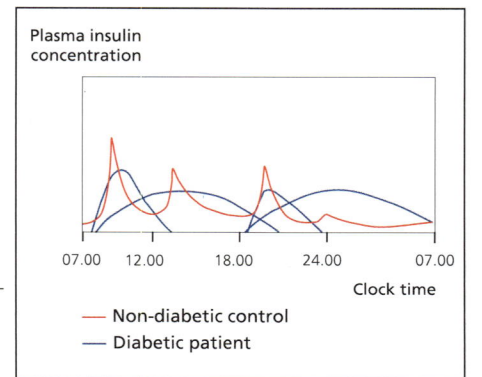

For recurrent or unexplained episodes
Plasma insulin and c-peptide analysis.
Blood and urine screening: for sulphonylureas.
Urea, creatinine, liver function, insulin antibody tests.
Thyroid and adrenal function tests, gastric emptying studies, growth hormone measurement: to investigate recurrence in treated diabetic patients.

Plasma insulin concentrations over 24 h from a patient on twice-daily injections of mixed exogenous insulins and an approximation of the plasma insulin profile of a non-diabetic person eating 3 meals daily, showing times of risk of hypoglycaemia.

For suspected insulinoma
Fasting glucose, insulin, c-peptide, and pro-insulin measurement: repeated during 72-h fast or until hypoglycaemia documented; care needed in children, in whom other metabolites should be measured; high c-peptide and insulin suggest insulinoma, sulphonyl-ureas, or insulin autoantibodies (rare); high insulin with low c-peptide indicates exogenous insulin.
CT, coeliac axis or mesenteric angiography, laparotomy, and perioperative ultrasonography: to localize insulinoma.

For non-insulinoma, non-diabetes related hypoglycaemia
09.00 h cortisol and Synacthen test, growth hormone profile, insulin-like growth factors analysis, liver function tests.

For suspected 'reactive' hypoglycaemia
Home blood glucose testing: patients must be taught to collect capillary blood samples at home during episodes for later laboratory estimates of blood glucose concentration.

Complications
Trauma: while patient is hypoglycaemic.
Seizure.
Loss of subjective awareness of subsequent episodes.
Permanent neurological sequelae: usually only with large insulin overdosage.
Death.

Differential diagnosis

Acute
Other causes of coma or confusion, including the following:
Ketoacidosis, non-ketotic hyperosmolar coma, intoxication or poisoning, uraemia, epilepsy, stroke, intracranial haemorrhage, meningitis, head injury.

Recurrent
Epilepsy, arrhythmias, psychiatric disorder, phaeochromocytoma.

Aetiology
- Causes include the following:

Excess insulin action in diabetic patients
Missed, small, or late meals, error in time or dose, exercise (effect may last 18 h), alcohol (delayed effect), hypothyroidism, renal failure, gastroparesis: with pharmacological treatment of diabetes mellitus (insulin, sulphonylureas, rarely metformin).
Vigorous insulin response to rapidly absorbed glucose or gastric surgery: in 'reactive or post-prandial' hypoglycaemia.
Insulinoma, nesidioblastosis.

Excess insulin action in non-diabetic patients
Tumours secreting insulin-like growth factor.
Surreptitious or malicious administration of insulin or sulphonylurea.

Increased insulin sensitivity
Cortisol deficiency.
Growth hormone deficiency.
Hypopituitarism.

Defects of hepatic glucose production
Liver disease.
Alcohol toxicity.
Glycogen storage diseases.
Ketotic hypoglycaemia of childhood.
Prematurity.
Defective fatty acid oxidation.

Epidemiology
- 1.2% of the UK population have diabetes mellitus; 10% of these have the insulin-dependent form; 4–40% experience severe hypoglycaemia.

- 10% of insulinomas are multiple, 10% are malignant, 9% with multiple endocrine neoplasia.

Treatment

Diet and lifestyle
- In 'reactive hypoglycaemia', patients should eat small, regular meals with high complex carbohydrates and should avoid simple sugars.
- In childhood disorders of metabolism, frequent, high-carbohydrate, low-fat meals should be eaten.
- In patients with diabetes, regular meals and snacks are essential, with patient-led dosage adjustments for certain situations, e.g. excessive exercise.

Pharmacological treatment

For conscious patients
Rapidly absorbed carbohydrates (20 g, e.g. 4 glucose tablets, ½ glass orange juice or Lucozade), then snack.

Contraindicated for loss of gag reflex or severely impaired level of consciousness.

For confused patients
Oral glucose gel.

Contraindicated for loss of gag reflex or severely impaired level of consciousness.

For unconscious patients
50% glucose 50 ml or 20% glucose 100–150 ml i.v.

In children: 20% dextrose 2.5 ml/kg.

In infants: 10% dextrose 2.5 ml/kg.

Alternatively, glucagon 1 mg i.m., followed by 30 g complex carbohydrate orally on recovery.

- Extravasation of glucose must be avoided.
- If hypoglycaemia is due to sulphonylurea treatment, massive insulin overdose, or unknown cause, the patient should be admitted to hospital for observation and i.v. glucose infusion considered.
- Glucagon may not be effective in very undernourished or very alcohol-intoxicated patients.

Treatment aims
To achieve recovery from acute event.
To prevent further episodes.

Other treatments
Surgery for insulinomas, tumours secreting insulin-like growth factor, nesidioblastosis.

Prognosis
- For diabetes, the prognosis is that of the underlying disease, but the patient may be prone to further attacks.
- For tumours secreting insulin-like growth factor, prognosis is poor.

Follow-up and management

Prevention of further episodes
- The diabetes regimen should be adjusted.
- Diazoxide can be given for insulinoma, after the diagnosis is established, pending definitive surgical management.
- Diet regimens should be followed for metabolic defects.

Key references
Amiel SA: Glucose counterregulation in health and disease: current concepts in hypoglycaemia recognition and response. *QJM* 1991, **293**:707–727.

Amiel SA: Hypoglycaemia in diabetes mellitus. *Med Int* 1993, **21**:279–280.

Hypopituitarism — P. Jenkins

Diagnosis

Symptoms

- Symptoms may be due to an underlying cause or to hormone deficiencies, which usually have a gradual onset if secondary to an expanding pituitary lesion and tend to occur in a sequential order: growth hormone, luteinizing or follicle-stimulating hormone, thyroid-stimulating hormone, adrenocorticotrophic hormone.

Impotence or amenorrhoea, decreased libido: due to deficiency of gonadotrophins.
Poor growth and development: in children, due to deficiency of growth hormone.
Cold intolerance, weight gain, tiredness, lethargy: due to deficiency of thyroid-stimulating hormone.
Dizziness, nausea, vomiting: due to deficiency of adrenocorticotrophic hormone.
Urinary frequency, nocturia: due to deficiency of vasopressin.
Headache or visual disturbance: due to macroadenoma.
Galactorrhoea: due to prolactinoma or pituitary stalk compression by lesion.

Signs

Small soft testes, loss of pubic and axillary hair: due to deficiency of gonadotrophins.
Short stature: in children, due to deficiency of growth hormone.
Cool skin, absent or slow reflexes: due to deficiency of thyroid-stimulating hormone.
Postural hypotension, shock: due to deficiency of adrenocorticotrophic hormone.
Visual field defect, diplopia or cranial nerve palsies, papilloedema, CSF rhinorrhoea, excessive hormone production or galactorrhoea: indicating macroadenoma.
Signs of acromegaly.

Investigations

Cortisol measurement for adrenal axis: if 09.00 h cortisol >550 nmol/L, significant deficiency improbable; if <50 nmol/L, adrenocorticotrophic hormone (ACTH) deficiency very probable unless patient is taking steroids; intermediate values need insulin tolerance test to assess ACTH reserve.
Thyroid tests: thyroxine, free thyroxine (T_4), triiodothyronine, thyroid-stimulating hormone (TSH); secondary hypothyroidism suggested by low T_4 or free T_4 index unaccompanied by raised TSH.
Sex hormone measurement for gonadal axis: *in men:* 09.00 h testosterone, sex hormone-binding globulin (high level can give rise to high total bound testosterone, while free level remains low), luteinizing hormone (LH) or follicle-stimulating hormone (FSH); gonadotrophin deficiency suggested by low basal testosterone and no rise of LH/FSH; *in women:* oestradiol, sex hormone-binding globulin, LH/FSH, progesterone on day 21 (normal concentration implies normal gonadal axis).
Prolactin test: on 2–3 occasions; hyperprolactinaemia may suppress pulsatile gonadotrophin secretion in either sex in absence of absolute deficiency.
Growth hormone (GH) measurement: basal values usually undetectable and therefore unhelpful; insulin tolerance or glucagon test necessary to assess GH reserve.
Plasma and urine osmolality measurement for posterior pituitary: plasma osmolality >295 mOsm/L and urine:plasma osmolality ratio of <2:1 suggest diabetes insipidus.
Insulin tolerance test: to assess ACTH and GH reserve; must be done in a specialized unit; contraindicated in patients with ischaemic heart disease, epilepsy, or unexplained blackouts; particular caution in children and elderly patients.
Releasing hormone tests: thyrotrophin-releasing and luteinizing hormone-releasing hormone tests only assess 'readily releasable' pool of anterior pituitary hormones and cannot be used to diagnose normality of physiological secretion of the hormone.
Radiography: may show double floor of pituitary fossa due to pituitary enlargement.
MRI or CT of pituitary gland: to visualize macroadenomas and most microadenomas.

Complications

Cardiovascular collapse: resulting from adrenocortical insufficiency.
Expanding pituitary mass: with optic chiasm compression and local invasion of brain.
Hydrocephalus: with third ventricular compression by tumour.
Temporal-lobe epilepsy: with temporal extension of tumour.

Differential diagnosis

Primary adrenal or thyroid insufficiency.
Anorexia nervosa.

Aetiology

- Causes include the following:

Pituitary tumours: most common.
Iatrogenic disorders: previous surgery or radiotherapy.
Secondary deposits: especially breast, lung.
Infectious disease: e.g. tuberculosis.
Vascular disease: e.g. Sheehan's syndrome, postpartum necrosis.
Severe exercise or malnutrition: may cause reversible loss of luteinizing-hormone-releasing hormone release.

Epidemiology

- The incidence of panhypopituitarism is difficult to determine, but ~1 in 10 000 patients each year develops a pituitary tumour.

P. Jenkins **Hypopituitarism**

Treatment

Diet and lifestyle
- Patients need a steroid card, Medicalert bracelet or necklace, and emergency pack of parenteral hydrocortisone (for deficiencies of pituitary–adrenal axis).

Pharmacological treatment

For deficiencies of pituitary–adrenal axis

Standard dosage	Hydrocortisone 20 mg on waking, 10 mg with evening meal (variable). Prednisolone (non-enteric coated) 5 mg and 2.5 mg or dexamethasone 0.5 mg and 0.25 mg may also be used.
Contraindications	None.
Special points	Response monitored by clinical assessment and hydrocortisone day curve. With severe illness, especially vomiting or diarrhoea, or for perioperative cover, parenteral treatment is needed (hydrocortisone 100 mg i.m. every 6 h).
Main drug interactions	Oestrogens increase cortisol-binding globulin and thus hydrocortisone concentration.
Main side effects	Iatrogenic Cushing's syndrome due to over-replacement.

For thyroid deficiencies

Standard dosage	Thyroxine 100–150 µg daily.
Contraindications	None.
Special points	Response monitored by clinical assessment and serum thyroxine and triiodothyronine measurement (if patient taking the latter); 09.00 h cortisol must be >100 nmol/L before replacement; for severe hypothyroidism, initially low doses of triiodothyronine (2.5 µg; short half-life), increased gradually to 20 µg 2–3 times daily; can precipitate angina, and replacement in patients with ischaemic heart disease must be commenced in hospital.
Main drug interactions	Oestrogens increase thyroid-binding globulin and raise total thyroxine; free thyroxine should be used for monitoring.
Main side effects	None.

For growth hormone deficiencies
- Children should be given growth hormone 2–4 units s.c. daily (0.5 units/kg/week).
- In adults, replacement is controversial and of uncertain benefit.

For deficiencies of pituitary–gonadal axis

Standard dosage	*Men:* testosterone enanthate or propionate 250–500 mg i.m. every 3–4 weeks or testosterone undecanoate 40–80 mg orally 3 times daily. *Women:* ethinyl oestradiol 30 µg daily and medroxyprogesterone acetate 5–10 mg on days 1–14 of calendar month.
Contraindications	Prostatic cancer, breast cancer.
Special points	Response monitored by potency and serum testosterone, menses, and symptoms of oestrogen deficiency.
Main drug interactions	Oestrogen increases many binding globulins and thus total hormone concentrations.
Main side effects	Aggression due to over-replacement of testosterone.

For posterior pituitary deficiencies

Standard dosage	Desmopressin 10–20 µg at night by intranasal spray; dose may also be needed in morning.
Contraindications	None.
Special points	Response monitored by plasma and urine osmolality.
Main drug interactions	None.
Main side effects	Dilutional hyponatraemia due to over-replacement.

Treatment aims
To achieve patient's clinical well-being.
To achieve normal target gland hormone concentrations.
To remove underlying cause.

Other treatments
- Surgery is indicated for the following.
Pituitary tumours.
Visual field defects.
Cranial nerve palsies.
CSF rhinorrhoea.

Prognosis
- Accurate and careful hormone replacement restores a normal life expectancy.

Follow-up and management
- Initial close supervision is necessary to ensure the correct dosage.
- Thereafter, patients should be reviewed every 6–12 months.

Key references
Cuneo RC *et al.*: The growth hormone deficiency syndrome in adults. *Clin Endocrinol* 1992, **37**:387–397.

Jones SL *et al.*: An audit of the insulin tolerance test in adult subjects in an acute investigation unit over one year. *Clin Endocrinol* 1994, **41**:123–128.

Littley MD *et al.*: Hypopituitarism following external radiotherapy for pituitary tumours in adults. *AJM* 1989, **70**:145–160.

Hypothyroidism   J.A. Franklyn

Diagnosis

Symptoms
Weight gain, fatigue, cold intolerance, neck swelling, hoarseness.
Angina, shortness of breath.
Aches and pains, depression, carpal tunnel syndrome.
Dry skin.
Menorrhagia, infertility, galactorrhoea secondary to hyperprolactinaemia.
Constipation.
Poor growth, mental retardation, delayed puberty: in children.

Signs
Bradycardia, pericardial effusion (rare), cardiac failure.
Hoarseness, deafness, cerebellar ataxia, delayed relaxation of tendon reflexes, psychosis ('myxoedema madness').
Anaemia: iron-deficiency, normochromic, normocytic, macrocytic, pernicious.
Goitre: small firm diffuse (Hashimoto's thyroiditis), nodular or diffuse (iodine deficiency).
Dry skin, myxoedema, vitiligo, erythema *ab igne*.

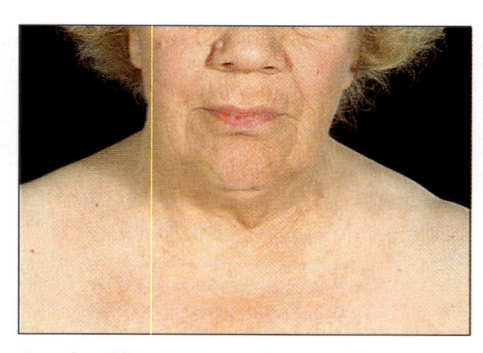

Hypothyroid appearances of an elderly patient with severe untreated Hashimoto's thyroiditis.

Investigations
Serum thyroid hormone measurement: reduction in free or total thyroxine indicates severity of hypothyroidism; serum triiodothyronine usually normal except in severely ill patients, so measurement not helpful.
Serum thyroid-stimulating hormone (TSH) measurement: elevation indicates primary thyroid failure; raised TSH with normal thyroxine is termed 'subclinical' hypothyroidism; TSH within or below normal range, with low serum thyroxine, suggests secondary hypothyroidism (hypothalamic/pituitary; same picture seen in 'non-thyroidal' illness and treatment by certain drugs, e.g. glucocorticoids).
Autoantibody measurement: antithyroid peroxidase and antithyroglobulin antibodies often present in high titre in Hashimoto's thyroiditis.

Complications
Hypothermia and coma: in severely ill patients, typically in the elderly in cold weather
Hyperlipidaemia and ischaemic heart disease: associated with longstanding hypothyroidism.

Differential diagnosis
- Middle-aged, overweight, depressed women often appear mildly hypothyroid and should always be screened.

Neurasthenia.
Menstrual disorders.
Weight change.
Anaemia.
Unexplained heart failure (unresponsive to digoxin).
Hyperlipidaemia.
Unexplained ascites.
Primary amyloidosis.
Depression, primary psychosis, cerebral disorders (arteriosclerosis, tumour).

Aetiology

Causes of primary thyroid failure

Autoimmune thyroiditis: Hashimoto's thyroiditis.
Previous treatment by radioiodine or thyroidectomy.
Idiopathic atrophy.
Iodine deficiency.
Antithyroid drugs or excess iodine.
Subacute and silent thyroiditis.
Poor compliance with thyroxine replacement.
Dyshormonogenesis, agenesis, infiltrative disease (uncommon).

Causes of secondary thyroid failure

Disease of pituitary or hypothalamus.

Epidemiology
- The prevalence of hypothyroidism is ~15 in 1000 females, ~1 in 1000 males.
- In the UK, >90% of cases are due to autoimmune thyroiditis, idiopathic atrophy, or previous treatment for hyperthyroidism.

Congenital hypothyroidism
Prevalence: 1 in 4000 infants in UK.
Detection: routine screening of all infants.
Possible causes: thyroid agenesis, ectopic or hypoplastic thyroid tissue, inherited disorders or hormonogenesis, transplacental passage of thyroid-stimulating hormone receptor blocking antibodies (such cases resolve spontaneously within 2 months).

Iodine-deficient hypothyroidism
- Iodine deficiency is the major cause of hypothyroidism worldwide. It is typically found in mountainous regions.
- Iodine supplementation programmes are effective in abolishing symptoms.

Treatment

Diet and lifestyle
- Long-term ingestion of iodine-containing compounds, e.g. kelp preparations or expectorants, can result in hypothyroidism in adults.

Pharmacological treatment
- Thyroxine for patients with symptomatic hypothyroidism; triiodothyronine is used occasionally in patients with myxoedema coma to produce more rapid effect.
- Symptoms begin to resolve within 2–3 weeks of commencing treatment, but treatment at full dose for 8 weeks may be needed to restore serum thyroid-stimulating hormone to normal.

Standard dosage	Thyroxine 100–150 µg daily as single dose. Triiodothyronine 20 µg orally 2–3 times daily.
Contraindications	Caution in severe ischaemic heart disease (patient should be admitted to hospital).
Main drug interactions	None.
Main side effects	Generally none; exacerbation of ischaemic heart disease may follow initiation of treatment; can precipitate acute adrenal failure in patients with subclinical adrenal disease.

Treatment aims
To relieve symptoms.
To restore serum thyroid-stimulating hormone and thyroxine to normal values.

Prognosis
- Life expectancy is not adversely affected by long-term thyroxine treatment.
- Thyroxine treatment (in doses that reduce serum thyroid-stimulating hormone to below normal) may reduce bone density and may increase risk of osteoporotic fractures.
- Up to 25% of patients in the community prescribed thyroxine have biochemical evidence of undertreatment that may be associated with hyperlipidaemia and increased risk of ischaemic heart disease.

Follow up and management
- Serum thyroid-stimulating hormone should be measured 8 weeks after starting treatment to check whether the dose needs to be increased and should be measured annually in patients on established treatment to ensure continuing compliance.
- Treatment is for life, except in mild cases occurring within the first 6 months after radioiodine treatment, pregnancy, or partial thyroidectomy (possibly temporary) and in patients who are hypothyroid secondary to subacute or silent thyroiditis.

Key references
Anonymous: Hypothyroidism? *Lancet* 1990, **335**:1316.

Lazarus JH, Hall R (eds): Hypothyroidism and goitre. *Ballières Clin Endocrinol Metab* 1988, **2**.

Toft AD: Thyroxine therapy. *N Engl J Med* 1994, **331**:174–180.

Utiger RD: Therapy of hypothyroidism. When are changes needed? *N Engl J Med* 1990, **323**:126–127.

Obesity J. Garrow

Diagnosis

Symptoms
Social embarrassment.

Shortness of breath on mild exercise.

Pain in back, hips, or knees: especially in middle-aged women.

Infertility, menstrual irregularity.

Pain associated with angina, gallstones, varicose veins.

Heat-intolerance.

Signs
Weight:height ratio >30 kg/m^2: definitive diagnosis.

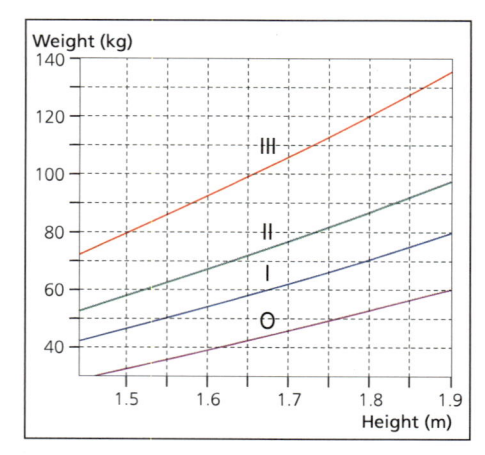

Relation of weight and height for desirable range (O) and mild (I), moderate (II), and severe (III) obesity.

Differential diagnosis
Genetic disorders in children of short stature.

Hyperphagia caused by hypothalamic damage (in adults) or depressive illness.

Cushing's syndrome: alters fat distribution.

Hypothyroidism.

Aetiology
- Obesity is caused by greater energy intake than output.
- Familial clustering is seen, partly due to genetic factors and partly to lifestyle.

Epidemiology
- In the UK population aged 16–64 years, the prevalence is 13% in men, 16% in women; it is inversely related to social class.
- The prevalence is higher in southern and eastern Europe, lower in Scandinavia and Japan.
- The worldwide prevalence is increasing.

Investigations
- Often no investigation is needed; elaborate endocrine tests are counterproductive because they wrongly imply a probable metabolic basis for obesity.

24-h urine cortisol measurement: for Cushing's syndrome.

Measurement of thyroid-stimulating hormone or free thyroxine: for hypothyroidism if clinically indicated.

Complications
Hypertension, impaired glucose tolerance or non-insulin-dependent diabetes mellitus: common in grade II (moderate) and III (severe) obesity; risk of hypertension or diabetes greater with positive family history or central fat distribution (waist:hip circumference ratio >0.93 in men, >0.83 in women).

Myocardial infarction.

Gallstones.

Hiatus hernia.

Osteoarthritis.

Varicose veins.

Infertility.

Increased liability to cancer: colon, rectum, prostate in men; breast, endometrium, ovary in women.

Treatment

Diet and lifestyle
- The mainstay of treatment is a reduction in dietary energy, especially from fat, sugar, and alcohol.
- The loss of 1 kg/week of adipose tissue requires an energy deficit of 4.2 MJ/day (1000 kcal/day).
- Physical exercise promotes fitness but is ineffective alone in causing weight loss.
- The help of a dietitian should be sought, and regular (monthly) supportive counselling is essential.

Pharmacological treatment
- Long-term results of drug treatment are disappointing; a short course of anorectic drugs does not assist subsequent weight loss.
- Drugs designed to inhibit the absorption of energy from the gut or stimulate the metabolic rate have not yet been shown to be clinically useful.

Treatment aims
To maintain an average rate of weight loss of 0.5–1 kg/week until 'desirable' ratio of weight:height is achieved.
To maintain reduced weight indefinitely.
To restore patient's self-esteem.

Other treatments
Gut bypass surgery: intended to cause malabsorption; not generally used because metabolic complications can be severe and prolonged.
Gastric stapling or jaw wiring: to restrict intake; can cause massive weight loss.
'Apronectomy': useful to remove excess skin after weight loss but not an effective primary treatment.
Psychotherapy: role unclear; obese people have no specific psychopathology but often have exogenous depression and eating disorders caused by ill advised 'crash' diets.

Prognosis
- Substantial weight loss can be achieved by well supervised dieting in 1–2 years and brings great health benefits, especially in young patients.
- Maintenance of weight loss requires constant vigilance: a nylon waist cord provides a warning of unwanted weight regain.

Follow-up and management
- A reasonable target weight (i.e. in grade I) and rate of weight loss (i.e. 0.5–1.0 kg/week) should be set.
- The following errors must be avoided: unrealistic expectations about targets; dietetic incompetence by doctor or patient; misinformation about 'wonder cures'; mutual recrimination between doctor and patient from failure to appreciate that dieting is tedious and difficult.

Key references
Anonymous: Gastrointestinal surgery for severe obesity. NIH Consensus Development Conference; March 25–27, 1991. Washington: National Institutes of Health, 1991.
Garrow JS: Treatment of obesity. *Lancet* 1992, **340**:409–413.
Manson JE *et al.*: A prospective study of obesity and risk of coronary heart disease in women. *N Engl J Med* 1990, **322**:822–829.

Phaeochromocytoma — P.M. Stewart

Diagnosis

Symptoms
- Symptoms are usually paroxysmal, resulting from tumour release of catecholamines with stimulation of adrenergic receptors.
- If asked, patients often report a feeling of 'impending doom'; up to 20%, however, are asymptomatic; flushing is not typical.

Headache: in 80% of patients.
Sweating: in 70%.
Palpitations: in 70%.
Pallor: in 40%.
Nausea: in 40%.
Tremor: in 30%.
Weakness: in 30%.
Anxiety: in 20%.
Epigastric pain: in 20%.
Chest pain: in 20%.
Dyspnoea: in 20%.
Constipation: in 10%

Signs
Hypertension: in >90% of patients (sustained in 60% or paroxysmal in 30%); malignant hypertension possible, retinopathy common, paradoxically postural hypotension (secondary to reduction in plasma volume) frequent.

Supraventricular tachycardia, myocardial ischaemia and infarction, cardiomyopathy, and heart failure.

Fever, weight loss.

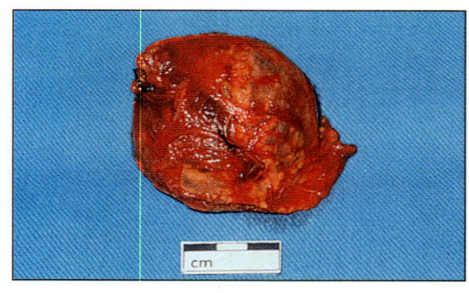

Operative specimen of a phaeochromocytoma.

Differential diagnosis
Thyrotoxicosis, hypoglycaemia, migraine.
Labile 'essential' hypertension, tachyarrhythmia, angina.
Anxiety neurosis.
Cerebellar tumours (rare).

Aetiology
- Phaeochromocytomas are tumours of chromaffin tissue, secreting predominantly noradrenaline (85%).
- The cause of sporadic cases is unknown.
- Familial causes include the following:

Multiple endocrine neoplasia type II: hyperparathyroidism, medullary thyroid cancer.
Neurofibromatosis.
Von Hippel–Lindau disease: cerebellar or retinal haemangioblastoma, renal carcinoma.

Epidemiology
- Phaeochromocytoma is found in 0.1% of hypertensive patients.

Investigations

To establish the diagnosis
- Plasma catecholamines and provocative tests are of limited value.

Urinalysis: to measure metanephrines, free catecholamines (adrenaline, noradrenaline), vanillylmandelic acid; 24-h collection using an acid-containing bottle mandatory (30 ml 6N HCl); possible false-positive results due to interfering medications (propranolol, labetalol, methyldopa, clonidine withdrawal).

To localize the disorder
- These investigations should be done only after biochemical diagnosis has been made.

CT or MRI of abdomen: >95% specificity, >55% sensitivity.

^{131}I-meta-iodobenzylguanidine scintigraphy, imaging of other regions (thorax, head and neck): to detect extra-abdominal tumours; can be considered if imaging of abdomen negative; successful localization after scintigraphy with ^{131}I-somatostatin has been reported.

Complications
Diabetes mellitus.

Hypercalcaemia: suggesting a malignant phaeochromocytoma or multiple endocrine neoplasia.

Malignant phaeochromocytoma: in 10% of patients.

Myocardial infarction.

Pulmonary oedema.

Cerebrovascular accident.

Paralytic ileus.

Treatment

Diet and lifestyle
- No special precautions are necessary.

Pharmacological treatment

Alpha blockade
- Alpha blockers should always precede beta blockers.

Standard dosage	Phenoxybenzamine 20 mg orally twice daily, increasing by 20 mg every second day to 200 mg daily maximum.
Contraindications	None.
Special points	Control of hypertension and paroxysms with abolition of postural hypotension monitored to assess response. Hypertensive crises can be treated by phentolamine 2–5 mg i.v.
Main drug interactions	None.
Main side effects	Postural hypotension, tachycardia, inhibition of ejaculation, nasal congestion, gastrointestinal irritation, fatigue.

Beta blockade
- Tachycardia can be treated by propranolol. Unopposed beta blockade, however, should be avoided, as should combined alpha and beta blockade preparations.
- Alpha-methyl-tyrosine is usually reserved for patients with malignant phaeochromocytomas or those who have failed to respond to surgery.

Standard dosage	Propranolol 40 mg 3 times daily, increased as needed to 240 mg daily maximum. Alpha-methyl-tyrosine 250 mg initially 4 times daily, increasing to 4 g daily.
Contraindications	*Propranolol*: severe asthma, heart failure (possibility of catecholamine-induced cardiomyopathy). *Alpha-methyl-tyrosine*: hypersensitivity.
Special points	*Alpha-methyl-tyrosine*: dose monitored by titrating with clinical features and catecholamine excretion.
Main drug interactions	*Propranolol*: verapamil reduces myocardial contractility; phenytoin or rifampicin increases clearance; cimetidine reduces clearance. *Alpha-methyl-tyrosine*: phenothiazines or haloperidol.
Main side effects	*Propranolol*: bradycardia, atrioventricular block, claudication, tiredness, vivid dreams, bronchospasm, gastrointestinal disturbances. *Alpha-methyl-tyrosine*: sedation, diarrhoea in 10% of patients, anxiety, vivid dreams, extrapyramidal side effects, crystalluria (reduced by high fluid intake).

For malignant disease
- Patients can be given therapeutic doses of ^{131}I meta-iodobenzylguanidine, chemotherapy, alpha or beta blockade, or alpha-methyl-tyrosine.

Treatment aims
To normalize blood pressure.
To eradicate tumour.

Other treatments
Resection of metastatic deposits, when possible, for patients with malignant disease. Adrenalectomy for patients with an adrenal tumour.
- Inadequate surgical preparation can result in precipitous hypertension during induction for surgery and severe hypotension after removal of the tumour; this is minimized by alpha and beta blockade for at least 2 weeks before surgery and the use of plasma volume expanders if needed.
- During surgery, patients can be given i.v. phentolamine or nitroprusside for hypertensive episodes.

Prognosis
- Blood pressure is restored in 70% of patients postoperatively.
- Failure to lower blood pressure may reflect a second tumour, operative damage to renal vasculature, or secondary haemodynamic changes in a hypertensive patient.
- The 5-year survival rate for patients with malignant disease is 35%.

Follow-up and management
- Urinary catecholamine excretion should be measured 1 week postoperatively and, if normal, annually for 5 years.

Key references
Kaplan NM: Phaeochromocytoma. In *Clinical Hypertension* edn 6. Edited by Kaplan NM. Baltimore: Williams and Wilkins, 1994, pp 367–387.

Orchard T *et al.*: Phaeochromocytoma – continuing evolution of surgical therapy. *Surgery* 1993, **114**:1153–1158.

Young WF Jr: Phaeochromocytoma: 1926–1993. *Trends Endocrinol Metab* 1993, **4**:122–127.

Polycystic ovarian disease
R. Fox and D. Cahill

Diagnosis

Symptoms
Heavy menstruation, oligomenorrhoea or amenorrhoea: endometrium remains oestrogenized, in contrast with other causes of anovulation.
Infertility: anovulatory.
Recurrent miscarriage: associated with hypersecretion of luteinizing hormone.
Mild androgenism: hirsutism, acne, seborrhoea.
Severe virilization: alopecia, voice change, clitoromegaly.

Signs
- The syndrome associated with polycystic ovaries is extremely variable; in most women with polycystic ovaries, the endocrine disturbance is subtle and the disorder has no outward signs.

Obesity.
Central adiposity.
Mild hypertension.
Hirsutism: documented by photography or Ferriman–Gallway score.
Acanthosis nigricans and pseudo-acromegaly: features of severe insulin resistance.
- Abdominal and pelvic examinations are rarely helpful but should be done to exclude ovarian masses.

Investigations
- The aims are to make a positive diagnosis, to exclude other causes of anovulation, infertility, recurrent miscarriage and virilization as appropriate, and to screen for features of insulin resistance (syndrome X).
- Diagnosis of polycystic ovarian disease should incorporate both an endocrine and a morphological assessment.

For the disorder
Endocrine tests: non-raised follicle-stimulating hormone (<10 IU/L; all patients); raised luteinizing hormone (>10 IU/L; <30% on single sample); positive progestogen challenge.
Transvaginal ovarian ultrasonography: increased follicularity with expanded stromal compartment.

For other causes
Ultrasonography: to examine endometrium, possibly with endometrial biopsy (menstrual disorder); to diagnose small intra-ovarian tumours (virilization).
Full blood count: to rule out anaemia (menstrual disorder).
Serum testosterone measurement: tumour more likely if concentration >6 nmol/L (virilization).
Serum ferritin measurement: low concentration contributes to alopecia (virilization).

For features of insulin resistance (risk factors for cardiovascular disease)
Blood pressure measurement.
Glucose tolerance test: especially during pregnancy and sex-steroid therapy.
Serum lipid measurement.

Complications
Endometrial cancer: despite anovulation, ovaries continue to secrete oestradiol.
Diabetes mellitus, myocardial infarction, stroke: related to insulin resistance.

Differential diagnosis
Classic syndrome
Hypothyroidism.
Cushing's syndrome.
Acromegaly.
Androgen-secreting tumour.
Oestrogenized amenorrhoea
Granulosa cell tumour.

Aetiology
- Causes include the following:
Insulin receptor dysfunction.
Adrenal hyperandrogenaemia.

Epidemiology
- 10–20% of apparently normal women are found to have polycystic ovaries on ultrasonography.
- 1% of young women (15–40 years) have clinically evident disease.
- Family studies show the prevalence of polycystic ovaries to be high among asymptomatic close relatives (80%).
- 50–60% of women with anovulation are found to have polycystic ovaries on ultrasonography (30% in amenorrhoea, 90% in oligomenorrhoea).
- The disease is a factor in ~10% of couples with infertility and ~50% of cases of recurrent abortion.

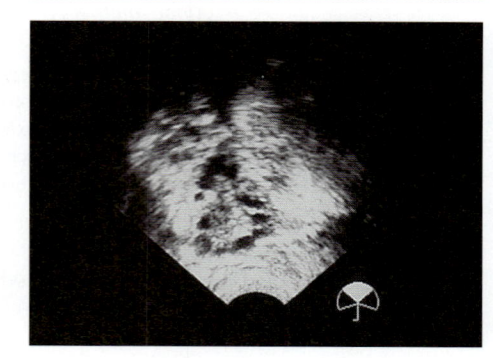

Transvaginal ultrasound scan of polycystic ovary showing multiple small follicles and echodense stroma.

Treatment

Diet and lifestyle
- In view of the increased risk of cardiovascular disease, advice should be given about diet, smoking, and exercise.
- An energy-restricted diet may help by improving ovarian function.
- Women with oligo- or amenorrhoea not wishing to conceive should be warned of the small risk of conception.

Pharmacological treatment
- Pregnancy must be ruled out before treatment begins.

For menstrual disorder
Combined oral contraceptive to improve regularity or reduce flow.

Cyclical progestogen or combined oral contraceptive to prevent endometrial neoplasia in women with oligo- or amenorrhoea.
- Treatment is contraindicated in patients with undiagnosed abnormal menstruation.

For anovulatory infertility
- Each treatment should be tried in turn, starting with the simplest.
- After ovulation has been established, an adequate trial of treatment is needed (9 months).

Anti-oestrogen treatment (clomiphene): acts through the hypothalamus.

Laparoscopic ovarian surgery.

Exogenous gonadotrophin treatment involves direct ovarian stimulation with human menopausal gonadotrophin (hMG) or human follicle stimulating hormone (hFSH), with human chorionic gonadotrophin (hCG) to trigger ovulation.

Standard dosage	*Anti-oestrogen:* clomiphene 100 mg orally daily on days 2–6 of cycle for up to 3 cycles. *Exogenous gonadotrophin:* hMG or hFSH 75 units s.c. daily.
Contraindications	Pregnancy, hormone-dependent tumours, undiagnosed abnormal menstruation.
Special points	*Anti-oestrogen:* near-normal conception rates expected; low risk of high-order multiple pregnancy (8% twin rate) and ovarian hyperstimulation; minimal monitoring needed (midluteal serum progesterone measurement). *Gonadotrophin:* risk of multiple pregnancy and ovarian hyperstimulation; detailed monitoring mandatory (serial follicle scanning and oestradiol measurement); no clear benefit of pure hFSH over hMG.
Main drug interactions	None.
Main side effects	*Anti-oestrogen:* hot flushes, mild abdominal discomfort, visual disturbance (rare). *Gonadotrophin:* nausea, abdominal discomfort, allergy.

For recurrent miscarriage
Luteinizing hormone-releasing hormone agonist, with superovulation (hMG/hCG); risks of multiple pregnancy and ovarian hyperstimulation.

Laparoscopic ovarian surgery.

For virilization
Combined oral contraceptive containing cyproterone acetate.

Combined oral contraceptive and high-dose cyproterone acetate: reduces libido; liver function must be checked; feminization of male fetus.

Flutamide: gastric upset common; possible feminization of male fetus.

Cimetidine: modest effect only.

Low-dose nocturnal corticosteroids: relatively ineffective, promote weight gain.

Spironolactone.

Ferrous sulphate: may improve alopecia if ferritin level is low.

Treatment aims
To prevent long-term health risks (syndrome X).
To alleviate symptoms.
To restore fertility.

Other treatments
Shaving, bleaching, electrolysis: for hirsutism.
Laparoscopic ovarian surgery: electrodiathermy or laser drilling; 80% ovulation rate; near-normal conception rate; normal twin rate and low miscarriage rate; effect lasts about 9 months on average.

Prognosis
- Acne and seborrhoea respond within a few weeks, but the duration of the hair cycle means that improvement in hair growth may take many months.
- Symptoms generally return quickly after withdrawal of treatment.

Follow-up and management
- Follow up varies according to the disorder.

Key references
Conway GS *et al.*: Risk factors for coronary artery disease in lean and obese women with polycystic ovary syndrome. *Clin Endocrinol* 1992, **37**:119–125.

Fox R *et al.*: Oestrogen and androgen states in oligo-amenorrhoeic women with polycystic ovaries. *Br J Obstet Gynaecol* 1991, **98**:294–299.

Fox R *et al.*: Polycystic ovarian disease: diagnostic methods. *Contemp Rev Obstet Gynaecol* 1992, **4**:84–89.

Pubertal abnormalities — M.O. Savage

Diagnosis

Symptoms

Precocious puberty
Pubertal development <8 years in girls, <9 years in boys.
Rapid growth.
Menstruation in girls.
Advanced skeletal maturation.
Behavioural disturbance.

Delayed puberty
Lack of pubertal development >14 years in girls, >15 years in boys.
Lack of pubertal growth spurt.
Small external genitalia in boys.
Possible anosmia.
Emotional disturbance, lack of confidence.

Signs

Precocious puberty
Secondary isosexual sexual development.
Tall stature.
Gynaecomastia in boys.
Cutaneous pigmentation: McCune–Albright syndrome.
Acne, clitoromegaly: indicating virilization in girls.

Delayed puberty
Lack of secondary sexual development.
Short stature.
Signs of Turner's syndrome in girls.
Chronic paediatric illness: e.g. Crohn's disease, thalassaemia.
Family history of delayed puberty.

Investigations

Precocious puberty
Hormone measurement: for gonadotrophin and sex steroid concentrations.
CT of hypothalamic–pituitary region: to exclude structural lesion.
Ovarian ultrasonography: to assess ovarian development.
Adrenal CT: for gonadotrophin-independent precocious puberty.

Delayed puberty
Full blood count, ESR and electrolytes analysis, liver function tests: to exclude chronic disease.
Hormone measurement: for gonadotrophin and sex steroid concentrations.
Karyotyping: in girls.
Clomiphene test: in older patients, to exclude gonadotrophin-releasing hormone deficiency.
Ovarian ultrasonography: to assess ovarian development.
Test of smell: to exclude Kallmann's syndrome.
CT of hypothalamic–pituitary region: to exclude structural lesion.

Complications

Precocious puberty
Progression of pubertal development.
Menstruation.
Advance of skeletal maturation.
Adult tall stature.

Delayed puberty
No secondary sexual development.
Absent pubertal growth.
Adult short stature.
Emotional, physical immaturity.
Psychological disturbance.
Infertility.

Differential diagnosis

Not applicable.

Aetiology

- Causes include the following:

True precocious puberty (gonadotrophin-dependent)
Idiopathic (principally girls).
Structural lesions of hypothalamic region (tumours).
Post-cranial irradiation.
Hydrocephalus.
Hypothyroidism.

Pseudoprecocious puberty (gonadotrophin-independent)
McCune–Albright syndrome.
Adrenal tumours.
Congenital adrenal hyperplasia.
Gonadal tumours.
Testotoxicosis.
Human chorionic gonadotrophin secreting tumours.
Exogenous sex steroids.

Delayed puberty
Constitutional.
Chronic paediatric illness.
Malnutrition.
Hypopituitarism (idiopathic, tumours).
Isolated gonadotrophin-releasing hormone deficiency and anosmia (Kallmann's syndrome).
Hyperprolactinaemia.
Exercise (gymnasts).
Turner or Klinefelter syndromes.
Radiotherapy, surgery, chemotherapy, autoimmunity.

Epidemiology

- No data have been published.

Treatment

Diet and lifestyle
- No special precautions are necessary.

Pharmacological treatment

For true precocious puberty
- Primary CNS lesions, e.g. tumours, must be treated.

Gonadotropin-releasing hormone analogue (e.g. goserelin) fixed dose s.c. injection monthly or cyproterone acetate 50–100 mg daily; treatment continued until appropriate age for puberty to progress.

- Long-term cyproterone treatment may induce adrenal insufficiency.

For pseudoprecocious puberty
- The primary cause or congenital adrenal hyperplasia must be treated.

Cyproterone acetate 50–100 mg daily.

Testolactone up to 40 mg/kg/day for McCune–Albright syndrome.

For delayed puberty
- The primary cause must be treated, e.g. chronic illness, pituitary tumour, hyperprolactinaemia.

For boys: oxandrolone 1.25–2.5 mg orally daily for 6–12 months; depot testosterone from 50 mg 2-weekly to 500 mg monthly i.m. depending on age.

For girls: ethinyloestradiol 2–10 µg daily, increasing to 30 µg daily with norethistone or medroxyprogesterone acetate 5 mg daily on days 1–14 of each calendar month.

Treatment aims
To replace hormones.

Prognosis
- Prognosis is always good unless the disorder is caused by a tumour.

Follow-up and management
- Patients should be checked every 3–6 months to ensure that treatment is effective.

Key references
Bridges NA, Brook CDG: Premature sexual development. In *Clinical Endocrinology*. Edited by Grossman A. Oxford: Blackwell Scientific Publications, 1992, pp 837–846.

Stanhope R, Albanese A, Shalet S: Delayed puberty. *BMJ* 1992, **305**:790.

Syndrome of inappropriate antidiuresis — P.H. Baylis

Diagnosis

Symptoms
- Mild chronic hyponatraemia (serum sodium concentration 125–135 mmol/L) may be asymptomatic.
- More profound hyponatraemia (serum sodium concentration <120 mmol/L) can cause the following:

Headache.*	Confusion.	Seizures.
Malaise.	Depression.	Coma.
Nausea and vomiting.	Cramps.	Death.
Irritability.	Drowsiness.	

*The severity of the symptoms depends on the rate of fall of serum sodium as much as on the absolute value.

Signs
- Mild chronic hyponatraemia usually has no specific signs.
- Severe hyponatraemia may cause the following:

Diminished reflexes.
Extensor plantar responses.

Cardinal features
Dilutional hyponatraemia: plasma osmolality appropriately low for serum sodium.
Urine osmolality greater than plasma osmolality.
Persistent renal sodium excretion.
Absence of hypotension, hypovalaemia, or oedema-forming states.
Normal thyroid, renal and adrenal function.

Investigations
- Laboratory tests are not specific for the diagnosis but help to exclude other causes of hyponatraemia and to identify underlying causes.

Chest radiography: to check for lung cancer.
Serum sodium measurement: low concentration.
Plasma osmolality measurement: <270 mOsm/kg.
Blood glucose measurement: to exclude spurious hyponatraemia in hyperglycaemia.
Serum protein and lipoprotein measurement: to exclude pseudohyponatraemia.
Serum uric acid measurement: low concentration.
Urine osmolality measurement: usually >300 mOsm/kg.
Renal function tests: creatinine clearance rate or serum creatinine concentration.
Thyroid function tests: thyroxine, thyroid-stimulating hormone; to exclude hypothyroidism.
Adrenocortical tests: short Synacthen test; to exclude cortisol deficiency.
Plasma vasopressin measurement.
Pituitary function tests: to exclude adrenocorticotrophic hormone deficiency.
Pituitary fossa radiography.

Complications
Permanent neurological deficit, high neurological morbidity and mortality: caused by prolonged profound hyponatraemia or aggressive treatment leading to rapid rise in serum sodium concentration..

Differential diagnosis

Hyponatraemia associated with hypervolaemia
Cardiac failure.
Cirrhosis.
Nephrotic syndrome.
Renal failure.

Hyponatraemia associated with hypovolaemia
Gastrointestinal fluid loss.
Severe burns.
Mineralocorticoid deficiency (i.e. Addison's disease).
Salt-losing nephritis.

Aetiology
- Causes include the following:

Neoplastic disease: e.g. lung cancer, pancreatic cancer, lymphoma.
Chest disorders: e.g. pneumonia, tuberculosis, abscess.
Neurological disorders: e.g. head injury, infections, haemorrhage.
Drugs: e.g. thiazides, cytotoxic agents, carbamazepine.

Epidemiology
- Hyponatraemia is the most common electrolyte disturbance seen in hospitals (~10% of patients have serum sodium concentrations of <130 mmol/L).
- ~50% of all hyponatraemia is due to the syndrome of inappropriate diuresis.

Treatment

Diet and lifestyle
- Fluid should be restricted to 0.5–1.0 L daily.
- Patients must eat a well balanced diet.

Pharmacological treatment
- The underlying cause of the syndrome should be treated (e.g. cancer of the bronchus).
- Specific V_2-receptor antagonists to block the antidiuretic effect of vasopressin are awaited.

Induction of partial nephrogenic diabetes insipidus
Standard dosage	Demeclocycline 1.2 g in divided doses. Lithium carbonate 0.4–1.2 g daily.
Contraindications	*Demeclocycline*: renal failure, pregnancy, children. *Lithium carbonate:* renal and cardiac disease.
Special points	*Demeclocycline:* full effect may need up to 3 weeks of treatment. *Lithium carbonate:* plasma concentrations must be measured.
Main drug interactions	*Demeclocycline:* warfarin. *Lithium carbonate:* diuretics, antibiotics, antihypertensives, sumtriptan.
Main side effects	*Demeclocycline:* nausea, diarrhoea, photosensitivity. *Lithium carbonate:* gastrointestinal disturbances, goitre, CNS dysfunction.

Inhibition of neurohypophysial vasopressin secretion
Standard dosage	Phenytoin 300 mg daily.
Contraindications	Renal and hepatic dysfunction, porphyria.
Main drug interactions	Antibacterials, anxiolytic, hypnotics, calcium antagonists.
Main side effects	Drowsiness, ataxia.

Induction of diuresis and natriuresis
Standard dosage	Frusemide 40–80 mg daily and slow sodium chloride 3 g orally daily.
Contraindications	Decompensated liver cirrhosis; caution in prostatism.
Main drug interactions	Antifungals, potassium-losing drugs.
Main side effects	Hypokalaemia, gastrointestinal disturbances.

Treatment aims
To relieve symptoms of hyponatraemia. To increase serum sodium concentration to 125–140 mmol/L.

Prognosis
- This depends on the underlying cause.
- Patients with serum sodium concentrations <110 mmol/L have high morbidity and mortality (~50%).
- Development of osmotic demyelination syndrome indicates poor prognosis (~50% mortality).

Follow-up and management
- Depending on the underlying condition, fluid restriction or drug treatment may be needed indefinitely.
- Serum sodium concentrations must be checked monthly.

Osmotic demyelination syndrome
- This occurs after rapid correction of chronic severe hyponatraemia, irrespective of the means of increasing serum sodium concentrations.
- It is found in central pontine and intracerebral structures.
- It is clinically evident 2–4 days after correction of serum sodium concentrations.
- It can be avoided by increasing serum sodium by <0.5 mmol/L/h.

Key references
Arieff AI: Management of hyponatraemia. *BMJ* 1993, **307**:307–308.

Ayus JC, Arieff AI: Pathogenesis and prevention of hyponatraemic encephalopathy. *Endocrinol Metab Clin North Am* 1993, **22**:425–446.

Baylis PH, Thompson CJ: Osmoregulation of vasopressin and thirst in health and disease. *Clin Endocrinol* 1988, **29**:549–576.

Berl T *et al.*: Clinical disorders of water metabolism. *Kidney Int* 1976, **10**:117–132.

Robertson GL: Syndrome of inappropriate antidiuresis. *N Engl J Med* 1989, **321**:538–539.

Sterns RH, Riggs, J, Achochet SS: Osmotic demyelination syndrome following correction of hyponatraemia. *N Engl J Med* 1986, **314**:1535–1542.

Testicular disorders
D.C. Anderson

Diagnosis

Symptoms and signs

Delayed puberty and hypogonadism
Failure to gain sufficient weight: in children (picky eaters or anorexic).
Severe weight loss and malnutrition: in adults.
Poor virilization, tall stature with long limbs, gynaecomastia, failure to develop sex drive, nocturnal emissions or masturbation; small firm testes, partial puberty, azoospermia: indicating Klinefelter's syndrome.
Hypergonadotrophic gonadism, progressive decline in sperm count: azoospermia within months, with later progressive decline in Leydig cell function; after testicular irradiation or chemotherapy.
Failure of puberty, and eunuchoidism: indicating isolated gonadotrophin deficiency.
Anosmia: indicating Kallmann's syndrome.
Evidence of pituitary tumour or past damage, hormonal deficiencies, absence of secondary sexual hair: indicating pituitary failure.
Mild hypogonadism with Turner's features, pulmonary stenosis: indicating Noonan's syndrome.
Obesity, micropenis, hypotonia, mental retardation, moderate hypogonadism: indicating Prader–Willi syndrome.

Adult male infertility
Diminished sperm count, defective sperm motility.
Absent or obstructed epididymis or vas deferens, post-epididymitis or seminal vesiculitis: indicating obstruction.
Post-orchitis, torsion, incomplete testicular descent: indicating tubular damage.
Swelling: sometimes painful; empties on lying down; indicating varicocoele.
Dystrophia myotonica-myotonia, cataracts, frontal alopecia, mental impairment, testicular atrophy with generally normal virilization, peritubular fibrosis.
Mental retardation, mild dysmorphic features, large testes as adults: indicating fragile X syndrome.

Male pseudohermaphroditism
Normal female genitalia, primary amenorrhoea: indicating failure of testis to develop.
Inguinal testes, female external genitalia with short, blind vagina, female breasts at puberty, scant secondary sexual hair: indicating defective androgen receptor.

Investigations
Hormone tests: single clotted blood for serum luteinizing hormone, follicle-stimulating hormone, prolactin and testosterone; 17-hydroxyprogesterone in well virilized patients possibly with early puberty with small testes and suppressed gonadotrophins (congenital adrenal hyperplasia); raised follicle-stimulating hormone with oligo- or azoospermia indicates almost certain irreversible primary testicular damage; dynamic tests add little more.
Serum oestradiol measurement: for gynaecomastia.
Karyotyping: for Klinefelter's syndrome in hypergonadotrophic hypogonadism.
Semen morphology, count, motility, and post-coital test.
Immunology: mixed agglutination reaction, to detect anti-sperm antibodies.
Testicular biopsy: not often indicated.
Ultrasonography: for testicular masses or prostatic disease.
Pituitary CT or nuclear MRI: for possible tumours.

Complications

Delayed puberty and hypogonadism
Major psychological damage: if untreated at puberty.
Long-term increased risk of fracture: especially vertebral and hip.

Infertility
Androgen deficiency: in severe disorders or spermatogenesis.
Psychosocial problems.

Male pseudohermaphroditism
Psychological damage: without effective and sympathetic handling at outset.
Malignancy: in XY patients with streak gonads.

Differential diagnosis
Delayed puberty and hypogonadism
Growth-hormone deficiency.

Male pseudohermaphroditism
Female pseudohermaphroditism.

Aetiology
- Causes include the following:
Genetic factors: X-linked in testicular feminization, microdeletion, chromosome 15 abnormality in Prader–Willi syndrome.
Hormone or enzyme deficiencies.
Testicular irradiation or chemotherapy.

Epidemiology
- Male pseudohermaphroditism is rare.
- Testicular feminization occurs in 1 in 60 000 males.
- Kallmann's syndrome occurs in 1 in 10 000 males.
- Prader–Willi syndrome occurs in 1 in 10 000–20 000 births.
- Congenital adrenal hyperplasia occurs in 1 in 7000 people.
- All other enzyme deficiencies are much rarer.
- Delayed puberty, oligospermia, and azoospermia are all common.
- Gynaecomastia occurs in one-third of boys in puberty; it is common later in life.

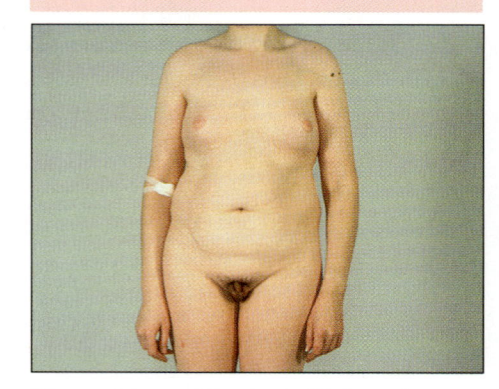

26-year-old man with untreated Kallmann's syndrome.

D.C. Anderson | **Testicular disorders**

Treatment

Diet and lifestyle
- Most phenotypic female patients with androgen-receptor disorders (male pseudo-hermaphroditism, testicular feminization, pure XY gonadal dysgenesis) are raised as females.
- Patients with 5α-reductase deficiency generally identify as male.

Pharmacological treatment
- For each patient, the relative importance of androgen deficiency and infertility and practicability of treatment must be defined clearly.

For androgen deficiency
Standard dosage	Testosterone undecanoate 80 mg orally twice daily. Primoteston depot 250 mg i.m. every 2–3 weeks. Sustanon (mixed testosterone esters) 250 mg i.m. every 2–3 weeks. *For gonadotrophin deficiency, when fertility is desired:* pulsatile gonadotrophin-releasing hormone 15 µg s.c. every 90 min by pump, or human chorionic gonadotrophin 2000 IU s.c. twice weekly or 5000 IU s.c. weekly, with subsequent menotrophin 225 IU 3 times weekly.
Contraindications	Caution if history of violent behaviour.
Special points	*Gonadotrophin replacement:* sperm count should rise for 6 months; sperm may be stored in sperm bank for future use; menotrophin very expensive.
Main drug interactions	None.
Main side effects	Secondary sexual characteristics, balding, stimulation of prostatic hyperplasia; gynaecomastia with human chorionic gonadotrophin therapy.

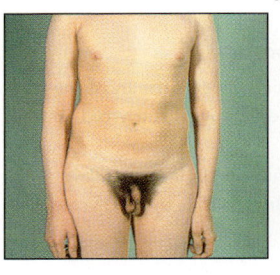

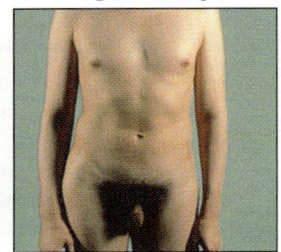

Hypogonadal patient with partial gonadotrophin deficiency (fertile eunuch syndrome) before (left) and after (right) 1 year's treatment with twice-weekly human chorionic gonadotrophin.

For male congenital adrenal hyperplasia
Standard dosage	Glucocorticosteroid, e.g. hydrocortisone 15–30 mg daily in divided doses. *For salt-losers:* mineralocorticosteroid replacement (fludrocortisone 50 µg twice daily).
Contraindications	None.
Special points	Adrenocorticotrophic hormone suppression should restore normal gonadotrophins and spermatogenesis.
Main drug interactions	With hepatic enzyme inducers (e.g. rifampicin), more glucocorticosteroid and mineralocorticosteroid are needed.
Main side effects	Hypercortisolism with excessive glucocorticosteroid.

For 5α-reductase deficiency
- Patients should be treated by high-dose testosterone, e.g. Sustanon 250 mg weekly.

For gynaecomastia
- The cause should be removed if possible.
- Danazol in low doses is worth a therapeutic trial.
- Surgery (mastectomy through peri-areolar incision) is indicated for severe cases.

Treatment aims
To restore virilization and normal sex drive and potency.
To prevent long-term risk of osteoporotic fracture.

Prognosis
- Androgen deficiency itself does not adversely affect life-expectancy.
- Prader–Willi syndrome and dystrophia myotonica do adversely affect life expectancy.

Follow-up and management
- Regular attendance is necessary for testosterone treatment.
- Patients with germ-cell damage should have annual measurement of serum luteinizing hormone, follicle-stimulating hormone, and testosterone, with onset of androgen replacement early rather than late.

Key references
Anderson DC: Endocrine diseases. In *Textbook of Medicine* edn 2. Edited by Souhami RL, Moxham J. London: Churchill Livingstone, 1994, pp 706–718.

Anderson DC, Large DM: Endocrine function of the testis: normal and abnormal. In *Scientific Foundation of Urology* edn 3. Edited by Chisholm GD, Fair WR. Oxford: Heinemann, 1990, pp 379–390.

Griffen JE, Wilson JD: Disorders of the testes and male reproductive tract. In *Williams Textbook of Endocrinology* edn 8. Edited by Wilson JD, Foster DW. Philadelphia: WB Saunders, 1992, pp 799–852.

Grumbach MM, Conte FA: Disorders of sex differentiation. In *Williams Textbook of Endocrinology* edn 8. Edited by Wilson JD, Foster DW. Philadelphia: WB Saunders, 1992, pp 853–951.

Thyroid carcinoma — M.C. Sheppard

Diagnosis

Symptoms
- Patients can be asymptomatic (thyroid swelling is noted by someone else).

Neck swelling: rapid increase in size (particularly important symptom if patient is taking thyroid hormone).

Pain in neck, radiating to jaw or ear.

Dysphagia.

Dyspnoea.

Dysphonia.

Symptoms of thyrotoxicosis: rare.

Bone pain, haemoptysis, abdominal discomfort: indicating metastases.

Signs
Thyroid swelling (goitre): single nodule, multinodular, diffuse.

Cancer: most common in single nodules, least in diffuse goitre.

Fixation of thyroid swelling to local structures.

Cervical lymphadenopathy.

Spinal-cord compression, spastic paraparesis.

Hepatomegaly, bone swellings, tenderness: indicating metastases.

Investigations
- No laboratory test distinguishes malignant from benign lesions of the thyroid.

Thyroid function tests: serum free thyroxine and thyroid-stimulating hormone to exclude hyperthyroidism and hypothyroidism.

Thyroid autoantibody tests.

Serum calcitonin measurement: raised concentration (basal or stimulated) in medullary thyroid cancer.

Fine-needle aspiration cytology: routine preoperative evaluation of most patients with thyroid nodules.

Ultrasonography: to detect solid, solitary nodules (with greater risk of malignancy).

Isotope scanning: to detect hypofunctioning, solitary nodules (with greater risk of malignancy).

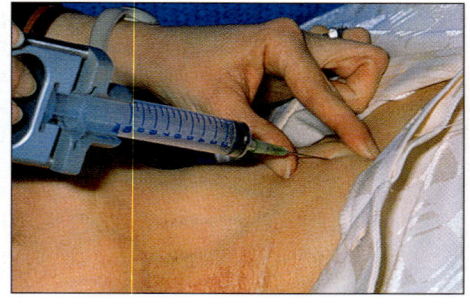

Fine-needle aspiration of a thyroid nodule, allowing rapid cytological examination of aspirated material.

Serum thyroglobulin evaluation: of no use for diagnosis; great value in monitoring treated patients.

Complications
Local infiltration of trachea, oesophagus, nerves.

Metastases of bone, liver, lung.

Differential diagnosis
Benign thyroid disease: diffuse goitre, single or multiple nodules.
Hashimoto's disease.
Other causes of lymphadenopathy.

Aetiology
- Causes include the following:
External irradiation of head and neck.
Iodine deficiency.
Proto-oncogene expression (ptc oncogene unique to papillary thyroid cancer).
Genetic: medullary cancer in multiple endocrine neoplasia syndrome.

Epidemiology
- Thyroid cancer accounts for <0.5% of new malignancies and <0.5% of cancer deaths.
- Goitre, including thyroid nodules, is present in up to 10% of the population.
- The female:male ratio is 3:1.
- The risk of malignancy is increased when nodules develop in people aged >60 years.

Tumour pathology
- Papillary thyroid cancer is the most frequently diagnosed malignant thyroid tumour.
- Follicular thyroid cancer is a relatively unusual malignancy (~15% of all thyroid cancers).
- Hurthle cell cancer occurs in 3–6% of patients.
- Anaplastic cancer accounts for <10% of patients.

Treatment

Diet and lifestyle
- No evidence indicates that environmental factors affect the prognosis of established thyroid cancer.
- An iodine-replete diet and avoidance of external irradiation to head and neck reduces the risk of developing thyroid cancer.

Pharmacological treatment
- After surgery, patients can be considered for radioiodine treatment.
- No consensus has been reached on ^{131}I ablation of the thyroid in patients with small solitary papillary lesions.
- Routine ablation of thyroid remnant is indicated in patients with follicular thyroid cancer.
- Ablation has a clear role in the management of residual disease or established metastases.
- All patients with differentiated thyroid cancer need suppressive thyroxine treatment after definitive treatment; thyroxine is necessary in all patients rendered hypothyroid after treatment.

Non-pharmacological treatment
- The extent of surgery (simple lobectomy, near-total thyroidectomy, total thyroidectomy) depends on pathology and surgical preference.
- Anaplastic thyroid cancer is resistant to treatment; best results are achieved with a combination of surgery, external irradiation, and chemotherapy.
- Surgery is the primary mode of treatment for papillary, follicular, and medullary thyroid cancers.
- Surgical removal of involved lymph nodes is indicated.

Treatment aims
To minimize morbidity and mortality of disease.
To minimize morbidity of diagnostic and therapeutic interventions.

Prognosis
- Prolonged survival is usual.
- Patients with localized papillary or follicular thyroid cancers have an excellent prognosis, (10–20-year recurrence rates of 5–10% and death rates of 2–5%).
- Adverse prognostic factors include older age, greater degree of invasiveness, distant metastases, and abnormal chromosomal number within tumour tissue.
- Anaplastic cancer is very aggressive, with a 5-year survival rate of 7%.

Follow-up and management
- After radioablation of the thyroid, total-body radioiodine scans can detect recurrent or metastatic disease and may be performed at 12-monthly intervals.
- Serum thyroglobulin is a valuable tumour marker; patients with differentiated papillary or follicular thyroid cancers have normal or undetectable concentrations in the absence of tumour but raised concentrations in the presence of residual, recurrent, or metastatic disease.

Key references
DeGroot LJ et al.: Natural history, treatment, and course of papillary thyroid carcinoma. *J Clin Endocrinol Metabol* 1990, **71**:414–424.

Kaplan MM (ed): Thyroid carcinoma. *Endocrinol Metab Clin North Am* 1990, **19, No. 3**.

Samaan NA et al.: The results of different modalities of treatment of well differentiated thyroid carcinoma: a retrospective review of 1599 patients. *J Clin Endocrinol Metab* 1992, **75**:714–720.

Index

A

acarbose for non-insulin-dependent diabetes mellitus 13
acidosis, lactic 30
acne 6, 26, 48, 50
acromegaly 2, 12, 40, 48
ACTH see adrenocorticotrophic hormone
Addison's disease 4, 52
adenomectomy for Cushing's disease 7
adrenal
    adenoma 7
    insufficiency 2, 4, 40
adrenalectomy
    for Cushing's disease 7
    for phaeochromocytoma 47
adrenocorticotrophic hormone
    deficiency 40
    syndrome, ectopic 6
adrenocorticotrophic hormone-dependent Cushing's syndrome 6
alfacalcidol
    for hypoparathyroidism 37
    for renal failure 37
alopecia 48, 54 see also hair loss
alpha
    blockers for phaeochromocytoma 47
    methyl tyrosine for phaeochromocytoma 47
amenorrhoea 2, 20, 22, 32, 40, 48, 54
aminoglutethimide for Cushing's syndrome 7
androgen
    deficiency 54
    for tall stature 27
androgen-secreting tumour 48
androgenism 48
anorexia nervosa 40 see also eating disorders
anosmia 22, 50, 54
antibiotics for infection 19, 31
anticoagulation for hyperglycaemic emergencies 31
antidiuresis, syndrome of inappropriate 52
antidiuretic hormone concentration, raised 4
antihypertensive treatment for diabetic nephropathy 10, 12
antioestrogens
    for anovulatory infertility 49
    for infertility 23
'apronectomy' for obesity 45
arachnodactyly 26 see also Marfan syndrome
arginine vasopressin for diabetes insipidus 9
ataxia, cerebellar 42
atenolol for hyperthyroidism 35
atresia, uterine 22
atrophy
    optic 32
    testicular 54
azoospermia 54

B

balanitis 12
Basedow's disease see Graves' disease
behaviour
    altered 38
    disorder 26
    irrational 38
behavioural disturbances 50
Besnier–Boeck disease see sarcoidosis
beta blockers
    for hyperthyroidism 35
    for phaeochromocytoma 47
biguanide for non-insulin-dependent diabetes mellitus 13
bisphosphonates for hypercalcaemia 29
bladder
    distension 8
    outflow obstruction 8
Boeck's disease see sarcoidosis
breathing see respiration
bromocryptine
    for acromegaly 3
    for hyperprolactinaemia 33

C

cabergoline for hyperprolactinaemia 33
calciferol for vitamin D deficiency 37
calcification
    basal ganglia 36
    corneal 28
    soft-tissue 28
calcitriol
    for hypoparathyroidism 37
    for renal failure 37
calcium gluconate for hypocalcaemia 37
calculi see stones
cancer see also malignancy
    breast 44
    colon 44
    endometrium 44, 48
    ovary 44
    prostate 44
    rectum 44
carbamazepine for diabetes insipidus 9
carbimazole for hyperthyroidism 35
cardiac see also heart
    arrest 14, 30
    failure 2, 34, 42, 52
cardiomyopathy 46
cardiovascular
    collapse 40
    disease 20, 22
carpal tunnel syndrome 2, 42
cataracts 10, 36, 54
cerebrovascular
    accident 32, 46 see also stroke
    disease 6, 10, 12, 30

chemosis 34
chlorpropamide for diabetes insipidus 9
Chvostek's sign 36
cimetidine for virilization 49
cliteromegaly 26, 48, 50
clodronate for hypercalcaemia due to malignancy 29
clomiphene for anovulatory infertility 49
clumsiness 26
cold intolerance 40, 42
coma 10, 38, 42
    hyperglycaemic non-ketotic 12
    hyperosmolar 30
    non-ketotic hyperosmolar 38
compression
    optic chiasma 2, 22, 40
    optic nerve 34
    spinal-cord 56
consciousness
    reduced level 10, 38
    variable level 30
contraceptives, oral
    for menstrual disorders 49
    with cyproterone acetate for virilization 49
convulsions 32 see also epilepsy, seizures
coronary
    artery disease 2, 12
    vascular disease 10, 12
corticosteroids
    for hypercalcaemia due to sarcoidosis 29
    for male congenital adrenal hyperplasia 55
    for sarcoidosis 9
    for virilization 49
cryptomenorrhoea 22
Cushing's
    disease 6, 12
    syndrome 44, 48
        adrenal 6
        adrenocorticotrophic hormone-dependent 6
cyproterone acetate
    for precocious puberty 51
    for pseudoprecocious puberty 51

D

danazol for gynaecomastia 55
DDAVP
    for diabetes insipidus 9
    for posterior pituitary deficiencies 41
dehydration 8, 10, 12, 14, 18, 28, 30
demeclocycline for induction of partial nephrogenic diabetes insipidus 53
desmopressin see DDAVP
desogestrel for female hypogonadism
    hypergonadotrophic 21
    hypogonadotrophic 23
dexamethasone
    for Addison's disease 5
    for deficiencies of pituitary–adrenal axis 41

Index

dextrose
  for diabetic management
    in pregnancy 17
    in surgery 19
  for hyperglycaemic emergencies 31
  for hypoglycaemia 39
diabetes 6
  bronze *see* haemochromatosis
  insipidus 8
  mellitus 2, 6, 8, 46, 48
    adult-onset *see* non-insulin-dependent diabetes mellitus
    gestational 16
    insulin-dependent 10
    juvenile-onset *see* insulin-dependent diabetes mellitus
    ketosis-resistant *see* non-insulin-dependent diabetes mellitus
    non-insulin-dependent 12, 44
    stable *see* non-insulin-dependent diabetes mellitus
    type 1 *see* insulin-dependent diabetes mellitus
    type 2 *see* non-insulin-dependent diabetes mellitus
diabetic
  acidosis *see* diabetic ketoacidosis
  ketoacidosis 10
  ketosis *see* diabetic ketoacidosis
  management in children 14
  management in pregnancy 16
  management in surgery 18
  nephropathy 10, 12, 14, 16
  neuropathy 10, 12, 14
  retinopathy 10, 12, 14, 16
dialysis, continuous ambulatory peritoneal, for diabetic nephropathy 10, 12
diplopia 32, 40
dopamine agonists for hyperprolactinaemia 23, 33
dwarfism *see* short stature
dysmorphic features 24, 26, 54
dysphonia 56 *see also* speech, slurred
dystrophia myotonica–myotonia 54

E

eating disorders 22 *see also* anorexia nervosa
emotional disturbance 50
epididymis, absent or obstructed 54
epilepsy 32, 36, 38, 40 *see also* seizures
ethinyloestradiol
  for deficiencies of pituitary–gonadal axis 41
  for delayed puberty 51
  for female hypogonadism
    hypergonadotrophic 21
    hypogonadotrophic 23
  for short stature 25
  for tall stature 27
etidronate for hypercalcaemia 29
eunuchoidism 54
eyelid retraction 34

F

ferrous sulphate for virilization 49
fibrosis
  peritubular 54
  vitreous 10, 12
fludrocortisone for male congenital adrenal hyperplasia 55
flutamide for virilization 49
follicle-stimulating hormone
  deficiency 40
  human, for anovulatory infertility 49
fracture
  atraumatic 20
  long-term increased risk of 54
  osteoporotic 34
fragile X syndrome 54
frusemide for induction of diuresis and natriuresis 53

G

galactorrhoea 2, 22, 32, 40, 42
gallstones 44
gastric stapling for obesity 45
genitalia
  female, in males 54
  small external, in boys 50
gigantism *see* tall stature
glibenclamide for non-insulin-dependent diabetes mellitus 13, 19
gliclazide for non-insulin-dependent diabetes mellitus 13, 19
glipizide for non-insulin-dependent diabetes mellitus 13
glucagon for hypoglycaemia 11, 39
glucose
  for Addison's disease 5
  for hypoglycaemia 11, 39
  insulin infusion for diabetic management in surgery 19
  tolerance, impaired 44
goitre 2, 24, 34, 42, 56
  exophthalmic *see* Graves' disease
gonadectomy, laparoscopic, for female hypergonadotrophic hypogonadism 21
gonadism, hypergonadotrophic 54
gonadotrophin
  deficiency 2, 54
  for hyperprolactinaemia 23
  for infertility 23
    anovulatory 49
  human
    chorionic
      for androgen deficiency 55
      for anovulatory infertility 49
    menopausal for anovulatory infertility 49
gonadotrophin-releasing hormone
  analogue for precocious puberty 51
  for androgen deficiency 55
goserelin for precocious puberty 51
Graves'
  disease 34
  hyperthyroidism 35
  ophthalmopathy 34
growth
  abnormalities
    short stature 20, 22, 24, 40, 50
    tall stature 26, 50, 54
  disproportionate 24
  hormone
    deficiency 40, 54
    for deficiencies in children 41
    for short stature 25
  poor 40, 42
  rapid 50
  retardation, intrauterine 24
guar gum for non-insulin-dependent diabetes mellitus 13
gut bypass surgery for obesity 45
gynaecomastia 50, 54

H

haemochromatosis 4
haemorrhage, vitreous 10, 12
hair
  absence of secondary sexual 54
  loss 20, 22 *see also* alopecia
    androgenic 6
    axillary 40
    pubic 40
Hashimoto's
  disease 56
  thyroiditis 42
heart *see also* cardiac
  disease
    congenital 16
    ischaemic 6, 42
  failure 42, 46
hemianopia, bitemporal 32
heparin for hyperglycaemic emergencies 31
hiatus hernia 44
hirsutism 6, 48
hormone
  adrenocorticotrophic
    deficiency 40
    syndrome, ectopic 6
  antidiuretic, raised concentration 4
  deficiencies 40, 54
  follicle-stimulating
    deficiency 40
    human, for anovulatory infertility 49
  gonadotrophin-releasing
    analogue for precocious puberty 51
    for androgen deficiency 55
  growth
    deficiency 40, 54
    for deficiencies in children 41
    for short stature 25

Index

hormone *cont.*
  luteinizing
    deficiency 40
    hypersecretion 48
  luteinizing hormone-releasing
    agonist for recurrent miscarriage 49
    pulsatile
      for hyperprolactinaemia 23
      for infertility 23
  thyroid-stimulating, deficiency 40
hydramnios 16
hydrocephalus 32, 40
hydrocortisone
  for Addison's disease 5
  for pituitary–adrenal axis deficiencies 41
  for male congenital adrenal hyperplasia 55
hydronephrosis 8
hydroureter 8
hypercalcaemia 2, 4, 28, 30, 46
hypercalciuria 2
hyperglycaemia 12, 16, 30
hyperkalaemia 4, 14
hyperlipidaemia 42
hyperosmolality 12
hyperparathyroidism 28
hyperplasia
  male congenital adrenal 54
  prostatic 12
hyperprolactinaemia 2, 22, 32
hypertension 2, 6, 14, 44, 46, 48
hyperthyroidism 26, 34 *see also* thyrotoxicosis
hypertrophy, nasopharyngeal soft-tissue 2
hyperventilation 30
hypocalcaemia 16, 36
hypoglycaemia 4, 10, 11, 14, 16, 38, 46
hypogonadism 54
  female
    hypergonadotrophic 20
    hypogonadotrophic 22
hypokalaemia 14
hypomagnesaemia 36
hyponatraemia 4, 52
hypoparathyroidism 4, 36
hypopituitarism 2, 32, 40
hypotension 4, 12, 18, 30
  postural 4, 32, 40, 46
hypothyroidism 2, 4, 24, 32, 42, 44, 48
  congenital 42
  iodine-deficient 42

I

^{131}I meta iodobenzylguanidine for malignant phaeochromocytoma 47
IDDM *see* insulin-dependent diabetes mellitus
immaturity
  emotional 50
  physical 50
impotence 2, 32, 40
infarction, myocardial 18, 30, 44, 46, 48
infection 6, 18, 30
  chest 30
  ear 14
  foot 12
  lung 14
  throat 14
  urinary tract 12, 14
infertility 20, 22, 32, 42, 44, 48, 50, 54
insulin
  for diabetic management
    in children 15
    in pregnancy
    in surgery 19
  for hyperglycaemic emergency 31
  for non-insulin-dependent diabetes mellitus 13
  intermediate-acting for diabetes mellitus 11
  longer-acting for diabetes mellitus 11
  ready-mixed for diabetes mellitus 11
  resistance 48
  short-acting
    for diabetes mellitus 11
    for diabetic management in surgery 19
iodine deficiency 42
ischaemia, myocardial 46

J

jaw wiring for obesity 45
joint
  degeneration 2
  hypermobility 26

K

Kallmann syndrome 22, 54
keratitis, ulcerative *see* corneal ulceration
ketoacidosis 30, 38
  diabetic 10
ketoconazole for Cushing's syndrome 7
ketosis 16, 18
  diabetic *see* diabetic ketoacidosis
kidney *see* renal
Klinefelter syndrome 26, 54
Kussmaul's respiration 10, 14, 30

L

laser treatment for diabetic retinopathy 10, 12
lens dislocation 26
libido
  decreased 32, 40
  impaired 2
liothyronine *see* triiodothyronine
lisuride for hyperprolactinaemia 33
lithium for induction of partial nephrogenic diabetes insipidus 53
lobectomy for thyroid carcinoma 57
luteinizing hormone
  deficiency 40
  hypersecretion 48
luteinizing hormone-releasing hormone
  agonist for recurrent miscarriage 49
  pulsatile
    for hyperprolactinaemia 23
    for infertility 23
lypressin *see* lysin vasopressin
lysin vasopressin for diabetes insipidus 9

M

macroadenoma 32, 40
macroglossia 2
macrosomia 16
malformation
  congenital 16
  uterine 22
malignancy 10, 34 *see also* cancer
  testicular 54
Marfan syndrome 26
mastectomy for gynaecomastia 55
McCune–Albright syndrome 50
medroxyprogesterone
  for pituitary–gonadal axis deficiencies 41
  for delayed puberty 51
menorrhagia 42
menotrophin for androgen deficiency 55
menstruation 50
  erratic 20
  heavy 47
mental impairment 28, 42, 54
metformin for non-insulin-dependent diabetes mellitus 13
metyrapone for Cushing's syndrome 7
micropenis 54
mineralocorticoid
  deficiency 52
  for male congenital adrenal hyperplasia 55
miscarriage, recurrent 48
mitotane for Cushing's syndrome 7
'moon' face 6, 36
myxoedema 42
  'madness' 42
  pretibial 34

N

nadolol for hyperthyroidism 35
neck
  swelling 34, 42, 56
  webbed 20
neoplasia
  gonadal 20
  multiple endocrine 46
nephritis, salt-losing 52
nephropathy, diabetic 10, 12, 14, 16
nephrotic syndrome 52

Index

neuropathy, diabetic 10, 12, 14
NIDDM *see* non-insulin-dependent diabetes mellitus
nitroprusside for phaeochromocytoma 47
nocturnal
  emissions 54
  masturbation 54
Noonan's syndrome 54
norethisterone for delayed puberty 51

O

o,p'DDD *see* mitotane
obesity 6, 12, 36, 44, 48, 54
octreotide for acromegaly 3
oedema
  cerebral 14
  lower limb 6
  pulmonary 46
oestradiol for female hypogonadism
  hypergonadotrophic 21
  hypogonadotrophic 23
oestrogen
  deficiency 20, 22
  for female hypogonadism
    hypergonadotrophic 21
    hypogonadotrophic 23
oligomenorrhoea 20, 22, 32, 48
ophthalmopathy, Graves' 34
ophthalmoplegia 34
osteoarthritis 26, 44
osteoporosis 6, 20, 22, 32
ovarian
  disease, polycystic 6, 32, 48
  surgery, laparoscopic
    for anovulatory infertility 49
    for recurrent miscarriage 49
oxandrolone for delayed puberty 51

P

palmidronate for hypercalcaemia 29
palsy, cranial nerve 32, 40
panhypopituitarism 22
papilloedema 40
paralysis, oculomotor *see* ophthalmoplegia
paraparesis, spastic 56
pergolide for hyperprolactinaemia 33
phaeochromocytoma 34, 38, 46
phenoxybenzamine for phaeochromocytoma 47
phentolamine for hypertensive crises 47
phenytoin for inhibition of neurohypophysial vasopressin secretion 53
pigmentation 4
  buccal 4
  cutaneous 50
  scar 4
pitressin *see* arginine vasopressin

pituitary
  damage 54
  failure 54
  irradiation for Cushing's syndrome 7
  mass, expanding 40
  radiotherapy
    for acromegaly 3
    for hyperprolactinaemia 33
  tumour 22, 54
pituitary–adrenal axis deficiencies 41
pituitary–gonadal axis deficiencies 41
polycystic ovarian disease 6, 32, 48
polydipsia 8, 10, 12, 28, 30
polyneuropathy, symmetrical sensory 10, 12
polyp, colorectal 2
polyuria 8, 10, 12, 14, 18, 28, 30
post-epididymitis 54
post-orchitis 54
potassium chloride
  for hyperglycaemic emergencies 31
  with dextrose for diabetic management in surgery 19
Prader–Willi syndrome 54
prednisolone
  for Addison's disease 5
  for pituitary–adrenal axis deficiencies 41
  for hypercalcaemia due to sarcoidosis 29
progestogen
  for female hypogonadism
    hypergonadotrophic 21
    hypogonadotrophic 23
  for menstrual disorders 49
  for short stature 25
  for tall stature 27
prolactinoma 32, 40
prolapse, vaginal 12
propranolol
  for hyperthyroidism 35
  for phaeochromocytoma 47
proptosis 34
propylthiouracil for hyperthyroidism 35
pruritus vulvae 12
pseudoacromegaly 2, 48
pseudohermaphroditism
  male 54
  female 54
pseudohypoparathyroidism 36
pseudoprolactinoma 32
psychological disturbance 50, 54
psychosis 42
psychotherapy for obesity 45
pubertal
  abnormalities 50
  growth, absent 50
  maturation, incomplete 20, 22
puberty
  arrested 32
  delayed 20, 22, 24, 32, 42, 50, 54
  failure of 54

puberty *cont*.
  partial 54
  precocious 50
  pseudoprecocious 50

Q

quinagolide for hyperprolactinaemia 33

R

radioiodine
  after surgery for thyroid carcinoma 57
  for hyperthyroidism 35
radiotherapy
  for ectopic adrenocorticotrophic hormone syndrome 7
  pituitary
    for acromegaly 3
    for hyperprolactinaemia 33
reflexes
  diminished 40, 52
  tendon, delayed relaxation of 42
rehydration
  for hypercalcaemia 29
  for hyperglycaemic emergencies 31
renal
  failure 30, 36, 52
  impairment, progressive 10
  stones 2, 28
resistant ovary syndrome 20
respiration, Kussmaul's 10, 14, 30
respiratory
  disease 2
  distress, fetal 16
retinopathy 46
  diabetic 10, 12, 14, 16

S

saline
  for Addison's disease 5
  for hyperglycaemic emergencies 31
sarcoidosis 9, 29
Schmidt's syndrome 4
seizures 38, 52 *see also* epilepsy
sex steroids
  for female hypogonadism
    hypergonadotrophic 21
    hypogonadotrophic 23
  for short stature 25
sexual
  development
    lack of 50
    secondary isosexual 50
  hair, secondary, absence of 54
  infantilism *see* hypogonadism
short stature 20, 22, 24, 40, 50
SIADH *see* syndrome of inappropriate antidiuresis
Simmond's disease *see* hypopituitarism

Index

sodium
  bicarbonate for hyperglycaemic emergency 31
  chloride in induction of diuresis and natriuresis 53
somatostatin analogues for tall stature 27
speech
  irrational 38
  slurred 38 see also dysphonia
sperm
  count, diminshed 54
  motility, defective 54
spironolactone for virilization 49
Stein–Leventhal syndrome see polycystic ovarian disease
steroids see corticosteroids, sex steroids
stones, renal 2, 28
stroke 38, 48 see also cerebrovascular accident
sulphonylureas for non-insulin-dependent diabetes mellitus 13, 19
swelling
  around eyes 34
  neck 34, 42, 56
  testicular 54
  thyroid 56
synchiae, uterine 22
syndrome
  of inappropriate antidiuresis 52
  X 48

T

tachyarrhythmia 46
tachycardia 18, 30, 38
  sinus 34
  supraventricular 46
tall stature 26, 50, 54
tan, persistent 4
terguride for hyperprolactinaemia 33
testes
  failure to develop 54
  inguinal 54
  large as adult 54
  small
    firm 54
    soft 40
testicular
  atrophy 54
  descent, incomplete 54
  malignancy 54
  torsion 54
testolactone for pseudoprecocious puberty 51
testosterone
  for androgen deficiency 55
  for delayed puberty 51
  for pituitary–gonadal axis deficiencies 41
  for short stature 25
  for tall stature 27
tetany 36
thionamides for hyperthyroidism 35

thirst 8, 14, 18, 30
  sensation, loss of 8
thyroid
  carcinoma 56
  disease, benign 56
  insufficiency, primary 40
  swelling 54
thyroidectomy
  for Graves' disease 35
  for thyroid carcinoma 57
thyroiditis, Hashimoto's 42
thyroid-stimulating hormone deficiency 40
thyrotoxicosis 10, 12, 26, 30, 46, 56 see also hyperthyroidism
thyroxine
  after treatment for thyroid carcinoma 57
  for hyperprolactinaemia 23
  for hypothyroidism 43
  for thyroid deficiencies 41
  for short stature 25
toxaemia, pre-eclamptic 16
transplantation for diabetic nephropathy 10, 12
trans-sphenoidal
  microadenectomy for hyperprolactinaemia 33
  surgery
    for acromegaly 3
    for Cushing's disease 7
triiodothyronine for hypothyroidism 43
Trousseau's sign 36
tumour
  androgen-secreting 48
  cerebellar 46
  cerebral 42
  granulosa-cell 48
  pituitary 22, 54
Turner's syndrome 20, 24, 50, 54
twitching, facial 36

U

ulceration
  corneal 34
  foot 10, 12
uraemia 38
urinary
  frequency 40
  tract infection 12, 14
uterine
  atresia 22
  malformation 22
  synchiae 22

V

vaginal
  dryness 20, 22
  mucosa, atrophic 20, 22
  prolapse 12
varicocoele 54

varicose veins 44
vas deferens, absent or obstructed 54
vascular disease
  coronary 10, 12
  peripheral 6, 10, 12
vasodilatation, peripheral 30
vasopressin
  arginine for diabetes insipidus 9
  lysin for diabetes insipidus 9
vesiculitis, seminal 54
virilization 26, 48, 50
  poor 54
vision, double see diplopia
visual
  deterioration 2
  disturbance 40
  field defect 32, 40
  impairment 22
vitamin deficiency
  B12 4
  D 36
vitiligo 4, 42
voice change 48

W

weight gain 6, 40, 42

CURRENT DIAGNOSIS & TREATMENT

in

Gastroenterology

Edited by
Roy Pounder
Mark Hamilton

A **QUICK** Reference for the Clinician

Contributors

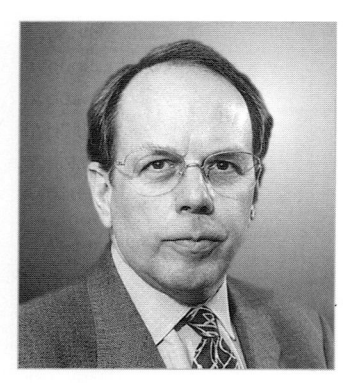

EDITOR

R E Pounder

Professor Roy Pounder is Professor of Medicine at the Royal Free Hospital, London. His research interests include the pharmacological control of gastric acid secretion and the pathogenesis of Crohn's disease and ulcerative colitis. He is the editor of 15 textbooks of medicine and gastroenterology and has written more than 130 research articles.

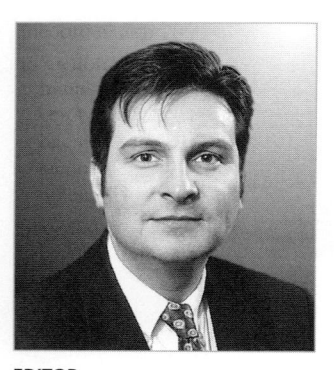

EDITOR

M Hamilton

Dr Mark Hamilton is currently senior registrar in the University Department of Medicine at the Royal Free Hospital, London. His research interests have been the role of autoimmunity, vascular factors and microvascular injury in ulcerative colitis.

REFEREES

Professor Christopher J Hawkey
Gastroenterology Division
University Hospital
Nottingham, UK

Professor Rodney H Taylor
Royal Naval Hospital of Medicine
Gosport, UK

AUTHORS

ACHALASIA
Dr Robert Heading
Department of Medicine
Royal Infirmary
Edinburgh, UK

ANAEMIA, PERNICIOUS
Dr Mark Hamilton
University Department of Medicine
Royal Free Hospital
London, UK

BACTERIAL OVERGROWTH OF THE SMALL INTESTINE
Dr Ray G Shidrawi
Gastroenterology Unit
The Rayne Institute
St Thomas's Hospital
London, UK

Professor Paul Ciclitira
Gastroenterology Unit
The Rayne Institute
St Thomas's Hospital
London, UK

COELIAC DISEASE
Professor Paul Ciclitira
Gastroenterology Unit
The Rayne Institute
St Thomas's Hospital
London, UK

COLORECTAL DISEASE
Mr Mark Winslet
Department of Academic Surgery
Royal Free Hospital
London, UK

CROHN'S DISEASE
Dr Mark Hamilton
University Department of Medicine
Royal Free Hospital
London, UK

DIVERTICULAR DISEASE OF THE COLON
Dr David G Maxton
Department of Gastroenterology
Royal Shrewsbury Hospital North
Shrewsbury, UK

DUODENAL ULCER
Professor Roy Pounder
Department of Medicine
Royal Free Hospital
London, UK

ENTERIC INFECTIONS
Dr Gordon Cook
Department of Clinical Sciences
Hospital for Tropical Diseases
London, UK

GALLSTONES, CHOLESTEROL
Dr Riadh P Jazrawi
Division of Biochemical Medicine
St George's Hospital
London, UK

Professor Tim Northfield
Division of Biochemical Medicine
St George's Hospital
London, UK

GASTRIC CANCER
Dr Paul Swain
Department of Gastroenterology
Royal London Hospital
London, UK

GASTRIC ULCERATION
Dr Mark Hamilton
University Department of Medicine
Royal Free Hospital
London, UK

GASTROINTESTINAL BLEEDING
Dr Paul Swain
Department of Gastroenterology
Royal London Hospital
London, UK

IRRITABLE BOWEL SYNDROME
Dr David G Maxton
Department of Gastroenterology
Royal Shrewsbury Hospital North
Shrewsbury, UK

OESOPHAGEAL CARCINOMA
Dr Mounes Dakkak
Department of Gastroenterology
Hull Royal Infirmary
Hull, UK

Professor John R Bennett
Department of Gastroenterology
Hull Royal Infirmary
Hull, UK

OESOPHAGITIS AND HIATUS HERNIA
Dr Mounes Dakkak
Department of Gastroenterology
Hull Royal Infirmary
Hull, UK

Professor John R Bennett
Department of Gastroenterology
Hull Royal Infirmary
Hull, UK

PANCREATIC CANCER
Professor John P Neoptolemos
Department of Surgery
Queen Elizabeth Hospital
Birmingham, UK

PANCREATITS, ACUTE
Professor John P Neoptolemos
Department of Surgery
Queen Elizabeth Hospital
Birmingham, UK

PANCREATITS, CHRONIC
Professor John P Neoptolemos
Department of Surgery
Queen Elizabeth Hospital
Birmingham, UK

ULCERATIVE COLITIS
Dr Ian A Finnie
Department of Gastroenterology
Glan Clwyd Hospital
Bodelwyddan, UK

Professor Jonathan Rhodes
Gastroenterology Research Unit
University of Liverpool
Liverpool, UK

ZOLLINGER–ELLINSON SYNDROME
Professor Roy Pounder
Department of Medicine
Royal Free Hospital
London, UK

Contents

2 Achalasia

4 Anaemia, pernicious

6 Bacterial overgrowth of the small intestine

8 Coeliac disease

10 Colorectal cancer

12 Crohn's disease

14 Diverticular disease of the colon
 diverticulitis
 diverticulosis

16 Duodenal ulcer

18 Enteric infections

20 Gallstones, cholesterol

22 Gastric cancer

24 Gastric ulceration

26 Gastrointestinal bleeding
 peptic ulcer
 bleeding varices

28 Irritable bowel syndrome

30 Oesophageal carcinoma

32 Oesophagitis and hiatus hernia

34 Pancreatic cancer

36 Pancreatitis, acute

38 Pancreatitis, chronic

40 Ulcerative colitis

42 Zollinger-Ellison syndrome

44 Index

Achalasia — R.C. Heading

Diagnosis

Symptoms
Dysphagia: usually perceived with both solid food and liquids.
Retrosternal chest pain: intermittent and variable duration, often related to eating.
Weight loss.
Regurgitation.
Nocturnal cough: related to regurgitation and aspiration.

Signs
- Usually no signs are manifest.

Evidence of weight loss.

Investigations
Radiography (plain film, erect): may show absence of air in gastric fundus or dilated oesophagus with fluid contents.
Radiography (barium swallow): shows delayed passage of contrast through cardia, absence of peristalsis (although 'tertiary waves' may be prominent), or oesophageal dilatation in 60% of patients.
Upper gastrointestinal endoscopy: often normal; retained food or fluid may be encountered; increased resistance to passage of endoscope through cardia may be apparent.
Oesophageal manometry: shows impaired relaxation of lower oesophageal sphincter and absent peristalsis; may show prominent non-peristaltic (synchronous) contractions in oesophageal body or elevated tonic pressure of lower oesophageal sphincter.

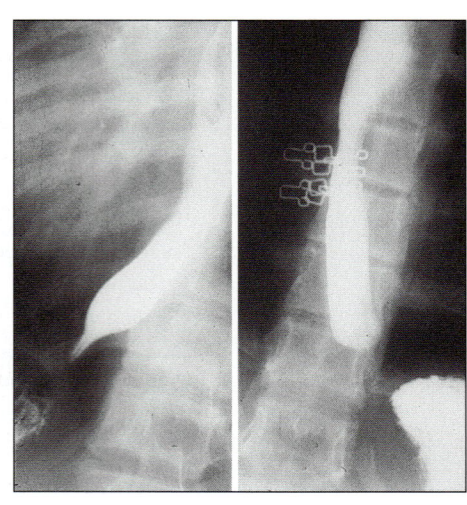

Delay of barium swallow due to spasm.

Complications
Respiratory complications: e.g. cough, aspiration pneumonitis, in 10% of patients.
Oesophageal carcinoma: possibly a late complication; very unusual.

Differential diagnosis
Benign or malignant oesophageal stricture.
Gastric or other malignancy at cardia.
Aortic aneurysm compressing cardia.
Diffuse oesophageal spasm.
Chagas' disease.
Hollow visceral neuropathy.

Aetiology
- The underlying cause of the defect in the inhibitory innervation of the oesophageal body and lower sphincter is unknown.

Epidemiology
- The annual incidence of achalasia is 1 in 100 000 adults.
- The male:female ratio is equal; achalasia may appear at any age in adult life.
- It is rare in children (incidence, 0.1 in 100 000 annually).

Diagnostic pitfalls
- The clinical features and radiography of 'classic' achalasia are so characteristic that the existence of less typical presentations is not always appreciated; awareness of the following helps to minimize diagnostic errors:
- Early symptoms in some patients resemble those of gastroesophageal reflux.
- Abnormalities on barium swallow are sometimes subtle, so the diagnosis of achalasia is easily missed.
- Minor inflammation of the mucosa may be diagnosed as oesophagitis at endoscopy when food retention in the oesophagus is significant.
- In children especially, achalasia may be manifest with its respiratory complications.
- Despite clinical features and radiographs typical of achalasia, carcinoma or a peptic stricture should always be suspected when an endoscope cannot be passed through the cardia.

Treatment

Diet and lifestyle
- No special precautions are necessary.

Pharmacological treatment
- Nitrates and calcium antagonists (e.g. nifedipine) reduce the lower oesophageal sphincter pressure and may give short-term benefit before dilatation or surgery.

Non-pharmacological treatment

Dilatation of the cardia
- Dilatation is the procedure of choice in most centres.
- Dysphagia is relieved in about two-thirds of patients after one attempt.
- A second attempt is usually worth while if the first attempt was unsuccessful.
- Complications include oesophageal perforation in 2–10% of patients; surgical repair is not always needed.

Surgery
- Cardiomyotomy through the thorax or abdomen or as a 'minimal-access' procedure can be done.

Treatment aims
To restore acceptable swallowing.

Prognosis
- Treatment cannot restore normal oesophageal function; patients may have to eat more slowly and carefully than they did before the condition developed.
- 50% of patients continue to experience some intermittent retrosternal pain.

Follow-up and management
- Symptomatic gastroesophageal reflux occurs in 5–10% of patients after successful dilatation or cardiomyotomy; treatment with an H_2 receptor antagonist or proton pump inhibitor is usually successful.

Key references
Howard PJ et al.: Five year prospective study of the incidence, clinical features and diagnosis of achalasia in Edinburgh. Gut 1992, **33**:1011–1015.

Parkman HP et al.: Pneumatic dilatation or esophagomyotomy treatment for idiopathic achalasia: clinical outcomes and cost analysis. Dig Dis Sci 1993, **38**:75–85.

Spencer J: Achalasia cardia: dilatation or operation? Gut 1993, **34**:148–149.

Anaemia, pernicious — M. Hamilton

Diagnosis

Symptoms
- Possibly no symptoms are apparent (vitamin B_{12} deficiency or atrophic gastritis may be an incidental finding).
- Symptoms are usually due to anaemia or complications of vitamin B_{12} deficiency.

Shortness of breath, lethargy.

Sore tongue: glossitis in 50% of patients.

Parasthesiae: due to peripheral neuropathy.

Gait disturbance: due to myelopathy (subacute combined degeneration of spinal cord).

Depression.

Impaired memory.

Signs
Mucosal pallor: reflecting anaemia.

Glossitis.

Mild splenomegaly.

Signs of other organ-specific autoimmune disease: e.g. hypothyroidism.

Peripheral sensory neuropathy with absent reflexes.

Pyramidal or long-tract signs.

Extensor plantars.

Loss of joint position sense.

Investigations
Haematology: for macrocytic anaemia (mean corpuscular volume >100 fl), leucopenia or thrombocytopenia, hypersegmented neutrophils on blood film.

Bone-marrow analysis: megaloblastic changes with maturation arrest.

Liver function test: increased bilirubin due to ineffective erythropoiesis.

Serum vitamin B_{12} measurement: to detect low concentrations (normal, >160 ng/L).

Schilling test: abnormal part I test using ^{58}Co-labelled vitamin B_{12} (<10% urinary excretion); part II corrects to normal after administration of intrinsic factor.

Serum gastrin measurement: raised concentration in pernicious anaemia (normal <100 pmol/L).

Pentagastrin or histamine-fast analysis: shows achlorhydria.

Endoscopy and biopsy: for atrophic gastritis on endoscopy and histological assessment of stage of gastritis.

Complications
Gastric carcinoid and enterochromaffin cell hyperplasia: associated with marked reflex rise in serum gastrin due to intragastric anacidity; 2–9% prevalence of gastric carcinoid in patients with pernicious anaemia.

Gastric carcinoma: 1–7% increased risk in patients with pernicious anaemia.

Peripheral sensory neuropathy, subacute combined degeneration of spinal cord: affects pyramidal tracts, causing spastic paraparesis and bladder involvement, and dorsal columns, causing sensory ataxic and impaired joint position sense.

High-output cardiac failure, myocardial ischaemia: in severe anaemia.

Differential diagnosis
Type B chronic gastritis related to *Helicobacter pylori* infection.

Other causes of vitamin B_{12} deficiency: e.g. dietary deficiency in vegans, terminal ileitis (Crohn's disease), terminal ileal resection, blind loop syndromes, small bowel diverticula or bacterial overgrowth, postgastrectomy states, pelvic irradiation.

Aetiology
- Pernicious anaemia is an organ-specific autoimmune disease, with a strong association with other organ-specific autoimmune diseases, especially thyroid disease.

Epidemiology
- Pernicious anaemia occurs more often in female patients than in male.
- Pernicious anaemia is common in all races and countries.

Immunology
- Antigastric parietal-cell antibodies (probably involved in pathogenesis) occur in 70–90% of patients, anti-intrinsic factor antibodies in 50–70%.
- Antibodies have been shown to be directed against membrane-bound hydrogen/potassium ATPase pump, resulting in blockade of hydrochloric acid secretion and correlating with concentrations of gastric parietal-cell antibodies.

Treatment

Diet and lifestyle
- No special precautions are necessary for uncomplicated disease.

Pharmacological treatment

Standard dosage	Hydroxycobalamin 1 mg i.m. 6 times in 2–3 weeks, then 1 mg every 3 months.
Contraindications	None.
Special points	Can cause initial hypokalaemia and folate deficiency in patients with marked vitamin B_{12} deficiency; chloride and folic acid supplements are advisable.
Main drug interactions	None.
Main side effects	None.

Treatment aims
To prevent neurological complications.
To correct anaemia.

Prognosis
- Despite the small risk of gastric carcinoid or carcinoma, life expectancy is little altered in patients with uncomplicated disease.
- Gastric carcinoids have a good prognosis, with no reported cases of carcinoid syndrome in these patients and a low reported incidence of local or regional spread.

Follow-up and management
- The cost of endoscopic surveillance has been shown to outweigh the benefit of screening for the few patients who are found to have unsuspected malignancy; it should probably be reserved for patients who develop symptoms.
- Regular vitamin B_{12} supplementation in outpatients must be ensured.

Key references
Born K *et al.*: Gastric endocrine cell hyperplasia and carcinoid tumors in pernicious anaemia. *Gastroenterology* 1985, **88**:638–648.

Lechago J, Correa P: Prolonged achlorhydria and gastric neoplasia: is there a causal relationship? *Gastroenterology* 1993, **104**:1554–1557.

Bacterial overgrowth of the small intestine
R.G. Shidrawi and P.J. Ciclitira

Diagnosis

Definition
- This disorder is also known as bacterial contamination of the small intestine or blind loop syndrome.
- Normally, the microflora of the small intestine consists of aerobic, Gram-positive organisms derived from the upper gastrointestinal tract. In bacterial overgrowth, these are replaced by anaerobic, facultative Gram-negative organisms, especially *Escherichia coli, Bacteroides,* and *Clostridium* spp. at >10^5 colony-forming units/ml on culture.

Symptoms
- Many patients are asymptomatic and suffer no adverse effects.
- Bacterial overgrowth of the proximal small intestine tends to produce more marked symptoms than overgrowth of the distal small bowel.

Diarrhoea, abdominal pain, weight loss, nausea and vomiting.

Signs
Steatorrhoea: bulky, offensive stools.

Anaemia: megaloblastic, secondary to vitamin B_{12} deficiency.

Erythema *ab igne*: using hot water bottles to relieve abdominal pain, often postprandial (rare).

Ataxia, neuropathy: due to vitamin B_{12} deficiency.

Pouchitis: in ileal reservoirs and ileo-anal anastomoses, with occult or obvious blood loss.

Investigations
Full blood count: 60% of patients have macrocytic anaemia.

Vitamin B_{12} measurement: concentration low or normal.

Serum or erythrocyte folate measurement: concentration high or normal; 'inverted' profile, useful but nonspecific marker.

Schilling test with intrinsic factor: absorption not corrected; also found in terminal ileal disease.

Spot test with Sudan red: marker for neutral stool fat.

3-day faecal fat collection: useful but unpopular test to quantify steatorrhoea.

Barium follow-through: for jejunal diverticulosis, strictures, and fistulae; delayed transit of barium through small intestine indirect evidence of impaired motility.

Duodenal aspiration: for culture and strain identification; gold standard; presence of detectable concentrations of unconjugated bile acids and short chain fatty acids can provide useful adjunct, although these tests are not widely available; false-negative results do not exclude bacterial overgrowth distal to ligament of Treitz.

Duodenal biopsy: to assess villous architecture and exclude parasitic infestation (compared with giardiasis, Whipple's disease).

Breath tests: simple and noninvasive and increasingly available; early rise of breath hydrogen after lactulose or glucose ^{14}C D-xylose or ^{14}C glycocholic acid.

Complications
- In patients with long-standing symptoms, complications result in chronic debility.

Secondary eating disorders: if food exacerbates abdominal pain.

Subacute combined degeneration of spinal cord: after profound vitamin B_{12} deficiency.

Skin rashes, liver, kidney, and joint involvement: from immune complex phenomena (rare).

Differential diagnosis
Coeliac disease.
Chronic pancreatitis.
Crohn's disease
Infections: *Yersinia* or *Campylobacter* spp. (bacterial); *Giardia lamblia* (protozoan); *Ascaris* or *Strongyloides* spp. (helminthic); AIDS enteropathy (viral).

Aetiology
- Causes are often multifactorial and poorly understood; they include the following:

Structural abnormalities
Jejunal diverticulosis.
Blind loop.
Adhesions.

Motility disorders
Autonomic neuropathy, as in insulin-dependent diabetes mellitus.
Progressive systemic sclerosis.
Postoperative ileus.

Excessive bacterial load
Diminished gastric acid production.
Incompetent ileocaecal valve.
Ileocolic fistula (Crohn's).
Seeding from infected biliary tree.

Impaired immunity
Raised intraluminal pH.
Gastric surgery or vagotomy.
Drugs: proton pump inhibitors.
Hypochlorhydria and associated states: e.g. autoimmune gastritis, pernicious anaemia, primary immunodeficiencies (especially IgA), protein or energy deficiency.
Acquired: e.g. intensive chemo- or radiotherapy, malignancy, HIV infection.

- Malnutrition can cause bacterial overgrowth by impairing mucosal immunity, diminishing gastric acid production, altering goblet cell mucus production, and reducing the bacteriostatic properties of pancreatic exocrine secretions.

Epidemiology
- Prevalence studies are difficult because of the lack of a suitable screening test.
- Children and elderly people are particularly susceptible.

Treatment

Diet and lifestyle
- A high-protein, high-energy, high-fat diet is recommended.
- Vitamin supplementation, especially injections of vitamin B_{12} and fat-soluble vitamins (A, D, K), or oral iron may be beneficial.
- Total parenteral nutrition may be necessary.

Pharmacological treatment
- Treatment is often empirical, the diagnosis being made by observing improvement in symptoms and biochemical abnormalities after treatment.

Antibiotics

Standard dosage	Trimethoprim 200 mg twice daily. Metronidazole 400 mg 3 times daily. Tetracycline 250 mg 4 times daily. Ciprofloxacin 500 mg twice daily (1-week course usually adequate). 2-week course may be adequate, but maintenance with alternating courses of two agents may be needed.
Contraindications	*Trimethoprim:* haematological disorders. *Metronidazole:* pregnancy, lactation. *Tetracycline:* renal insufficiency, children <12 years, lactation. *Ciprofloxacin:* children or adolescents, glucose 6-phosphate dehydrogenase deficiency, epilepsy, lactation.
Special points	*Metronidazole:* Antabuse (disulfiram-like) effect with alcohol. *Tetracycline:* permanent tooth discoloration if used during dental development. *Ciprofloxacin:* causes arthropathy in immature animals.
Main drug interactions	*Trimethoprim:* potentiates anticoagulant effect of warfarin, prolongs half-life of phenytoin and sulphonylureas. *Metronidazole:* potentiates warfarin. *Tetracyclines:* calcium, magnesium, iron, and aluminum salts (e.g. milk, antacids) impair absorption. *Ciprofloxacin:* magnesium, aluminium salts inhibit absorption; theophylline levels raised; anticoagulants potentiated.
Main side effects	*Metronidazole:* metallic taste (meteorism), furred tongue, peripheral neuropathy with prolonged use. *Tetracyclines:* gastrointestinal disturbances, photosensitive rash, hypersensitivity (rare). *Ciprofloxacin:* gastrointestinal symptoms, rashes, restlessness, dizziness, pruritus, tremor, convulsions.

Prokinetic agents

Standard dosage	Cisapride 10 mg 3 times daily or 20 mg twice daily, 15–30 min before meals for maximum effect. Octreotide 100–200 µg s.c. 3 times daily.
Contraindications	*Cisapride:* pregnancy, gastrointestinal haemorrhage, perforation, or obstruction. *Octreotide:* gallstones.
Main drug interactions	*Cisapride:* alters absorption of anticonvulsants, alcohol. *Octreotide:* reduces absorption of cyclosporine, cimetidine.
Main side effects	*Cisapride:* abdominal cramps, borborygmi, diarrhoea, headaches.

Treatment aims
To clear and prevent recurrence of bacterial overgrowth.
To improve general well-being.
To correct haematological abnormalities and secondary nutritional deficiencies.

Other treatments
Surgery to correct underlying anatomical abnormality; may cause prolonged post-operative ileus.

Prognosis
- The prognosis depends on the underlying disease: motility disorders have the worse prognosis.

Follow-up and management
- Regular infrequent outpatient follow-up may be needed to monitor for symptoms and to detect relapses early.
- Long-term maintenance antibiotic treatment is only rarely needed, and surgical treatment may be definitive.

Key references
Cook GC: Hypochlorhydria and vulnerability to intestinal infection. *Eur J Gastroenterol Hepatol* 1994, **6**:693–695.

Fried M *et al.*: Duodenal bacterial overgrowth during treatment in outpatients with omeprazole. *Gut* 1994, **35**:23–26.

Kirsch M: Bacterial overgrowth. *Am J Gastroenterol* 1990, **85**:231–237.

Larner AJ, Hamilton MIR: Infective complications of therapeutic gastric inhibition. *Aliment Pharmacol Ther* 1994, **8**:579–584.

Coeliac disease — P.J. Ciclitira

Diagnosis

Symptoms
- Only 50% of patients present with the classic symptoms of diarrhoea associated with malabsorption. Many are detected because of anaemia (especially iron with folate deficiency).

Symptoms of steatorrhoea: foul-smelling bulky motions, difficult to flush away.

Failure to thrive, vomiting or diarrhoea: in infants.

Short stature, lassitude, irritability: in children.

Diarrhoea, malabsorption, lassitude, infertility, constipation: in adults.

Pallor: due to anaemia.

Weight loss: in patients with insulin-dependent diabetes mellitus or thyroid disease.

Signs
Short stature, fine skin, clubbing, evidence of weight loss.

Iron or folic acid deficiency: causing anaemia.

Calcium deficiency.

Tetany: due to hypocalcaemia and hypomagnesaemia.

Investigations

Initial
Full blood count, serum iron, ferritin, or folate, and erythrocyte folate measurement: to identify microcytic (iron deficiency) or macrocytic (folic acid deficiency) anaemia or a dimorphic pattern of anaemia due to both.

Vitamin B_{12} measurement: concentration frequently low normal but rarely depressed.

Serum calcium and magnesium measurement: concentration possibly depressed.

Specific
Circulating antibody measurement: concentrations always raised; may be used as a screening test, particularly in children.

Faecal fat estimation: 3-day faecal fat excretion >17 mmol/day in patients receiving at least 100 g fat daily (infrequently used).

Upper gastrointestinal endoscopy, peroral suction biopsy of proximal jeunum: for unequivocal diagnosis; normal macroscopic haustration in duodenum may be lost; at least three biopsies should be taken; villus flattening over Brunner's glands normal; suction biopsy if diagnostic probability strong or to aid interpretation of duodenal biopsy.

Contrast radiography: small-bowel follow-through to assess small intestine.

Histology: shows villous atrophy in severe cases, 'crazy paving' on dissecting microscopy.

Gastrointestinal permeability tests: lactulose rhamnose hypertonic test; decreased values in untreated coeliac patients return to normal with treatment.

Complications

Anaemia: due to iron or folic acid deficiency.

Osteomalacia, tetany and fits, osteoporosis: due to hypocalcaemia (tetany and fits due to exacerbation by magnesium deficiency).

Ulcerative jejunitis: rare, possibly early manifestation of malignancy.

Small-intestinal lymphoma: T-cell lymphoma complicating 5–10% of cases; may be manifest as unexplained small intestinal perforation.

Wernicke's encephalopathy or Korsakoff's psychosis: due to acute or prolonged vitamin B_1 (thiamine) deficiency.

Differential diagnosis

Diarrhoea
Irritable bowel syndrome.
Giardiasis.
Inflammatory bowel disease.
Laxative abuse.
Chronic pancreatitis.
Tropical sprue.
Zollinger–Ellison syndrome.

Failure to thrive
Cow's milk allergy.
Cystic fibrosis.
Postinfective mucosal damage.
Shwachman's syndrome (inherited pancreatic insufficiency).

Nutritional deficiencies
Inadequate dietary intake.
Small-bowel bacterial overgrowth syndrome.

Aetiology
- In the UK, 98% of cases of coeliac disease are associated with the extended haplotype HLA B8, DR3, DQ2, although, in southern Europe, HLA DR5/7, DQ2 accounts for one-third of cases.
- 10–20% of first-degree relatives of probands are similarly affected.
- Family history often reveals a Celtic ancestry.

Epidemiology
- The prevalence of coeliac disease in the UK is 1 in 1200 people, rising to 1 in 300 around Galway Bay in Ireland.
- Slightly more women than men suffer from coeliac disease; an association with anaemia due to menstruation and pregnancy is possible.
- The incidence of presentation has three peaks:
infancy (9–36 months), on introduction of foods containing gluten;
third decade, frequently manifest as severe anaemia of pregnancy;
fifth decade, normally manifest with a specific nutritional deficiency e.g. iron, folic acid, or calcium.

Treatment

Diet and lifestyle

- A gluten-free diet is the mainstay of treatment and involves avoiding products containing wheat, rye, barley, or oats. Care should be taken to avoid any food contaminated by these cereals or their partial hydrolysates, including beer. Women of childbearing age who experienced amenorrhoea due to nutritional deficiencies will probably have a return of regular menstruation and may become pregnant. Men who have had long-standing disease may complain of impotence and infertility. These problems normally resolve within 2 years of starting a gluten-free diet.
- Specific nutritional deficiencies should be treated by replacement: iron, calcium, vitamin B_{12}, folic acid, or magnesium.

Pharmacological treatment

- For most patients, a gluten-free diet is sufficient; extremely ill patients can be given systemic steroids.

Standard dosage	Prednisolone 20–40 mg daily initially, usually rapidly reduced to 5–10 mg daily.
	Hydrocortisone 50–100 mg i.v. 6-hourly in patients who need i.v. fluid replacement.
Contraindications	Caution in diabetes mellitus, peptic ulcers, or pregnancy.
Special points	Care should be taken to avoid high-dose (>10 mg/day), long-term steroid treatment because of side effects.
Main drug interactions	Mild antagonism to thiazide diuretics.
Main side effects	Weight gain, fluid retention, osteoporosis, cushingoid facies, diabetes mellitus.

Treatment aims

To improve general well-being, small intestinal mucosal structure, and associated nutritional deficiencies.

To reduce the risk of development of small intestinal lymphoma.

Prognosis

- With a gluten-free diet, general health is improved within a few weeks.
- Untreated patients are at a 5–10% risk of developing a small intestinal T-cell lymphoma, the incidence of which progressively falls if they maintain a strict diet.
- Failure to improve suggests incorrect initial diagnosis, failure to adhere strictly to a gluten-free diet, or concurrent disorder.

Follow-up and management

- Outpatients must be reassessed 6–8 weeks and 3–4 months after starting a gluten-free diet, when repeat peroral jejunal biopsy should be done.
- A further jejunal biopsy should be done 1 year after starting treatment, when continued improvement in the structure of the small-intestinal mucosa should be expected.
- Annual haematological screening is recommended to exclude development of specific nutritional deficiencies.
- When the diagnosis is doubtful, a gluten challenge, with 40 g gluten or 4 slices of normal bread daily for 2 weeks (adults) or 6 weeks (children), should be followed by a further jejunal biopsy.

Key references

Ciclitira PJ: Coeliac disease and related disorders and the malignant complications of coeliac disease. In *Gastroenterology: Clinical Science and Practice*. Edited by Bouchier I, Hodgson H. London: Baillière Tindall, 1993.

Ferguson A, Arranz E, O'Mahony S: Clinical and pathological spectrum of coeliac disease: active, silent, latent, potential. *Gut* 1993, **34**:150–155.

Kagnoff MF: Celiac disease: a gastrointestinal disease with environmental, genetic, and immunologic components. *Gastroenterol Clin North Am* 1992, **21**:405–425.

Colorectal cancer — M. Winslet

Diagnosis

Symptoms
- Symptoms may be related to primary tumour, secondary disease, or general effects of malignancies.

Change of bowel habit.
Blood or mucus in stools.
Tenesmus: rectal lesions.
Abdominal pain or swelling.
Loss of weight.

Signs
- Signs may be related to primary tumour, secondary disease, or general effects of malignancies.

Anaemia.
Abdominal mass or distension.
Mass or blood *per rectum*.
Peritonitis: perforation.
Hepatomegaly.
Ascites.
Cachexia.

Investigations

Assessment of primary tumour
Haemoglobin analysis.
Serum carcinoembryonic antigen estimation: to establish baseline for monitoring recurrence.
Endoscopy: rigid or flexible sigmoidoscopy, colonoscopy.
Double-contrast barium enema.
Endoluminal ultrasonography: for rectal lesion; not widely available.

Assessment of disseminated disease
Liver function tests.
Chest radiography.
Liver ultrasonography: in absence of CT; inexpensive but lower sensitivity than CT.
Abdominal CT: high sensitivity for liver metastases (>95%); low sensitivity for pelvis (50%) and retroperitoneum (30%).
Abdominal MRI: higher sensitivity than CT for assessing pelvis and retroperitoneum.
Intravenous urography: rarely necessary.
Immunoscintigraphy: useful in identifying recurrent disease.

Screening for prevention
Faecal occult blood testing: benefits not yet proven.
Colonoscopy: for high-risk groups, e.g. with familial colon cancer; controversial.

Complications
Obstruction: usually left-sided lesions.
Perforation.
Acute haemorrhage.
Fistula formation.

Differential diagnosis

Colonic
Diverticular disease.
Inflammatory bowel disease.
Irritable bowel syndrome.

Rectal
Solitary rectal ulcer.

Aetiology
- Causes include the following:

Familial polyposis coli.
Gardner's syndrome.
Chronic ulcerative colitis or Crohn's disease.
Genetic: hereditary non-polyposis colo-rectal cancer.
Ureterosigmoidostomy.
Colorectal polyps.
Diet: low unrefined fibre, high animal fat.

Epidemiology
- The peak incidence is at 60–69 years.
- Colon cancer occurs more often in women than in men (ratio, 1.5:1).
- It is the second most frequent cause of death due to malignancy in developed countries (17 000 deaths annually in UK).

Pathology
Microscopic: adenocarcinoma.
Macroscopic: polypoidal, ulcerative, annular, diffuse, colloidial.

Site
Caecum and ascending colon: 25%.
Transverse colon: 10%.
Descending colon: 15%.
Sigmoid colon: 20%.
Rectum: 30%.

Spread
Direct, lymphatic, venous.

Stage (Dukes' classification)
A: confined to mucosa/submucosa.
B: invasion of muscularis propria.
C: local node involvement.
D: distant metastases.

Treatment

Diet and lifestyle
- For primary prevention, fat intake should be reduced to 30% of energy intake, and dietary unrefined fibre and fruit and vegetable consumption should be increased.

Pharmacological treatment
- Adjuvant chemotherapy (5-fluorouracil and levamisole) is advocated in the USA for Dukes' stage B and C lesions; no evidence indicates material benefit in disseminated disease.

Non-pharmacological treatment

Elective surgery
Curative resection: right hemicolectomy, left hemicolectomy, anterior resection, abdominoperineal excision.

Palliative resection or bypass.

Local treatment for rectal lesions: local transanal resection (open or endoscopic), diathermy fulgeration, cryotherapy or laser therapy, alcohol instillation, intracavity radiation.

Emergency surgery
- 20% of patients present with obstruction, possibly with perforation.
- Management is controversial but may include one of the following:

Primary resection and anastomosis.

Primary resection and secondary anastomosis.

Primary defunction and secondary resection and anastomosis.

Adjuvant radiotherapy
- For rectal carcinoma, radiotherapy may be used preoperatively to reduce tumour fixity, but no evidence exists of material survival benefit.

Management of recurrence
- Management depends on the site, size, and number of metastases.
- Serial carcinoembryonic antigen estimation may predict recurrence by an average of 6 months in 50% of patients.
- ~20% of patients with recurrence after a 'curative' resection are suitable for re-resection.

Site of recurrence: local (20%; related to Dukes' stage), hepatic (30%), abdominal (20%), pulmonary (20%), retroperitoneal (10%).

For local disease: 50% amenable to further ablative surgery, with potential cure in 25%; radiotherapy effective palliation for rectal recurrence but limited by myelotoxicity.

For hepatic metastases: 20% (solitary or unilobar) amenable to curative resection, with 5-year survival >25%; possible short-term benefit from hepatic artery infusion of 5-fluoroxyuridine; possible symptomatic relief for capsular distension with fractionated radiotherapy.

Treatment aims
To remove primary tumour and loco-regional nodes, including mesorectum for rectal lesions (curative resection).

To remove or bypass the primary lesion with advanced local or metastatic disease, in order to ameliorate symptoms (palliative resection or bypass).

To control local disease in patients unfit for resection.

Prognosis
- 25% of patients have metastases at the time of presentation.
- In-hospital postoperative mortality (5–7%) is related to intra-abdominal sepsis, obstruction, age, or cardiopulmonary complications.
- Overall 5-year survival rates are 80–90% for Dukes' stage A, 50–60% for stage B, 30% for stage C, and 5% for stage D.

Follow-up and management
- A widespread policy in the UK is 6-monthly examination and sigmoidoscopy with annual colonoscopy for 2 years, followed by yearly examination and sigmoidoscopy with triannual colonoscopy or barium enema until the age of 75 years.

Key references
Hall C et al.: Haemoccult does not reduce the need for colonoscopy in surveillance after curative resection for colorectal cancer. Gut 1993, 34:227–229.

Moertel CG: Drug therapy: chemotherapy for colorectal cancer. N Engl J Med 1994, 330:1136–1142.

Selby JV et al.: A case–control study of screening sigmoidoscopy and mortality from colorectal cancer. N Engl J Med 1992 326:653–657.

Crohn's disease — M. Hamilton

Diagnosis

Symptoms
Malaise, anorexia, weight loss.

Growth retardation and failure of normal development: in children.

Diarrhoea, intermittent colicky pain: from subacute obstruction in the terminal ileum.

Pain: from oral or duodenal ulceration; abdominal pain due to inflammation, infection, or obstruction.

Tenesmus or rectal bleeding: with distal disease.

Bloody diarrhoea: with Crohn's colitis.

Recurrent perianal abscesses: with local pain.

Signs
Aphthous ulceration in mouth.

Atrophic glossitis: beefy-red tongue, due to vitamin B_{12} malabsorption.

Pallor of mucous membranes: indicating anaemia.

Growth retardation, weight loss: signs of malabsorption.

Right iliac fossa mass.

Perianal skin tags and abscesses.

Erythema nodosum, pyoderma gangrenosum, clubbing.

Investigations
Full blood count: to check for normochromic anaemia of chronic disease, microcytic anaemia of iron deficiency, macrocytic anaemia (B_{12} and folate deficiency); increased platelets, leucocyte count markers of infection or inflammation.

ESR or CRP measurement: inflammatory indices useful as marker of disease activity.

Vitamin and mineral measurements: magnesium, vitamin B_{12}, folate, iron, calcium, albumin deficiencies useful markers of absorptive function of small bowel.

Sigmoidoscopy and rectal biopsy: allow histological confirmation in rectal disease.

Colonoscopy: allows assessment of colonic disease and possibly visualization of terminal ileum and appropriate biopsy.

Upper gastrointestinal endoscopy: if relevant symptoms; lesions must be biopsied to confirm that they are due to Crohn's disease.

Barium imaging: follow-through allows assessment of small-bowel mucosal disease; useful in assessing stricture formation and defining anatomy for surgery; barium enema may complement colonoscopy, particularly in checking for fistulae.

Ultrasonography and CT: useful when checking for intra-abdominal collections.

Labelled leucocyte scans: may be of use in localizing inflammation and sepsis.

Radiography: features depend on site of disease; rose-thorn ulceration, string sign, skip lesions, cobblestone mucosa, stricture, fistulous tracts.

Complications
Intestinal obstruction or perforation, intra-abdominal sepsis: directly related to disease.

Amyloid: related to inflammation; rare.

Renal oxalate stones: rare.

Fistula formation: to bowel, bladder, vagina, or skin.

Differential diagnosis
Terminal ileal disease
Tuberculosis.
Yersinia spp. infection.
Lymphoma.

Colonic disease
Ulcerative colitis.
Bacterial infections (*Salmonella*, *Shigella*, *Campylobacter* spp.)
Amoebic infection.
Pseudomembranous colitis.
Colonic carcinoma.

Aetiology
- Crohn's disease is caused by multifocal granulomatous vasculitis.

Histological hallmark: non-caseating intravascular granulomata.

Possible genetic influences: studies have shown familial clustering, suggesting a genetic predisposition.

Possible viral infections: measles virus identified in vascular endothelium.

Epidemiology
- The prevalence of Crohn's disease is 1 in 1000 (50 000 cases in the UK).
- Ethnic clustering has been found.
- Onset may be in childhood.
- The disease is common in the third decade.
- The male : female ratio is equal.

Histology
Macroscopic
Discontinuous disease with skip lesions.
Transmural inflammation.

Microscopic
Non-caseating intravascular granuloma.
Lymphocytic infiltrate.
Transmural inflammation.

Treatment

Diet and lifestyle
- Nutritional supplementation is needed in patients with severe illness, with total parenteral nutrition in acute disease.
- Elemental diets may be effective but are poorly tolerated because of unpalatability; remission induced by elemental diets does not continue after diets have been stopped.

Pharmacological treatment
- Disease activity must be monitored using inflammatory markers (CRP and ESR).

Corticosteroids
Standard dose	Prednisolone 30–60 mg orally (i.v. in severe relapse); topical steroids for rectal or perineal disease.
Contraindications	Overt sepsis; caution in hypertension and diabetes.
Special points	May exacerbate growth retardation by premature fusion of epiphyses. Many patients are on long-term low-dose steroids, possibly with more potent immunosuppressive drugs. Long-term use should be avoided if possible, especially in young patients.
Main drug interactions	Significant immunosuppression with azathioprine: risk of opportunistic infections increased.
Main side effects	Fluid retention and hypertension, induction of glucose intolerance, osteoporosis, cushingoid features.

5-aminosalicylic acid preparations
- Sulphasalazine, mesalazine, or olsalazine may be of some benefit in extensive ileocolonic disease and in Crohn's colitis.

Standard dosage	Mesalazine 800 mg twice daily.
Contraindications	Salicylate hypersensitivity, sulphonamide sensitivity with sulphasalazine, renal impairment with mesalazine.
Special points	Sulphasalazine causes reversible oligospermia, may cause haemolysis; slow-release preparation of mesalazine of particular benefit in small-bowel Crohn's disease.
Main drug interactions	None of importance.
Main side effects	Nausea, rashes, occasional diarrhoea.

Antibiotics
- Antibiotics are effective in acute relapse, particularly in perianal disease; they are of some benefit in small bowel disease but mainly of use in colonic disease.

Standard dosage	Metronidazole 400 mg orally 3 times daily.
Contraindications	Previous hypersensitivity, peripheral neuropathy.
Special points	Crossover trials with 5-aminosalicylic acid drugs have shown a significant fall in clinical and laboratory parameters of disease on switching to metronidazole.
Main drug interactions	Enhances effects of warfarin; inhibits metabolism of phenytoin.
Main side effects	Nausea, metallic taste, risk of neuropathy (long-term use).

Other immunosuppressive drugs
- These are useful as steroid-sparing agent and for additional immunosuppression in resistant disease.

Standard dosage	Azathioprine 1–1.5 mg/kg once daily.
Contraindications	Neutropenia.
Special points	Risk of myelotoxicity maximal on starting treatment; whole blood count must be monitored closely, particularly in first few weeks, monthly thereafter.
Main drug interactions	Additive immunosuppressive effect with steroids.
Main side effects	Rashes, nausea, myelosuppression, increased risk of opportunistic infection, pancreatitis.

Treatment aims
To suppress disease activity.
To restore quality of life.
To prevent complications.
To correct nutritional deficiencies.

Other treatments
- Conservative surgery (stricturoplasty rather than resection, to avoid short-bowel syndromes) is indicated for the following:

Acute: acute ileitis with signs of acute abdomen at presentation, fulminating colitis, uncontrolled or severe rectal haemorrhage (rare), intra-abdominal collections (abscesses), ruptured viscus with peritonism.

Chronic: subacute intestinal obstruction from fibrosis or scarring, fistulae, chronic debilitating disease unresponsive to medical treatment.

Prognosis
- Modern medical treatment, improved immunosuppressive regimens, and conservative surgery have greatly decreased the incidence of long-term complications.
- The risk of carcinoma has increased slightly.

Follow-up and management
- Close outpatient follow-up, especially during relapse, is recommended.
- Open and rapid access to a specialist centre is essential in order to institute early treatment.
- Disease activity correlates closely with elevations of the acute-phase reactant, CRP, although this is similarly raised in infective complications.

Key references
Griffiths A *et al.*: Slow-release 5-aminosalicylic acid therapy in children with small intestinal Crohn's disease. *J Pediatr Gastroenterol Nutr* 1993, **17**:186–192.

Reynolds PD *et al.*: Pharmacotherapy of inflammatory bowel disease. *Dig Dis* 1993, **11**:334–342.

Riordan AM *et al.*: Treatment of active Crohn's disease by exclusion diet: East Anglian multicentre controlled trial. *Lancet* 1993, **342**:1131–1134.

Diverticular disease of the colon
D.G. Maxton

Diagnosis

Symptoms
- Most patients are asymptomatic.

Uncomplicated disease (diverticulosis)
- This may be due simply to irritable bowel syndrome (*see* Irritable bowel syndrome *for further details*).

Cramping lower abdominal pain: often relieved by opening bowels; may be localized to left iliac fossa.

Altered bowel habit, hard pellet or ribbon-like stools.

Complicated disease (diverticulitis)
Pain, altered bowel habit, fever: indicating inflammation due to abscess formation; pain often in left iliac fossa or radiating into lower back.

Shock, peritonitis: indicating inflammation due to perforation.

Fresh rectal bleeding: indicating haemorrhage.

Colicky lower abdominal pain: indicating stricture, subacute obstruction.

Signs

Uncomplicated disease
- Few signs are manifest.

Tender sigmoid colon: possible but nonspecific.

Complicated disease
Fever, tenderness, guarding, palpable inflammatory mass: indicating inflammation due to abscess.

Shock, acute abdomen, paralytic ileus: indicating inflammation due to perforation.

Anaemia, shock, fresh blood *per rectum*: indicating haemorrhage.

Abdominal distension, obstruction: indicating stricture.

Investigations
- Laboratory tests are usually normal in uncomplicated diverticular disease but can help to exclude other diagnoses.
- The diagnosis is made by demonstration of diverticula on barium enema or colonoscopy.

General
Full blood count: to identify iron deficiency due to bleeding.

Liver function tests: to exclude biliary disease (gallstones associated with diverticular disease).

Sigmoidoscopy: may reproduce pain and give diagnosis of low colonic carcinomas missed on barium enema.

Complicated disease
Leucocyte count and ESR measurement: elevation indicates abscess or perforation.

Plain abdominal radiography: may show features of ileus or perforation.

Contrast enema: may show obstruction or stricture.

Ultrasonography or CT of abdomen and pelvis: may show abscess cavity.

Colonoscopy: may be needed for biopsy of stricture to exclude malignancy.

Complications
- Most patients have no complications, but complications can be life threatening.

Acute haemorrhage.

Abscess formation or perforation: leading to subphrenic or pericolic collections.

Intestinal obstruction.

Stricture formation.

Fistula: connection to bladder or vagina.

Differential diagnosis

General
Carcinoma of colon.
Inflammatory bowel disease.

Uncomplicated disease
Drug-induced colonic symptoms.
Genitourinary disease, e.g. ovarian carcinoma, hydronephrosis.

Abscess or perforation
Pelvic inflammatory disease.
Pyelonephritis.
Perforated peptic ulcer.
Ischaemic colitis.

Haemorrhage
Polyp in colon.
Angiodysplasia.
Upper gastrointestinal tract bleeding.

Stricture
Radiation damage.
Ischaemic colitis.
Endometriosis.

Aetiology
- Factors believed to be implicated include the following:

Low stool weight, leading to excessive intracolonic pressure.
Dietary fibre deficiency, reducing stool weight and colonic transit time.
Exaggerated colonic pressure due to abnormal colon muscular motility.
Weakness and poor elasticity of colon wall.

Epidemiology
- Colonic diverticula occur in 33% of people >40 years and 50% of people >70 years.
- The disease is common in developed countries, rare in Africa, the Middle East, and India.
- Population groups in the same region vary, probably because of dietary factors.

Irritable bowel syndrome or diverticular disease?
- The possibility of substantial overlap must be considered.
- Long-standing constipation (in irritable bowel syndrome) may predispose to diverticula formation.
- Disordered motility may be important in both conditions.
- Clinical management is very similar in uncomplicated cases.

Treatment

Diet and lifestyle
- Increased dietary fibre intake may help some patients, especially those with marked constipation.
- Excessive bran or fruit may worsen symptoms.
- Small regular meals, with no excess of fatty foods, are generally advised.
- Regular exercise improves bowel function.

Pharmacological treatment
- Drugs should be used judiciously and can often be given 'as required'.
- Constipation is the most common complaint.
- Antibiotics for acute diverticulitis include penicillin (or ampicillin), gentamicin and metronidazole, cefuroxime and metronidazole, and co-amoxiclav.

Bulking agents
- These are indicated for constipation.
- The full effect may not be apparent for several days.

Standard dosage	Bran 2.4 g, ispaghula husk 3.5 g, or sterculia 7 g, twice daily. Lactulose 15 ml twice daily, increased as needed, or stimulant laxatives may be needed for intractable cases.
Contraindications	Intestinal obstruction.
Special points	Patients must take adequate fluid.
Main drug interactions	None.
Main side effects	Distension, flatulence, worsening of pain.

Antispasmodics
- Antispasmodics, either with anticholinergic properties or direct muscle relaxants, are given for pain relief.

Standard dosage	*Anticholinergics:* dicyclomine 10–20 mg up to 3 times daily or hyoscine 20 mg up to 4 times daily. *Direct relaxants:* mebeverine 135 mg, alverine 60 mg, or peppermint oil 1 capsule; each up to 3 times daily.
Contraindications	Paralytic ileus, ulcerative colitis. *Anticholinergics:* glaucoma.
Special points	Dosage times should be varied to suit the individual.
Main drug interactions	*Anticholinergics:* disopyramide, cisapride, antidepressants.
Main side effects	*Anticholinergics:* dry mouth, blurring of vision, palpitations, constipation. *Direct relaxants:* heartburn.

Non-pharmacological treatment

For acute diverticulitis: may be a medical emergency; parenteral antibiotics and consideration of defunctioning colostomy can be required.

For perforated diverticular disease of the colon: emergency decompression of the colon by colostomy, followed by elective resection of the diseased segment.

For life-threatening haemorrhage from diverticular disease: possible surgical control, perhaps after selective mesenteric arteriography.

Treatment aims
To relieve acute symptoms.
To improve bowel function.
To reduce incidence of further symptom attacks.

Prognosis
- Uncomplicated diverticular disease is a chronic condition, with relapses and remissions.
- Most sufferers have good symptom control, but a few become intractable.
- Complicated diverticular disease occurs frequently in elderly and frail people and can be life-threatening; attention to other medical conditions is important.

Follow-up and management
- Recurrent symptoms are common, but new or different symptoms need further investigations.
- If symptoms are relieved by fibre supplementation, long-term treatment must be continued.

Key references

Campbell K, Steele RJC: Non-steroidal anti-inflammatory drugs and complicated diverticular disease. *Br J Surg* 1992, **78**:190–191.

Cheskin LJ, Bohlman M, Schusler MM: Diverticular disease in the elderly. *Gastro Clin North Am* 1990, **19**:391–403.

Jones DJ: Diverticular disease. *BMJ* 1992, **304**:1435–1437.

Kronberg O: Treatment of perforated sigmoid diverticulitis: a prospective randomized trial. *Br J Surg* 1993, **80**:505–507.

McKee RF, Deignan RW, Krukowski ZH: Radiological investigation in acute diverticulitis. *Br J Surg* 1993, **80**:560–565.

Duodenal ulcer — R.E. Pounder

Diagnosis

Symptoms

Uncomplicated ulcer

Epigastric pain: sometimes described as dull or burning, often occurring 1–4 h after eating and relieved quickly by antacids or food.

Waking at night because of pain.

Complicated ulcer

Haematemesis or melaena: indicating bleeding ulcer.

Vomiting: sometimes indicating gastric outflow obstruction.

Severe pain: indicating pancreatitis or peritonitis, but 50% of patients with fatal complications present without ulcer pain.

Signs

Uncomplicated ulcer

- Few signs are manifest.

Epigastric tenderness: usually midline or to right of midline.

Complicated ulcer

Acute haemorrhage: indicating shock, melaena.

Anaemia: indicating chronic haemorrhage.

Peritonitis: indicating perforation.

'Succussion splash': indicating gastric outflow obstruction.

Investigations

- Laboratory tests are not diagnostic but can be used to identify complications and exclude other abnormalities.

Full blood count: to identify iron-deficiency anaemia.

Serum amylase measurement: raised concentration indicates penetration into pancreas or acute pancreatitis.

Serum gastrin measurement: can be considered in patients with recurrent or multiple ulcers.

Fibreoptic endoscopy: allows direct view of ulcer, assessment of scarring or deformity, assessment of *Helicobacter pylori* status (by CLOtest, culture, or histology), photographic documentation, and assessment of coincidental disease; identifies small lesions; treatment of bleeding ulcers possible; not tolerated by all patients (e.g. young men).

Contrast radiography: less accurate than endoscopy, small lesions may be missed, detection of *H. pylori* not possible, and does not allow tissue diagnosis; relatively cheap, and sedation not needed.

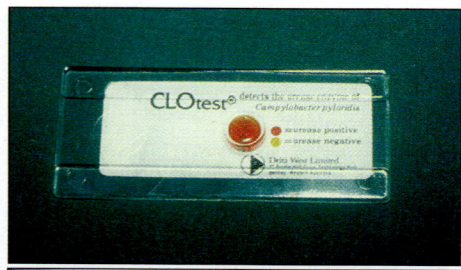

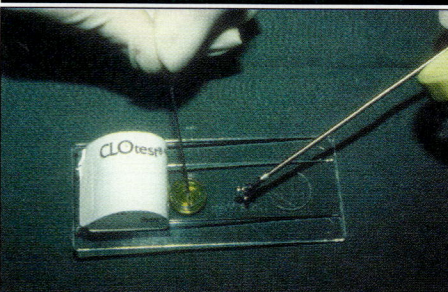

CLOtest detects urease activity in gastric biopsy.

Complications

Acute haemorrhage: in 10% of patients.

Perforation: in 1% (who may have been asymptomatic).

Pyloric channel obstruction: may cause weight loss due to vomiting and food aversion.

Differential diagnosis

Chronic pain

Gastroesophageal reflux disease.
Gastric ulcer.
Carcinoma of stomach.
Gallbladder disease.
Chronic pancreatitis.
Irritable bowel syndrome.

Acute severe pain

Acute pancreatitis.
Biliary colic.
Aortic dissection.
Acute myocardial infarction.

Aggressive ulceration

Zollinger–Ellison syndrome.
Crohn's disease.
Lymphoma.
Carcinoma.
Cytomegalovirus in imunosuppressed patients.

Aetiology

- Causes include the following:

Helicobacter pylori: in 95% of patients.

Increased basal acid secretion: in 30% of patients.

Increased nocturnal acid secretion.

Smoking.

Aspirin, NSAIDs.

Blood group O association: in non-secretors.

Genetic: familial clustering.

Epidemiology

- 10% of the population have a duodenal ulcer at some point in their lives.
- Duodenal ulcers occur almost as often in women as in men.

Treatment

Diet and lifestyle
- Bland or milk diets have not been shown to decrease acidity, promote healing, or relieve symptoms.
- Patients should restrict alcohol consumption, eat three well balanced meals daily, with no bedtime snacks, avoid aspirin and NSAIDs, and stop cigarette smoking.

Pharmacological treatment

Antacids
- Antacids are effective for duodenal ulcer, taken 1 and 3 h after meals; some patients may find complying with this regimen difficult.

H_2-receptor antagonists
- These produce symptomatic relief in days and ulcer healing in 80% of patients at 4 weeks and 95% at 8 weeks; they are also used as maintenance treatment to prevent recurrence at half the usual dose.

Standard dosage	Ranitidine 300 mg, cimetidine 800 mg, famotidine 40 mg, or nizatidine 300 mg at bedtime.
Contraindications	Rare hypersensitivity; avoided in pregnancy and lactation.
Main drug interactions	*Cimetidine:* oral anticoagulants, theophylline, phenytoin, warfarin.
Main side effects	Constipation, headache, diarrhoea (all rare). *Cimetidine:* gynaecomastia.

Proton-pump inhibitors
- These are indicated for unresponsive ulcers.
- They produce 93% healing after 4 weeks of treatment.
- They are not recommended for long-term treatment.

Standard dosage	Omeprazole 20 mg or lansoprazole 30 mg once daily.
Contraindications	Pregnancy and lactation.
Main drug interactions	*Omeprazole:* diazepam, phenytoin, warfarin.
Main side effects	Diarrhoea, headache, rash (all rare); increased risk of enteric infection.

Triple therapy for *Helicobacter pylori* eradication
- Triple therapy has been shown to decrease the chance of duodenal ulcer relapse, but the optimal regimen remains uncertain.

Standard dosage	Tripotassium dicitrato bismuthate 1 tablet, tetracycline 500 mg, and metronidazole 200 mg; all taken 4 times daily before food for 2 weeks, with ranitidine 300 mg at bedtime. *Or* clarithromycin 500 mg and metronidazole 400 mg 3 times daily, with ranitidine 300 mg at bedtime for 10 days. *Or* amoxycillin 750 mg and metronidazole 400 mg 3 times daily, with omeprazole 20 mg daily for 10 days.
Contraindications	Pregnancy.
Special points	Patients should avoid alcohol.
Main drug interactions	Warfarin.
Main side effects	Nausea, darkening of stool.

Treatment aims
To relieve pain.
To heal ulcer.
To prevent recurrence and complications.
To eradicate *Helicobacter pylori* infection.

Other treatments
Surgery: for uncontrollable bleeding, second major bleed, perforation or penetration, pyloric stenosis, or antibiotic-resistant *Helicobacter pylori* in young adults.
- Elective surgery is very rarely necessary.

Prognosis
- Untreated, most patients with duodenal ulcers relapse within 1–2 years of initial healing, particularly the elderly, NSAID users, and smokers.

Follow-up and management
- If symptoms continue after 8 weeks of full-dose H_2 blockade, patients should be checked with endoscopy, and the ulcer and antrum should be biopsied.
- Maintenance with half-dose H_2 antagonist should be considered to prevent recurrence for patients with a history of aggressive ulcer (e.g. previous bleeding), the elderly, or those with other illnesses.

Key references
Feldman M, Burton ME: Histamine 2-receptor antagonists: standard therapy for acid-peptic diseases. *N Engl J Med* 1991, **323**:1672–1678, 1749–1755.

Maton PN: Omeprazole. *N Engl J Med* 1991, **324**:965–975.

Penston JA: *Helicobacter pylori* eradication– understandable caution but no excuse for inertia. *Ailment Pharmacol Ther* 1994, **8**:369–390.

Peterson WL: *Helicobacter pylori* and peptic ulcer disease. *N Engl J Med* 1991, **324**:1043–1048.

Tytgat GNJ: Treatments that impact favourably upon the eradication of *Helicobacter pylori* and ulcer recurrence. *Ailment Pharmacol Ther* 1994, **8**:359–368.

Enteric infections — G.C. Cook

Diagnosis

Symptoms
Dysphagia: due to *Candida* spp. infection.
Flatulence, colic, distension, large-volume diarrhoea (watery, fatty, or bloody stools).
Anorexia, nausea, vomiting, colicky abdominal pain, fever: sometimes.
Acute diarrhoea: watery or bloody.
Chronic diarrhoea, weight loss.
Constipation: due to *Salmonella typhi* or *paratyphi* infection.
Lower abdominal colic.
Pruritus ani: due to *Enterobius vermicularis* infection.

Signs
Raised temperature: sometimes.
Splenomegaly, rose spots: due to *Salmonella typhi* or *paratyphi* infection.
Borborygmi.
Large-volume, watery, fatty, or bloody stools.
Weight loss, loss of muscle bulk.
Anaemia.
Anal rash or excoriation: due to infection by *Enterobius vermicularis* or *Strongyloides stercoralis*.

Investigations
Haematology: peripheral blood eosinophilia suggests helminthic infection.
Faecal microscopy, parasitology, culture: fresh warm specimens yield highest positivity rate for *Entamoeba histolytica*.
HIV serology.
Small-intestinal biopsy: morphology, parasitology, culture, disaccharidase assay.
Upper gastrointestinal endoscopy, including duodenal biopsy.
Small-intestinal radiography: to check for ileocaecal tuberculosis.
Blood tests: for blood glucose response to oral lactose.
Hydrogen breath test.
Rectal scrape or biopsy.
Serological tests: for *Entamoeba histolytica* or *Schistosoma* spp.
Colonoscopy.
Colorectal radiography.

Complications
Dehydration, electrolyte disturbance.
Renal failure: due to cholera or other severe enterotoxigenic diarrhoeas.
Anaemia: due to haemorrhage.
Gram-negative septicaemia: rare.
'Hyperinfection syndrome': due to *Strongyloides stercoralis* infection.
Ileal perforation, haemorrhage: due to salmonellosis.
Mesenteric adenitis or ileitis, non-suppurative arthritis, ankylosing spondylitis, erythema nodosum, Reiter's syndrome: due to *Yersinia enterocolitica* infection.
Perforation, haemorrhage, Reiter's syndrome, haemolytic uraemic syndrome: due to shigellosis.
Acute necrotising colitis, appendicitis, amoeboma, haemorrhage, stricture: due to amoebic colitis.
Colorectal polyp formation: due to schistosomiasis.

Differential diagnosis
'Spurious diarrhoea'.
Drug-induced diarrhoea: laxatives, magnesium compounds, methyldopa, diuretics, para-aminosalicylic acid, herbal remedies.
Excessive alcohol intake.
Diabetic autonomic neuropathy.
Endocrine-associated diarrhoea.
Phaeochromocytoma.
Other noninfective causes of bulky, fatty stools (malabsorption): Mediterranean lymphoma (alpha-chain disease), severe malnutrition, intestinal resection, chronic pancreatitis, chronic hepatocellular dysfunction.
Idiopathic diarrhoea.
Inflammatory bowel disease (usually ulcerative colitis).

Aetiology
- Causes include the following:

Travellers' diarrhoea: clinical syndrome with many causes including viruses, bacteria, and protozoa.
Food poisoning.
Post-infective malabsorption.
Immunosuppression.
Bacteria: *Aeromonas* spp., *Campylobacter* spp., *Clostridium difficile*, *Cryptosporidium* spp., *Escherichia coli*, *Mycobacterium tuberculosis*, *Plesiomonas shigelloides*, *Salmonella* spp., *Shigella* spp., *Vibrio* spp., *Yersinia enterocolitica*.
Viruses: adenovirus, astrovirus, caliivirus, coronavirus, Norwalk virus, rotavirus.
Protozoa: *Balantidium coli*, *Blastocystis hominis*, *Cyclospora cayetanensis*, *Entamoeba histolytica*, *Giardia lamblia*, *Isospora belli*, *Sarcocystis* spp.
Helminths: *Capillaria philippinensis*, *Enterobius vermicularis*, *Fasciolopsis buski*, *Schistosoma mansoni*, *S. japonicum*, *Strongyloides stercoralis*, *Taenia* spp., *Trichuris trichiuria*.

Epidemiology
- Intestinal infection occurs worldwide.
- Travellers' diarrhoea occurs more often in people who have travelled to an area where socioeconomic standards and hygiene are imperfect (including most tropical and subtropical countries), although great geographical variations are found in prevalence rates.

Treatment

Diet and lifestyle
- Food hygiene must be strictly observed: most intestinal infections result from a contaminated environment, commonly food or drink (especially drinking water).
- Avoidance of milk and dairy products frequently diminishes symptoms due to secondary hypolactasia complicating an intestinal infection of any cause.

Pharmacological treatment

Indications
Cholera, watery (enterotoxigenic) diarrhoeas: oral rehydration (i.v. in extreme cases, e.g. infection by *Vibrio cholerae*).

Post-infective malabsorption: tetracycline, folic acid, dietary support, vitamin supplements.

Travellers' diarrhoea, food poisoning, most acute bacterial infections: possibly quinolones (usually self-limiting).

Cryptosporidium spp. infection: possibly hyperimmune bovine colostrum (no cure proved).

Mycobacterium tuberculosis infection: antituberculous chemotherapy for at least 9 months.

Balantidium coli infection: tetracycline.

Capillaria philippinensis infection: albendazole.

Clostridium difficile infection: vancomycin or metronidazole.

Entamoeba histolytica infection: metronidazole or tinidazole and diloxanide furoate.

Enterobius vermicularis infection: albendazole or mebendazole.

Fasciolopsis buski infection: praziquantel.

Giardia lamblia infection: metronidazole or tinidazole.

Isospora belli infection: co-trimoxazole.

Salmonella typhi or *paratyphi* infection: ciprofloxacin, chloramphenicol, co-trimoxazole, or amoxycillin.

Schistosoma mansoni, japonicum, mekongi, intercalatum, or *matthei* infection: praziquantel.

Strongyloides stercoralis infection: albendazole or thiabendazole.

Taenia spp. infection: praziquantel.

Trichuris trichiuria infection: albendazole or mebendazole.

Selected regimens
Amoxycillin 500 mg 3 times daily for 14 days (in *S. typhi* infection, reduced after defervescence).

Ampicillin 1 g 6-hourly for 14 days.

Chloramphenicol 50 mg/kg daily in 4 divided doses for 14 days.

Ciprofloxacin 500–750 mg twice daily for 3 days for severe travellers' diarrhoea; for 14 days for *Salmonella* spp.

Co-trimoxazole 960 mg twice daily for 14 days (longer for *I. belli* infection).

Tetracycline 500 mg 3 times daily for 10 days.

Vancomycin 125 mg 6-hourly for 10 days.

Metronidazole 2 g for 3 days for *G. lamblia* infection; 800 mg 3 times daily for 5–10 days for *E. histolytica* infection.

Tinidazole 2 g initially for *G. lamblia* infection; 2 g for 5–6 days for *E. histolytica* infection.

Diloxanide furoate 500 mg 3 times daily for 10 days.

Albendazole 400 mg twice daily for 1–3 days; with *S. stercoralis* infection, 3-day course repeated after 3 weeks.

Mebendazole 100 mg initially (second dose may be needed).

Thiabendazole 25 mg/kg twice daily for 3 days (longer in 'hyperinfection syndrome').

Praziquantel 40–50 mg/kg initially; for *S. japonicum* infection, 60 mg/kg in three divided doses on a single day.

See drug data sheets for further details.

Treatment aims
To relieve diarrhoea, abdominal colic, and other intestinal symptoms.

To rehydrate patient as rapidly as possible, preferably orally.

To ensure bacteriological or parasitic cure.

To return patient's nutritional status to normal, especially when clinically overt malabsorption has accompanied infection.

To prevent recurrences, especially of *Salmonella typhi* or *paratyphi* infections.

To relieve symptoms in untreatable immunosuppressed patients.

Prognosis
- In some severe infections (e.g. shigellosis, *Entamoeba histolytica* colitis), specific chemotherapy results in complete recovery in almost all patients.
- If surgery is necessary for complications, the prognosis is less favourable.

Follow-up and management
- Most intestinal infections are acute; follow-up is unnecessary.
- *Salmonella typhi* or *paratyphi* infections should be followed up in order to establish that the carrier state has not ensued.
- Patients with overt malabsorption as a secondary manifestation of an intestinal infection should be followed up for maintenance therapy and ascertainment of ultimate cure.

Key references
Cook GC: *Parasitic Disease in Clinical Practice.* London: Springer-Verlag, 1990.

DuPont HL, Ericsson CD: Prevention and treatment of travelers' diarrhea. *N Engl J Med* 1993, **328**:1821–1827.

Gorbach SL, Bartlett JG, Blacklow NR (eds): *Infectious Diseases.* Philadelphia: WB Saunders, 1992.

Gracey M (ed): *Diarrhea.* Boca Raton: CRC Press, 1991.

Gallstones, cholesterol — R.P. Jazrawi and T.C. Northfield

Diagnosis

Symptoms
- Up to 70% of patients are asymptomatic or have nonspecific dyspeptic symptoms.

Uncomplicated
Biliary colic: sudden-onset severe epigastric or upper right quadrant abdominal pain, lasting for several hours, usually radiating to back, sometimes associated with nausea and vomiting.

Complicated
Fever, abdominal pain, nausea and vomiting: indicating acute cholecystitis.
Fever, pain, jaundice: indicating acute cholangitis.
Abdominal and back pain, collapse, vomiting: indicating acute pancreatitis.

Signs

Uncomplicated
- Few signs are manifest.

Tenderness in right upper quadrant: usually during or after episodes of biliary colic.

Complicated
Jaundice: indicating stone impaction in common bile duct.
Murphy's sign: indicating acute cholecystitis.
Hypotension: indicating acute pancreatitis.

Investigations
- Gallstones are frequently found incidentally by ultrasonography or abdominal radiography (if calcified).
- Laboratory tests are not diagnostic but are useful for identifying complications and excluding other abnormalities.

Serum amylase measurement: >1000 IU/L indicates acute pancreatitis.
Serum alkaline phosphatase and bilirubin measurement: elevation indicates biliary tract disease.
Leucocyte count: for cholecystitis and biliary colic.
Antimitochondrial antibody tests: to exclude primary biliary cirrhosis.
Plain abdominal radiography: identifies calcified stones.
Oral cholecystography: identifies radiolucent stones, good for determining gallbladder contraction and cystic duct patency and for identifying anatomical abnormalities in gallbladder; not sensitive for detecting small stones and invalid in case of non-opacifying gallbladder.
Ultrasonography: more sensitive for detecting small stones and biliary sludge; no exposure to radiation; detects dilated bile ducts and can identify disease in other organs.
CT: more sensitive than radiography in detecting calcification; prerequisite for selecting patients for non-surgical treatment.
Cholescintigraphy: using ^{99M}Tc-HIDA or ^{131}I-rose bengal; helpful in suspected acute cholecystitis.

Complications
Acute cholecystitis.
Acute cholangitis.
Acute pancreatitis.
Hydrops, white bile, empyema of gallbladder.
Malignancy of gallbladder.
Perforation.
Internal and external biliary fistulas.
Gallstone ileus.
Haemobilia.
Porcelain gallbladder.

Differential diagnosis
- Few patients with gallstones have typical biliary colic (<10%).

Obstructive jaundice
Pancreatic neoplasm.
Bile-duct stricture.
Cholestatic hepatitis

Biliary colic
Pancreatitis.
Oesophagitis.
Peptic ulcer.
Irritable bowel syndrome.

Aetiology
- No unifying cause has been found, but the following may have a role:

Pathogenesis
Cholesterol supersaturation of bile.
Sluggish gallbladder emptying.
Rapid cholesterol nucleation.

Predisposing factors
Obesity.
Diet.
Disease: cirrhosis of liver, ileal dysfunction.
Drugs: e.g. octreotide.

Epidemiology
- 10–15% of the adult population have cholesterol gallstones.
- The incidence is 0.6% of the population.
- Gallstones occur more often in women, and their occurrence increases with age.

Treatment

Diet and lifestyle
- No evidence indicates that high-cholesterol diet promotes gallstones, nor that diet high in fibre and low in cholesterol dissolves stones or prevents their recurrence.
- Patients at risk of gallstones should avoid obesity and not miss meals.
- Rapid weight reduction should also be avoided.

Pharmacological treatment
- Drugs are indicated for patients with infrequent or mild symptoms, radiolucent stones, and functioning gallbladder or for those not fit for or not wanting surgery.
- Bile-acid treatment is used for patients with small stones (<15 mm diameter); bile acids dissolve cholesterol gallstones by micellar solubilization or liquid crystal formation; they also reduce cholesterol absorption by intestine or secretion by liver.

Standard dosage	Chenodeoxycholic acid (CDCA) 15 mg/kg daily. Ursodeoxycholic acid (UDCA) 10 mg/kg daily. UDCA and CDCA 5 mg/kg each daily. All as single bedtime dose for up to 2 years.
Contraindications	Pregnancy and lactation. *CDCA:* chronic liver disease or diarrhoea. *UDCA:* active peptic ulcers.
Special points	UDCA or combination better than CDCA alone.
Main drug interactions	Sex hormones, oral contraceptives, blood cholesterol-lowering agents.
Main side effects	*CDCA:* diarrhoea, hypertransaminasaemia (reversible and dose-dependent). *UDCA:* gallstone calcification resulting in treatment failure.

Non-pharmacological treatment

Surgery
- Open cholecystectomy is the traditional treatment.
- Laparoscopic cholecystectomy is less invasive and has rapid discharge but a higher risk of serious complications (bile duct strictures), and the risk of morbidity multiplies with age.

Extracorporeal shock-wave lithotripsy
- Lithotripsy is indicated for 1–3 stones <30 mm in diameter.
- Dissolution is quicker with bile acids.
- Expensive equipment is needed.
- The incidence of biliary colic and haematuria is higher.
- It is contraindicated in haemolytic disorders.

Contact dissolution with methyl tert-butyl ether (MTBE)
- MTBE is a powerful cholesterol solvent (dissolves stones in a few hours).
- The procedure is invasive (percutaneous, transhepatic gallbladder cannulation).
- Leakage causes drowsiness, nausea, and duodenitis.
- The risk of recurrence is higher because of undissolved debris.
- It is contraindicated in haemolytic disorders.

Strategy for the management of gallstones. CDCA, chenodeoxycholic acid; MTBE, methyl tert-butyl ether; UDCA, ursodeoxycholic acid.

Treatment aims
To dissolve stones, with consequent relief of symptoms and prevention of complications.

Prognosis
- Gallstone recurrence occurs in 50% of patients within 5 years but not after that.
- If recurrent stones are detected early and treated, >80% of patients remain gallstone-free in the long term.

Follow-up and management
- Regular ultrasonography is needed every 6–12 months to detect early recurrence.
- Bile acid treatment (full dose) is needed for recurrent stones.

Causes of treatment failure
Patients' non-compliance with treatment. Presence of radiolucent pigment stones or subradiographic calcification of stones. Development of nonfunctioning gallbladder. Inadequate dose (especially in obese patients).

Key references
Cuschieri A *et al.*: The European experience with laparoscopic cholecystectomy. *Am J Surg* 1991, 161:385–387.

Jazrawi RP *et al.*: Optimum bile acid therapy for rapid gallstone dissolution. *Gut* 1992, 33:381–386.

Jonston DE, Kaplan MM: Pathogenesis and treatment of gallstones. *N Engl J Med* 1993, 328:412–421.

Sauerbruch T, Paumgartner G: Gallbladder stones: management. *Lancet* 1991, 338:1121–1124.

Gastric cancer — C.P. Swain

Diagnosis

Symptoms
Epigastric pain, 'ulcer-like dyspepsia'.
Dyspepsia: lasting more than a few weeks, in middle-aged or older patients.
Rapid satiety, fullness.
Dysphagia.
Vomiting.
Haematemesis or melaena.
Weight loss.
Malaise.

Signs
- Often no signs are manifest.

Pallor: due to anaemia.
Koilonychia: iron deficiency (rare).
Abdominal epigastric mass: palpable gastric tumour.
Knobbly hard enlarged liver: due to metastases.
Succussion splash: due to pyloric stenosis.
Ascites.
Pleural effusion.
Hard fixed node: sentinel node of Virchow; in left supraclavicular fossa. *[sentinel: one who keeps watch.]*
Left anterior axillary node.
Mass: rectal shelf of Blumer; on rectal examination.
Infiltration of the umbilicus: Sister Joseph's nodule.
Palpable ovarian secondary: Krukenberg tumour.

Investigations
- Laboratory tests are not diagnostic but can hint at the presence of bleeding or liver metastases.

1. Full blood count: to identify iron-deficiency anaemia.
2. Liver function tests: raised alkaline phosphatase may suggest metastases.
3. Fibreoptic endoscopy: allows direct view of cancer and assessment of extent of cancer; allows biopsy (eight should be taken, if suspicious), especially from the edge, and cytology (infiltrating cancer [linitis plastica] and lymphoma may need deep or large biopsy at repeat endoscopy to make diagnosis); allows assessment of obstruction to cardia or pylorus; superficial cancers may be difficult to recognise.
4. Double-contrast barium meal: blunting, fusion, clubbing, or tapering of mucosal folds suggests cancer; less accurate than endoscopy.
5. Ultrasonography: conventional abdominal ultrasonography to assess liver metastases and presence of lymph nodes; endoscopic ultrasonography superior but not widely available.
6. CT: to assess local spread, metastases (liver, ovaries).

Complications
Tumour spread: lymphatic, haematogenous (liver, lungs, bone, adrenals), local dissemination into oesophagus, invasion of adjacent organs (pancreas, mesocolon, liver).

Differential diagnosis
Ulcer or non-ulcer dyspepsia.
Reflux oesophagitis.
Anaemia of other causes.
Depression.

Aetiology
- Causes include the following:

Smoked foods, salt fish, pickled foods, high salt and starch intake (inverse association with refrigeration, vitamin C, fresh fruit and vegetable intake).
Genetic factors: including blood group A, family history, and Lynch syndrome II.
Helicobacter pylori infection (an important cause of gastritis).

Epidemiology
- Gastric cancer occurs in 6 men in 100 000 in the UK; the male:female ratio is 2:1.
- It occurs more often in middle-aged, elderly, and poor patients (social class V).
- Patients with early gastric cancer are, on average, 8 years younger than those with advanced disease.

Pathology
Malignant neoplasm of stomach
90% adenocarcinoma; 5% lymphoma; 5% others (carcinoid, leiomyosarcoma, adenoacanthoma, squamous, hepatoid, liposarcoma).
- Advanced cancer may be polypoidal or fungating, ulcerating with a raised border, or diffusely infiltrating (linitis plastica).

Early gastric cancer
Confined to gastric mucosa or submucosa, irrespective of lymph-node invasion. Three types: protruded (type I), superficial (type II, most common), excavated (type III).

Associated conditions
1. Chronic atrophic gastritis.
2. Achlorhydria: in 65% of gastric cancer patients. — *absence of HCl in stomach.*
3. Dysplasia.
4. Adenomatous polyps.
5. Pernicious anaemia: 8% may develop gastric tumours (cancers and carcinoids).
6. Hypertrophic gastropathy (Menetrier's disease): 10% may develop gastric cancer.
7. Previous gastrectomy (especially 10–20 years after Billroth II with gastrojejunostomy).

Treatment

Diet and lifestyle
- After gastrectomy, patients should eat a good, balanced diet, with smaller frequent meals, reduction of sweet or starchy food, and drinking before but not during or after meals.
- Patients with dysphagia should have a semi-liquid diet, with enteral feeding supplements.
- Patients should be encouraged to lead a normal lifestyle.

Pharmacological treatment
- Chemotherapy has not been shown in trials to produce increased survival; it can produce effective reduction in tumour size and has been used for palliation.
- Symptoms may respond to treatment, as follows:

Ulcer-type pain: H_2 blockers.
Oesophageal pain: nystatin if candida is present.
Infiltrative pain: opiate analgesics.
Constipation: purgatives.
Vomiting (infiltrative: incompetence of cardiac sphincter): metoclopramide or cisapride (rarely responds).

Non-pharmacological treatment
Curative resection: for the 30–50% of patients without evidence of distant metastases.
Total gastrectomy: if tumour is extensive or close to cardio-oesophageal junction; higher mortality and morbidity than partial gastrectomy; side effects include small reservoir or bilious vomiting, diarrhoea, and malabsorption.
Partial gastrectomy: for early gastric cancer or infiltrative advanced cancer with 5 cm distance clear of cancer from the cardia; side effects include weight loss and altered eating ability.
Dissection of lymph glands draining stomach: important even in early gastric cancer.
Palliation of symptoms, as follows:
For obstructive pain or obstructive vomiting due to pyloric stenosis: bypass surgery.
For dysphagia: laser treatment or intubation.
For bleeding: surgery, endoscopic laser or electrocautery treatment, iron.
For depression, anxiety, or anger: careful discussion, enlistment of family, family doctor, and palliative care team support.
- Palliative surgery for locally advanced disease involving adjacent organs may benefit patients with bleeding or pyloric obstruction even with metastatic spread.
- Complications after surgery include anastomotic leakage and small gastric residue.

Treatment aims
To provide curative resection when still possible.
To provide effective symptomatic palliation when cure not possible.

Prognosis
- In patients having an 'open and close' laparotomy confirming unresectability, mean survival is 4–12 months, with almost no 5-year survivors.
- In patients having apparent curative resection, mean survival is 28 months, and the 5-year survival rate is 40%.
- The 5-year survival rate is 15% overall, 50% in patients without lymph-gland involvement, and 30% in those with lymph-gland involvement.
- The prognosis of early gastric cancer is much better, with a 5-year survival rate of 80%, compared with 20% for advanced gastric cancer after resection (types I and II better prognosis than type III).

Follow-up and management
- Gastrectomy patients may need iron and vitamin B_{12} or D supplements.
- Some total gastrectomy patients need careful nutritional support, with energy supplementation.
- Endoscopy, ultrasonography, or CT may be needed during follow-up to diagnose local or distant recurrence.

Key references
Cushieri A: Gastrectomy for gastric cancer: definitions and objectives. *Br J Surg* 1986, **73**:513–514.

Gouzi JL *et al.*: Total versus subtotal gastrectomy for adenocarcinoma of the gastric antrum. *Ann Surg* 1989, **2**:162–166.

Green PHR *et al.*: Increasing incidence and excellent survival of patients with early gastric cancer. *Am J Med* 1988, **85**:658–661.

Lechago J, Correa P: Prolonged achlorhydria and gastric neoplasia: is there a causal relationship? *Gastroenterology* 1993, **104**:1554–1557.

Takemoto T *et al.*: Impact of staging on treatment of gastric carcinoma. *Endoscopy* 1993, **25**:46–50.

Thompson GB, van Heerden JA, Sarr MG: Adenocarcinoma of the stomach: are we making progress? *Lancet* 1993, **342**:713–718.

Valen B *et al.*: Treatment of stomach cancer. A national experience. *Br J Surg* 1988, **75**:708–710.

Gastric ulceration   M. Hamilton

Diagnosis

Symptoms

Uncomplicated disease

- This is usually clinically indistinguishable from duodenal ulcer.

Epigastric pain: described as dull, burning discomfort; variably affected by food; relieved by antacids.

Nocturnal pain.

Complicated disease

Haematemesis or melaena.

Severe abdominal pain: when perforation occurs.

Nausea or vomiting and upper abdominal distension: with gastric outflow obstruction.

Marked anorexia, weight loss: suggesting malignant gastric ulceration.

Signs

Uncomplicated disease

Epigastric tenderness.

Complicated disease

Signs of haemodynamic compromise: in acute haemorrhage.

Local or generalized peritonism: if ulcer has perforated.

Upper abdominal distension, succussion splash, visible peristalsis: with gastric outflow obstruction.

Investigations

Full blood count: to detect iron-deficiency anaemia or decreased haemoglobin in acute bleeds.

Serum gastrin measurement: in recurrent or multiple ulceration, for Zollinger–Ellison syndrome.

Chest radiography: plain film may show subdiaphragmatic gas in perforation.

Contrast radiography: barium studies may make diagnosis.

Fibreoptic endoscopy: investigation of choice (biopsy and cytology essential to exclude malignancy); allows direct visualization of ulcer; may help to diagnose small lesions or mucosal abnormalities; allows histological confirmation of diagnosis; allows assessment of *Helicobacter pylori* status.

Complications

Perforation.

Haemorrhage.

Gastric outflow obstruction.

Differential diagnosis

Chronic pain

Duodenal ulceration.

Chronic gastritis.

Gastric carcinoma.

Chronic pancreatitis.

Irritable bowel syndrome.

Gastroesophageal reflux disease.

Acute pain

Acute pancreatitis.

Myocardial infarction.

Aortic dissection.

Biliary colic.

- Pain due to peptic ulceration is usually not severe enough to suggest the above diagnoses.

Aetiology

- Causes include the following:

NSAIDs inhibiting protective prostaglandin synthesis.

Basal and peak acid secretion usually within normal range; mucosal defences impaired, with subsequent back-diffusion of acid into mucosa.

Helicobacter pylori infection in 70% of patients, although role remains unproved.

Alcohol.

Epidemiology

- The incidence of gastric ulceration increases with age.
- The male:female ratio is equal.
- Gastric ulceration is more prevalent in low socioeconomic groups (IV, V).

Treatment

Diet and lifestyle
- In addition to specific pharmacological treatment, avoiding aspirin, NSAIDs, and alcohol excess is useful.
- Eating regular meals and discontinuing smoking may help.
- Smoking and NSAIDs are associated with delayed healing and early relapse.

Pharmacological treatment
- Despite the uncertain role of *Helicobacter pylori* in the pathogenesis, most clinicians would attempt eradication if present (*see* Duodenal ulcer *for further details*).

Antacids
- These may give temporary symptomatic relief if taken 3 h after meals; they do not speed ulcer healing.

H_2-receptor antagonists
- The mainstay of treatment, these produce symptomatic relief within days and have ulcer healing rates of 80% at 4 weeks and 96% at 8 weeks.

Standard dosage	Ranitidine 300 mg, cimetidine 800 mg, famotidine 400 mg, or nizatidine 300 mg; all given as single dose at night.
Contraindications	Known hypersensitivity (rare), pregnancy and lactation.
Main drug interactions	*Cimetidine:* oral anticoagulants, theophylline, phenytoin.
Main side effects	*Cimetidine:* headache, constipation or diarrhoea, gynaecomastia (all unusual).

Prostaglandins
- Prostaglandins are probably most useful with continuing predisposing factors, e.g. concomitant NSAID treatment. Healing rates are inferior to H_2 antagonists.

Standard dosage	Misoprostol 800 mg in 2–4 divided doses.
Contraindications	Pregnancy or planned pregnancy.
Special points	Small doses of synthetic prostaglandins have been shown to exhibit a cytoprotective effect and to inhibit gastric acid secretion.
Main drug interactions	None known.
Main side effects	Diarrhoea, abdominal pain, flushing, menorrhagia.

Proton-pump inhibitors
- The primary role is management of resistant ulceration or treatment of Zollinger–Ellison syndrome.

Standard dosage	Omeprazole 20 mg in morning.
Contraindications	None known.
Special points	Long-term treatment not indicated.
Main drug interactions	Diazepam, phenytoin, warfarin.
Main side effects	Headache, diarrhoea, nausea, skin rashes (all unusual).

Treatment aims
To relieve symptoms.
To heal ulcer.

Other treatments
- Surgery is indicated for uncontrolled ulcer-related haemorrhage (early operation important in elderly patients), second major bleed, perforation, or malignant ulceration or delayed healing.

Prognosis
- After completion of a healing course of H_2 antagonists, the chance of recurrence in 1 year is 50%.

Follow-up and management
- Endoscopic confirmation of mucosal healing at 8–12 weeks is essential, with repeated biopsy and further endoscopy if ulcer healing has not occurred.
- After ulcer healing, treatment is usually discontinued unless an obvious and continuing predisposing factor is present.
- Recurrence of symptoms must be reassessed with further endoscopy.
- Recurrent ulceration is managed by maintenance treatment with half-dose H_2 blockade.

Key references

Feldman M, Burton ME: Histamine 2-receptor antagonists: standard therapy for acid peptic disease. *N Engl J Med* 1991, **323**:1672, 1749–1755.

Maton PN: Omeprazole. *N Engl J Med* 1991, **324**:965–975.

McCarthy DM: Omeprazole. *N Engl J Med* 1991, **325**:1017–1025.

Peterson WL: *Helicobacter pylori* and peptic ulcer disease. *N Engl J Med* 1991, **324**:1043–1048.

Soll H: Pathogenesis of peptic ulcer and implications for therapy. *N Engl J Med* 1990, **322**:909–916.

Walt RP: Misoprostol for the treatment of peptic ulcer and antiinflammatory-drug-induced gastroduodenal ulceration. *N Engl J Med* 1992, **327**:1575–1580.

Gastrointestinal bleeding   C.P. Swain

Diagnosis

Symptoms
Haematemesis: fresh red blood or darker altered blood that may resemble ground coffee.
Melaena: passage of black, sticky, shiny, rich-smelling stool; fresh blood takes ~14 h to be altered to haematin and passed rectally.
Rectal bleeding (haematochezia): passage of fresh red blood or darker red 'maroon' from rectum; may be unaltered blood, blood mixed into the stool, blood clots, or bloody diarrhoea.
Collapse, loss of consciousness, angina, shortness of breath, malaise, headache: symptoms of hypotension or anaemia.

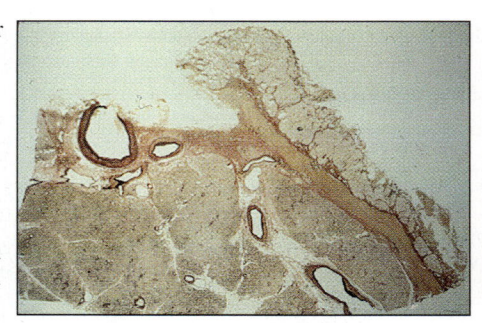

Large hole in an artery in the large duodenal ulcer in a patient who died.

Signs
Tachycardia: earliest sign of shock.
Hypotension: especially postural.
Splenomegaly, spider naevi, palmar erythema: stigmata of chronic liver disease (varices should be considered).
Mass, hepatomegaly, lymph-gland enlargement, Kaposi's sarcoma: signs of cancer.
Findings of telangiectasia: Osler–Weber–Rendu syndrome.
Lax skin: pseudoxanthoma elasticum.
Rubber joints: Ehler–Danlos syndrome.
Blue rubber bleb.
Abdominal tenderness: unusual.

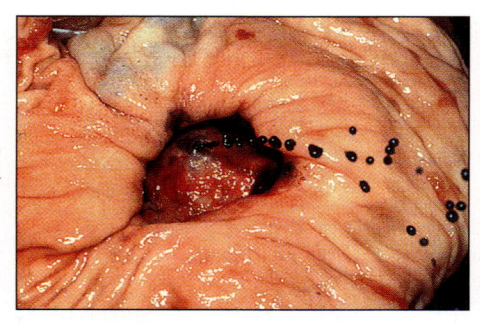

Bleeding gastric ulcer.

Investigations
Haemoglobin and haematocrit analysis: time needed for haemodilution, so initial haemoglobin may not reflect severity of bleeding.
Urea measurement: concentration can only double with ingested blood but may rise further in hypotensive patients.
Mean cell volume measurement: raised volume with alcohol-related disorders or may indicate a raised reticulocyte count.
Platelet count: raised with recent bleeding, may be low in liver or HIV-related disease.
Clotting screening: especially if patient has liver disease or easy bruising.
Fibreoptic endoscopy: stigmata of haemorrhage in peptic ulcers allow prediction of further bleeding (absence of stigmata suggests low chance of further bleeding); visible vessel in peptic ulcer indicates 50% chance of further haemorrhage and increased risk of death; large varices and cherry-red spots may predict increased risk of further bleeding; endoscopy superior to barium studies in making diagnosis in most situations.
Angiography: occasionally useful for difficult severe recurrent bleeding (needs bleeding rate of >5 ml/min); presence of barium may prevent angiography.
^{99m}Tc-labelled erythrocyte scanning: may detect bleeding rate of 1 ml/min.
Tc pertechnate scanning: useful for Meckel's diverticulum because isotope taken up by ectopic gastric mucosa in diverticulum.

Complications
Recurrent or continued bleeding.
Peptic ulcer: in 20–30% of patients.
Exsanguination.
Varices: in 50%.

Differential diagnosis

Haematemesis
Nose bleeds and haemoptysis, with subsequently swallowed blood.

Melaena
Ingestion of iron, bismuth-containing preparations, or Guinness, producing black stool.

Aetiology
History of previous bleeding, ulcer, or gastrointestinal disease (in <50% of patients).
Alcohol, NSAID, or anticoagulant intake.
Haematemesis preceded by retching (suggesting Mallory–Weiss tear).
Liver disease, coagulopathy, amyloid.
Family history of bleeding.
Previous surgery for peptic ulcer or arterial bypass grafts.
Nose bleeds before haematemesis.

Causes of upper gastrointestinal bleeding
Gastric erosions, duodenal ulcer, gastric ulcer, varices, oesophagitis, erosive duodenitis, Mallory–Weiss tear, neoplasm, oesophageal ulcer, stomal ulcer.
Osler–Weber–Rendu syndrome (autosomal dominant), pseudoxanthoma elasticum, Ehler–Danlos syndrome (autosomal dominant and recessive types).
Reflux oesophagitis and hiatus hernia.
Helicobacter pylori and AIDS-related disease.

Causes of lower gastrointestinal bleeding
Haemorrhoids, polyps, cancer, inflammatory bowel disease, angiodysplasia, diverticular disease, radiation enteritis, ischaemic colitis, drug-induced ulcer or solitary rectal ulcer. Meckel's diverticulum, leiomyoma, adenocarcinoma, lymphoma, aorto-enteric fistula (especially in the distal duodenum), mesenteric ischaemia.

- Haemorrhoids are the most usual cause of lower gastrointestinal bleeding. Bright blood unmixed with stool drips into pan or is seen on toilet paper; this is rarely a cause of major bleeding. Blood from haemorrhoids can reflux to splenic flexure. 25% of patients with prolapsing haemorrhoids have another cause of rectal bleeding.

Epidemiology
- The incidence of upper gastrointestinal bleeding is 50–150 hospital episodes in 100 000 population.

Treatment

Diet and lifestyle
- Patients should be warned not to take aspirin or NSAIDs and should be advised not to smoke.
- Alcoholic patients, especially with liver disease, should be advised to stop drinking alcohol and should be given medical, family, or non-medical support.
- Patients must not eat just before endoscopy or surgery; at other times, no evidence suggests that starving or feeding patients confers benefit.

Pharmacological treatment

For peptic ulcer
- Little evidence indicates that drug treatment affects outcome from bleeding peptic ulcer.
- Treatment by long-term H_2 blockade or eradication of *Helicobacter pylori* may reduce the incidence of readmission with peptic ulcer bleeding.

For bleeding varices
- Drug treatments are probably ineffective in the treatment of bleeding varices. Some clinicians claim that glypressin, a somatostatin analogue (octreotide), or propanolol may improve outcome.

Non-pharmacological treatment

Transfusion
Whole blood or packed cells; not for patients with minor bleeding or who are at low risk for further bleeding.

For peptic ulcer
Endoscopic treatment (laser, monopolar, bipolar, heater probe, and injection of adrenaline alone, adrenaline and a sclerosant, or alcohol): can reduce rebleeding rate, need for surgery, and mortality; repeat endoscopic treatment may be preferable to surgery in elderly patients.

Surgery: in patients with continued or recurrent bleeding in hospital; if surgery necessary, best done before repeated episodes of hypotension have impaired chances of recovery.

For bleeding varices
Endoscopic variceal injection sclerotherapy, using sclerosants such as ethanolamine, alcohol, sodium tetradecyl sulphate, and sodium morrhuate: has been shown to reduce the incidence of further bleeding and to reduce mortality in patients with recent bleeding from oesophageal varices, and it can stop bleeding from varices.

Endoscopic variceal band ligation: less invasive than surgery, may have lower complication rate than endoscopic sclerotherapy.

Balloon tamponade: stops bleeding in 85% of patients, but bleeding recurs in 21–60% and survival not improved; dangerous, causing oesophageal rupture, aspiration pneumonia, with lethal complications of 10%.

Percutaneous transhepatic cannulation of portal vein: with injection of sclerosant or obliterative substance, e.g. Gelfoam, thrombin, cyanoacrylate.

Transjugular intrahepatic portacaval shunt.

Surgery: for the few patients who do not respond to endoscopic treatment; options include portosystemic shunt, direct suture ligation, oesophageal transection, devascularization, hepatic transplantation.

Complications of treatment
After surgery: pneumonia, renal or cardiac failure, further bleeding.

With endoscopy for bleeding peptic ulcer: precipitation of acute bleeding, perforation, infarction of stomach or duodenum (with injection).

With endoscopy for bleeding varices: oesophageal ulceration, perforation, septicaemia, distant thrombosis, pleural effusion, aspiration.

Treatment aims
To reduce mortality, need for urgent surgery, and rebleeding rate.

Prognosis
- For peptic ulcer bleeding, the risk of rebleeding in hospital is 15–30%, of needing urgent surgery 15–20%, and of death 5–10%.
- The risk of death after admission with first variceal bleeding is 30%.
- 70% of patients with bleeding varices die within 1–4 years.
- Bleeding due to Mallory–Weiss tear, oesophagitis, gastritis, and duodenitis has excellent prognosis.
- Most patients with bleeding upper gastrointestinal cancer die within 1 year.

Follow-up and management
- Ulcer patients with major bleeding should have follow-up endoscopy to check healing and eradication of *Helicobacter pylori*.
- Patients with second major bleed should be considered for surgery.
- Patients with bleeding varices need repeat endoscopy and sclerotherapy until varices are eradicated.

Key references
Consensus Development Panel, National Institutes of Health 1990: Consensus statement on therapeutic endoscopy and bleeding ulcers. *Gastrointest Endosc* 1990, **36**:S62–S63.

Cook DJ et al.: Endoscopic therapy for acute nonvariceal upper gastrointestinal hemorrhage: a meta-analysis. *Gastroenterology* 1992, **102**:139–148.

Fleischer D: Endoscopic hemostasis in non-variceal bleeding. *Endoscopy* 1992, **24**:58–63.

Laine L: Upper gastrointestinal bleeding. *Alimentary Pharmacol Ther* 1993, **7**:207–232.

Laine L, Peterson WL: Medical progress: bleeding peptic ulcer. *N Engl J Med* 1994, **331**:717–727.

Wheatley KE, Dykes PW: Upper gastrointestinal bleeding: when to operate. *Postgrad Med J* 1990, **45**:926–936.

Irritable bowel syndrome
D.G. Maxton

Diagnosis

Symptoms
- Restrictive criteria for irritable bowel syndrome are continuous or recurrent symptoms for at least 3 months of abdominal pain and disturbed defaecation (at least 25% of time; at least three of altered stool frequency, form, or passage, passage of mucus, abdominal distension).

Abdominal pain: often intermittent, crampy lower abdominal pain; relieved by defaecation or flatus; associated with change in frequency or consistency of stool.
Straining, urgency, passage of mucus, feeling of incomplete evacuation.
Diarrhoea: often in morning or after meals, rarely nocturnal.
Constipation: small, hard stools, difficult to pass.
Abdominal distension: bloating worse after meals and at end of day.
Functional abdominal bloating.
Functional constipation.
Painless diarrhoea.
Chronic functional abdominal pain.
Nausea, heartburn, early satiety.
Urinary frequency, urgency.
Dyspareunia.
Tiredness, backache.

Signs
Variable abdominal tenderness: often over palpable sigmoid colon; frequently present but nonspecific.

Investigations

Screening tests
Full blood count: anaemia or nutritional deficiency needs investigation.
Liver function tests: abnormal tests may indicate biliary disease.
Thyroid function tests: for myxoedema manifest as constipation, or thyrotoxicosis as diarrhoea.
Colonic imaging: barium enema or colonoscopy; for new or different symptoms in patients aged >40 years to detect colonic carcinoma or inflammatory bowel disease.

Further tests
Small-bowel contrast studies, gastroscopy, abdominal ultrasonography or CT, duodenal or jejunal biopsy or aspiration: e.g. for Crohn's disease, peptic ulcer, biliary or pancreatic disease.
Colonic biopsy, faecal fat analysis, breath hydrogen test, lactose tolerance test, ^{75}Se-HCAT absorption measurement, laxative screening: in patients with diarrhoea predominantly; e.g. for collagenous colitis, steatorrhoea, small-bowel overgrowth, bile-acid malabsorption.
Plain abdominal radiography, colonic transit timing, full-thickness colonic biopsy, defaecography: in patients with constipation predominantly; e.g. for megacolon, idiopathic slow-transit constipation, neuromuscular gut disorders, obstructed defaecation.

Complications
Increased incidence of colonic diverticulosis: caused by prolonged constipation.
Major physical and psychological morbidity: frequent in intractable cases.

Differential diagnosis
- Colonic malignancy.
- Inflammatory bowel disease: Crohn's and ulcerative colitis.
- Diverticular or coeliac disease.
- Infections: e.g. by *Giardia* spp.
- Pancreatic disorder: e.g. chronic pancreatitis.
- Gastric disorders: e.g. peptic ulcer.
- Biliary and liver disease: e.g. gallstones.
- Congenital or acquired motility disorder, bile-acid malabsorption, bacterial overgrowth, laxative abuse (rarer).
- Endometriosis, ovarian malignancy.
- Hydronephrosis.
- Thyroid disease.

Aetiology
- Possible causes include the following:
Abnormal gut motility.
Enhanced visceral sensitivity.
Abnormal central pain perception.
Psychological or psychiatric disorder.
Food allergy or intolerance.

Epidemiology
- Irritable bowel syndrome is common and occurs world wide (10–20% of population in industrialized countries).
- It occurs more frequently in women.
- Up to 50% of gastroenterological referrals are for irritable bowel syndrome.

Organic or functional bowel disease
- The following features should not be considered part of irritable bowel syndrome without investigation:
Change of bowel habit: new gastrointestinal symptoms in patients aged >40 years.
Weight loss.
Rectal bleeding or nocturnal diarrhoea.
Fever.
Abnormal haematology or biochemistry results.

Psychological factors
- 50% of patients have a psychiatric abnormality.
- Anxiety, depression, and personality disorders are common.
- Adverse life events may precede symptoms.
- Psychological factors may determine who consults doctors rather than cause the condition.

Treatment

Diet and lifestyle
- Patients should be encouraged to eat small frequent meals, throughout the day.
- Bran or fruit may exacerbate pain and distension when eaten in excess.
- Regular exercise improves bowel function.

Pharmacological treatment
- Placebo response rates are high (range, 20–70%).
- Few drugs have been proved to be of unequivocal benefit; many patients, however, find drugs helpful in controlling symptoms, often preferring 'as-required' medication to long-term usage.
- Treatment should be targeted to predominant complaint.
- Dosage should be as low as possible because patients often report side effects.

Bulking agents
- These are mostly useful for constipation.
- The full effect may not be apparent for several days.

Standard dosage	Bran 2.4 g, ispaghula husk 3.5 g, or sterculia 7 g, twice daily. Lactulose 15 ml twice daily, increased as needed, or stimulant laxatives may be needed for intractable cases.
Contraindications	Intestinal obstruction.
Special points	Patients must take adequate fluid.
Main drug interactions	None.
Main side effects	Distension, flatulence, abdominal pain.

Antispasmodics
- Antispasmodics, either with anticholinergic properties or direct muscle relaxants, are given for pain relief.

Standard dosage	*Anticholinergics:* dicyclomine 10–20 mg up to 3 times daily or hyoscine 20 mg up to 4 times daily. *Direct relaxants:* mebeverine 135 mg, alverine 60 mg, or peppermint oil 1 capsule; each up to 3 times daily.
Contraindications	Paralytic ileus, ulcerative colitis. *Anticholinergics:* glaucoma.
Special points	Dosage times should be varied to suit the individual.
Main drug interactions	*Anticholinergics:* disopyramide, cisapride, antidepressants.
Main side effects	*Anticholinergics:* dry mouth, blurring of vision, palpitations, constipation. *Direct relaxants:* heartburn.

Antimotility drugs
- The diarrhoea must be confirmed (not pseudodiarrhoea or faecal retention with overflow).

Standard dosage	Loperamide 2–8 mg daily in divided doses or codeine phosphate 30 mg 3–4 times daily; dose adjusted to control symptoms.
Contraindications	Intestinal obstruction, inflammatory bowel disease.
Special points	Night-time dosage might prevent morning diarrhoea.
Main drug interactions	*Codeine:* anxiolytics and hypnotics.
Main side effects	*Codeine:* constipation, dependence.

Other options
Motility stimulants: cisapride 10 mg 3 times daily may be useful in constipation.
Antidepressants: tricyclic antidepressants (e.g. amitriptyline 25 mg at night) can be helpful, but side effects and excess sedation limit use.
5-HT uptake inhibitors: e.g. fluoxetine 20 mg daily, effective and less sedating.

Treatment aims
To control or cure the most intrusive complaint.
To treat associated psychological disorders.

Other treatments
- Behavioural therapy (hypnotherapy, psychotherapy, relaxation techniques) is effective for some intractable cases.
- Benefit is seen especially in younger patients or those with identifiable psychological disease or stress and recent symptom onset.
- Behavioural therapy is ineffective for older patients or constant or chronic pain sufferers.

Prognosis
- This is a chronic relapsing condition.
- >75% of patients respond to treatment over 1 year.
- ~50% have a few symptoms after 5 years.
- Response is better in men, constipation-predominant sufferers, and those with a short history or symptoms after acute diarrhoea.

Follow-up and management
- Follow-up is not needed for mild or moderate cases.
- Patients must be monitored for change in symptoms; new or different complaints should be investigated; persistent symptoms do not need further tests.
- Regular, brief review of intractable cases may reduce inappropriate investigation and further referral.

Key references
Camilleri M, Prather CM: The irritable bowel syndrome: mechanisms and a practical approach to management. *Ann Int Med* 1992, **116**:1001–1008.

Heaton KW *et al.*: Symptoms of irritable bowel syndrome in a British urban community: consulters and non-consulters. *Gastroenterology* 1992, **102**:1962–1967.

Lynn RB, Friedman LS: Irritable bowel syndrome. *N Engl J Med* 1993, **329**:1940–1945.

Thompson WG: Irritable bowel syndrome: pathogenesis and management. *Lancet* 1993, **341**:1569–1572.

Oesophageal carcinoma — M. Dakkak and J.R. Bennett

Diagnosis

Symptoms and signs
Dysphagia: classic symptom but tends to occur when disease is advanced.

Inability to swallow saliva and regurgitation: due to luminal stenosis.

Pain: occasionally early symptom; usually manifestation of mediastinal extension.

Weight loss, anaemia, cervical lymphadenopathy, hepatomegaly: late symptoms; less specific.

Investigations
Blood count: may reveal iron-deficiency anaemia.

Biochemical analysis: may show raised alkaline phosphatase concentration with hepatic or bony metastases; low serum albumin concentration indicates malnutrition.

Barium swallow: shows lesion; endoscopy always needed for confirmation.

Endoscopy: offers direct examination of lesion and provides opportunity to obtain specimens for histology and cytology.

CT, MRI, endoscopic ultrasonography: to select patients with localized tumours for resection.

Complications
Oesophageal obstruction.
Malnutrition.
Bleeding.
Fistula to bronchial tree.
Invasion of mediastinum.
Aspiration.

Differential diagnosis
Benign oesophageal stricture.
Motility disorders, particularly achalasia.
Extrinsic compression of oesophagus: e.g. carcinoma of bronchus.

Aetiology
- Several factors have been identified in association with oesophageal cancer, including the following:

Poor nutrition: particularly shortage of vitamins.

Increased consumption of tobacco and alcohol.

Genetics and race: certain families in China are thought to carry a defective gene; blacks in America have a higher incidence.

Stasis: possibly the underlying factor in patients with achalasia who develop cancer.

Caustic injury: carcinoma occurs ~40 years later.

Barrett's oesophagus.

Epidemiology
- Oesophageal carcinoma is one of the most common cancers in the world, but wide geographic variations are found.
- It is relatively less frequent in western Europe and North America (incidence, 5 in 100 000).

Histological types
Tumours of upper and middle oesophagus: usually squamous cell carcinoma.

Tumours of lower oesophagus: mostly adenocarcinoma.

Treatment

Diet and lifestyle
- Adequate nutrition should be ensured, preferably orally.
- A fine-bore enteral feeding tube may be necessary.

Pharmacological treatment
- Simple analgesics are used for pain control in the early stages, but opiates are needed later.

Standard dosage	Morphine 10 mg every 4 h initially.
Contraindications	Raised intracranial pressure.
Special points	Concerns about side effects should not deter use.
Main drug interactions	None significant.
Main side effects	Constipation, nausea, drowsiness.

Non-pharmacological treatment
- Curative surgery or radiotherapy is attempted whenever possible, but most patients are suitable for only palliative treatment.

Surgical resection: suitable in only about one-third of patients; oesophagectomy with primary oesophagogastrostomy most frequently chosen.

Endoscopic palliation: to create a wider lumen to allow food and drink to pass; options include simple dilatation (by bougie or balloon), endoscopic intubations (various prosthetic stents available), laser therapy, thermal devices (e.g. bipolar coagulation), alcohol injection.

Radiotherapy: intracavitary irradiation with cobalt or iridium or external beam irradiation; can be beneficial for pain from mediastinal extension.

Nutritional support: alimentary support in selected patients; includes nasogastric tube, percutaneous endoscopic gastrostomy, and surgically placed jejunostomy.

Treatment aims
To delay physical deterioration by improving and maintaining swallowing and nutrition.
To diminish pain.
To avoid respiratory complications.

Prognosis
- Most patients die within a few months; in patients with successful surgical resection, the 5-year survival rate is 10–15%.
- After resection, mortality is 3–20% and complications are 5–12%.
- Causes of death from surgery include cardiopulmonary complications and sepsis due to anastomotic leaks; malnutrition is a contributing factor.

Follow-up and management
- Patients who had curative treatment should be monitored for features of relapse.

Key references
Cameron AJ: Barrett's oesophagus and adenocarcinoma. *Gastroenterology* 1993, **102**:1421–1424.

Cuschieri A: Treatment of carcinoma of the oesophagus. *Ann R Coll Surg Engl* 1991, **73**:1–3.

Griffin SM, Robertson CS: Nonsurgical treatment of cancer of the oesophagus. *Br J Surg* 1993, **80**:412–413.

Haller DG: Treatments for esophageal cancer. *N Engl J Med* 1992, **326**:1629–1630.

Kruse P et al.: Barrett's oesophagus and oesophageal adenocarcinoma. *Scand J Gastroenterol* 1993, **28**:193–196.

Oesophagitis and hiatus hernia — M. Dakkak and J.R. Bennett

Diagnosis

Symptoms

Oesophagitis
- Symptoms do not help to discriminate between reflux with and without oesophagitis.

Heartburn: the most common symptom.

Retrosternal pain: may resemble angina.

Odynophagia (painful swallowing).

Regurgitation of food, acid, or bitter juice: may be described as 'vomiting' (but without nausea).

Dysphagia: stricture or motility disorder.

Respiratory symptoms.

Hiatus hernia
- A common condition, this can be asymptomatic.
- The two varieties are sliding (more common) and rolling or para-oesophageal.

Reflux, cardiac and pulmonary symptoms (related to presence of hernia in thoracic cavity): symptoms of sliding hernia.

Cardiac and pulmonary symptoms, dysphagia, hiccough, volvulus, strangulation: symptoms of rolling hernia.

Signs
- Usually no signs are manifest.

Pulmonary consolidation or atelectasis: rarely, if aspiration has occurred as a result of regurgitation.

Investigations
- Blood tests are not helpful.

Radiography: not reliable for showing oesophagitis (particularly mild forms) or reflux; can be used to assess peristalsis and other structural abnormality, particularly if video recording obtained or if solid bolus used in addition to barium.

Endoscopy: preferred to radiography because it offers visualization of mucosa and option of obtaining cytology and histology; allows determination of severity of oesophagitis.

pH monitoring: for diagnosis of acid reflux without oesophagitis; for quantifying reflux to assess effectiveness of treatment or before antireflux surgery.

Manometry: useful only with associated motility disorder or before antireflux surgery.

Cardiac tests: in difficult cases.

Complications
Stricture.

Barrett's oesophagus.

Aspiration, leading to night cough, bronchospasm, pneumonia, asthma, hoarseness.

Differential diagnosis
Ischaemic heart disease.
Oesophageal motility disorder.
Peptic ulcer disease.
Gallstone disease.

Aetiology
- Oesophagitis is mucosal damage caused by gastroesophageal reflux, which occurs when the lower oesophageal sphincter is incompetent or oesophageal clearance is impaired.
- The damage is caused by prolonged exposure of oesophageal mucosa to gastric juice and is more intense if the mucosa is compromised or if gastric emptying is delayed.

Epidemiology
- Two-thirds of the population may suffer from reflux at some time, but only a small proportion seek medical advice; of these, only 38–75% have oesophagitis.
- Mechanical and hormonal factors make reflux common during pregnancy.

Savary–Miller endoscopic classification
Grade I: non-confluent mucosal lesions.
Grade II: confluent mucosal lesions.
Grade III: circumferential mucosal lesions.
Grade IV: deep ulcer, stricture, or Barrett's oesophagus.

Treatment

Diet and lifestyle
- Reducing weight, stopping smoking, eating small meals, avoiding certain foods (e.g. fat, chocolate, spices, citrus juices, coffee), and raising the head of the bed are measures that decrease reflux.
- NSAIDs, slow-release potassium chloride, nitrates, and calcium antagonists must be avoided.

Pharmacological treatment

Antacids
- Antacids provide reasonable but short-lasting relief and have no effect on mucosal inflammation.
- They combine with alginates to form a floating raft, creating a barrier between gastric juice and oesophageal mucosa.

Standard dosage	Antacids 10 ml 3–4 times daily.
Contraindications	Hypophosphataemia.
Main drug interactions	Iron, phenytoin, penicillamine, tetracycline.
Main side effects	Constipation, diarrhoea.

Acid antisecretory agents
- These diminish gastric juice production, thus decreasing exposure of the oesophageal mucosa.
- Proton-pump inhibitors (omeprazole) are more powerful than H_2 antagonists (ranitidine) and are favoured in severe cases.

Standard dosage	Ranitidine 150–300 mg twice daily. Omeprazole 20–40 mg daily. Lansoprazole 30 mg daily. Dose can be titrated against symptoms.
Contraindications	*Ranitidine:* known hypersensitivity; caution in renal and hepatic impairment.
Main drug interactions	*Omeprazole, lansoprazole:* warfarin, phenytoin, diazepam.
Main side effects	*Ranitidine:* altered bowel habits, reversible liver damage, headache, blood disorders. *Omeprazole:* skin reactions, diarrhoea, headache, enteric infections.

Motility-enhancing agents
- These are not widely used, with the exception of cisapride, which is as effective as some H_2 antagonists.

Standard dosage	Cisapride 10–20 mg 3–4 times daily, 30 min before meals.
Contraindications	Gastrointestinal haemorrhage or perforation, mechanical bowel obstruction.
Main drug interactions	Anticoagulants: effect possibly enhanced.
Main side effects	Abdominal cramp, diarrhoea.

Mucosal-protecting agents
- Only sucralfate has proved reasonably effective.

Standard dosage	Sucralfate 1 g 4 times daily.
Contraindications	Caution in renal impairment.
Main drug interactions	Decreased bioavailability of tetracycline, phenytoin, cimetidine (avoided by separating administration from sucralfate by 2 h).
Main side effects	Constipation.

Treatment aims
To control symptoms.
To prevent complications, especially for stricture formation.

Other treatments

Antireflux surgery
- Nissen fundoplication and its modifications are the most popular techniques; they are sometimes done laparascopically.
- Surgery is indicated for the following:
Failure to respond to or comply with medical treatment.
Regurgitation as predominant feature.
Severe respiratory symptoms.
Stricture needing frequent dilatation.
- In hiatus hernia, surgical repair is indicated only when symptoms or complications are severe.

Prognosis
- This is a chronic and relapsing condition, but up to 40% of patients remain in remission.

Follow-up and management
- Permanent reflux-reducing measures (particularly weight reduction) must be implemented in order to avoid relapse. Some form of treatment may be necessary to maintain remission. Achievement of oesophagitis healing may not be necessary; the simple aim of symptom control may be sufficient.
- Long-term treatment is indicated in patients who have had frequent relapse, particularly if they are unfit for or unwilling to have surgery or in those with respiratory complications of reflux, if surgery is inappropriate.

Key references
Blum AL, Armstrong D, Fraser R (Guest Editors): Gastro-oesophageal reflux in the 1990's. *Gullet* 1993, **3**:1–98.

Marks AD, Richter JE: Peptic strictures of the oesophagus. *Am J Gastroenterol* 1993, **88**:1160–1173.

Pope CE: Acid-reflux disorders. *N Engl J Med* 1994, **331**:656–660.

Sontag SJ: Gastro-oesophageal reflux disease. *Aliment Pharmacol Ther* 1993, **7**:293–312.

Pancreatic cancer — J.P. Neoptolemos

Diagnosis

Symptoms
Weight loss: in 90% of patients.
Pain: in 80%.
Jaundice: in 70% when tumour is in head of pancreas; in 5% when in body.
Anorexia: in 60%.
Lethargy: in 40%.
Pruritus: in 40%.
Diabetes mellitus: in 15%.
Acute pancreatitis: in 5%.
Ascites: in 5%.
Acute cholangitis: in 2%.
Psychiatric illness: in 1%.
Deep-vein thrombosis: in 1%.

Signs
Jaundice: in 85% of patients.
Cachexia: in 70%.
Hepatomegaly: in 60%.
Palpable gallbladder: Courvoisier's sign in 40%.
Epigastric mass: in 15%.
Ascites: in 10%.
Abdominal tenderness: in 5%.
Trousseau's syndrome: migratory thrombophlebitis in <1%.
Troissier's syndrome: Virchow's node in 1%.
Splenic-vein thrombosis: gastric fundus varices in <1%.

Investigations
Full blood count: to detect anaemia or sepsis.
Clotting studies: results often abnormal but should correct after vitamin K 10 mg i.m.
Liver function tests: to confirm 'obstructive' jaundice; proteins often low.
Ultrasonography: to confirm dilated bile ducts and to localize disease (75% accuracy); increased detection of small tumours with endoluminal ultrasonography (90–100% accuracy).
Endoscopic retrograde cholangiopancreatography: 90–95% accuracy; brush or pancreatic juice cytology positive in 60–70% of cases.
Contrast-enhanced CT: 80–90% accuracy.
Laparoscopy: to detect small metastatic lesions otherwise missed.
Percutaneous biopsy: 80–93% accuracy; must not be used in patients with potentially resectable tumours because cure is improbable because of seeding along biopsy track.
Serum marker analysis: e.g. CA-19-9, CA-125; many influenced by jaundice and have poor sensitivity for 'early' pancreatic cancer.

Complications
- The symptoms and signs are complications in themselves.

Massive gastrointestinal haemorrhage: caused by erosion into duodenum.

Differential diagnosis

Obstructive jaundice
Bile-duct stones, ampullary tumour, tumours of the biliary tract, benign bile duct strictures, metastatic disease, duodenal cancer.

Hepatic jaundice
Chronic hepatitis, sclerosing cholangitis, congestive heart failure.

Cachexia
Gastric, colorectal, or ovarian cancer.

Other pancreatic disease
Chronic pancreatitis (may coexist), non-functioning endocrine tumours, metastases to pancreas.

Aetiology
- The cause is largely unknown, but the following may have a role:

Smoking: relative risk, ~2.0 (compared with relative risk of lung cancer, ~20).
Diets high in total or animal fat.
Genetic predisposition (rare): familial colonic and pancreatic cancer, hereditary chronic pancreatitis, familial adenomatous polyposis, Peutz–Jeghers disease, von Hippel–Lindau disease, Lynch II, ataxic telangiectasia.
Long-standing chronic pancreatitis (possibly).

Epidemiology
- The incidence varies widely according to country and ethnicity, the highest incidences being in central and northern Europe, North America, and Australasia.
- The incidence standardized by age is 8–11 in 100 000 women and 10–12.5 in 100 000 men.
- Pancreatic cancer occurs less in premenopausal women, but the difference between men and women decreases with age.
- The mean age of presentation is 67 years for women and 63 years for men.

Pathology
- 70–80% of pancreatic cancers arise in the head of the gland, the rest in the body or tail or diffusely located; <6% are multicentric.

Duct cell origin: 95%.
Acinar cell origin: 2%.
Uncertain histogenesis: 2%.
Non-epithelial tumours: 1%.

Treatment

Diet and lifestyle
- No special precautions are necessary.

Pharmacological treatment

Before surgery or endoscopy
- Relief of jaundice is possible in 60–80% of patients, with a 7–20% 30-day mortality.
- The following are needed initially before resection or relief of jaundice (surgical or nonsurgical):

Correction of anaemia and hypoproteinaemia.

Vitamin K 10–20 mg i.v. or i.m.

Crystalloid solution 1–2 L i.v. for at least 24 h before any procedure.

Mannitol 20 g i.v. over 20 min if urinary output <60 ml/h after rehydration (assessed by catheterizaton).

Antibiotic cover for any interventional procedure.

Lactulose for 3–5 days before resection (reduces endotoxin load).

Preparation of 4–6 units of blood and fresh frozen plasma for surgery.

For pain
- In up to 30% of patients, the disease is so advanced that conservative management is more appropriate (i.e. pain relief and palliative care).
- NSAIDs must be avoided because they can precipitate acute renal failure.
- Patients can be given morphine slow-release orally, i.v., or epidural infusion using a portable pump; this may cause constipation, nausea, and drowsiness.

Non-pharmacological treatment
- The choice of treatment to relieve jaundice depends on age, tumour burden, and local expertise.
- In-hospital mortality figures are comparable for the different techniques, although endoscopic methods are probably superior.
- Patients who are fit for surgery (50–60%) must be appropriately staged (ultrasonography, CT, laparoscopy), with the help of a specialist radiologist and surgeon.

Surgical resection
- Resection is possible in 10–30% of patients, with a hospital mortality of 3–10%.

Endoscopic stents
- Stents can be used in elderly patients.
- Expandable metal stents need fewer changes and are recommended for patients with an expected better survival rate.

Percutaneous internal stenting
- The complication rate is higher than for endoscopic stents.
- Permanent external drainage is contraindicated.

Surgical bypass
- Bypass is indicated for young patients with low tumour burden.
- Duodenal bypass may also be used to avoid obstruction from growth into duodenum (10–15%).

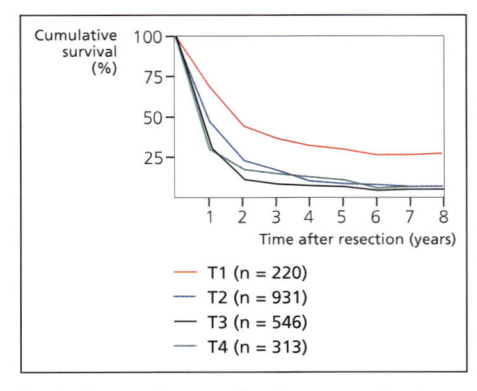

Survival rates after resection for pancreatic cancer stages T1–T4, based on data from the Japanese Pancreatic Cancer Registry.

Treatment aims
To relieve jaundice, duodenal obstruction, weight loss, and pain.

Prognosis
- Cure is rarely possible, but resection often results in the best palliation.
- After palliative treatment, mean survival is 3–6 months.
- After resection, mean survival is 12–18 months, and the 5-year survival rate is 5–15%; the survival rate may be increased by adjuvant radiochemotherapy.

Follow-up and management
- Patients who have had resection may be suitable for postoperative adjuvant external beam radiotherapy followed by chemotherapy for 6–24 months.
- After palliative treatment, stents may need to be changed, gastric bypass may be needed for duodenal obstruction, and patients may need pain control.
- Localized recurrence may be worth re-resecting in some patients.

Key references

Cotton PB: Management of malignant bile duct obstruction. *J Gastroenterol Hepatol* 1990, **Suppl 1**:63–67.

Klöppel G, Maillet B: Classification and staging of pancreatic non-endocrine tumors. *Radiol Clin North Am* 1989, **27**:105–115.

Lowenfels AB *et al.*: Pancreatitis and the risk of pancreatic cancer. *N Engl J Med* 1993, **328**:1433–1437.

Russell RCG: Surgical resection for cancer of the pancreas. *Clin Gastroenterol* 1990, **4**:889–916.

Warshaw AL: Implications of peritoneal cytology for staging of early pancreatic cancer. *Am J Surg* 1991, **161**:26–30.

Pancreatitis, acute
J.P. Neoptolemos

Diagnosis

Symptoms
Epigastric pain: sudden onset; radiation into back; may become increasingly severe.
Anorexia, nausea, vomiting.
Abdominal pain: severe, generalized, often with pyrexia; coma possible.

Signs
Tachycardia, perspiration, peritonitis: mild; usually in upper abdomen.
Generalized peritonitis, shock, respiratory failure, 'septic' picture.
Grey Turner's sign, Cullen's sign: on flanks and peri-umbilical, respectively; signs of intra-abdominal haemorrhage.
Peripheral fat necrosis: occasionally (more frequent in alcohol-induced pancreatitis).
Jaundice: especially in gallstone-induced pancreatitis.

Investigations
Serum or urine amylase measurement: serum concentration >1000 IU/L or urine concentration >3000 IU/L indicates acute pancreatitis (urine measurement if >48h after attack).
Chest radiography (erect): to exclude gastrointestinal perforation.
Peritoneal tap or lavage with Gram stain: in doubtful cases; bacteria suggest alternative diagnosis.
Ultrasonography: in severe pancreatitis to determine as soon as possible whether gallstones are causative (~80% sensitive); useful in following course of acute fluid collections, pseudocysts, and abscesses.
Serum transaminase or bilirubin measurement: concentrations on admission of >60 IU/L or >40 µmol/L, respectively (the latter indicating bile-duct stones).
Coma severity assessment: using modified Glasgow coma score (severe, 3 factors or more) or APACHE II score (severe, 8–10).
Arterial blood gases: hypoxia indicates poor prognosis.
Contrast-enhanced CT: extent of necrosis (>50 Houndsfield units) accurately determined in 85–90% of cases; only for clinically severe or suspected 'silent' pancreatitis.
Fine-needle aspiration: for biopsy of necrotic tissue and Gram stain and culture to ascertain presence of infected necrosis.
Endoscopic retrograde cholangiopancreatography: to ascertain presence of gallstones and other causes in biliary tree or pancreas; in severe pancreatitis, disruption of main pancreatic duct suggests significant central necrosis (communicating pseudocysts unusual, 6%).
Bile collection: during convalescence to ascertain presence of cholesterol crystals, indicating microlithiasis or cholesterolosis.

Complications
- At least one systemic complication occurs in 25–30% of patients.

Cardiovascular, respiratory, and renal failure.
Uraemia, hyperglycaemia, hypocalcaemia.
Acute cholangitis: may coexist with gallstone pancreatitis in 5–10%.
Disseminated intravascular coagulation, major haematological abnormalities: in 1–5%.
Acute fluid collections: occur early, in 30–50% with severe disease and often in patients with mild disease.
Pancreatic necrosis: clinically significant in 3–5%; up to 70% are infected necroses; lesser degrees (<30% of the gland) often occur in clinically mild pancreatitis.
Pseudocysts: in 15–20%, although only 33–50% of these become clinically significant; develop 4 weeks after attack.
Abscess: in 1%.
Death: in 8–20%.

Differential diagnosis
Abdominal catastrophe: any perforation of gastrointestinal tract, ruptured aneurysm, ectopic pregnancy, mesenteric infarction, ovarian cyst torsion.
Myocardial infarction.
Acute cholecystitis.
Hyperamylasaemia.
Complication of endoscopic retrograde cholangiopancreatography.
- Serum amylase concentrations may be raised in most of the above.
- Other conditions include intestinal obstruction, salpingitis, Crohn's disease, afferent loop obstruction after gastrectomy, appendicitis, pregnancy, protein-bound hyperamylasaemia (macroamylasaemia, lymphoma, AIDS), various tumours, salivary gland disease, renal failure, diabetic ketoacidosis.

Aetiology
- Causes include the following.

Biliary disorders in 60–70% of patients: gallstones, cholesterolosis, 'sludge', ascariasis, sclerosing cholangitis, choledochocoele, tumours.
Alcohol in 30–40%.
Hyperlipidaemia in 1–5%: types I (30%), IV (15%), and V (30–40%).
Unusual causes in 1–5%: obstructive (pancreas divisum, strictures, tumours), trauma, ischaemia, infections (viruses, bacteria, parasites), drugs (azathioprine, L-asparaginase, warfarin), vasculitides, transplantation, hypercalcaemia, scorpion bites.

Epidemiology
- Gallstone-induced pancreatitis occurs more often in elderly people and women.
- Typically, 30–60 in 10^5 population are affected annually.
- The incidence is increasing.

Treatment

Diet and lifestyle
- Patients must eat regular meals; prolonged starvation followed by large meals must be avoided.

Pharmacological treatment
- Supportive care involves the following:

Intravenous fluid: crystalloid and colloid (up to 12 L may be sequestered in the first 24–48 h).

Pain relief (morphine should be avoided if possible).

Albumin and calcium as needed.

Monitoring and treatment of diabetes mellitus as needed.

Inotropic support: if systolic blood pressure <100 mmHg or renal perfusion inadequate despite fluid replacement.

Antibiotics: for patients with gallstone pancreatitis or severe pancreatitis.

- Glucagon, antiproteases (e.g. aprotinin), somatostatin, and peritoneal lavage are of no value.

Non-pharmacological treatment

Oxygen administration: by mask if partial pressure of oxygen in arterial blood <9 kPa; ventilation if <8 kPa despite this; patients should be given chest physiotherapy, and large pleural effusions should be tapped.

Haemofiltration: for renal failure despite fluid replacement and inotropic support.

Endoscopic retrograde cholangiopancreatography and endoscopic sphincterotomy: for patients with severe pancreatitis (as soon as possible), those with 'mild' disease that does not resolve, or those needing surgery for complications; an option in elderly patients.

Necrosectomy: usually from second week of attack of pancreatic necrosis; for continued clinical deterioration, with objective evidence of extensive necrosis; infected necrosis is a strong indication for surgery.

Drainage: for large pseudocysts (>6 cm), persisting in size, expanding, or causing symptoms; repeated percutaneous tapping increases risk of infection and abscess; percutaneous or endoscopic drainage can be used for pseudocysts, although surgical internal drainage is preferred in many patients; abscess can be effectively treated by external drainage; abscess must not be confused with infected pancreatic necrosis and expansive retroperitoneal spread of necrosis and infection.

Treatment aims
To provide supportive care.
To prevent further attacks.
To reduce complications and underlying disorders (e.g. hyperlipidaemia).

Prognosis
- The mortality is 8–20% overall, <2% for endoscopic sphincterotomy for gallstones, <20% for necrosectomy, <5% for pseudocysts, <5% for abscess.
- Most patients recover after management on a regular ward or high-dependency unit with fluid replacement and oxygen by mask.
- Recurrent attacks are highly probable if alcohol abuse continues or if hyperlipidaemia is not treated.
- Unless cholecystectomy or endoscopic sphincterotomy is performed in patients with gallstones, 10–40% suffer recurrent attacks.

Follow-up and management
- Further attacks can be prevented by laparoscopic cholecystectomy (for gallstones) or endoscopic sphincterotomy, stopping alcohol intake, treating hyperlipidaemia and other underlying disorders, and eating regular meals.
- Follow-up is only needed in patients in whom the cause has not been identified or treated or who have had extensive surgery for necrosis.

Key references
Bradley EL III: A clinically based classification system for acute pancreatitis. *Arch Surg* 1993, **128**:586–590.

Fernandez del Castillo C, Rattner DW, Warshaw AL: Acute pancreatitis. *Lancet* 1993, **342**:475–479.

Poston GJ, Williamson RCN: Surgical management of acute pancreatitis. *Br J Surg* 1990, **77**:5–12.

Warshaw AL: Damage prevention versus damage control in acute pancreatitis. *Gastroenterology* 1993, **104**:1216–1219.

Pancreatitis, chronic J.P. Neoptolemos

Diagnosis

Symptoms
- Chronic pancreatitis usually evolves over 5–20 years; symptoms, signs, and complications vary during this period.

Abdominal pain: in 90% of patients.
Weight loss: in 80%.
Diarrhoea or steatorrhoea: in 40%.
Diabetes mellitus: in 40%.
Acute pancreatitis: in 40%.
Vomiting: in 10%.
Drug abuse: in 10%.
Jaundice: in 5%.
Haematemesis: in 5%.
Abdominal distension: in 1%.

Signs
Marked weight loss: in 40% of patients.
Erythema abigne: in 10% over lumbar spine or epigastrum.
Greasy stool: in 10% on rectal examination.
Epigastric mass: in 10%.
Anaemia: in 5%.
Jaundice: in 5%.
Gastric splash: in 5%.
Splenomegaly: in 1%.
Pleural effusion: in 1%.
Pericardial effusion: in 1%.

Investigations
Chest radiography: for effusion, mediastinal pseudocyst.
Abdominal radiography: for pancreatic calcification.
Upper gastrointestinal endoscopy: for peptic ulcer, gastric fundal varices, duodenal obstruction.
Barium swallow: for compression of oesophagus, stomach, or duodenum due to pseudocyst or inflammatory mass.
Ultrasonography: for parenchymal changes, duct dilatation, calcification, pseudocysts, ascites.
Contrast-enhanced CT: highly sensitive for calcification; for inflammatory mass, state of the duct, pseudocysts, ascites.
Endoscopic retrograde cholangiopancreatography: for changes in main duct and side branches ('minimal change pancreatitis'), stones (calcified and non-calcified) and protein plugs in duct, necrotic cysts, pseudocysts, fistulas.
Blood glucose measurement and glucose tolerance test.
'Tube' test: pancreatic juice collection and measurement of enzymes and bicarbonate after stimulation by creatine kinase-secretin or Lundh meal to assess exocrine function.
'Tubeless' tests: faecal fat and enzyme measurements to assess exocrine function.
Serum enzymes measurement: raised only in acute exacerbation or pancreatitis.
Pancreatic biopsy or cytology: to distinguish from pancreatic cancer.

Complications
Pancreatic exocrine insufficiency.
Pancreatic endocrine insufficiency.
Acute pancreatic pancreatitis and sequelae.
Duodenal ulcer.
Common bile duct obstruction: secondary biliary cirrhosis.
Liver disease: usually subclinical.
Duodenal obstruction.
Colonic stricture.
Pseudocysts: pancreatic, intra-abdominal, mediastinal.
Pancreatic ascites.
Pleural effusion.
Pancreatic abscess.
Pancreatic pseudoaneurysm.
Splenic vein thrombosis: gastric fundus varices.
Complications of alcohol and drug abuse.
Complications of smoking.
Bleeding into the pancreatic duct.
Exocrine pancreatic cancer: long-standing.

Differential diagnosis
Recurrent acute pancreatitis without chronic pancreatitis.
Idiopathic hypertrophy of head of pancreas.
Secondary pancreatic inflammation (duodenal ulceration).
Pancreatic cancer.

Aetiology
- Causes include the following:
Alcohol in 60–80% of patients.
Obstruction in 10%: ampullary stenosis, pancreas divisum, annular pancreas, stricture (trauma, tumour), irradiation, pancreatitis.
Idiopathic in 10%.
Hereditary (chronic familial pancreatitis).
Smoking.
Malnutrition (tropical pancreatitis).
Cystic fibrosis.
Coeliac disease.
Hypercalcaemia.
- Many of these causes are associated with decreased pancreatic stone protein (reducing calcium-protein precipitation).

Epidemiology
- In industrialized countries, the incidence largely depends on alcohol consumption (other factors have a modifying effect): 1–10 in 10^5 population are affected annually.
- Chronic pancreatitis occurs more often in men than in women; the ratios vary from 10:1 to 2:1.
- The incidence is increasing in all countries.

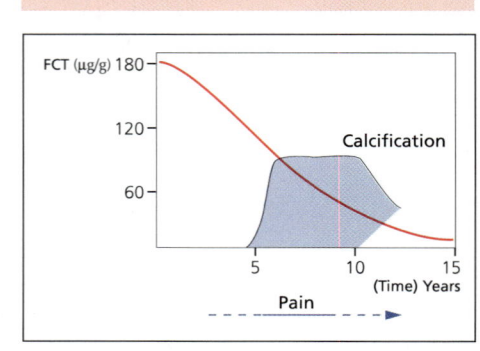

Relationship between pancreatic function (in this case faecal chymotrypsin [FCT]), evolution of calcification, and pain. Onset and resolution of pain are unpredictable.

Treatment

Diet and lifestyle
- Patients should eat regular meals and abstain from alcohol.
- If alcohol is the cause, patients must participate in drug-addiction programmes and, if necessary, change occupation from alcohol-related industry or high-pressure employment.
- Restriction of fat intake or use of medium-chain triglycerides is rarely needed.

Pharmacological treatment

For the underlying cause
See Peptic ulceration and Diabetes mellitus *for details*.
- For exocrine insufficiency, pancreatic enzyme therapy (2–6 capsules 3 times daily with meals) should be titrated to symptoms (steatorrhoea, weight); concomitant H_2-receptor antagonists may improve the activity of enzyme supplements.

For pain
- Self-titration of pancreatic supplements (1–2 capsules 3 times daily with meals) may reduce mild or moderate pain (in the absence of overt steatorrhoea).
- Simple analgesics or NSAIDs can be used.
- Coeliac plexus block with steroids can be considered, repeated if necessary.
- Sclerosing agents should be avoided because effects are limited and may make subsequent surgery difficult.

Non-pharmacological treatment

Main pancreatic duct drainage
- Endoscopic sphincterotomy and stone extraction are suitable in only a few patients; stenting of strictures for excessive periods should be avoided.
- Pancreaticojejunostomy or transduodenal sphincteroplasty are alternatives to endoscopic treatment and for strictures preferable to long-term stenting; draining alone is usually insufficient in the presence of extensive parenchymal calcification, inflammation, and pain.

Surgery for pain
- Surgery is indicated for complications and intractable pain.
- For non-diabetic patients or those having an operation for the first time, treatment should be conservative, and only 'dominant' disease is resected.
- For patients with diabetes or previous surgery patients, radical treatment is indicated.
- Preservation of the stomach, pylorus, duodenum, and spleen is almost always possible.
- The Beger operation produces excellent results for patients with small or large duct disease with inflammatory mass in head of pancreas; it preserves the duodenum and tail of the pancreas with prograde duct drainage.

Treatment aims
To eliminate cause.
To relieve pain.
To delay disease progression (duct drainage).
To treat malabsorption.

Prognosis
- The disease is not always progressive.
- Pain and calcification occur after 5–10 years, and both may subsequently regress, but this is unpredictable.
- The long-term survival may be poor: up to 50% of patients die within 7 years.
- Causes of late death include chronic pancreatitis itself (40%), malignancy (20%), sudden death (suicide, cardiovascular disease; 20%).

Follow-up and management
- All patients must be followed up to control endocrine and exocrine function and pain and to ascertain the need for operation or reoperation.

Key references

Beger HG, Büchler M, Bittner R: The duodenum preserving resection of the head of the pancreas (DPRHP) in patients with chronic pancreatitis and an inflammatory mass in the head. *Acta Chir Scand* 1990, **156**:309–315.

Gold EB, Cameron JL: Chronic pancreatitis and pancreatic cancer. *N Engl J Med* 1993, **328**:1485–1486.

Greenen JE, Rolny P: Endoscopic management of pancreatic disease. *Baillières Clin Gastroenterol* 1991, **5**:155–182.

Ihse I, Permerth J: Enzyme therapy and pancreatic pain. *Acta Chir Scand* 1990, **156**:281–283.

Malfertheiner P, Dominquez-Munoz JE, Büchler M: Diagnosis and staging of chronic pancreatitis. In *Standards in Pancreatic Surgery*. Edited by Beger HG *et al*. Berlin: Springer-Verlag, 1993, pp 297–313.

Nealon WH, Thompson JC: Progressive loss of pancreatic function in chronic pancreatitis is delayed by main pancreatic duct decompression. *Ann Surg* 1993, **217**:458–466.

Watanapa P, Williams RC: Pancreatic sphincterotomy and sphincteroplasty. *Gut* 1992, **33**:865–867.

Ulcerative colitis — I.A. Finnie and J.M. Rhodes

Diagnosis

Symptoms

General
- Diarrhoea usually indicates that disease extends above the rectosigmoid junction.

Mucus and blood *per rectum*.
Urgency to defaecate.
Constitutional upset.

Mild attack
Diarrhoea up to 4 times daily or passage of small amounts of macroscopic blood *per rectum*: without appreciable constitutional symptoms.

Moderate attack
Diarrhoea >4 times daily: without severe bleeding or severe constitutional symptoms.

Severe attack
Diarrhoea >4 times daily.
Large amounts of blood mixed with faeces.
Fever >37.5°C, heart rate >100 beats/min, abdominal pain, anorexia or weight loss.

Signs

Mild or moderate attack
- Typically no signs are manifest.

Severe attack
Pallor.
Fever >37.5°C.
Hypoalbuminaemia: <30 g/L.
Diffuse abdominal tenderness.
- Any signs of severe disease warrant emergency admission, intensive therapy, and daily monitoring to exclude toxic dilatation.

Investigations

Stool culture: should always be done even in established ulcerative colitis.
Full blood count, ESR, CRP measurement.
Rigid sigmoidoscopy and rectal biopsy.
Plain abdominal radiography: allows exclusion of dilatation and gives good guide to disease extent (bowel containing faeces is probably not severely inflamed).
Colonoscopy: allows accurate assessment of extent of disease and histological confirmation of presence of disease or dysplasia.
Barium enema: less frequently used because of inability to obtain histology.
- Colonoscopy and barium enema should be avoided in an acute attack because they may cause exacerbation; a single-contrast 'instant' barium enema without bowel preparation may help to assess extent before surgery if response to medical treatment has been poor.

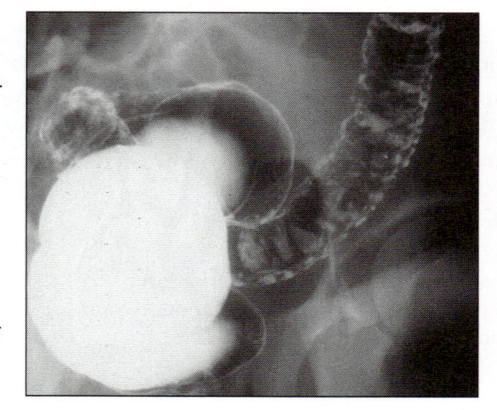

Double-contrast barium enema in severe ulcerative colitis, showing submucosal ulceration producing 'tramline' effect in sigmoid and descending colon.

Complications

Haemorrhage: chronic blood loss causing anaemia common, severe acute bleeding rare.
Perforation: 50% mortality; avoidable with careful management and surgical referral.
Fibromuscular strictures: colonoscopy and biopsy needed to exclude malignancy.
Colon cancer.

Differential diagnosis

Microscopic (lymphocytic) colitis.
Collagenous colitis.
Drug-associated disorders: oral contraceptives have been associated with a Crohn's-like colitis; NSAIDs and purgatives may cause microscopic colitis.
Diversion colitis.
Crohn's colitis.
Irradiation proctitis: associated with vascular ectasia.
Ischaemic colitis: rarely affects rectum.
Bacterial or amoebic infection (dysentery).
Irritable bowel syndrome: should not cause bleeding or nocturnal diarrhoea.
Cytomegalovirus, herpes simplex, cryptosporidia in immunosuppressed patients.
Colon cancer.

Aetiology

- The cause is unknown, but the following may have a role:
Autoimmunity.
Defective mucosal barrier: e.g. mucus.
Altered neutrophil function.

Epidemiology

- The prevalence of ulcerative colitis in Jewish people is higher than in non-Jews, and more whites than blacks are affected.
- Patients present at any age; the highest prevalence is in the 2nd and 3rd decades, but a second peak in the 5th and 6th decades has been reported.
- The prevalence in northwestern Europe and the USA is 1 in 1500; it is rarely diagnosed in developing countries.
- An unexplained association with non-smoking exists (95% of sufferers are non-smokers or ex-smokers).
- No convincing association with diet or stress has been found.
- The risk in first-degree relatives increases 15-fold.

Clinical patterns

Acute fulminant.
Relapsing/remitting: in ~66% of patients.
Chronic continuous: more often in patients who are elderly at first presentation.
Single attack of colitis (stool culture negative): in <1%.
Rectum involved in >90%, extending proximally for variable length.

I.A. Finnie and J.M. Rhodes **Ulcerative colitis**

Treatment

Diet and lifestyle
- No special precautions are necessary.

Pharmacological treatment

For mild attacks

Standard dosage	*Initially:* sulphasalazine 1 g twice daily, mesalazine 1.2–2.4 g daily, or olsalazine 1.5–3 g daily, with rectal corticosteroid as foam or rectal 5-aminosalicylic acid preparation. *Maintenance:* sulphasalazine 1.5–4 g daily, mesalazine 1.2–2.4 g daily, or olsalazine 1.5–3 g daily.
Contraindications	Salicylate intolerance, renal failure.
Special points	Regular full blood counts and urea measurement advised. *Olsalazine:* increasing dose gradually and taking with food may reduce diarrhoea.
Main drug interactions	*Sulphasalazine:* warfarin, anticonvulsants.
Main side effects	Occasional nephrotoxicity. *Sulphasalazine:* nausea, headaches, malaise, dyspepsia, reversible male infertility. *Mesalazine:* occasional nausea, diarrhoea, interstitial nephritis. *Olsalazine:* diarrhoea in 10–20% of patients.

For moderate attacks

Standard dosage	Prednisolone 40 mg orally once daily, with oral 5-aminosalicylic acid preparation.
Contraindications	Systemic infections, hypersensitivity.
Special points	Weekly review essential; hospital admission if no improvement within 2 weeks. Corticosteroids used in short courses; response should occur within 1–4 weeks then tail off over 6–8 weeks; if response poor, more severe attack should be assumed; corticosteroids of no value in maintaining remission.
Main drug interactions	None.
Main side effects	Occasional steroid-psychosis; steroid-related side-effects uncommon if long-term treatment avoided.

For severe attacks
- Treatment includes admission to hospital for close observation, bed-rest, high-dose i.v. corticosteroids, i.v. feeding if patient is vomiting or malnourished, antiembolism stockings, and s.c. heparin.
- The colonic diameter should be monitored by plain radiography daily until it has settled.

For toxic dilatation
- Dilatation of the transverse colon to a diameter of >5.5 cm accompanied by signs of fever or tachycardia may be treated intensively for up to 48 h, but any clinical or radiographic deterioration during this period or failure to respond to treatment necessitates immediate surgery.

Treatment aims
To achieve and maintain remission, with good quality of life.
To avoid life-threatening complications by prompt, effective treatment.

Other treatments
- 20% of patients need colectomy at some time; surgery is indicated for the following:
Failed full medical treatment for severe colitis (after ~2 weeks as inpatient).
Toxic megacolon or perforation.
Chronic ill health due to persistent mild or moderate colitis, with poor quality of life.
Cancer or raised dysplastic lesion.
Dilatation in patients already on systemic prednisolone >40 mg daily or who deteriorate or do not respond to medical treatment.

Prognosis
- Most patients have relapses interspersed with periods of prolonged remission; 90% are capable of full-time work.
- Life expectancy is normal.
- The risk of colon cancer is significantly increased but counterbalanced by reduced risk of ischaemic heart disease or lung cancer.

Follow-up and management
- After a single mild attack, patients should continue taking 5-aminosalicylic acid preparations for 1 year or, for severe or multiple attacks, until they have been free of disease for at least 5 years.
- Patients should be screened by colonoscopy for dysplasia or early colon cancer (2–yearly for patients with colitis proximal to splenic flexure and lasting >7 years).

Patient support
National Association for Colitis and Crohn's disease, 98A London Rd, St Albans, Herts, AL1 1NX, tel/fax 01727 44296.

Key references
Crotty B, Jewell DP: Drug therapy of ulcerative colitis. *Br J Clin Pharmacol* 1992, **34**:189–198.

Podolsky DK: Inflammatory bowel disease (parts 1 and 2). *N Engl J Med* 1991, **325**:928–937, 1008–1016.

Zollinger–Ellison syndrome   R.E Pounder

Diagnosis

Symptoms
Simple duodenal ulcer: especially if multiple or delayed healing, also if patient has neither *Helicobacter pylori* infection nor history of NSAID ingestion.

Recurrent peptic ulcer: after surgery.

Oesophagitis and duodenal ulcer: in the same patient.

Peptic ulcer and diarrhoea or malabsorption.

Diarrhoea or malabsorption alone.

Signs
- No typical physical signs are manifest, apart from those of complicated duodenal ulceration (haemorrhage, perforation, pyloric stenosis).

Investigations
Fasting plasma gastrin measurement: ideally when patient has not taken antisecretory drugs for 48 h: normal concentration <100 pg/ml; Zollinger–Ellison syndrome (ZES) is probable if hypergastrinaemia occurs with increased gastric acid secretion.

Gastric acid secretion measurement: basal secretion measured for 1 h; output >50 mmol/h or >5 mmol/h if patient has had gastric surgery are diagnostic.

Secretin test: i.v. bolus of secretin causes rise of fasting plasma gastrin (>200 pg/ml).

Gastric pH measurement: fasting pH >3.5 indicates hypergastrinaemia due to hypo- or achlorhydria not to ZES.

CT of pancreas or arteriography: to check for primary tumour or metastases (only 40% and 20% positive, respectively, in ZES).

Transhepatic portal-vein sampling: to localize gastrin release (rarely used).

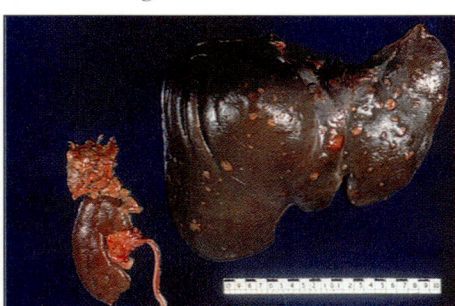

An islet cell tumour secreted gastrin and adreno-corticotrophic hormone. Post-mortem examination showed hyperplastic adrenals and liver metastases. The patient died from perforated jejunal peptic ulceration before omeprazole treatment.

Complications
- Complications are those of severe peptic ulceration, often manifest as the following:

Non-healing ulceration.

Surgical problems: after emergency ulcer surgery.

Differential diagnosis
Severe or refractory peptic ulceration. Hypergastrinaemia due to pernicious anaemia, *Helicobacter pylori* infection, or profound hypoacidity secondary to acid antisecretory drugs (especially proton pump blockers: omeprazole, lansoprazole, pantoprazole).

Retained gastric antrum after Billroth II partial gastrectomy (now extremely rare).

Aetiology
- Zollinger–Ellison syndrome is caused by uncontrolled gastric acid hypersecretion, driven by plasma gastrin released by a gastrinoma (50% malignant).
- 75% of gastrinomas are localized in a triangle defined by the junction of the cystic and common bile ducts, the junction of the second and third parts of the duodenum, and the head and body of the pancreas.
- 15% of gastrinomas occur in the wall of the duodenum, 10% in extraintestinal locations.

Epidemiology
- Hypercalcaemia, due to hyperparathyroidism in the multiple endocrine neoplasia syndrome type I, accounts for 25% of patients.
- Zollinger–Ellison syndrome can coexist with phaeochromocytoma or ectopic adrenocorticotrophic hormone production from tumour.

Treatment

Diet and lifestyle
- No special precautions are necessary.

Pharmacological treatment
- As soon as Zollinger–Ellison syndrome is suspected, blood must be taken for fasting plasma gastrin concentration, ideally when the patient is not on antisecretory treatment.

Emergency control of gastric acid secretion

Standard dosage	Ranitidine 300 mg or omeprazole 20 mg orally 4 times daily; if patient cannot take oral treatment, ranitidine 100 mg i.v. as slow bolus and infusion of 0.5 mg/kg/h.
Contraindications	Hypersensitivity.
Special points	Basal acid secretion must be measured every 4 h, and rate of infusion increased until <10 mmol/h.
Main drug interactions	None.
Main side effects	None.

Long-term control of gastric acid secretion
- Omeprazole 20–120 mg daily is the treatment of choice (titrated to control basal acid secretion rate <10 mmol/h).
- Large doses of H_2-blockers may be needed because they are competitive antagonists.
- Lansoprazole 30–120 mg daily is an alternative proton-pump inhibitor.

Treatment aims
To control gastric acid secretion and thereby heal aggressive peptic ulceration.
To identify and remove primary tumour, if possible.

Other treatments
For hyperparathyroidism: parathyroidectomy may decrease gastrin release and acid secretion.
For localized tumours: laparotomy to search for primary tumour; if no hepatic metastases detected on CT or arteriogram, after initial control of acid secretion by drugs.
Partial gastrectomy or vagotomy: no longer recommended.

Prognosis
- All complications of peptic ulceration should be avoided by pharmacological control of gastric acid secretion.
- ~20% of patients may be cured by surgical resection of the primary tumour.
- Death is usually from metastatic tumour, with survival prolonged by the usual chemotherapy for disseminated adenocarcinoma.

Follow-up and management
- Fasting plasma gastrin concentration should be measured and basal acid secretion assessed.

Causes of treatment failure
Hypercalcaemia associated with multiple endocrine neoplasm syndrome type I.
Insufficient dose of medication.
Spread of the primary tumour.

Key references
Maton PN: The management of Zollinger–Ellison syndrome. *Aliment Pharmacol Ther* 1993, **7**:467–475.
Norton J, Jensen R: Unresolved surgical issues in the management of patients with Zollinger–Ellison syndrome. *World J Surg* 1991, **15**:151–159.

Index

A

abdominal
 bloating 28
 distension 10, 14, 24, 28, 38
 mass 10
 pain 6, 10, 14, 18, 24, 28, 36, 38, 40
 swelling 10
abscess
 colonic 14
 pancreatic 36, 38
 perianal 12
 skin 12
achalasia 2, 30
acid antisecretory agents for oesophagitis and hiatus hernia 33
albendazole for enteric infections 19
albumin for acute pancreatitis 37
alverine
 for diverticular disease of the colon 15
 for irritable bowel syndrome 29
5-aminosalicylic acid preparations
 for Crohn's disease 13
 for ulcerative colitis 41
amitriptyline for irritable bowel syndrome 29
amoxycillin
 for duodenal ulcer 17
 for enteric infections 19
ampicillin
 for diverticular disease of the colon 15
 for enteric infections 19
anaemia 6, 8, 10, 12, 14, 16, 18, 22, 26, 30, 38, 40
 megaloblastic 6
 pernicious 4, 22, 42
analgesics
 for chronic pancreatitis 39
 for oesophageal carcinoma 31
antacids
 for duodenal ulcer 17
 for gastric ulceration 25
 for oesophagitis and hiatus hernia 33
antibiotics
 for acute pancreatitis 37
 for bacterial overgrowth of the small intestine 7
 for Crohn's disease 13
 for diverticulitis 15
antidepressants for irritable bowel syndrome 29
antimotility agents for irritable bowel syndrome 29
antispasmodics
 for diverticular disease of the colon 15
 for irritable bowel syndrome 29
antituberculous chemotherapy for *Mycobacterium tuberculosis* infection 19
anxiety 28
appendicitis 18, 36
ascites 10, 22, 34, 38
ataxia 4, 6
azathioprine for Crohn's disease 13

B

bacterial
 infection 6, 12, 40
 overgrowth 4, 28
  of the small intestine 6
  syndrome, small-bowel 8
Beger operation for chronic pancreatitis 39
behavioural therapy for irritable bowel syndrome 29
bile-acid
 malabsorption 28
 treatment for cholesterol gallstones 21
bile-duct
 obstruction 38
 stone 34
 stricture 20, 34
bleeding 30 *see also* haemorrhage
 gastrointestinal 14, 26
 into pancreatic duct 38
 nose 26
 rectal 12, 26
 ulcer 16
 varices 26
blind loop syndrome 4 *see also* bacterial overgrowth of the small intestine
blood
 in stools 10
 per rectum 10, 14, 40
 poisoning *see* septicaemia
 pressure, low *see* hypotension
 transfusion for gastrointestinal bleeding 27
bowel *see also* intestinal
 disease, inflammatory 8, 10, 14, 18, 28
bran
 for diverticular disease of the colon 15
 for irritable bowel syndrome 29
bulking agents
 for diverticular disease of the colon 15
 for irritable bowel syndrome 29

C

calcium
 antagonists for achalasia 3
 deficiency 8
 for acute pancreatitis 37
calculi *see* stones
cancer 26 *see also* malignancy
 colonic 40
 colorectal 10, 34
 duodenal 34
 gastric 22, 34
 ovarian 34
 pancreatic 34, 38
carcinoid, gastric 4
carcinoma 16
 colonic 12, 14
 gastric 4, 16, 24
 oesophageal 2, 30
 of the bronchus 30
cardiac *see* heart
cardiomyotomy for achalasia 3
cefuroxime for diverticular disease of the colon 15
Chagas' disease 2
cheodeoxycholic acid for cholesterol gallstones 21
chest pain, retrosternal 2
chloramphenicol for enteric infections 19
cholangitis 20
 acute 34, 36
 sclerosing 34
cholecystectomy for cholesterol gallstones 21
cholecystitis 20, 36
cholelithiasis *see* gallstones
cholera 18
cimetidine
 for duodenal ulcer 17
 for gastric ulceration 25
ciprofloxacin
 for bacterial overgrowth of the small intestine 7
 for enteric infections 19
cirrhosis, biliary 38
cisapride
 for bacterial overgrowth of the small intestine 7
 for gastric cancer 23
 for oesophagitis and hiatus hernia 33
 for irritable bowel syndrome 29
clarithromcyin for duodenal ulcer 17
clubbing 8, 12
coagulation, disseminated intravascular 36
co-amoxyclav for diverticular disease of the colon 15
codeine phosphate for irritable bowel syndrome 29
coeliac disease 6, 8, 28
colic 18
 biliary 16, 20, 24
colitis
 acute necrotizing 18
 collagenous 40
 Crohn's 12, 28, 40
 diversion 40
 granulomatous *see* Crohn's disease
 ischaemic 14, 40
 pseudomembranous 12
 ulcerative 12, 18, 28, 40
colon
 diverticular disease of the 14
 polyp 14
 tender sigmoid 14
colonic
 abscess 14
 cancer 40
 carcinoma 12, 14
 malignancy 28
 perforation 40
 stricture 38

Index

colorectal *cont.*
   cancer 10, 34
   perforation 40
   polyp 18
colostomy for diverticulitis 15
constipation 8, 14, 18, 28
corticosteroids
   for chronic pancreatitis 39
   for coeliac disease 9
   for Crohn's disease 13
   for ulcerative colitis 41
co-trimoxazole for enteric infections 19
Courvoisier's sign 34
Crohn's
   colitis 12, 28, 40
   disease 4, 6, 12, 16, 36
Cullen's sign 36

D

defaecation, disturbed 28
degeneration of spinal cord, subacute combined 4, 6
dehydration 18
depression 4, 22, 28
diabetes mellitus 8, 34, 37, 38
diabetic
   acidosis *see* diabetic ketoacidosis
   ketoacidosis 36
   ketosis *see* diabetic ketoacidosis
   neuropathy 18
diarrhoea 12, 6, 8, 18, 28, 38, 40, 42
   bloody 12
   drug-induced 18
   endocrine-associated 18
   idiopathic 18
   spurious 18
   travellers' 18
dicyclomine
   for diverticular disease of the colon 15
   for irritable bowel syndrome 29
dietary
   deficiency in vegans 4
   intake, inadequate 8
dilatation
   of the cardia 3
   toxic 41
diloxanide for enteric infections 19
dissection
   aortic 16, 24
   of lymph glands for gastric cancer 23
disseminated intravascular coagulation 36
dissolution of cholesterol gallstones with methyl tert-butyl ether 21
diverticula, small-bowel 4
diverticular disease 10, 28
   of the colon 14
diverticulitis 14
diverticulosis 14, 28
duodenal
   cancer 34

duodenal *cont.*
   obstruction 38
   perforation 16, 42
   ulcer 12, 16, 24, 38, 42
dyspareunia 28
dyspepsia 22
   'ulcer-like' 22
dysphagia 2, 18, 22, 30, 32
dsyplasia 22

E

eating disorder 6
effusion
   pericardial 38
   pleural 22, 37, 38
Ehlers–Danlos syndrome 26
empyema, gallbladder 20 *see also* cholecystitis
encephalopathy, Wernicke's 8
endometriosis 14, 28
enteritis
   granulomatous *see* Crohn's disease
   regional *see* Crohn's disease
epigastric
   mass 22, 34, 38
   pain 16, 22, 24, 36
   tenderness 24
erythema
   ab igne 6, 38
   nodosum 12, 18
   palmar 26
exsanguination 26

F

famotidine
   for duodenal ulcer 17
   for gastric ulceration 25
faecal evacuation, feeling of incomplete 28
fibrosing disease of the pancreas *see* fibrosis, cystic
fibrosis, cystic 8
fistula 10, 12, 14, 20, 30
flatulence 18
5-fluorouracil for colorectal cancer 11
fluoxetine for irritable bowel syndrome 29
folate deficiency 8
folic acid for postinfective malabsorption 19
fundoplication, Nissen, for oesophagitis and hiatus hernia 33

G

gallbladder
   disease 16
   empyema 20 *see also* cholecystitis
   malignancy 20
   palpable 34
   porcelain 20
gallstones 28, 32

gallstones *cont.*
   cholesterol 20
   ileus 20
gastrectomy for gastric cancer 23
gastric
   cancer 22, 34
   carcinoid 4
   carcinoma 4, 16, 24
   fundus varices 34, 38
   outflow obstruction 16, 24
   perforation 24
   regurgitation *see* gastroesophageal reflux
   splash 38
   tumour 22
   ulcer 16, 24
gastritis
   atrophic 4, 22
   chronic 4, 24
gastroduodenal ulcer *see* peptic ulcer
gastroesophageal reflux 16, 24
gastrointestinal
   bleeding 14, 26
   haemorrhage 34
   perforation 36
gastropathy, hypertrophic 22
gastrostomy, percutaneous endoscopic, for oesophageal carcinoma 31
gentamicin for diverticular disease of the colon 15
glossitis 4, 12
glypressin for bleeding varices 27

H

H_2 blockers
   for bleeding peptic ulcer 27
   for chronic pancreatitis 39
   for duodenal ulcer 17
   for gastric cancer 23
   for gastric ulceration 25
   for oesophagitis and hiatus hernia 33
   for Zollinger–Ellison syndrome 43
haematemesis 16, 22, 24, 26, 38
haematochezia 26
haemobilia 20
haemofiltration for acute pancreatitis 37
haemolytic uraemic syndrome 18
haemoptysis 26
haemorrhage 10, 14, 16, 18, 24, 40, 42 *see also* bleeding
   gastrointestinal 34
   ileal 18
heart
   disease, ischaemic 32
   failure
      congestive 34
      high-output 4
heartburn 28, 32
Helicobacter pylori infection 4, 16, 24, 42
heparin for ulcerative colitis 41

Index

hepatitis
   cholestatic 20
   chronic 34
hepatocellular dysfunction 18
hiatus hernia 32
   para-oesophageal 32
   rolling 32
   sliding 32
5-HT reuptake inhibitors for irritable bowel syndrome 29
hydrocortisone for coeliac disease 9
hydronephrosis 14, 28
hydrops 20
hydroxocobalamin for pernicious anaemia 5
hyoscine for irritable bowel syndrome 29
hyperamylaesaemia 36
hypergastrinaemia 42
hyperglycaemia 36
hyperimmune bovine colostrum for enteric infections 19
hyperinfection syndrome 18
hyperparathyroidism 43
hyperplasia, enterochromaffin cell 4
hypertrophy of head of pancreas 38
hypnotherapy for irritable bowel syndrome 29
hypoacidity 42
hypoalbuminaemia 40
hypocalcaemia 8, 36
hypomagnesaemia 8
hypotension 20, 26
hypothyroidism 4

I

ileal
   haemorrhage 18
   obstruction, terminal 12
   perforation 18
   resection, terminal 4
ileitis
   mesenteric 18
   regional *see* Crohn's disease
   terminal 4 *see also* Crohn's disease
ileocolitis *see* Crohn's disease
ileus *see also* intestinal obstruction, volvulus
   gallstone 20
   paralytic 14
infarction
   mesenteric 36
   myocardial 16, 24, 36
infection 12, 28
   amoebic 12, 40
   bacterial 6, 12, 40
   Bacteroides 6
   Candida 18
   Clostridium 6
   cytomegalovirus 16, 40
   enteric 18
   Enterobius 18
   Escherichia coli 6

infection *cont*.
   Helicobacter pylori 4, 16, 24, 42
   helminthic 6
   herpes simplex 40
   protozoan 6
   Salmonella 18
   Strongyloides 18
   viral 6
   Yersinia 12, 18
inflammation 12, 14
   pancreatic 38
inflammatory bowel disease 8, 10, 14, 18, 28
ingestion
   of bismuth-containing preparations 26
   of Guinness 26
   of iron 26
intestinal *see also* bowel
   obstruction 12, 14, 36 *see also* volvulus
   perforation 12, 20
   resection 18
   strangulation 32
iron
   deficiency 8
   ingestion of 26
irritable bowel syndrome 8, 10, 14, 16, 20, 24, 28, 40
islet-cell tumour, ulcerogenic *see* Zollinger–Ellison syndrome
ispaghula husk
   for diverticular disease of the colon 15
   for irritable bowel syndrome 29
itching *see* pruritus

J

jaundice 20, 34, 36, 38
   hepatic 34
   obstructive 20, 34
jejunitis, ulcerative 8

K

Kaposi's sarcoma 26
karaya gum *see* sterculia
ketoacidosis, diabetic 36
ketosis, diabetic *see* diabetic ketoacidosis
kidney *see* renal

L

lactulose
   before surgery or endoscopy for pancreatic cancer 35
   for diverticular disease of the colon 15
   for irritable bowel syndrome 29
lansoprazole
   for duodenal ulcer 17
   for oesophagitis and hiatus hernia 33
   for Zollinger–Ellison syndrome 43
laparotomy for Zollinger–Ellison syndrome 43
laxatives *see also* purgatives
   abuse 8, 28
   for diverticular disease of the colon 15
levamisole for colorectal cancer 11

ligation, endoscopic variceal band, for bleeding varices 27
lithotripsy, extracorporeal shock-wave, for cholesterol gallstones 21
loperamide for irritable bowel syndrome 29
lymphoma 12, 16
   Mediterranean 18
   small-intestinal 8
   T-cell 8

M

macroamylasaemia 36
malignancy 2, 8, 10 *see also* cancer
   colonic 28
   gallbladder 20
   gastric 2
   ovarian 28
mannitol before surgery or endoscopy for pancreatic cancer 35
mebendazole for enteric infections 19
mebeverine
   for diverticular disease of the colon 15
   for irritable bowel syndrome 29
melaena 16, 22, 24, 26
Menetrier's disease 22
mesalazine
   for Crohn's disease 13
   for ulcerative colitis 41
methyl tert-butyl ether dissolution of cholesterol gallstones 21
metoclopramide for gastric cancer 23
metronidazole
   for bacterial overgrowth of the small intestine 7
   for Crohn's disease 13
   for diverticular disease of the colon 15
   for duodenal ulcer 17
   for enteric infections 19
misoprostol for gastric ulceration 25
morphine
   for oesophageal carcinoma 31
   for pancreatic cancer 35
motility stimulants for irritable bowel syndrome 29
mucus
   in stools 10
   passage of 28
   per rectum 40
Murphy's sign 20
muscle
   bulk, loss of 18
   relaxants
      for diverticular disease of the colon 15
      for irritable bowel syndrome 29

N

naevi, spider 26
narcotics *see* opiates
necrosectomy 37

Index

necrosis
    pancreatic 36
    peripheral fat 36
neoplasm, pancreatic 20
neuropathy 6
    diabetic 18
    hollow visceral 2
    peripheral sensory 4
nifedipine for achalasia 3
nitrates for achalasia 3
nizatidine
    for duodenal ulcer 17
    for gastric ulceration 25
node
    left anterior axillary 22
    Virchow's 22, 34
nodule, Sister Joseph's 22
nonsteroidal anti-inflammatory drugs see NSAIDs
nose bleeds 26
NSAIDs for chronic pancreatitis 39
nystatin for gastric cancer 23

O

obstruction
    afferent loop 36
    colorectal 10
    common bile duct 38
    duodenal 38
    gastric outflow 16, 24
    intestinal 12, 14, 36 see also volvulus
    oesophageal 30
    pyloric channel 16
    terminal ileal 12
octreotide for bacterial overgrowth of the small intestine 7
odynophagia 32
oesophageal
    carcinoma 2, 30
    obstruction 30
    reflux see gastroesophageal reflux
oesophageal cont.
    spasm 2
    stricture 2, 30, 32
    transection for bleeding varices 27
oesophagectomy for oesophageal carcinoma 31
oesophagitis 20, 32, 42
    reflux 22
oesophagogastrostomy for oesophageal carcinoma 31
oesophagus, Barrett's 32
olsalazine
    for Crohn's disease 13
    for ulcerative colitis 41
omeprazole
    for duodenal ulcer 17
    for gastric ulceration 25
    for oesophagitis and hiatus hernia 33
    for Zollinger–Ellison syndrome 43

opiates
    for gastric cancer 23
    for oesophageal carcinoma 31
opioids see opiates
Osler–Weber–Rendu syndrome 26
osteomalacia 8
osteoporosis 8
ovarian
    cancer 34
    carcinoma 14
    cyst torsion 36
    malignancy 28
oxygen for acute pancreatitis 37

P

pain
    abdominal 6, 14, 18, 24, 28, 36, 38, 40
    chest 2
    colicky 12
    epigastric 16, 22, 24, 36
    nocturnal 24
pancreas
    fibrosing disease of see cystic fibrosis
    hypertrophy of head of 38
pancreatic
    abscess 36, 38
    ascites 38
    cancer 34, 38
    enzyme therapy for chronic pancreatitis 39
    inflammation 38
    insufficiency 38
    necrosis 36
    neoplasm 20
    pseudoaneurysm 38
    supplements for chronic pancreatitis 39
    tumour 34
pancreaticojejunostomy for chronic pancreatitis 39
pancreatitis 16, 20
    acute 16, 20, 24, 34, 36, 38
    chronic 6, 8, 16, 18, 24, 28, 34, 38
pancreatitis cont.
    gallstone-induced 36
penicillin for diverticular disease of the colon 15
peppermint oil
    for diverticular disease of the colon 15
    for irritable bowel syndrome 29
peptic ulcer 14, 20, 24, 26, 28, 32, 39, 42
perforation
    colonic 40
    colorectal 10
    duodenal 16, 42
    gastric 24
    gastrointestinal 36
    ileal 18
    intestinal 12, 20
peristalsis, visible 24
peritonism 24
peritonitis 10, 14, 16, 36
personality disorders 28

phaeochromocytoma 18
pneumonia 32
pneumonitis, aspiration 2
polyp
    adenomatous 22
    colon 14
    colorectal 18
pouchitis 6
praziquantel for enteric infections 19
prednisolone
    for coeliac disease 9
    for Crohn's disease 13
    for ulcerative colitis 41
pregnancy, ectopic 36
proctitis, irradiation 40
propranolol for bleeding varices 27
prostaglandins for gastric ulceration 25
proton-pump inhibitors
    for duodenal ulcer 17
    for gastric ulceration 25
    for oesophagitis and hiatus hernia 33
pruritus 34
    ani 18
pseudoaneurysm, pancreatic 38
pseudocyst 36, 38
pseudoxanthoma elasticum 26
psychiatric
    abnormality 28
    illness 34
psychotherapy for irritable bowel syndrome 29
purgatives see also laxative
    for gastric cancer 23
pyelonephritis 14
pyloric
    channel obstruction 16
    stenosis 22, 42
pyoderma gangrenosum 12
pyrosis see heartburn

Q

quinolones for enteric infections 19

R

radiotherapy
    adjuvant, for colorectal cancer 11
    for oesophageal carcinoma 31
ranitidine
    for duodenal ulcer 17
    for gastric ulceration 25
    for oesophagitis and hiatus hernia 33
    for Zollinger–Ellison syndrome 43
rectal
    bleeding 12, 14, 26
    lesions 10
    ulcer 10
reflexes, absent 4

Index

reflux
   gastroesophageal 16, 24
   oesophageal *see* gastroesophageal reflux
   oesophagitis 22
regurgitation 2, 30, 32
   gastric *see* gastroesophageal reflux
rehydration for diarrhoea due to enteric infections 19
Reiter's syndrome 18
relaxation techniques for irritable bowel syndrome 29
renal
   failure 18, 36
   oxalate stones 12
resection, terminal ileal 4
respiratory failure 36
rose spots 18

S

saliva, inability to swallow 30
salpingitis 36
sarcoma, Kaposi's 26
satiety
   early 28
   rapid 22
schistosomiasis 18
Schwachman's syndrome 8
sclerotherapy, endoscopic variceal injection, for bleeding varices 27
sepsis, intra-abdominal 12
septicaemia, Gram-negative 18
serotonin *see* 5-HT
shock 14, 16, 26, 36
short stature 8
shunt, transjugular intrahepatic portacaval, for bleeding varices 27
skin
   abscess 12
   rashes 6
   tag 12
small
   bowel *see also* small intestine
      bacterial overgrowth syndrome 8
      diverticula 4
   intestine *see also* small-bowel
      bacterial overgrowth of the 6
spasm, oesophageal 2
spasmophilia *see* tetany
sphincteroplasty, transduodenal, for chronic pancreatitis 39
sphincterotomy, endoscopic, for pancreatitis
   acute 37
   chronic 39
spinal-cord degeneration 4, 6
spondylarthritis *see* spondylitis, ankylosing
spondylitis
   ankylosing 18
   rheumatoid *see* spondylitis, ankylosing
sprue, tropical 8

stagnant loop syndrome *see* bacterial overgrowth of the small intestine
steatorrhoea 6, 8, 38
stenosis
   luminal 30
   pyloric 22, 42
stents for pancreatic cancer
   endoscopic 35
   percutaneous internal 35
sterculia
   for diverticular disease of the colon 15
   for irritable bowel syndrome 29
steroids *see* corticosteroids
stomach *see* gastric
stones
   bile duct 34
   renal oxalate 12
stool, greasy 38
straining to defaecate 28
strangulation, intestinal 32
stricture 14, 18
   bile-duct 20, 34
   colonic 38
   fibromuscular 40
   oesophageal 2, 30, 32
stricturoplasty for Crohn's disease 12
succussion splash 16, 22, 24
sucralfate for oesophagitis and hiatus hernia 33
sulphasalazine
   for Crohn's disease 13
   for ulcerative colitis 41

T

tachycardia 26, 36
telangiectasia 26
tenesmus 10, 12
tetany 8
tetracycline
   for bacterial overgrowth of the small intestine 7
   for duodenal ulcer 17
   for enteric infections 19
thiabendazole for enteric infections 19
thrombophlebitis *see* thrombosis, venous
thrombosis, venous
   deep 34
   splenic 34, 38
tinidazole for enteric infections 19
transection, oesophageal, for bleeding varices 27
trimethoprim for bacterial overgrowth of the small intestine 7
tripotassium dicitrato bismuthate for duodenal ulcer 17
Troissier's syndrome 34
Trousseau's syndrome 34
trypanosomiasis, South American *see* Chagas' disease

tuberculosis 12
tumour 10
   ampullary 34
   biliary tract 34
   gastric 22
   endocrine 34
   islet-cell, ulcerogenic *see* Zollinger–Ellison syndrome
   Krukenberg 22
   pancreatic 34
Turner's sign 36

U

ulcer
   aphthous 12
   bleeding 16
   deep 32
   duodenal 12, 16, 24, 38, 42
   dyspepsia 22
   gastric 16, 24
   gastroduodenal *see* peptic ulcer
   nonhealing 42
   oral 12
   peptic 14, 20, 24, 26, 28, 32, 39, 42
   rectal 10
uraemia 36
urgency
   to defaecate 28, 40
   urinary 28
urinary
   frequency 28
   urgency 28
ursodeoxycholic acid for cholesterol gallstones 21

V

vancomycin for enteric infections 19
varices
   bleeding 26
   gastric fundus 34, 38
vitamin
   B12 deficiency 4, 6, 12
   K before surgery or endoscopy for pancreatic cancer 35
   supplements for enteric infections 19
volvulus 32 *see also* intestinal obstruction

W

Wernicke's encephalopathy 8

Z

Zollinger–Ellison syndrome 8, 16, 25, 42

CURRENT DIAGNOSIS & TREATMENT

in

Haematology

Edited by
Grant Prentice

Series editors
Roy Pounder
Mark Hamilton

A QUICK Reference for the Clinician

Contributors

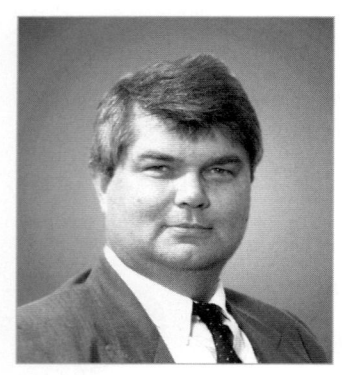

EDITOR

H G Prentice

Professor Grant Prentice is Professor of Haematological Oncology at the Royal Free Hospital, London. His clinical research interests are in the treatment of leukaemia, including bone-marrow transplantation. The prevention and treatment of infection in the immunosuppressed patient is a major interest.

REFEREES

Professor Adrian Newland
Royal London Hospital
London, UK

Professor David Linch
Department of Haematology
University College Hospital
London, UK

AUTHORS

ANAEMIA, APLASTIC

Dr Judith Marsh
Department of Haematology
St George's Hospital
London, UK

ANAEMIA, MEGALOBLASTIC

Professor A Victor Hoffbrand
Professor of Haematology
Royal Free Hospital
London, UK

DISSEMINATED INTRAVASCULAR COAGULATION

Dr John Pasi
Department of Haematology
Royal Free Hospital
London, UK

HAEMOPHILIA AND VON WILLEBRAND'S DISEASE

Dr Christine Lee
Haemophilia Centre and
Haemostasis Unit
Royal Free Hospital
London, UK

Dr John Pasi
Department of Haematology
Royal Free Hospital
London, UK

HODGKIN'S DISEASE

Dr Adele Fielding
Department of Haematology
University College Hospital
London, UK

Dr Anthony Goldstone
Department of Haematology
University College Hospital
London, UK

INFECTIONS IN HAEMATOLOGICAL MALIGNANCY

Professor H Grant Prentice
Professor of Haematological Oncology
Royal Free Hospital
London, UK

Dr Christopher C Kibbler
Department of Medical Microbiology
Royal Free Hospital
London, UK

LEUKAEMIA, ACUTE LYMPHOBLASTIC IN ADULTS

Dr Adele Fielding
Department of Haematology
University College Hospital
London, UK

Dr Anthony Goldstone
Department of Haematology
University College Hospital
London, UK

LEUKAEMIA, ACUTE LYMPHOBLASTIC IN CHILDREN

Dr Ian Hann
Department of Haematology
Great Ormond Street Hospital
London, UK

LEUKAEMIA, ACUTE MYELOID

Professor Alan K Burnett
Department of Haematology
University of Wales College of Medicine
Cardiff, UK

LEUKAEMIA, CHRONIC LYMPHOCYTIC

Professor TJ Hamblin
Department of Pathology
Royal Victoria Hospital
Bournemouth, UK

LEUKAEMIA, HAIRY CELL

Professor TJ Hamblin
Department of Pathology
Royal Victoria Hospital
Bournemouth, UK

MULTIPLE MYELOMA

Dr Atul B Mehta
Department of Haematology
Royal Free Hospital
London, UK

MYELOPROLIFERATIVE DISORDERS

Professor John Goldman
Department of Haematology
Royal Postgraduate Medical School
Hammersmith Hospital
London, UK

NON-HODGKIN'S LYMPHOMA

Dr Adele Fielding
Department of Haematology
University College Hospital
London, UK

Dr Anthony Goldstone
Department of Haematology
University College Hospital
London, UK

PLATELET DISORDERS

Dr Justin Harrison
Consultant Haematologist
Hemel Hempstead General Hospital
Hemel Hempstead, UK

PROTHROMBOTIC STATES

Professor Samuel J Machin
Department of Haematology
University College Hospital
London, UK

SICKLE CELL DISEASE

Dr Sally Davies
Department of Haematology
Central Middlesex Hospital
London, UK

THALASSAEMIA

Dr Beatrix Wonke
Department of Haematology
Whittington Hospital
London, UK

TRANSFUSION MEDICINE

Dr Mary Brennan
National Blood Transfusion Service
North London Blood Transfusion Centre
London, UK

Dr Marcela Contreras
National Blood Transfusion Service
North London Blood Transfusion Centre
London, UK

WALDENSTRÖM'S MACROGLOBULINAEMIA

Professor TJ Hamblin
Department of Pathology
Royal Victoria Hospital
Bournemouth, UK

Contents

2 **Anaemia, aplastic**

4 **Anaemia, megaloblastic**

6 **Disseminated intravascular coagulation**

8 **Haemophilia and von Willebrand's disease**

10 **Hodgkin's disease**

12 **Infections in haematological malignancy**

14 **Leukaemia, acute lymphoblastic in adults**

16 **Leukaemia, acute lymphoblastic in children**

18 **Leukaemia, acute myeloid**

20 **Leukaemia, chronic lymphocytic**

22 **Leukaemia, hairy cell**

24 **Multiple myeloma**

26 **Myeloproliferative disorders**
   chronic myeloid leukaemia
   essential thrombocythaemia
   polycythaemia rubra vera
   primary myelofibrosis

28 **Non-Hdgkin's lymphoma**

30 **Platelet disorders**
   alloimmune thrombocytopenia (neonatal, post-transfusion)
   platelet function defect
   immune thrombocytopenia
   thrombotic thrombocytopenic purpura

32 **Platelet disorders**
   alloimmune thrombocytopenia (neonatal, post-transfusion)
   platelet function defect
   immune thrombocytopenia
   thrombotic thrombocytopenic purpura

34 **Sickle cell disease**

36 **Thalassaemia**

38 **Transfusion medicine**
   erythrocytes
   fresh frozen plasma
   platelets

40 **Waldenström's macroglobulinaemia**

42 **Index**

Anaemia, aplastic
J.C.W. Marsh

Diagnosis

Symptoms
- Symptoms and signs are due to and relate to the severity of the peripheral blood pancytopenia.

Fatigue, shortness of breath on exertion, headache, palpitation: symptoms of anaemia.

Easy bruising and petechiae, gum bleeding, buccal haemorrhage, visual disturbance due to retinal haemorrhage: symptoms of thrombocytopenia.

Mouth and tongue ulcers: symptoms of infection due to leucopenia.

History of jaundice: may indicate post-hepatitic aplasia or associated paroxysmal nocturnal haemoglobinuria.

Signs
- Bleeding manifestations are usually more common than infection.

Pallor.

Ecchymoses, petechiae of skin and mouth, retinal haemorrhage.

Fever.

Mouth and tongue ulceration.

Pharyngitis, pneumonia.

Skin and perianal sepsis.

Skeletal, skin, and nail anomalies, short stature: may occur in congenital aplastic anaemia.

- Spleen, liver, and lymph nodes are not enlarged.

Investigations

Full blood count and examination of blood film: shows pancytopenia (isolated cytopenias may occur in early stages), macrocytosis, toxic granulation of neutrophils.

Reticulocyte count: shows absolute reticulocytopenia.

Bone-marrow aspiration and biopsy: shows hypocellular bone marrow, no abnormal infiltration, no increase in reticulin, colony-forming cells low or absent; cytogenetic studies to exclude pre-leukaemia; in Fanconi anaemia, cultured peripheral blood lymphocytes show increased chromosomal breaks with DNA cross-linking agent (e.g. diepoxybutane).

Ham's test and urine haemosiderin analysis: classically negative in aplastic anaemia and positive in paroxysmal nocturnal haemoglobinuria (PNH), but a small proportion of PNH cells can be detected in up to 30% of patients with aplastic anaemia.

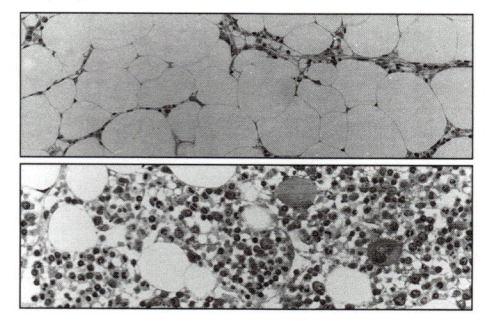

Aplastic anaemia bone marrow (top), normal bone marrow (bottom).

Liver function tests and viral studies: to detect antecedent hepatitis; test for hepatitis A, B, and non-A, non-B (hepatitis C), Epstein–Barr virus, cytomegalovirus, and parvovirus B19 (parvovirus classically causes pure erythrocyte aplasia and can also cause pancytopenia associated with haemophagocytosis).

Chest and sinus radiography.

Hand and forearm radiography: may be abnormal in congenital aplastic anaemia.

Abdominal ultrasonography: to exclude splenomegaly; anatomically displaced or abnormal kidneys in Fanconi anaemia.

Complications

Failure of random donor platelet transfusions to increase recipient's platelet count, increased bone-marrow graft rejection potential: due to sensitization to non-HLA antigens from multiple blood transfusions.

Late clonal evolution to myelodysplastic syndrome or acute myeloid leukaemia in 10% or paroxysmal nocturnal haemoglobinuria in 10% of untransplanted patients.

Differential diagnosis

Hypoplastic myelodysplastic syndrome or hypoplastic acute myeloid leukaemia in adults.

Hypoplastic acute lymphoblastic leukaemia in children.

Hairy cell leukaemia.

Other bone-marrow infiltration: e.g. lymphoma, carcinoma, myelofibrosis.

Anorexia nervosa.

Severe infection: e.g. tuberculosis, overwhelming Gram-negative or Gram-positive sepsis.

Aetiology

Congenital causes
E.g. Fanconi anaemia, dyskeratosis congenita.

Acquired causes
Idiopathic: in 75% of patients.

Drugs: e.g. NSAIDs, gold, chloramphenicol, sulphonamides.

Chemicals: benzene, organic solvents, aniline dyes.

Viruses: hepatitis A, B, or non-A, non-B (hepatitis C) and other as yet unidentified viruses, Epstein–Barr virus.

Paroxysmal nocturnal haemoglobinuria: 25% of patients later develop aplastic anaemia.

Rare causes
SLE, pregnancy.

Epidemiology

- The annual incidence in Europe is 2–3 in one million; 100–150 new cases are expected annually in the UK.
- The male:female ratio is equal.
- Two peaks are seen in the age incidence for men: 15–25 years and >60 years; one peak for women: >60 years.

Treatment

Diet and lifestyle
- If neutrophils are <0.5×10⁹/L, food should be well cooked and fresh fruit washed before consumption.

Pharmacological treatment
- Drugs are indicated for patients ineligible for bone-marrow transplantation.
- High-dose corticosteroids should be avoided because of toxicity (infection, hypertension, diabetes, avascular necrosis of bone) and lack of convincing benefit in aplastic anaemia.
- Drugs that affect platelet function (aspirin, NSAIDs) or that may cause aplastic anaemia must be avoided.

Antilymphocyte globulin (ALG) or antithymocyte globulin (ATG)
- Horse ALG (lymphoglobuline) should be used initially; then, if patient shows no response or later relapse, rabbit ATG (thymoglobuline) should be tried.

Standard dosage	ALG 0.1 vial i.v. over 1 h test dose, followed by 1.5 vials/10 kg body weight i.v. over 12–18 h for 5 days.
Contraindications	Hypersensitivity or severe systemic reaction to test dose, active infection, haemolytic paroxysmal nocturnal haemoglobinuria, SLE.
Special points	Central line infusion to prevent thrombophlebitis; platelet transfusion before each dose; low-dose prednisolone to prevent serum sickness.
Main drug interactions	None.
Main side effects	Anaphylaxis or allergic reactions (during infusion); serum sickness (7–14 days after starting treatment).

Cyclosporin
- Cyclosporin can be used after ALG or as a single agent.

Standard dosage	Cyclosporin 2.5 mg/kg orally twice daily for 3–6 months.
Contraindications	Renal or liver impairment, breast feeding.
Special points	Drug blood concentration, blood pressure, renal and liver function must be monitored regularly.
Main drug interactions	Erythromycin, ketoconazole, aminoglycosides, vancomycin, amphotericin B, rifampicin, phenytoin.
Main side effects	Nephrotoxicity, nausea, tremor, hypertension, hypertrichosis, gum hypertrophy, hepatotoxicity.

Oxymetholone
- Oxymetholone is now used after ALG rather than as a single agent.

Standard dosage	Oxymetholone 2.5 mg/kg orally daily (0.5–1 mg/kg daily for Fanconi anaemia).
Contraindications	Liver impairment, breast and prostate cancer, pregnancy; caution in children (behavioural problems) and elderly men (prostatic hypertrophy).
Special points	Serum cholesterol concentration must be monitored.
Main drug interactions	Other potentially hepatotoxic drugs, e.g. erythromycin, rifampicin, ketoconazole, cyclosporin.
Main side effects	Reversible cholestatic jaundice, liver tumours, and peliosis hepatitis with long-term use, virilization in females, acne.

Treatment aims
To provide good supportive care (critical for survival of patient).
To treat fever promptly (broad-spectrum i.v. antibiotics), routine oral antifungal prophylaxis.

Other treatments
Allogeneic bone-marrow transplantation: treatment of choice for patients who have severe aplastic anaemia, are <45 years, and have an HLA-identical sibling donor.
Bone-marrow transplantation from an HLA-matched volunteer donor: if patient has very severe aplastic anaemia, is <30 years, and has no HLA-identical sibling
- Haemopoietic growth factors such as granulocyte-colony stimulating factor (CSF), granulocyte macrophage-CSF, interleukin-3 and interleukin-6 have little effect in aplastic anaemia, apart from a transient increase in neutrophil count in some patients. Serious toxicity may occur in aplastic anaemia patients.

Prognosis
- After bone-marrow transplantation from an HLA-identical identical sibling, at least 70–80% of patients are long-term survivors and can be considered cured of their disease.
- Response to antilymphocyte globulin or cyclosporin occurs in 50–70% (rarely before 3–6 months), but relapse and later clonal disorders may occur.

Follow-up and management
- Long-term monitoring is needed for clonal disorders and relapse.

Key references
Marsh JCW et al.: Haemopoietic growth factors in aplastic anaemia: a cautionary note. Lancet 1994, **344**:172–173.

Soutar RL, King DJ: Bone marrow transplantation. BMJ 1995, **310**:31–36.

Storb R, Champlin RE: Bone marrow transplantation for severe aplastic anaemia. Bone Marrow Transplant 1991, **8**:69–72.

Anaemia, megaloblastic — A.V. Hoffbrand

Diagnosis

Symptoms
- Many patients have no symptoms; the disease is suspected on routine blood count.

Dyspnoea on exertion, tiredness, headache.

Painful tongue.

Paraesthesiae in feet, difficulty walking: vitamin B_{12} deficiency only.

Infertility.

Signs
Pallor of mucous membranes: if haemoglobin concentration <9 g/dl.

Mild jaundice.

'Beefy red' glossitis.

Signs of vitamin B_{12} neuropathy: if present.

Investigations

General
Blood count: raised mean cell volume (>100 fl), reduced erythrocyte count, haemoglobin, and haematocrit, low reticulocyte count, reduced leucocyte and platelet counts (in severely anaemic patients).

Blood film: shows oval macrocytes, hypersegmented neutrophils (>5 nuclear lobes).

Bone-marrow analysis: in severely anaemic patients; shows hypercellular, increased proportion of early cells, many dying cells, megaloblastic erythroblasts, giant and abnormally shaped metamyelocytes, hypersegmented megakaryocytes.

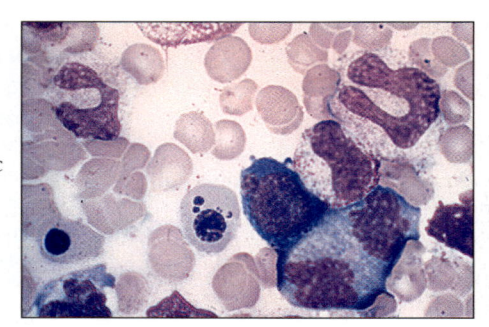

Bone marrow with megaloblastic anaemia.

Serum indirect bilirubin and lactic dehydrogenase measurement: concentrations raised.

Direct Coombs test: complement only, positive in some patients.

Tests for disseminated intravascular coagulation or intravascular haemolysis: positive in some patients.

Tests for vitamin B_{12} (B_{12}) or folate deficiency: serum B_{12} low in B_{12} deficiency, normal or slightly low in folate deficiency; serum folate normal or raised in B_{12} deficiency, low in folate deficiency; erythrocyte folate normal or low in B_{12} deficiency, low in folate deficiency.

Deoxyuridine suppression, serum homocysteine and methylmalonic acid measurement: additional tests performed in some laboratories for B_{12} or folate deficiency.

Special
Diet history: to exclude veganism, low folate intake.

Schilling test: for B_{12} absorption.

Serum analysis: for intrinsic factor and parietal cell antibodies.

Fibreoptic endoscopy: for gastric biopsy, exclusion of gastric polyps, carcinoma in pernicious anaemia.

Contrast radiography: to detect gastric atrophy, neoplasm (pernicious anaemia), or small intestinal lesions.

Endoscopy and jejunal biopsy: if gluten-induced enteropathy is suspected in patients with folate deficiency.

Complications
Neuropathy: due to vitamin B_{12} deficiency.

Neural tube defects in fetus: risk reduced by folate treatment.

Carcinoma of stomach: in pernicious anaemia.

Differential diagnosis

Other causes of macrocytosis
Alcohol, liver disease, hypothyroidism, aplastic anaemia, myelodysplasia, acute myeloid leukaemia, myeloma, reticulocytosis.

Other causes of megaloblastic anaemia
Nitrous oxide anaesthesia.

Transcobalamin II deficiency.

Antifolate drugs: methotrexate, pyrimethamine (reversed by folinic acid), co-trimoxazole.

Drugs inhibiting DNA synthesis: cytosine arabinoside, hydroxyurea, 6-mercaptopurine, azathioprine, 5-fluorouracil.

Congenital abnormalities of vitamin B_{12} or folate metabolism.

Congenital abnormalities of DNA synthesis: e.g. orotic aciduria.

Aetiology

Causes of vitamin B_{12} deficiency
Diet deficiency: e.g. in vegans.

Pernicious anaemia.

Congenital intrinsic factor deficiency.

Total or subtotal gastrectomy.

Sclerosing gastritis, gastric bypass.

Stagnant-loop syndrome.

Ileal resection or abnormality: e.g. Crohn's disease.

HIV infection.

Drugs: e.g. metformin.

Specific malabsorption with proteinuria.

Fish tapeworm.

Causes of folate deficiency
Dietary deficiency: poor-quality diet, goat's milk, specialized diets.

Malabsorption: gluten-induced enteropathy, tropical sprue, congenital.

Increased turnover: pregnancy, prematurity, haemolytic anaemias, myelofibrosis, widespread inflammatory or malignant diseases.

Increased losses: congestive heart failure, haemodialysis or peritoneal dialysis.

Uncertain: anticonvulsant treatment.

Epidemiology
- The occurrence of megaloblastic anaemia relates to diet (e.g. Hindu communities, where veganism is common, poor people, in whom dietary folate intake is reduced).
- For pernicious anaemia, the peak age of incidence is 60 years.
- The female : male ratio is 1.6:1.

Treatment

Diet and lifestyle
- The quality of the diet must be increased in patients with dietary folate deficiency.

Pharmacological treatment

For vitamin B_{12} (B_{12}) deficiency

Standard dosage	Hydroxocobalamin 1 mg i.m. 6 times in 2–3 weeks, then 1 mg every 3 months.
Contraindications	Rare hypersensitivity.
Special points	No evidence suggests that more frequent doses are needed for B_{12} neuropathy.
Main drug interactions	None.
Main side effects	Gout and significant hypokalaemia a few days after commencing treatment.

For folate deficiency

Standard dosage	Folic acid 5 mg orally daily for 4 months, then 5 mg daily or weekly as needed.
Contraindications	B_{12} deficiency, malignancy (unless deficiency is clinically important).
Special points	B_{12} deficiency must be excluded because B_{12} neuropathy could be precipitated or aggravated.
Main drug interactions	None.
Main side effects	None.

- Folic acid should be used as prophylaxis in pregnancy (300–400 μg daily; 5 mg daily if previous neural defect in fetus), and also in renal dialysis.
- In women of child-bearing age, folate intake should be increased to at least 400 μg daily by diet or folate supplement.
- For premature babies (<1500 g birth weight), folic acid 1 mg daily is indicated.

Treatment aims
To correct anaemia by replenishing body stores of vitamin.
To correct underlying disease.
To restore normal neurological status (vitamin B_{12} deficiency).

Other treatments
- Packed erythrocyte transfusion should be used only if essential: removal of equivalent volume of plasma in patients with congestive heart failure.

Prognosis
- Prognosis depends mainly on the underlying cause.
- Life expectancy is reduced slightly in patients with pernicious anaemia because of the risk of carcinoma of the stomach.

Follow-up and management
- Patients with pernicious anaemia should have annual clinical review and blood count.
- Routine endoscopy is not recommended.
- Patients having total gastrectomy or ileal resection need prophylactic hydroxocobalamin 1 mg every 3 months from the time of surgery for life.

Key references
Anthony AC: Megaloblastic anaemias. In *Hematology. Basic Principles and Practice*. Edited by Hoffman R *et al*. New York: Churchill Livingstone, 1991, pp 392–422.

Hoffbrand AV, Jackson BFA: The deoxyuridine suppression test and cobalamin–folate interrelations. *Br J Haematol* 1993, **85**:232–237.

Savage DG, Lindenbaum J: Folate–cobalamin interactions. In *Folate in Health & Disease*. Edited by Baily L. New York: Marcel Dekker, 1994, pp 237–285.

Disseminated intravascular coagulation — K.J. Pasi

Diagnosis

Symptoms
- Disseminated intravascular coagulation occurs in a spectrum of guises from a chronic syndrome, diagnosed on laboratory tests, with no symptoms or signs (compensated), to an acute florid clinical bleeding state (uncompensated).
- It is always associated with an underlying disorder.
- The major symptoms are those of the underlying disorder.

Generalized bruising: especially over dependent areas.

Bleeding at surgical sites and incisions, around venepuncture sites, indwelling lines, and drainage tubes.

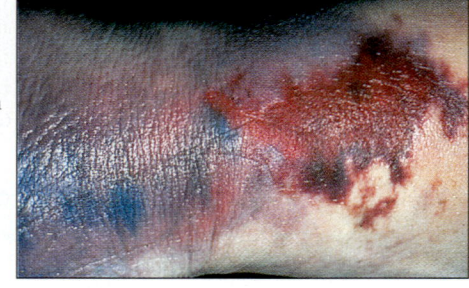

Haematemesis, melaena, haemoptysis, haematuria, and vaginal bleeding.

Gangrene of fingers and toes, purpura fulminans, haemorrhagic bullae: microthrombotic lesions in 5–10% of patients.

Purpura fulminans, with surrounding extensive subcutaneous haemorrhage.

Signs
Evidence of bleeding: as detailed under symptoms, when present.

Investigations
- Simple screening tests show reduced levels of clotting factors and platelets.
- Disseminated intravascular coagulation cannot be ruled out by a single set of normal results; serial values may be needed to show consumption.

Measurement of prothrombin time, activated partial thromboplastin time, thrombin time: all times prolonged; prolongation of thrombin time best guide to clinical significance of raised fibrinogen degradation products and low fibrinogen; thrombin time twice normal control value indicates impending overt clinical bleeding.

Fibrinogen measurement: concentration low.

Fibrinogen degradation products and D-dimers measurement: concentrations raised; fibrinogen degradation products sensitive but not specific for disseminated intravascular coagulation; D-dimer specific but not as sensitive.

Platelet count: low.

Blood film: many patients have associated microangiographic haemolytic anaemia; erythrocytes fragmented by passing through deposited fibrin strands.

Complications
Uncontrollable haemorrhage.
Microvascular blockage and tissue necrosis of heart, liver, kidney, and brain.
Adult respiratory distress.

Differential diagnosis
- Simple screening tests and the clinical picture are usually diagnostic.

Vitamin K deficiency: normal platelet count.
Liver disease: raised factor VIII concentrations.
Lupus anticoagulant and thrombocytopenia: normal fibrinogen, inhibitor present.
Thrombotic thrombocytopenic purpura: clotting tests usually normal, florid microangiopathic changes on blood film.
Massive transfusion: clinical history.

Aetiology

Causes and associated disorders

Infections: meningococcal septicaemia, Gram-negative septicaemia, malaria, viral (purpura fulminans).
Malignancy: disseminated metastatic carcinomas, myeloid leukaemia, promyelocitic leukaemia.
Obstetric complications: septic abortion, amniotic fluid embolism, placental abruption, eclampsia, retained dead fetus and placenta.
Tissue injury: severe burns or trauma, extensive surgery, hypo- or hyperthermia, shock.
Immunological phenomena: anaphylaxis, incompatible transfusion, allograft rejection.
Miscellaneous: liver disease and ascitic fluid shunts, extracorporeal circuits, certain snake and insect bites, vascular malformations.

Pathogenesis
- Disseminated intravascular coagulopathy is triggered by inappropriate and continued activation of clotting pathways.
- This leads to excessive thrombin generation, coagulation factor consumption, and platelet aggregation.
- Thrombin also activates protein C and fibrinolytic systems via secondary generation of plasmin.
- Natural inhibitors of the clotting cascade are overwhelmed.
- Coagulation factor consumption, consumptive thrombocytopenia, and hyperfibrinolysis lead to bleeding.
- Uncontrolled fibrin deposition leads to microthrombosis.

Epidemiology
- 60% of clinical cases of disseminated intravascular coagulation are associated with septicaemic infection, usually due to Gram-negative bacteria.
- Most acute cases are encountered in severely ill patients in intensive care.

Treatment

Diet and lifestyle
- No special precautions are necessary.

Pharmacological treatment

Anticoagulants
- Although controversial, anticoagulants may have a role in acute promyelocytic leukaemia (M3), acute intravascular haemolysis (incompatible blood transfusion), and purpura fulminans.

Standard dosage	Heparin 5–10 units/kg/h continuous i.v. infusion.
Contraindications	Florid bleeding
Special points	Requires antithrombin III for its action, which is often low in patients with disseminated intravascular coagulation; fresh frozen plasma may also be needed to supply antithrombin III to maintain effective heparinization. Partial thromboplastin time should be kept at 1.5–2 times control. May increase bleeding tendency; close monitoring and specialist advice needed.
Main drug interactions	Other anticoagulants.
Main side effects	Bleeding (with overdose).

Fibrinolytic inhibitors
- Because of increased deposition, fibrinolysis is protective against microvascular organ damage in disseminated intravascular coagulation; inhibitors of fibrinolysis are therefore generally contraindicated. In special circumstances of predominant fibrinolysis, however, they may be useful.
- Specialist advice must be sought before use.

Non-pharmacological treatment
See Transfusion medicine *for further details*.

Fresh frozen plasma
- Fresh frozen plasma supplies all clotting factors and naturally occurring inhibitors of coagulation.
- Initially, 10–15 ml/kg should be given.
- It may cause fluid overload.

Cryoprecipitate
- Cryoprecipitate supplies fibrinogen and factor VIII.
- It is used, at a rate of 1 unit/5 kg, when substantial fibrinogen replacement is needed.

Platelet concentrates
- Platelet concentrates are needed when consumptive thrombocytopenia is present.
- They are given, at a rate of 4 units/m² body surface area, if the platelet count falls below 50×10^9/L and overt bleeding occurs.

Packed erythrocytes
- Packed erythrocytes are needed to treat associated haemolysis or anaemia at a rate sufficient to maintain haematocrit >0.3.
- Virus transmission is a risk with any blood product.
- Fluid overload may also be a problem.

Treatment aims

To treat the underlying disorder.

To reverse the coagulopathy (by replacement of clotting factors and platelets or use of pharmacological inhibitors of coagulation).

To provide general supportive care for acutely ill patients.

Prognosis
- The mortality in severe disseminated intravascular coagulation is high and may exceed 80%.
- Death is usually due to progression of the underlying disease; elimination or amelioration of the cause is of utmost importance.

Follow-up and management
- Coagulation screening tests should be repeated to assess the effect of replacement therapy; the aim is a prothrombin time within 3 s of control, partial thromboplastin time within 10 s of control, and fibrinogen >1.0 g/L.
- The need for further replacement should be judged by the results of screening tests and degree of clinical bleeding.
- Laboratory abnormalities correct with successful treatment of the underlying disorder.

Key references

Bick R: Disseminated intravascular coagulation and related syndromes: a clinical review. *Semin Thromb Hemost* 1988, **14**:299–307

Levi M *et al*.: Pathogenesis of disseminated intravascular coagulation in sepsis. *JAMA* 1993, **270**:975–979.

Haemophilia and von Willebrand's disease — C.A. Lee and K.J. Pasi

Diagnosis

Symptoms

Haemophilia
Episodic spontaneous haemorrhage: into joints and muscles.
Deep-tissue haematoma: particularly after trauma or surgery.

Von Willebrand's disease
Bruising.
Epistaxis and melaena.
Excessive bleeding after dental extraction or surgery.
Post-partum bleeding, rarely haemarthroses and muscle haematomas.

Signs

Haemophilia
Hot swollen painful joint, unexpected bleeding after surgery: acute.
Crippling joint deformity: chronic.

Investigations

Haemophilia
Activated partial thromboplastin time measurement: prolonged.
Haemophilia A, factor VIII:C, haemophilia B, factor IX, and haemophilia C, factor XI assays: all three show low values.
Coagulation factor activity measurement: correlated with disease severity in haemophilia A and B (normal range, 50–150 units/dl):
<2 units/dl indicates severe disease, manifest as frequent spontaneous bleeding episodes, joint deformity, and crippling;
2–5 units/dl indicates moderate disease, manifest as post-traumatic bleeding, occasional spontaneous episodes;
5–20 units/dl indicates mild disease, manifest as post-traumatic bleeding.

Von Willebrand's disease
Bleeding time measurement: prolonged.
Factor VIII clotting activity, von Willebrand factor antigen and activity measurement: low values.
Platelet function tests: reduced aggregation of platelets with ristocetin.
• Von Willebrand's disease is classified on the basis of the type of protein abnormality; this is important for deciding treatment.

Complications

Transfusion-transmitted disease
Hepatitis A: has been a problem with a solvent detergent sterilized product; all patients with bleeding disorders should be vaccinated.
Hepatitis B: although all blood donors are tested for this, sterilization processes for clotting factor concentrate cannot be regarded as 100% safe; vaccination mandatory in patients with bleeding disorders.
Hepatitis C: all patients treated by unsterilized clotting factor concentrates have been infected (sterilization introduced in 1985); some patients progress to chronic liver disease; treatment by interferon may normalize transaminases; HIV co-infection results in faster progression of hepatitis C liver disease.
HIV infection: occurred in patients receiving concentrates between 1979 and 1985.

Inhibitors
Neutralizing antibodies: occurring after infusion of concentrates.

Chronic arthropathy
Chronic disabling arthritis: caused by recurrent haemarthroses.

Differential diagnosis
Other clotting factor deficiencies or platelet function disorders.

Aetiology

Causes of haemophilia
Quantitative deficiency of clotting factors.
Factor VIII: haemophilia A (most common).
Factor IX: haemophilia B.
Factor XI: haemophilia C.

Causes of von Willebrand's disease
Quantitative or qualitative deficiency of von Willebrand factor, important in primary platelet haemostasis, acting as an adhesive protein and a carrier protein for factor VIII.

Genetics
Haemophilia A and B: X-linked (men affected, but women carriers may need concentrate for surgery or trauma).
Von Willebrandœs disease: autosomal-dominant.
Haemophilia C (severe disease): autosomal-recessive or compound heterozygote.

Epidemiology
• 1 in 5000 men is affected by haemophilia A or B; 1 in 6 patients with haemophilia has haemophilia B.
• Haemophilia C is common in Ashkenazi Jews; it may occur in any ethnic group.
• Von Willebrand's disease is the most common inherited bleeding disorder if all grades of severity are considered; clinically significant disease occurs in ~125 in one million population.

Carrier detection and antenatal diagnosis
• Carrier status and presence of the disorders in fetuses can be detected by the following:
Restriction fragment length polymorphisms.
Variable-number repeat sequences.
Direct mutational analysis (research).
Chorionic villus sampling before 10 weeks (for carriers with a molecular marker).
Fetal sexing and choriocentesis (for carriers without a molecular marker).

Treatment

Diet and lifestyle
- Patients should avoid contact sports, but regular exercise, e.g. swimming, should be encouraged.

Pharmacological treatment
- Intramuscular injections must be avoided in patients with bleeding disorders.
- Aspirin or NSAIDs that impair platelet function must also be avoided.

Indications
For haemophilia A: factor VIII concentrate or DDAVP (desmopressin).
For haemophilia B: factor IX concentrate.
For haemophilia C: factor XI concentrate.
For von Willebrand's disease: factor VIII concentrate rich in von Willebrand's factor or DDAVP.

Clotting factor preparations
Recombinant: Recombinate (VIII), Kogenate (VIII).

Extracted by immunoaffinity chromatography: Hemofil M (VIII), BPL 8SM (VIII), Monoclate P (VIII), Mononine (IX), CRTS (von Willebrand's factor).

Extracted by conventional separation:
very high purity (>100 units/mg): Octavi (VIII), Alphanine (IX);
intermediate purity; (<50 units/mg): BPL 8Y, Haemate P (von Willebrand's factor), BPL 9A (IX), BPL factor XI.

- The units of clotting factor needed, x, can be calculated by the following equation:
$x = (\text{rise in clotting factor required (\%)} \times \text{weight (kg)}) \div K$
where $K = 1.5$ for factor VIII, 1 for factor IX, and 2 for factor XI.

- Approximate levels for haemostasis are as follows:

15–20 units clotting factor/dl plasma for minor spontaneous haemarthroses and haematomas.

20–40 units clotting factor/dl plasma for severe haemarthroses and muscle haematomas, minor surgery.

80–100 units clotting factor/dl plasma for major surgery.

DDAVP
- DDAVP releases factor VIII:C and von Willebrand's factor from endothelial cells.
- It is used to cover minor procedures in patients with mild haemophilia and von Willebrand's disease.
- It is not indicated for severe haemophilia or severe and variant types of von Willebrand's disease.

Standard dosage	DDAVP 0.3 µg/kg in 100 ml normal saline solution i.v. infusion over 20 min.
Contraindications	Vascular disease.
Special points	Response should be monitored using factor assays.
Main drug interactions	None.
Main side effects	Hyponatraemia and seizures (in children <2 years), coronary occlusion (in patients >60 years).

Tranexamic acid
- This inhibitor of fibrinolysis reduces blood loss, particularly in mucosal bleeding, e.g. oral surgery, epistaxis, and tonsillectomy.

Standard dosage	Tranexamic acid 1 g orally or i.v. 3–4 times daily; in children, 25 mg/kg 3 times daily.
Contraindications	Haematuria, risk of 'clot colic'.
Special points	Dose should be reduced in patients with renal impairment.
Main drug interactions	None.
Main side effects	Nausea, dizziness.

Treatment aims
To prevent spontaneous bleeds and make surgery safe.

Prognosis
- With the advent of virally safe blood products and home-treatment programmes, many severely haemophiliac patients can lead a relatively normal life.
- Mild disease, whether haemophilia or von Willebrand's disease, may impinge little unless an injury occurs or surgery is planned.

Follow-up and management
- All patients with bleeding disorders should be registered and regularly reviewed at a designated haemophilia centre; regular review and access to treatment is of paramount importance for the successful long-term management of these patients.

Key references
Bolton-Maggs PHB *et al.*: Production and therapeutic use of a factor XI concentrate from plasma. *Thromb Haemostas* 1992, **67**:314–319.

Goerdert JJ *et al.*: A prospective study of human immunodeficiency virus type I infection and the development of AIDS in subjects with haemophilia. *N Engl J Med* 1989, **321**:1141–1148.

Lee CA, Dusheiko G: Hepatitis and haemophilia. In *Viral Hepatitis*. Edited by Zuckerman AJ, Thomas HC, 1993.

Lee CA *et al.*: Progression of HIV disease in a haemophilic cohort followed for 11 years and the effect of treatment. *BMJ* 1991, **303**:1093–1094.

Mannucci PM: Modern treatment of haemophilia: from shadows towards light. *Thromb Haemostas* 1993, **70**:17–23.

Vermylen J, Briet E: Factor VIII preparations: need for prospective pharmacovigilance. *Lancet* **342**:693–694.

Hodgkin's disease
A.K. Fielding and A.H. Goldstone

Diagnosis

Symptoms
- The usual presentation is with a lymph-node mass noticed by the patient.
- Fluctuation in size is not unusual.
- ~25% of patients have other symptoms.

'B' symptoms: unexplained fever >38°C, loss of >10% body weight in 6 months, night sweats.

Pruritis: may lead to extensive excoriation from scratching.

Alcohol-induced nodal pain: rare and nonspecific.

Anorexia, lethargy.

Signs
Palpable lymphadenopathy: usually; careful examination of all node-bearing areas essential.

Extranodal involvement: e.g. bone-marrow, liver, CNS; in 10–20% of patients.

Investigations
- Initially, a good biopsy specimen must be carefully examined to make the diagnosis. Reed–Sternberg cells are the hallmark of Hodgkin's disease and the putative malignant cell.
- Investigation is then systematic to 'stage' the disease.

Full blood count: possible neutrophilia, eosinophilia, lymphopenia, leucoerythroblastic picture if bone-marrow is involved.

ESR measurement: rate sometimes raised; can be useful disease marker and prognostic feature.

Liver function tests: abnormalities raise possibility of liver involvement.

Lactate dehydrogenase measurement: useful disease marker and prognostic feature.

Chest radiography: to look for nodal and pulmonary disease.

CT of chest and abdomen: to detect nodes; poor at detecting hepatic and splenic disease.

Lymphangiography: in centres with expertise, better than CT for assessing retroperitoneal nodes.

Bone-marrow examination: with trephine; rarely reveals unsuspected bone-marrow involvement.

Staging laparotomy: controversial now and rarely performed in the UK; in theory, might detect unsuspected splenic disease and change treatment plan.

Complications
Infection related to underlying defect in cell-mediated immunity: herpes zoster seen in 20%, and tuberculosis not unusual.

Differential diagnosis
Non-Hodgkin's lymphoma.
Infections, e.g. Epstein-Barr virus, toxoplasma, cytomegalovirus.
Angioimmunoblastic lymphadenopathy.

Aetiology
- The origin of the Reed–Sternberg cell, the putative malignant cell, is still debated; cell surface marker CD15 is usually expressed; T- or B-lymphocyte markers are also sometimes expressed.
- Recent evidence implicates Epstein–Barr virus (EBV) in the cause of some cases of Hodgkin's disease; the EBV genome has been found incorporated into DNA in Reed–Sternberg cells, and serological evidence links EBV with Hodgkin's disease.

Epidemiology
- Hodgkin's disease has a bimodal distribution, with a first peak at 15–40 years, then increasing incidence with increasing age.
- Male patients are more frequently affected than female patients.
- The incidence is higher in whites.

Classification
Based on the Rye system:
1. Nodular sclerosing (>80% of patients): dense bands of collagen with nodules of tumour.
2. Lymphocyte predominant: infiltrate of small lymphocytes.
3. Mixed cellularity: pleomorphic infiltrate.
4. Lymphocyte depleted: few Reed–Sternberg cells seen.

Staging
Hodgkin's disease appears to start unifocally and spread to adjacent lymph nodes in an orderly fashion. Staging (based on the Ann Arbor Scheme) is important for rational planning of treatment.

Stage I: involvement of single lymph-node region.
Stage II: two or more lymph-node regions on same side of diaphragm.
Stage III: lymph-node involvement on both sides of diaphragm, including spleen.
Stage IV: diffuse involvement of extranodal sites.
Suffix A: no systemic symptoms.
Suffix B: 'B' symptoms as described above.

Treatment

Diet and lifestyle
- Some patients continue a normal lifestyle during chemotherapy; others feel quite unwell.

Pharmacological treatment
- Hodgkin's disease is a chemo- and radiosensitive disease.
- Treatment decision depends on accurate staging and should also take account of current clinical trials (e.g. by the British National Lymphoma Investigation).

Radiotherapy
- Patients with stage I and IIA disease and no other adverse prognostic features can be cured by radiotherapy alone.
- This is usually given to an extended field beyond the area of overt nodal disease over 1 month.
- Initial treatment with combined chemo- and radiotherapy provides no survival advantage in early-stage disease but may lead to increased toxicity.

Chemotherapy
- For more advanced disease, several standard four-drug combinations are used, e.g. MOPP (mustine, vincristine, procarbazine, prednisolone), LOPP (chlorambucil, vincristine, procarbazine, prednisolone), ABVD (adriamycin, bleomycin, vinblastine, dacarbazine), or EVAP (etoposide, vincristine, adriamycin, prednisolone).
- Precise details of treatment should always be decided by an experienced haematologist or oncologist.
- Good intravenous access is needed because some drugs, particularly vinca alkaloids and anthracyclines, are vesicant.
- Admission to the hospital is not usually required for treatment, although treatment should commence as soon as practical after initial diagnosis and staging.

Treatment after relapse
- Relapse after initial treatment may still be compatible with long-term survival.
- Patients who relapse after radiotherapy can be 'salvaged' with chemotherapy with similar overall survival to those who were initially treated with both modalities; the converse is rarely true.
- The longer the duration of first remission, the greater is the chance of obtaining a second remission on standard treatment.
- Increasing dose intensity of treatment is of benefit in Hodgkin's disease; ~50% of patients resistant to standard treatment can still achieve long-term survival with high-dose chemotherapy regimens such as BEAM (BCNU, etoposide, cytarabine, melphalan) and autologous haematopoietic stem cell support.

Complications of treatment
Skin reactions and pneumonitis after radiotherapy.

Myelosuppression, emesis, hair loss, and neurotoxicity after chemotherapy.

Second malignancy: lung cancer; acute myeloid leukaemia (~ 1%), peak incidence 4–11 years after initial treatment.

Impaired fertility after chemotherapy.

Pulmonary fibrosis.

Treatment aims
To cure the disease with minimal toxicity from the treatment.

Prognosis
- The overall survival at 10 years is ~60%.
- Poor prognostic features include the following:

Older age.
Presence of B symptoms.
Mixed cellularity/lymphocyte depleted histology.
Stage III or IV disease at presentation.
ESR >40 mm/h.
Lactic dehydrogenase >normal.
Mass >10 cm.
Failure to obtain complete remission after adequate first-line treatment.

Follow-up and management
- Regular review during treatment is essential to detect complications and assess response.
- Full blood count is mandatory before administration of each cycle of treatment.
- After treatment is finished, full re-staging is needed.
- Follow-up interval may gradually lengthen but should be continued indefinitely to detect late complications of treatment or relapse.

Key references
Collins RH Jr: The pathogenesis of Hodgkin's disease. *Blood Rev* 1990, **4**:61–68.

DeVita VT Jr, Hubbard SM: Drug treatment: Hodgkin's disease. *N Engl J Med* 1993, **328**:560–565.

Horwich A: The management of early Hodgkin's disease. *Blood Rev* 1990, **4**:181–186.

Linch DC *et al.*: Dose intensification with autologous bone marrow transplantation in relapsed and resistant Hodgkin's disease: results of a BNLI randomised trial. *Lancet* 1993, **341**:1051–1054.

Infections in haematological malignancy
H.G. Prentice and C.C. Kibbler

Diagnosis

Definition
- Infections in haematological malignancy are opportunistic infections that arise during the treatment of haematological malignancy due to the development of neutropenia. Patients are particularly vulnerable when the neutrophil count falls below $0.5 \times 10^9/L$.

Symptoms and signs
Fever: the only consistent indication of established infection.

Investigations
- Full examination should always be made, including mouth, pharynx, genitalia, perianal region, and central line sites.
- Surveillance cultures can be predictive of infection, e.g. with *Pseudomonas aeruginosa*, allowing planning of empirical treatment for individual patients, monitoring of prophylaxis, and facilitating infection control.
- Stool should be screened, e.g. for parasites, if patient comes from a high-risk area.

Blood cultures: from central line and peripheral vein, for bacteria and fungi.

Hickman swab: if inflamed or discharging.

Specimens from clinically suspicious sites.

Urinalysis and culture.

Chest radiography.

CT of thorax: invaluable in invasive aspergillosis.

Bronchoalveolar lavage: especially in bone-marrow transplant patients with dry cough or chest radiography lesions early on.

Skin lesion aspiration: valuable in diagnosis of disseminated fungal infection.

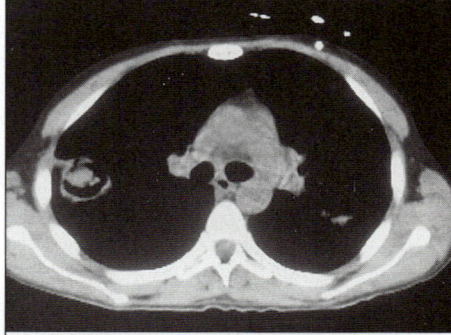

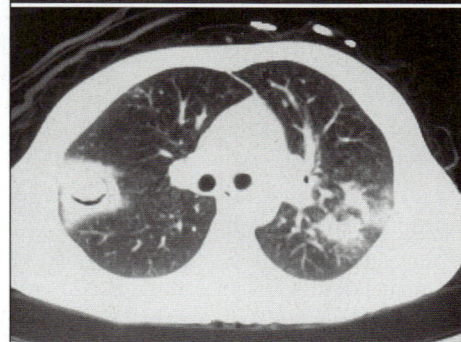

CT of lung with invasive aspergillosis. The mycotic lung sequestrum is usually pleural based and wedged shaped and often shows cavitation.

Complications
- Initially, complications may include those of septicaemia, e.g. acute tubular necrosis.

Increased risk of adult respiratory distress syndrome: in patients with *Streptococcus mitis* bacteraemia.

Ecthyma gangrenosum in patients with local or disseminated *Pseudomonas aeruginosa* infection.

Disseminated candidiasis: CT of liver or spleen can be helpful.

Pulmonary infarction or haemorrhage: especially in patients with invasive aspergillosis.

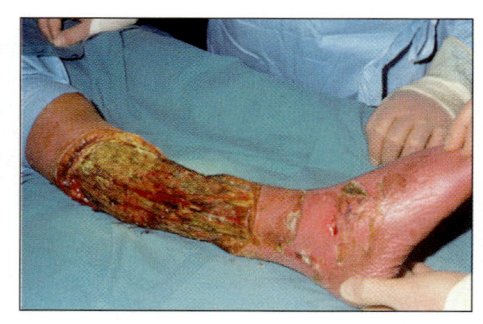

Extensive resection of necrotic tissue of the leg in a child with Pseudomonas septicaemia and ecthyma gangrenosum.

Differential diagnosis
Reaction to transfusion of blood products.
Drug fever.
Graft-versus-host disease.
Fever associated with underlying disease.

Aetiology
Causes of fever
Bacteraemia in 20–30% of patients.
Clinical or non-bacteraemic microbiologically documented infection in 30–40%.
Unexplained in 30–40%.

Documented focus of infection
Lower respiratory tract (50%).
Upper respiratory tract (20%).
Skin and soft tissue, including perianal (20–30%).
Urinary tract (<5%).

Predisposing factors for specific infections
Neutropenia: bacterial and fungal.
Lymphopenia: intracellular organisms, e.g. *Toxoplasma gondii*, *Pneumocystis carinii*, mycobacteria, herpes viruses.
Defects in humoral immunity and splenic hypofunction: encapsulated organisms.
Loss of physical barriers (mucosa, skin): bacteraemia, fungaemia.
Reservoir of infection (e.g. bronchiectasis): *Pseudomonas* spp.
Geographical considerations: mycobacteria, malaria, strongyloides.

Sources of major pathogens
Staphylococci: skin commensal, cross-infection.
Streptococcus mitis: oral commensal.
Enterobacteriaceae: gut.
Pseudomonas aeruginosa: environment, cross-infection.
Streptococcus pneumoniae: nasopharynx, cross-infection.
Mycobacterium tuberculosis: reactivation.
Pneumocystis carinii: reactivation, possibly cross-infection.
Toxoplasma gondii: reactivation, donor bone marrow.
Candida spp.: oropharynx or gut, cross-infection, parenteral feeding.
Aspergillus spp.: airborne (previous colonization).
Herpes simplex or varicella–zoster virus: reactivation (cross-infection).
Cytomegalovirus: reactivation, blood products.

Epidemiology
- ~1 febrile incident occurs per neutropenic episode (less with quinolone prophylaxis).

Treatment

Diet and lifestyle

- Neutropenic patients must eat a low-pathogen diet but maintain nutrition, e.g. by parenteral route if needed.
- Patients should be given a dental review.
- Hygiene is important for patients and attendants, e.g. hand-washing, cleaning of room and bedding, and i.v. catheter care.
- Water must be treated appropriately to prevent legionella infection.
- Patients must especially avoid exposure to measles and chickenpox; vaccination should be reviewed, but live vaccines must be avoided until immune recovery.

Pharmacological treatment

Empirical treatment for pyrexia of unknown origin in neutropenia

- Patients with a fever of 38.5°C or 38°C for 2 h should receive prompt empirical antibiotic treatment: e.g. vancomycin or teicoplanin and ceftazidime, or imipenem alone initially; aminoglycoside to be added after reinvestigation if deterioration after 24–72 h or no response after 72 h; amphotericin B to be added and vancomycin or teicoplanin stopped if fever persists at 96 h. Antibiotics should be rationalized according to isolates.

Standard dosage	Imipenem 500 mg i.v. 6-hourly (adults), vancomycin 1 g i.v. twice daily (adults), or teicoplanin 400 mg daily. Amikacin 7.5 mg/kg twice daily. Amphotericin B 1 mg/kg or AmBisome 3–5 mg/kg daily. Ceftrazidine 2 g i.v. 8-hourly (adults).
Contraindications	Hypersensitivity; caution in renal impairment; epilepsy, or known intracerebral lesion (imipenem).
Special points	Vancomycin and aminoglycoside dosages may need adjustment.
Main drug interactions	Ototoxicity when combined (uncommon with teicoplanin).
Main side effects	Nephrotoxicity (vancomycin, aminoglycosides, amphotericin). Ototoxicity (vancomycin, aminoglycosides).

Treatment of other specific infections

For most invasive fungal infection: amphotericin B 0.5–1.5 mg/kg i.v. daily, possibly with 5-flucytosine, or liposomal amphotericin B 1–4 mg/kg daily.
For herpes simplex infection: acyclovir 5 mg/kg 8-hourly for 7 days.
For varicella-zoster infection: acyclovir 10 mg/kg 8-hourly for 7 days.
For cytomegalovirus infection: ganciclovir 5 mg/kg i.v. 12-hourly for 2 weeks, maintained at 5 mg/kg daily for a further 2–3 weeks with immunoglobulin.
For *Pneumocystis carinii* pneumonitis: co-trimoxazole 120 mg/kg daily in divided doses, with steroids.

Prophylaxis

For Gram-negative bacteria: a 4-quinolone, e.g. ciprofloxacin 250–500 mg orally twice daily, with colistin 1.5 MU orally.
For Gram-positive bacteria: penicillin or macrolide antibiotic.
For mycobacteria (in cases of previous disease, family contact, endemic area): isoniazid 5 mg/kg daily or a 4-quinolone, e.g. ciprofloxacin 500 mg twice daily.
For legionella: a 4-quinolone, e.g. ciprofloxacin 500 mg twice daily.
For *Candida albicans* or *Cryptococcus neoformans*: fluconazole 100–200 mg orally daily.
For *C. glabrata*: amphotericin B suspension 500 mg orally 6-hourly.
For aspergillosis: air filtration, itraconazole, or amphotericin B 0.5–1 mg/kg i.v. daily.
For herpes simplex or varicella-zoster virus: acyclovir 5 mg/kg 8-hourly.
For cytomegalovirus: possibly acyclovir 10 mg/kg i.v. 8-hourly, ganciclovir (myelosuppression), or foscarnet.
For *Pneumocystis carinii*: co-trimoxazole 960 mg orally twice daily for 3 days weekly, or aerosolized pentamidine 150 mg every 2 weeks.
For strongyloides: thiabendazole 25 mg/kg orally twice daily for 3 days.
For toxoplasma: pyrimethamine 75 mg orally daily (loading dose, 100 mg), with folinic acid 15 mg 3 times daily, and possibly sulphadiazine 2 g i.v. or oral 3 times daily.

Treatment aims

To instigate antimicrobial therapy rapidly, using broad-spectrum cidal agents active against the most probable organisms.

Prognosis

- In patients with fever alone, mortality is <5%.
- In patients with fever and pulmonary infiltrates, mortality is 30–60%.

Follow-up and management

- Subsequent management should take into account the following:

Initial empirical treatment: patients may need addition of a glycopeptide.
Underlying disease and treatment: *Pneumocystis carinii* pneumonia and viral infection (especially cytomegalovirus) with lymphoid disease and bone-marrow transplantation.
Duration of neutropenia: invasive fungal infection increases with time.
Number of previous febrile episodes: increased risk of fungal infection with increased number.
Past history or evidence of latent infection: e.g. invasive aspergillosis, tuberculosis.
Foreign travel, ethnic origin: e.g. risk of malaria, tuberculosis, strongyloidiasis.

Key references

Hughes WT et al.: Guidelines for the use of antimicrobial agents in neutropenic patients with unexplained fever. *J Infect Dis* 1990, **161**:381–396.

Prentice HG, Kibbler CC, MacWhinney PH: Antimicrobial prophylaxis and treatment after chemotherapy or marrow transplantation. In *Recent Advances in Haematology* vol 6. Edited by Hoffbrand AV, Brenner M. London: Churchill Livingstone, 1991.

Leukaemia, acute lymphoblastic in adults
A.K. Fielding and A.H. Goldstone

Diagnosis

Symptoms
- Usually, acute lymphoblastic leukaemia has a short history of 2–3 months.

Tiredness and dyspnoea: due to anaemia.

Recurrent infections: due to leucopenia.

Bruising and bleeding: due to thrombocytopenia.

Symptoms of hyperviscosity: if leucocyte count is very high (e.g. $>200 \times 10^9$/L).

Joint and bone pain: less common than in children.

Signs
- Often no physical signs are manifest.

Pallor.

Evidence of infection.

Purpura or bruising.

Lymphadenopathy or hepatosplenomegaly.

Investigations

General
Full blood count (with Romanowsky stained film): diagnosis may be evident from careful morphological examination; leukaemic blasts not always seen in peripheral blood; platelet count and haemoglobin may be low or normal.

Bone-marrow aspiration: blasts should be >30% to make the diagnosis.

U&E, calcium, phosphate, urate measurement: important initial investigations before starting treatment particularly if leucocyte count is high.

Chest radiography: to look for mediastinal mass, seen in 70% of patients with T-cell acute lymphoblastic leukaemia (ALL; high risk of tumour lysis syndrome if this is present).

Lumbar puncture with CSF cytospin: important initial investigation to detect CNS involvement (unusual at presentation).

Special
- These tests help to confirm the diagnosis;: confirming that blasts are lymphoid in origin is occasionally difficult on light microscopy.
- They also help to categorize the disease more fully, giving additional prognostic information.

Cytochemistry: helps to differentiate ALL from acute myeloblastic leukaemia (e.g. negative reaction with Sudan black).

Immunophenotyping: identifies origin of blast cell using panel of cell-surface 'markers'; useful markers include TdT (all subtypes positive except B ALL), CD10 (identifies common ALL antigen), CD19 (positive in B-lineage ALL), CD2 (positive in T-lineage ALL).

Cytogenetics: direct examination of chromosomes at metaphase can identify translocations in ~70% of patients with ALL; this can identify poor-risk patients, e.g. those with t(9,22) or Philadelphia-positive ALL, which has bad prognosis; may provide a marker that can be used to detect early relapse.

Complications
- Most complications are related to bone-marrow failure (cytopenia) due to the disease or, more often, to the intensive treatment needed.

Differential diagnosis
Acute myeloid leukaemia:

Aplastic anaemia: diagnosis of acute lymphoblastic leukaemia might not be obvious initially if presenting leucocyte count is low and bone-marrow aspirate 'dry'.

Lymphoblastic lymphoma: predominantly lymphomatous presentation, with <25% blasts in bone marrow; distinction may be arbitrary in adults because treatment is often the same.

Aetiology
- The cause of acute lymphoblastic leukaemia is unknown; it is presumed to be due to genetic mutations, the risk of which is increased by DNA damage, e.g. due to radiation or DNA repair defects.
- Victims of exposure to ionizing radiation have a higher incidence of leukaemia, but this is more often myeloid than lymphoid in origin.

Epidemiology
- Acute lymphoblastic leukaemia is uncommon in adults, particularly in those aged >30 years.
- Patients aged >15 years are defined as adults because they constitute a separate group with much poorer remission and survival rates.

Classification

Morphological
- Based on appearance on light microscopy, the French–American–British (FAB) classification divides acute lymphoblastic leukaemia (ALL) into L1, L2, and L3.
- This has little correlation with prognosis or immunophenotype, except L3 morphology with B-cell ALL.

Immunological
- On the basis of expression of surface antigens by the blast cells, ALL is divided into T lineage (early T precursor and T cell ALL) and B lineage (early B precursor, common ALL, pre-B ALL, and B cell ALL).

Treatment

Diet and lifestyle
- Nutrition must be maintained.
- Psychological support should be provided to patients and their relatives, especially if a young family is involved; financial support should be considered if earnings are disrupted.
- Patients must take precautions against infection during neutropenia.

Pharmacological treatment

Principles
- Treatment should be given under specialist supervision, within the context of a clinical trial if possible to allow adequate evaluation and the development of new treatments.
- Initial treatment involves several blocks of inpatient treatment.

Induction: remission (i.e. <5% blasts in bone marrow) can be achieved in ~80% of adults usually within 1 month of starting treatment; agents include steroids, vincristine, and anthracyclines.

Consolidation: usually follows quickly after induction, and new chemotherapeutic agents should be introduced; optimum duration and intensity of treatment have not yet been established.

CNS-directed treatment: often described as 'CNS prophylaxis'; CNS leukaemia occurs in ~50% of patients in haematological remission if no specific treatment directed at the CNS is given; possible treatments include cranial irradiation, intrathecal methotrexate, or high-dose i.v. methotrexate (which crosses the blood–brain barrier).

Maintenance therapy: continuous treatment for ~2 years improves outcome; usual treatment involves weekly methotrexate and 6-mercaptopurine, with monthly courses of vincristine and steroids.

Supportive treatment: particularly important in the early stages of treatment; includes allopurinol, adequate hydration, blood-product support, and timely use of antimicrobial treatment.

General complications of treatment
Myelosuppression (inevitable).
Hair loss.
Compromise or loss of fertility.
Infection, particularly during neutropenia: empirical treatment is often needed for bacterial, viral, or fungal infection.
Nausea and vomiting: may be easy to control.

Complications of specific drugs
Vincristine: extravasation injury, alopecia, muscle and jaw pain, urinary retention, dysphagia, peripheral neuropathy.
Prednisolone: Cushing's syndrome and other steroidal side effects (including psychiatric).
L-Asparaginase: thrombotic episodes, pancreatitis, anaphylaxis.
Daunorubicin: extravasation injury, cardiomyopathy, bone-marrow suppression, vomiting, gut toxicity.
Cytarabine: gut and bone-marrow toxicity, erythema, cerebellar toxicity in high doses.
Thioguanine: hepatic and bone-marrow toxicity, rashes.
VP16 epipodophyllotoxin: gut and bone-marrow toxicity.
Methotrexate: renal, hepatic, and gut dysfunction, bone-marrow suppression, mucositis (depending on dose and mode of treatment); affects intellect.
Mercaptopurine: bone-marrow suppression, rashes, hepatic dysfunction.

Treatment aims
To maximize chance of cure, with minimal toxicity.

Other treatments

Allogeneic bone-marrow transplantation
- Adults should receive allograft in first complete remission if they have a matched sibling donor and are aged 20–50 years; this is particularly indicated in Philadelphia-positive disease (incurable by drugs alone).

Autologous bone-marrow transplantation
- The role is less well established; by definition, it is available to more patients but will probably be less effective because of lack of 'graft-versus-leukaemia effect'.

Prognosis
- Despite best available treatment, overall survival in adults is poorer than in childhood disease; studies indicate a 5-year leukaemia-free survival of 20–35% in unselected patients.
- Poor prognostic factors include increasing age, high leucocyte count at presentation (>30 × 10^9/L), t(9,22), and failure to reach complete remission after 1 month of treatment.

Follow-up and management
- After discharge the patient must be seen regularly for full blood count; if on maintenance therapy, the dose may need adjustment.
- Prophylactic co-trimoxazole is usually given during this time.

Relapsed disease
- ~70% of patients relapse; the risk varies from 40% for young adults to >80% for patients aged >50 years.
- Treatment depends on age, duration of initial remission, and previous treatment.
- Relapsed disease is not curable by conventional chemotherapy.

Key references
Bain BJ: *Leukaemia Diagnosis: A Guide to the FAB Classification.* London: Gower Medical Publishing, 1990.
Ramsay NKC, Kersey JH: Indications for bone marrow transplantation in acute lymphoblastic leukaemia. *Blood* 1990, **75**:815–818.

Leukaemia, acute lymphoblastic in children   I.M Hann

Diagnosis

Symptoms
- A constellation of symptoms is seen, many nonspecific and related to bone-marrow failure.

Easy bruising, bone pain, fevers, pallor, lethargy, anorexia, malaise: due to bone-marrow failure.

Abdominal distension: due to hepatosplenomegaly.

Shortness of breath, facial swelling: due to mediastinal mass; unusual.

Headache, vomiting: due to CNS disease; unusual.

Overt bleeding: due to bone-marrow failure; unusual.

Signs
Pyrexia, mucosal bleeding, skin purpura, pallor, congestive heart failure (rare): due to bone-marrow failure.

Hepatosplenomegaly, lymphadenopathy, upper trunk and facial oedema with distended superficial veins, skin infiltrates, testicular enlargement: due to leukaemic 'mass'.

Cranial nerve palsies (III, V, VI, VII), papilloedema, fundal haemorrhages, leukaemic infiltrates: due to CNS disease (rare).

Investigations
Full blood count: shows pancytopenia, normal counts, or isolated raised leucocyte count.

Blood film: shows possible presence of leukaemic blasts.

Bone-marrow morphology: confirms diagnosis in conjunction with cytochemistry and immunophenotyping (mature B cell varieties treated on lymphoma-type protocols).

Chest radiography: for mediastinal mass.

Lumbar puncture: for CNS disease.

U&E and urate analysis.

Liver function tests: for liver failure (rare).

Complications

Early
- Early complications are usually related to drug side effects or further bone-marrow suppression.

Tumour lysis syndrome, associated with hyperkalaemia, hyperuricaemia, hyperphosphataemia, renal dysfunction.

Infection of all types.

Bleeding.

Anaemia.

Vomiting, hair loss, peripheral neuropathy and myopathy, mucositis.

Late
Learning difficulties: e.g. problems with short-term memory or concentration; due to cranial radiation.

Cardiotoxicity: due to anthracycline treatment.

Cataracts, sterility, growth and hormone problems: due to cyclophosphamide treatment and total body irradiation for bone-marrow transplantation.

Second malignancies: due to epipodophyllotoxins.

Differential diagnosis

Lymphadenopathy
Infections: e.g. infectious mononucleosis.
Lymphomas or other tumours.

Hepatosplenomegaly
Leishmaniasis.
Macrophage, metabolic, storage, or auto-immune disorders.
Lymphomas.

Bone-marrow failure
Aplastic anaemia.
Myelodysplasia.
Macrophage disorders.
Autoimmune disorders.
Bone-marrow tumour: e.g. neuroblastoma.
Infections: e.g. tuberculosis, visceral leishmaniasis.

Aetiology
- The cause is unknown but is presumed to be a genetic mutation.
- Increased risk is associated with the following:

Down's syndrome.
Fanconi's anaemia.
Bloom's syndrome.
Ataxia telangiectasia and various immunodeficiency disorders.

- The effects of irradiation or electromagnetic fields are unconfirmed.

Epidemiology
- Acute lymphoblastic leukaemia is the most common malignant disease of childhood.
- A peak incidence at 2–5 years accounts for 20% of all leukaemia.
- Slightly more boys than girls are affected.
- 85% of childhood leukaemia is acute lymphoblastic.

Treatment

Diet and lifestyle
- Specialist support is needed for the children and their families, including siblings, both in hospital while having treatment and after discharge.
- Maintenance of nutrition is important.

Pharmacological treatment
- Treatment should be given under specialist supervision, in the context of a clinical trial if possible to allow adequate evaluation and the development of new treatments.

Treatment choice
For high-risk patients (slow remitters, near haploid, Philadelphia-chromosome positive, older boys with high leucocyte counts – usually $>100 \times 10^9/L$): transplantation in first remission.

For patients at high risk of CNS disease relapse (leucocyte count $>50 \times 10^9/L$): cranial irradiation or high-dose i.v. methotrexate.

For lower-risk patients (leucocyte count $<50 \times 10^9/L$): continuing intrathecal or high-dose methotrexate.

For patients with CNS disease at diagnosis: craniospinal or cranial irradiation and continuing intrathecal methotrexate.

For infants <6 months: intensive multiagent treatment.

Principles
Induction: usually vincristine, asparaginase, steroids; remission in 97% of patients.
Consolidation: intensive treatment with some different drugs from induction course to eradicate 'resistant clones'.
CNS-directed treatment: to eradicate disease in CNS sanctuary site.
Consolidation: as for second step; two or three consolidations may be needed.
Continuation treatment to 2 years: to eradicate minimal residue disease.

Complications of specific drugs
Vincristine: extravasation injury, alopecia, muscle and jaw pain, urinary retention, dysphagia, peripheral neuropathy

Prednisolone: Cushing's syndrome and other steroidal side effects (including psychiatric).

L-Asparaginase: thrombotic episodes, pancreatitis, anaphylaxis.

Daunorubicin: extravasation injury, cardiomyopathy, bone-marrow suppression, vomiting, gut toxicity.

Cytarabine: gut and bone-marrow toxicity, erythema, cerebellar toxicity in high doses.

Thioguanine: hepatic and bone-marrow toxicity, rashes.

VP16 epipodophyllotoxin: gut and bone-marrow toxicity.

Methotrexate: renal, hepatic, and gut dysfunction, bone-marrow suppression, mucositis (depending on dose and mode of treatment); affects intellect.

Mercaptopurine: bone-marrow suppression, rashes, hepatic dysfunction.

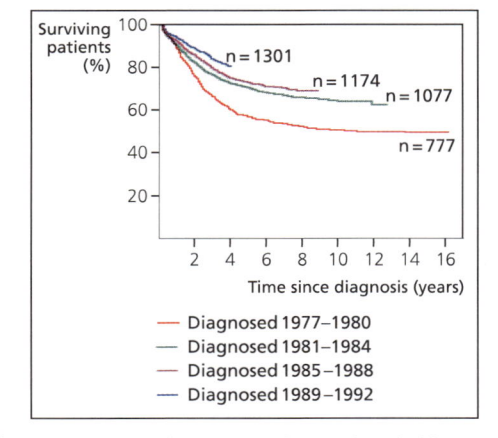

Survival rates of patients with acute lymphoblastic leukaemia 1977–1992.

Treatment aims
To cure patient at least cost (toxicity of specific drugs and complications).

Other treatments
Transplantation.
Cranial irradiation.
See Pharmacological treatment for indications.

Prognosis
- Adverse prognostic features include failure to remit after 1 month of treatment, Philadelphia-chromosome positive, near haploid, older age, male sex, high leucocyte count, infants <6 months.

Follow-up and management
- Patients on continuation treatment should be followed up every 1–2 weeks, depending on blood count.
- After completion of treatment, all patients should be followed indefinitely; for the first 6 years, they must be checked carefully for signs of relapse (organomegaly, testicular swelling, low blood count, blasts on film) and endocrine, growth, intellectual, and cardiac late effects.
- Prophylactic co-trimoxazole should be given for pneumocystis.
- Advice should be given on returning to school and when normal childhood immunization can be given.

Key references
Chessell JM: Treatment of childhood acute lymphoblastic leukaemia: present issues and future prospects. *Blood Rev* 1992, **6**:193–203.

Eden OB et al.: Report to the MRC: results of MRC UKALL VIII. *Br J Haematol* 1990, **78**:187–196.

Greaves MF: Speculations on the cause of childhood acute lymphoblastic leukaemia. *Leukaemia* 1988, **2**:120–125.

Hann IM: CNS directed therapy in childhood. *Br J Haematol* 1992, **82**:2–5.

Hann IM et al.: UKCCSG MACHO chemotherapy for B stages IV NHL & B-ALL. *Br J Haematol* 1990, **76**:359–364.

Leukaemia, acute myeloid — A.K. Burnett

Diagnosis

Symptoms
- Some patients are symptom-free.

Lethargy, irritability, fatigue, reduced exercise tolerance: symptoms of anaemia

Infection: due to leucopenia.

Spontaneous bleeding or bruising: symptom of thrombocytopenia.

Signs
Pallor, infections, bruises, petechiae.

Lymphadenopathy or hepatosplenomegaly: occasionally.

Gum hypertrophy, skin infiltration: features of monocytic leukaemia.

Haemorrhagic manifestations: feature of promyelocytic leukaemia.

Investigations
Full blood count: often shows reduced haemoglobin; thrombocytopenia frequent; leucocyte count $>100\times10^9$/L unusual, associated with poor response to treatment; presentation with count $<3.0\times10^9$/L common; differential leucocyte count usually abnormal, with neutropenia and presence of 'blast cells' (large cells, ~1.5–2 times diameter of erythrocytes; usually have large nuclear:cytoplasmic ratio (less common with acute myeloid leukaemia); nucleus may contain at least one nucleolus (usually large single nucleus in monoblast); blasts may show features of maturation, e.g. cytoplasmic granulation, auer rods, or monocytic features); numerical thrombocytopenia confirmed morphologically.

Bone-marrow analysis: increased proportion of blast cells; conventionally, >30% of bone-marrow cellularity to distinguish from the blastic forms of myelodysplasia.

Cytochemistry: useful to confirm myeloid or monocytic origin of blast cells; Sudan black, chloroacetate esterase, or myeloperoxidase stains.

Immunophenotyping: most reliable method of determining haemopoietic lineage of origin; expression of CD33 or CD15 indicates some myeloid maturation; CD34 and HLA DR earlier nonlymphoid markers, providing important objective methods for distinguishing myeloid from lymphoid leukaemia; antigens are expressed on normal cells, but 'leukaemia-specific' or aberrant phenotypes have been identified that will probably be useful for monitoring remission status when normal antigens are inappropriately expressed on leukaemic cells.

Cytogenetics: many structural chromosome abnormalities have been described; relationship between prognosis and cytogenic abnormality, e.g. better prognosis with FAB M3 (usually has 15:17 translocation), some M2s (8:21 translocation), and inverted 16; worse prognosis with abnormalities or deletions of chromosomes 5 and 7.

Molecular genetics: molecular probes for the 15:17 and 8:21 translocations now available; polymerase chain reaction detection of minor cell populations therefore possible; such technology will be important in assessing quality of remission.

Complications
Overwhelming infection.

Bleeding: especially intracranial or promyelocytic leukaemia.

Differential diagnosis
Any cause of pancytopenia.

Aetiology
- The risk is increased risk in the following:

Radiation exposure.

Chemotherapy for cancer, e.g. Hodgkin's disease.

Chronic myeloproliferative disorders or myelodysplasia.

Epidemiology
- Acute myeloid leukaemia is the most common form in adults.
- The median age of presentation is ~60 years.
- The male:female ratio is equal.
- The prevalence increases with age (e.g. 1 in 10^5 in children, up to 3 in 10^5 in patients >70 years).

Classification
- Based on morphological appearance, acute myeloid leukaemia is divided into FAB (French–American–British) types M0–7.
- The M3 type (promyelocytic) has a high chance of remission and a lower risk of relapse.
- Although valuable in standardizing terminology, this classification has limited prognostic power.

Treatment

Diet and lifestyle
- Nutrition must be maintained.
- Psychological support should be provided to patients and their relatives, especially if a young family is involved; financial support should be considered if earnings are disrupted.
- Patients must take precautions against infection during neutropenia.

Pharmacological treatment

Supportive
- Infection can be prevented by expert nursing care, isolation in a single room with air filtration, mouth care, gut decontamination, vigilance of temperature, mucous membranes, perineum, and central-line site.
- Infection can be treated, after appropriate bacteriological, fungal, and viral samples have been taken, by rapid introduction of i.v. antibiotics (usually aminoglycoside and ureidopenicillin).
- If a response occurs within 48 h, treatment should be continued for 3–5 days; in cases of no or incomplete response and no bacteriological guidance, vancomycin should be added; if further failure, i.v. amphotericin should be added. (See Infections in haematological malignancy for details.)

For coagulopathy
- Coagulation factor deficiency should be corrected by appropriate blood products or vitamin K supplements.
- Severe coagulopathy, including disseminated intravascular coagulation, can be a dominant feature in promyelocytic leukaemia (FAB M3), needing specific attention.
- All-trans-retinoic acid (ATRA) can be effective in correcting the defect (usually within 2–3 days).
- Blood-product support is essential, but fibrinolytic inhibition (tranexamic acid) and heparin have become less widely used.

Chemotherapy
- Treatment should be given under specialist supervision.
- If induction of remission and consolidation phases are sufficiently intense, maintenance should be of no benefit.
- Drugs include anthracyclines, cytosine arabinoside, thioguanine, and etoposide; side effects include cardiotoxicity.
- Intensive supportive care is needed during remission induction, but most patients achieve complete remission with one course.
- An extra course may be needed for less intensive approaches, and more supportive care may be needed overall in all patient groups.

Treatment aims
To restore normal bone-marrow function. To establish prolonged remission or cure.

Other treatments

Allogeneic bone-marrow transplantation
- The risk of relapse is reduced from 60% to 15%.
- Treatment-related mortality of 30% is due to toxicity, infection, pneumonitis, and graft-versus-host disease.
- Treatment may result in infertility and late cataracts (in 10–15% of patients).
- Allogeneic transplantation is available only to 10–15% of patients.

Autologous bone-marrow transplantation
- Autologous transplantation is indicated for patients <55 years without a sibling donor.
Advantages: less toxicity, no graft-versus-host disease, available to more patients, low procedure-related mortality (6–8%).
Disadvantages: potential for the harvested marrow to be contaminated, lack of graft-versus-leukaemia effect.

Prognosis
- Current schedules achieve remission in 80% of patients <55 years (range, 90% in children to 70% in those in fifth decade); in older patients, remission rates of 60% should be achieved.
- 30–40% of patients <55 years treated by chemotherapy alone and 20% of older patients remain in remission at 5 years.
- Allogeneic bone-marrow transplantation cures 50–60% of recipients; autologous transplantation cures 45–55% of recipients.
- Treatment failure >5 years is rare after bone-marrow transplantation but occurs in chemotherapy patients, although at a much lower rate than in the first 2–3 years.

Follow-up and management
- 2–3 weeks after recovery from hypoplasia induced by chemotherapy, the bone marrow should be checked for remission status.

Key references
Burnett AK, Lowenberg B: Treatment options for remission in acute myeloid leukaemia. In *Haematological Oncology* vol 1. Cambridge, Cambridge University Press, 1991.

Foon KA, Gale RP: Therapy for acute myelogenous leukaemia. *Blood Rev* 1992, **6**:15–25.

Leukaemia, chronic lymphocytic
T.J. Hamblin

Diagnosis

Symptoms
- 70% of patients are asymptomatic, the diagnosis being made on incidental blood count.

Enlarged lymph nodes or discomfort in left upper quadrant of abdomen: in 20%.

Symptoms of anaemia: uncommon.

Bruising or bleeding: rare.

Weight loss, fever unassociated with infection, night sweats: 'B' symptoms; very unusual and often signal transformation to high-grade lymphoma.

Signs
Lymphadenopathy in cervical, axillary, or inguinal regions: in 30% of patients.

Mild to moderate splenomegaly: in 10%.

Hepatomegaly: rare.

Anaemia: unusual.

Purpura: rare.

Investigations
Full blood count: shows lymphocytosis $>5 \times 10^9$/L, mature monomorphic small lymphocytes with smear cells.

Lymphocyte marker analysis: shows sparse surface immunoglobulin of a single light chain (κ or λ); CD5+, CD19+, CD20+, CD23+, CD37+, CD3-, CD10-, CD22-.

Serum immunoglobulin measurement: reduced concentration in all classes; IgM paraprotein in 5% of patients.

Direct antiglobulin test: positive in 10%.

Bone-marrow trephine analysis: interstitial, nodular, or diffuse infiltration by small lymphocytes.

Karyotyping: trisomy 12 in 30%, deletion 13q14 in 25%.

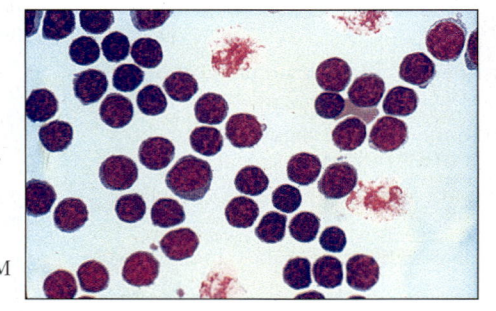

Leucapheresis specimen from chronic lymphocytic leukaemia, showing monomorphic small lymphocytes and smear cells.

Complications
Autoimmune haemolytic anaemia: in 10% of patients, more in stage C.

Autoimmune thrombocytopenia, neutropenia, pure erythrocyte aplasia: in <2%.

Infection: due to hypogammaglobulinaemia in a few patients.

Shingles: in 25%.

Transformation to prolymphocytic leukaemia or high-grade lymphoma: in 10% and 2% (Richter's syndrome), respectively.

Pneumococcal pneumonia.

Differential diagnosis
Prolymphocytic leukaemia.
Hairy cell leukaemia.
Splenic lymphoma with villous lymphocytes.
Large granular lymphocytic leukaemia.
Sezary syndrome and adult T-cell lymphoma/leukaemia.
Follicle centre cell lymphoma and mantle cell lymphoma.

Aetiology
- The cause is unknown.
- No association has been found with radiation or retroviruses.

Epidemiology
- Chronic lymphocytic leukaemia is the most common leukaemia in western Europe and North America.
- It is increasingly common with age, the median age at presentation being 69 years.
- The male:female ratio is 2:1, but, because women live longer, in the elderly population, ~50% of patients are female.
- A slight familial tendency has been found.

Staging

Binet (Europe)

Stage A: no anaemia or thrombocytopenia; <3 lymphoid areas* enlarged.

Stage B: no anaemia or thrombocytopenia; 3 or more lymphoid areas* enlarged.

Stage C: haemoglobin 100 g/L or platelets 100×10^9/dl.

*Cervical, axillary, or inguinal lymph nodes, spleen, and liver.

Rai (USA)

Stage 0: lymphocytosis alone.

Stage I: with lymphadenopathy.

Stage II: with spleno- or hepatomegaly.

Stage III: with anaemia; haemoglobin 110 g/L.

Stage IV: with thrombocytopenia; platelets 100×10^9/L.

Treatment

Diet and lifestyle
- Patients should be encouraged to lead a normal life.

Pharmacological treatment
- All treatment should be given under specialist supervision.
- Stage A patients should not receive chemotherapy.

Alkylating agents
- Chlorambucil is the mainstay of treatment.
- The response rate is 50%.

Standard dosage	Chlorambucil continuous oral dose or intermittently every 4 weeks. Cyclophosphamide orally or i.v. every 2–3 weeks.
Contraindications	None.
Main drug interactions	None established.
Main side effects	Nausea and bone-marrow suppression, drug rash (in 5% of patients on chlorambucil), alopecia (cyclophosphamide).

Nucleoside analogues
- Fludarabine is a purine analogue that produces responses in up to 50% of patients resistant to chlorambucil.
- 2-Chlorodeoxyadenosine is a similar, experimental agent.

Standard dosage	Fludarabine i.v. daily for 5 days every 28 days.
Contraindications	None.
Special points	Less bone-marrow suppression than chlorambucil, but profound T lymphocytopenia, which predisposes to infection by viruses, fungi, or protozoa.
Main drug interactions	None established.
Main side effects	Bone-marrow suppression, immunosuppression.

Other options
Prednisolone: for patients with autoimmune complications; effects a redistribution of lymphocytes from tissue to blood and may be useful in thrombocytopenic patients beginning treatment with alkylating agents.

CHOP chemotherapy (cyclophosphamide, doxorubicin, vincristine, prednisolone): may be more effective than chlorambucil in Stage C cases.

Immunoglobulin replacement therapy: for patients with recurrent infections whose serum immunoglobulin concentration is <4 g/L.

Treatment aims
To relieve symptoms.
To prolong life in stage B or C patients.

Other treatments
- Leucocytapheresis may be used to prevent or treat hyperleucostasis in patients with very high leucocyte counts (>500 × 10⁹/L) or to control the leucocyte count in drug-resistant patients.

Prognosis
- Stage A patients have the same prognosis as age- and sex-matched controls.
- Median survivals achieved with chlorambucil are 12 years for stage A, 5 years for stage B, and 2 years for stage C patients.

Follow-up and management
- Patients should be observed to determine whether the disease is progressive; patients whose disease is static and who are asymptomatic may safely be observed.
- Progressive disease should be treated by chlorambucil.
- All patients need long-term follow-up, the frequency being determined by the pace of the disease.

Key references
Binet JL: Treatment of chronic lymphocytic leukaemia. *Clin Haematol* 1993, 6:867–878.

Litz CE, Brunning RD: Chronic lymphoproliferative disorders: classification and diagnosis. *Clin Haematol* 1993, 6:767–783.

Leukaemia, hairy cell — T.J. Hamblin

Diagnosis

Symptoms
- 25% of patients are asymptomatic.

Fatigue, weight loss, weakness: in 25%.

Bruising or infections: in 25%.

Abdominal fullness or discomfort: in 25%.

Signs
Moderate to massive splenomegaly: in 75% of patients.

Lymphadenopathy: rarely.

Hepatomegaly: occasionally.

Signs of infection, bleeding, or bruising.

Investigations
Full blood count: shows normochromic, normocytic anaemia, neutropenia, monocytopenia, thrombocytopenia, 'hairy' leucocytosis. Hairy cells are large lymphocytes with open nucleus, with loose, lacy chromatin and one or two distinct nucleoli; the cytoplasm is pale blue-grey, with fine hair-like projections; usually few are found in blood, but they number $>10 \times 10^9/L$ in 10% of patients.

Bone-marrow trephine: shows diffuse or patchy infiltration of leukaemic cells, characteristic pale halos of cytoplasm surrounding monotonous, bland nuclei.

Cell marker analysis: moderately positive for surface immunoglobulin of a single light chain class; CD11c$^+$, CD19$^+$, CD20$^+$, CD25$^+$, CD37$^+$, CD3$^-$, CD15$^-$, CD10$^-$; tartrate-resistant acid phosphatase positive.

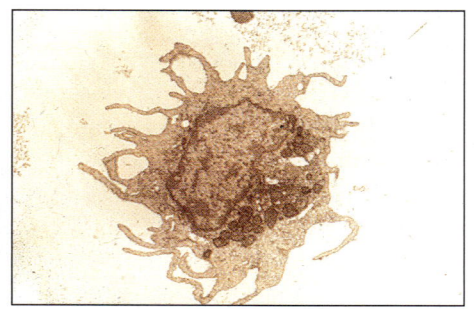

Hairy cell on transmission electron microscopy.

Complications
Infections: neutropenia and monocytopenia render patients susceptible to infection, so both bacterial and more atypical infections are seen; fungal, protozoan, and mycobacterial organisms are implicated.

Vasculitis: microscopic polyarteritis in 5% of patients.

Differential diagnosis
Tumours with similar 'hairy' cytoplasmic projections: e.g. splenic lymphoma with villous lymphocytes, hairy cell variant, and monocytoid B-cell lymphoma (may be distinguished by careful morphological examination and cell markers).
Other causes of isolated splenomegaly with hypersplenism.

Aetiology
- The cause is unknown, although, in one case of the rare T-cell hairy cell leukaemia, the human T-cell lymphotrophic virus II retrovirus was isolated.

Epidemiology
- This is a rare leukaemia, with an incidence of 1 in 500 000 population.
- The male:female ratio is 4:1.
- The median age at presentation is 55 years (range, 20–90 years).

Treatment

Diet and lifestyle
- Patients should be encouraged to live as normal a life as possible.

Pharmacological treatment
- Treatment should be given under specialist supervision.

Interferon-α

Standard dosage	Interferon-α 3 MU 3 times weekly usually for 2 years is effective in 80% of patients.
Contraindications	Hypersensitivity, severe renal failure, hepatic or myeloid dysfunction.
Special points	Early in treatment, cytopenias may be exacerbated, with risk of haemorrhage or infection. Antibodies to interferon-α occur in 50% of patients but only occasionally cause treatment failure.
Main drug interactions	No information available.
Main side effects	Mild influenza-like symptoms (improve with time).

2'Deoxycoformycin
- This inhibitor of adenosine deaminase produces a higher rate of complete remissions than interferon (up to 80%); early studies suggest that most remissions are prolonged beyond 4 years.

Standard dosage	2'Deoxycoformycin 4 mg/m^2 weekly for 3 weeks, then on alternate weeks for 6 weeks.
Contraindications	Low glomerular filtration rate; caution in renal dysfunction.
Main drug interactions	No information available.
Main side effects	Risk of fungal, viral, or protozoan infections due to CD4$^+$ T-cell suppression.

2-Chlorodeoxyadenosine
- This is currently for experimental use only.
- It may be capable of producing long-term complete remissions.
- Side effects include myelotoxicity (intense haematological support needed early in treatment to prevent death from haemorrhage or infection), and the risk of fungal, viral, or protozoan infection due to CD4$^+$ T-cell suppression (similar to 2'deoxycoformycin).

Treatment aims
To allow patient to lead symptom-free life. To attempt, particularly in younger patients, long-term remission, albeit at some early risk from increased pancytopenia.

Other treatments
- Splenectomy was the mainstay of treatment before effective drugs were available; it is still used in patients with the following: Important splenomegaly and cytopenias. Relatively little bone-marrow involvement. Intolerance of pharmaceutical intervention. Laparotomy for other reasons.

Prognosis
- With modern treatment, most patients have a normal lifespan.
- Only a few patients achieve complete remission after interferon treatment, but most achieve sufficient haematological improvement to make their disease of no consequence to them.
- Relapse occurs progressively 1–2 years off treatment.

Follow-up and management
- All patients should be followed up indefinitely.
- Treatment should be reintroduced if symptoms or blood count warrant it.

Key references
Lill MCC, Golde DW: Treatment of hairy cell leukaemia. *Blood Rev* 1990, **4**:238–244.

Multiple myeloma — A.B. Mehta

Diagnosis

Symptoms

- Up to 10% of patients are asymptomatic.

Anorexia, weight loss.
Bone pain, back pain, pathological fracture.
Anaemia, purpura, infection: symptoms of bone-marrow failure.
Polyuria, nocturia, pruritus: symptoms of renal failure.
Abdominal pain, anorexia, polyuria, polydipsia, constipation: symptoms of hypercalcaemia.
Infection: due to hypogammaglobulinaemia.
Visual symptoms, confusion, dyspnoea, bleeding manifestations, polyneuropathy: symptoms of hyperviscosity.
Cardiac failure and oedema: due to increased plasma oncotic pressure or viscosity.

Signs

Anaemia, purpura.
Bony tenderness: over sites of lytic deposits.
Infections: especially skin, respiratory tract, and urinary tract.
Skin and soft tissue deposits: particularly in IgD myeloma.
Proteinuria.
Peripheral neuropathy: due to paraprotein deposition.
Hepatosplenomegaly and lymphadenopathy: rare; suggest an IgM paraprotein or amyloidosis.

- Diagnosis requires the presence of >10% abnormal plasma cells in bone marrow and one of: bone lesions, serum paraprotein, and urine paraprotein.

Investigations

Full blood count: to check for anaemia or bone-marrow failure.
ESR measurement: characteristically raised, often exceeds 100 mm/h.
Complete biochemical screening: including creatinine, creatinine clearance, serum calcium (alkaline phosphatase usually normal), albumin.
Skeletal survey: preferred to isotope bone scan, to show osteolytic lesions, vertebral collapse or (rarely) osteoporosis.
Serum protein electrophoresis, immunoelectrophoresis, serum and urine analysis: to measure immunoglobulin concentrations, paraprotein quantification, and urinary Bence–Jones protein.
Beta 2 microglobulin and CRP measurement: to assess prognosis.
Bone-marrow aspiration and trephine biopsy: to show infiltration by malignant plasma cells and to assess normal bone-marrow reserve.
Microbiological cultures: if signs of infection.
Plasma cell labelling index, immunophenotype analysis, cytogenetic and DNA studies: if available, for further characterization of disease and prognosis.
MRI: a sensitive indicator of skeletal disease, especially good for detecting deposits around spine.

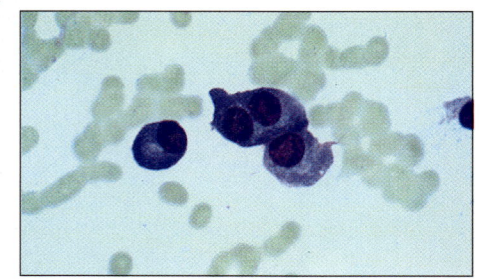

Plasma cells infiltrating bone marrow.

Complications

Renal failure, hypercalcaemia, hyperviscosity syndrome.
Infection: most common cause of death.
Pathological fracture and spinal-cord compression.
Polyneuropathy, cardiac and renal failure, macroglossia, skin infiltration: in 5–10% of patients, caused by amyloidosis.

Differential diagnosis

Metastatic carcinoma: hypercalcaemia, lytic lesions, but normal alkaline phosphatase differentiates.
Polymyalgia rheumatica, temporal arteritis: anaemia, high ESR, but no paraprotein.
Other causes of renal failure.
Benign monoclonal gammopathy: but paraprotein is <30 g/L, with normal concentrations of other immunoglobulins, anaemia, renal failure, lytic lesions all absent, little or no Bence-Jones proteinuria and no progression on follow-up.
Solitary plasmacytoma, primary amyloidosis, other lymphoproliferative disorders (e.g. Waldenström's macroglobulinaemia, non-Hodgkin's lymphoma).

Aetiology

- The cause is largely unknown, but risk factors include the following:
Ionizing radiation, organic chemical exposure, chronic antigenic stimulation, chronic inflammatory disease.
Genetic predisposition: acquired genetic mutations to oncogenes may promote tumour growth, and certain cytokines (e.g. interleukin-6) may function as growth factors.

Epidemiology

- Multiple myeloma forms ~1% of all malignancies, 10–15% of all haematological malignancies.
- The median age at diagnosis is 71 years.
- The incidence is rising gradually.
- The disease occurs more often in blacks.
- The male:female ratio is ~5:3.

Staging

Stage I: haemoglobin >10 g/dL, normal calcium, normal skeletal survey or solitary plasmacytoma, low paraprotein (IgG <50 g/L, IgA <30 g/L, urine Bence–Jones protein <4 g/24 h).
Stage II: neither stage I nor stage III.
Stage III: haemoglobin <8.5 g/dL, hypercalcaemia, advanced skeletal disease, high paraprotein (IgG >70 g/L, IgA >50 g/L, urinary Bence–Jones protein >12 g/24 h).
Subclassification: A, normal creatinine; B, raised creatinine.

Treatment

Diet and lifestyle
- Patients may need a diet appropriate for the degree of renal failure.
- Cooked or sterile food is needed for severely neutropenic patients.
- Patients should avoid bone damage, e.g. heavy lifting.

Pharmacological treatment

Supportive treatment
- Careful supportive care is important, e.g. the following:

Hydration and promotion of diuresis in renal failure and before chemotherapy.

Appropriate antibiotics or antifungal agents.

Adequate analgesia.

Blood component support.

Treatment of hypercalcaemia (e.g. biphosphonates): sodium clodronate may also reduce progression of bone disease and relieve pain.

Chemotherapy
- Oral chemotherapy is the simplest protocol and involves melphalan and prednisone for 4–7 days every 4–6 weeks.
- Intravenous combination chemotherapy generally leads to a more rapid response, with higher complete remission rates, but the survival advantage over melphalan and prednisone is marginal and probably only occurs in patients aged <70 years. Current regimens include the following:

ABCM (adriamycin, BCNU, cyclophosphamide, melphalan).
VBMCP (vincristine, BCNU, melphalan, cyclophosphamide, prednisone).
VAD (vincristine, adriamycin by continuous i.v. infusion over 4 days with oral dexamethasone; standard for relapsed patients, also has a place in induction).

- Alpha interferon s.c. 3 times weekly may improve combination therapy response rates and may prolong remission ('plateau' phase) and overall survival.
- Relapsed patients can be given cyclophosphamide orally or i.v. weekly, high-dose steroids (dexamethasone or methylprednisolone), and melphalan single i.v. dose (high or intermediate).
- VAD gives responses in up to 40% of patients, and cyclosporin (to block multiple drug resistance) combined with VAD may be even more effective. High-dose cyclophosphamide with etoposide and granulocyte–macrophage colony-stimulating factor is valuable in VAD-resistant myeloma.

Complications of treatment
- Chemotherapy is immunosuppressive and myelotoxic.
- Growth factor support (granulocyte- and granulocyte–macrophage colony-stimulating factor elevates the leucocyte count to reduce infective complications due to leucopenia, but also cause bone pain.
- Recombinant erythropoietin reduces erythrocyte transfusion requirement, particularly in renal failure.
- VAD and cyclophosphamide are preferred in renal failure because their metabolism is primarily by the liver.
- Antibacterial and antifungal prophylaxis with blood component support (principally platelets) are needed for myeloblative and intensive chemotherapy regimens.
- Hair loss, nausea, vomiting, mucositis (i.v. melphalan), and bone demineralization (prednisone) and fatigue, fever, and anorexia (alpha interferon) also occur.
- NSAID may accelerate renal failure if used for pain relief.

Treatment aims
To achieve normal immunoglobulin and blood counts and to relieve bone pain.

Other treatments
- The following are indicated for primary non-responders, relapsed patients, or those with local complications.

Radiotherapy: relieves pain from lytic lesions; systemic activity against tumour but often leads to prolonged pancytopenia.
Internal fixation of pathological fractures.
Allogeneic bone-marrow transplantation: after conditioning by high-dose cyclophosphamide and total-body radiotherapy; for patients <50 with histocompatible sibling.
Autologous bone-marrow transplantation or peripheral blood stem cell infusion: intensive treatment for patients <60 years, after high-dose chemotherapy.
Plasma exchange: for hyperviscosity syndrome.
Dialysis.

Prognosis
- In untreated patients, the median survival is <1 year; with treatment, it rises to 3–4 years.
- Beta-2 microglobulin concentrations correlate well with prognosis (<6 mg/L good, 6–12 mg/L intermediate, >12 mg/L poor prognosis).
- Raised CRP, poor response to treatment, age >75, skin or soft tissue involvement, and advanced stage indicate poor prognosis.
- Disappearance of paraprotein and restoration of normal immunoglobulin (complete remission) or normal blood counts with stable paraprotein ('plateau' phase) are achieved after 4–6 cycles of chemotherapy in >85% of patients.

Follow-up and management
- Full blood count, renal function, beta-2 microglobulin and serum and urine paraprotein concentrations should be assessed regularly (every 1–2 months) to monitor the disease and the effects of treatment.
- Patients should be checked for opportunistic infection and new skeletal abnormalities.

Key references
Alexanian R, Dimopoulos M: The treatment of multiple myeloma. *N Engl J Med* 1994, **330**:484–489.

Barlogie B (ed): Multiple myeloma. *Haematol Oncol Clin North Am* 1992, **6**:211–484.

Myeloproliferative disorders — J.M. Goldman

Diagnosis

Symptoms
- Chronic myeloid leukaemia is usually manifest in chronic phase; it transforms spontaneously to an accelerated phase and then to an acute blastic phase normally within 3–6 years of diagnosis (range 0–10 years).
- Polycythaemia rubra vera, essential thrombocythaemia, and primary myelofibrosis are manifest more insidiously and evolve more slowly.
- Symptoms are an incidental finding in many patients.

Abdominal pain and distension: also due to renal occlusive disease in polycythaemia rubra vera.

Spontaneous bleeding: including haematuria, bruising, visual disturbances.

Sweats, weight loss.

Priapism: in chronic myeloid leukaemia.

Pruritus: in chronic myeloid leukaemia.

Symptoms of hyperviscosity syndrome: in polycythaemia rubra vera.

Gout.

Peptic ulceration and hypertension: in polycythaemia rubra vera.

Signs
Splenomegaly.
Ecchymoses, retinal haemorrhages.
Weight loss.
Hepatomegaly: occasionally.

Investigations
Full blood count: raised leucocyte count (20 to >500 × 10^9/L); increased numbers of blasts, promyelocytes, neutrophils, eosinophils, basophils; low neutrophil alkaline phosphatase content in chronic myeloid leukaemia; variable anaemia; thrombocytosis especially in essential thrombocythaemia; raised haemoglobin, packed-cell volume, and erythrocyte mass in polycythaemia rubra vera.

Bone-marrow analysis: hypercellular, loss of fat spaces; increased megakaryocyte count, especially in essential thrombocythaemia; variable amounts of fibrosis in chronic myeloid leukaemia; increased reticulin and collagen in myelofibrosis; in chronic myeloid leukaemia, all dividing cells have a Philadelphia chromosomal translocation, designated t (9;22) (q34;q11), bringing into apposition parts of the *BCR* gene normally on chromosome 22q with the bulk of the *ABL* proto-oncogene normally present on chromosome 9q.

Biochemistry: uric acid raised, especially in myelofibrosis; increased vitamin B_{12} and vitamin B_{12}-binding protein.

Complications
'Blast' transformation: in chronic myeloid leukaemia; blast cells may be myeloid or lymphoid.

Changes between groups: e.g. polycythaemia rubra vera to myelofibrosis.

Vascular or thrombotic complications: in polycythaemia rubra vera.

Gout: especially in myelofibrosis.

Renal tubular obstruction.

Splenic infarction: in chronic myeloid leukaemia.

Retinal haemorrhages: in chronic myeloid leukaemia.

Gonadal failure: due to busulphan.

Differential diagnosis
Leucocytosis
Infections.
Allergic conditions.
Bone-marrow invasion by cancer.

Splenomegaly
Malaria, visceral leishmaniasis.
Acute leukaemia, lymphoma.
Gaucher's disease.
Thalassaemia syndromes.
Portal hypertension.

Aetiology
- Causes include the following:

Acquired abnormality in haemopoietic stem cells: such stem cells and their progeny carry a Philadelphia chromosome (22q-) with the *BCR-ABL* chimeric gene in chronic myeloid leukaemia.

Idiopathic disease.

Association with previous radiation exposure occasionally in chronic myeloid leukaemia.

Epidemiology
- Chronic myeloid leukaemia occurs in ~1 in 100 000 annually worldwide.

Treatment

Diet and lifestyle
- Patients may live normal lives during the chronic phase of chronic myeloid leukaemia.

Pharmacological treatment
- Drug treatment is indicated for polycythaemia rubra vera (hydroxyurea, radioactive phosphorus [^{32}P]), myelofibrosis (hydroxyurea, busulphan), and essential (primary) thrombocythaemia (hydroxyurea, busulphan, anagrelide, ^{32}P, supportive measures, e.g. dipyridamole, aspirin).
- Interferon-α (given daily or on alternate days by injection) controls haematological features in 70–80% of patients and induces some degree of Philadelphia chromosome negativity in the bone-marrow in 10–20%; it is the drug of first choice.
- Hydroxyurea is easier to tolerate.
- Busulphan should not be used in patients aged <50 years but can be used for older patients or those who cannot take hydroxyurea.

Non-pharmacological treatment

Bone-marrow transplantation
- Transplantation is indicated for chronic myeloid leukaemia; if applicable, it should be done within 1 year of diagnosis.
- Allogeneic bone-marrow transplantation is indicated for patients aged <55 years with HLA-identical siblings (~15% of all patients).

Treatment of other disorders
Polycythaemia rubra vera: venesection.

Myelofibrosis: splenic irradiation, splenectomy (in selected patients).

Treatment aims
To cure the patient.
To prolong life without cure.
To prevent or alleviate symptoms.
To maintain leucocyte count in normal range.
To re-establish Philadelphia chromosome-negativity with interferon treatment.

Prognosis
- The median duration of chronic phase diseases is 4 years and of survival with conventional treatment is 4.3 years.
- A few patients survive >10 years in chronic phase.
- The 5-year disease-free survival after bone-marrow transplantation is about 65%; most of these patients are cured; the procedure-related mortality is 15–20%, and the relapse rate 10–15%.

Follow-up and management
- Regular follow-up is needed if the patient is on chemotherapy or interferon.
- Bone marrow must be checked annually for progressive fibrosis or cytogenetic evolution.
- Patients should have the usual follow-up for bone-marrow transplantation.

Key references
Goldman JM: Management of chronic myeloid leukaemia. *Blood Rev* 1994, **8**:21–29.

Kantarjian HM *et al.*: Chronic myelogenous leukemia: a concise update. *Blood* 1993, **82**:691–703.

Soutar RL, King DJ: Bone-marrow transplantation. *BMJ* 1995, **310**:31–36.

Non-Hodgkin's lymphoma
A.K. Fielding and A.H. Goldstone

Diagnosis

Symptoms
Lymph node in neck, axilla, or groin, noticed by patient as unexplained 'lump': the most common presenting symptom.

- The disease may be seen in multiple sites at presentation.
- Systemic symptoms (e.g. the 'B' symptoms of Hodgkin's disease) are less common than in Hodgkin's disease.
- Symptoms may relate to the anatomical site of disease, e.g. superior vena cava obstruction due to mediastinal nodes or to primary lymphomas at extranodal sites (e.g. CNS, gastrointestinal tract).
- Primary extranodal non-Hodgkin's lymphoma occurs much more often than extranodal Hodgkin's disease.

Signs
Palpable lymphadenopathy: careful examination of all nodal areas essential.
Hepatomegaly and splenomegaly: possibly.
Signs of other organ involvement: e.g. pleural effusion as a result of pulmonary parenchymal involvement, skin involvement (rarely).

Investigations
- Initially, investigations must be directed at confirming the diagnosis.
- A good sample of tissue that has not been placed in formalin is needed.
- The diagnosis may be apparent on routine staining with haematoxylin and eosin or Giemsa.
- Immunohistochemistry, especially markers for T and B lymphocytes and leucocyte common antigen, is vital in subclassification and may help to distinguish undifferentiated lymphomas from carcinoma.
- Subsequent investigations must be systematic and thorough to enable accurate localization of disease and if possible to estimate disease volume.

Full blood count: usually normal.
U&E analysis: as a baseline.
Liver function tests: may be abnormal if liver is involved.
Lactate dehydrogenase measurement: useful marker of disease bulk and activity.
Chest radiography: to rule out hilar or mediastinal nodes or intrapulmonary disease.
CT of chest and abdomen: to rule out node or organ involvement.
Bone-marrow examination: trephine is particularly important.
Examination of postnasal space and tonsillar fossa.
Lumbar puncture with cytospin: in high-grade disease only.

Complications
Recurrent or atypical infections.
Autoimmune haemolysis and thrombocytopenia.
Bone marrow failure.
Gastrointestinal bleeding or perforation: obstructive jaundice.

Differential diagnosis
Other causes of lymphadenopathy: e.g. Hodgkin's disease.
Infective causes: e.g. toxoplasmosis, glandular fever, Epstein–Barr virus.

Aetiology
- The cause is unknown, but the following may have a role:

Epstein–Barr virus: associated with endemic Burkitt's lymphoma in Africa.
Adult T-cell leukaemia–lymphoma: associated in all cases with human T-cell lymphotrophic virus.
HIV infection: particularly primary CNS non-Hodgkin's lymphoma (rare in other settings).

Epidemiology
- The median age of onset is 50 years.
- Intermediate- or high-grade disease is more common in younger patients.

Classification
- Non-Hodgkin's lymphomas constitute a diverse group of disorders arising from different cell types, usually T and B lymphocytes; the wide spectrum of disease biology is reflected by the varying clinical presentations, responses to treatment, and overall outcomes.
- Various schemes for classification have been proposed and developed; the most useful are those that can be used to predict clinical behaviour and prognosis.
- Classifications include the following:

Rappaport.
Lukes and Collins.
Lennert: the Kiel classification.
The Working Formulation (used here): an international attempt to provide a translation from one classification to another, now widely used in its own right; non-Hodgkin's lymphoma is divided into low, intermediate, and high grades, each having different treatment and prognosis.

Staging
- Patients may be staged I–IV according to the Ann Arbor system originally developed for Hodgkin's disease.
- Staging is less useful than for Hodgkin's disease because, with the exception of stage 1 disease, all patients with non-Hodgkin's lymphoma should receive chemotherapy.

Treatment

Diet and lifestyle
- Many patients maintain a fairly normal lifestyle during treatment, but some are unwell and need multiple hospital admissions.

Pharmacological treatment
- Treatment should take place in the context of a clinical study whenever possible (e.g. the British National Lymphoma Investigation).
- It should be given by a specialist haematologist or oncologist.

For intermediate-grade non-Hodgkin's lymphoma
- Treatment should begin as soon as investigation is completed.
- These lymphomas are usually sensitive to many chemotherapy drugs, and many effective combination regimens may be curative.
- Stage 1 disease may be treated successfully by radiotherapy alone, but localized disease is very unusual in non-Hodgkin's lymphoma.
- The standard treatment is by CHOP (cyclophosphamide, adriamycin, vincristine, prednisolone), usually given on a monthly cycle for 6 months; other regimens including additional drugs, e.g. PACEBOM (prednisolone, adriamycin, cyclophosphamide, etoposide, bleomycin, vincristine, methotrexate) are given more intensively, reducing total time taken for treatment, but none has been shown to be superior to CHOP.
- Allopurinol 300 mg daily should be given for at least the first month.
- Main side effects include hair loss, nausea (often preventable) and myelosuppression (for which dose reductions may be needed during subsequent cycles).

For low-grade non-Hodgkin's lymphoma
- These lymphomas are also sensitive to chemotherapy, but, although they usually do not behave aggressively clinically, they are usually considered incurable by standard treatment.
- A conservative approach is often advocated, particularly in elderly asymptomatic patients, because early treatment has no survival advantage.
- 50% of patients may avoid treatment for up to 3 years.
- In truly localized low-grade disease, radiotherapy may give long-term remission.
- Patients may respond well to treatment and often may have considerable periods when no treatment is needed.
- Initial treatment is usually by oral chlorambucil, best used cyclically rather than continually.
- Combination chemotherapy, e.g. chlorambucil with prednisolone, vincristine, and possibly anthracycline, is sometimes used but has no proven advantage.
- Alpha interferon has just been licensed for low-grade disease, but its indications and benefits are not yet clear.
- The new agents fludarabine and 2-chlorodeoxyadenosine may be of value in relapsed disease.
- Main side effects of chlorambucil include myelosuppression and mild nausea.

For high-grade non-Hodgkin's lymphoma
- Lymphoblastic and Burkitt's lymphomas are very aggressive clinically and often manifest with widespread disease, including bone-marrow and CNS involvement; they need intensive leukaemia-style treatment, usually involving very myelosuppressive inpatient regimens and CNS-directed prophylaxis.

Treatment aims
To cure patient, with minimum toxicity.
To palliate if cure is not possible.

Other treatments
- High-dose treatment and autologous bone-marrow transplantation are indicated for the following:
Intermediate grade: age <60 years, relapsed disease still sensitive to chemotherapy.
Low grade: criteria difficult to define because long-term follow-up is needed to assess benefit because of the indolent nature of the disease.
- Allogeneic transplantation may have a role for young patients with high-grade disease.

Prognosis

Low grade
- At 5 years, ~70% of patients are still alive, but few are in complete remission; most patients eventually die of their disease.
- In many patients, the disease ultimately transforms to high grade and becomes refractory to chemotherapy.

Intermediate and high grades
- The complete remission rate is ~85% in patients with limited disease, ~55% with extensive disease.
- Overall disease-free survival is ~40% and depends on several factors; poor prognostic factors include stage III or IV disease, high lactate dehydrogenase concentration, failure to attain complete remission on first-line treatment, and older age.

Follow-up and management
- During treatment, regular follow-up is needed, including examination and full blood count before each course of chemotherapy; toxicity must be monitored, and complications treated.
- After treatment is completed, full re-staging should take place: if the patient is in complete remission, regular follow-up should be continued to detect early relapse.

Key references
Armitage JO: The place of third generation regimens in the treatment of adult aggressive non-Hodgkin's lymphoma. *Ann Oncol* 1991, **2** (suppl 1):37–41.

Falzon M, Isaacson PG: Histological classification of the non-Hodgkin's lymphoma. *Blood Reviews* 1990, **4**:111–115.

Platelet disorders J.F.M. Harrison

Diagnosis

Symptoms
- Platelet disorders may be manifest by bleeding or be discovered incidentally in an otherwise asymptomatic patient.

Bruising.

Bleeding: usually mucosal, e.g. gingival, nasal, gastrointestinal, menorrhagic; occasionally retinal (loss of vision) or intracranial (headache); after surgical procedures.

Deafness: in some familial disorders.

Signs
Petechiae, purpura, bruises.
Retinal haemorrhages.
Thrombosis and skin microinfarcts: in thrombotic thrombocytopenic purpura.
Capillary bleeding.

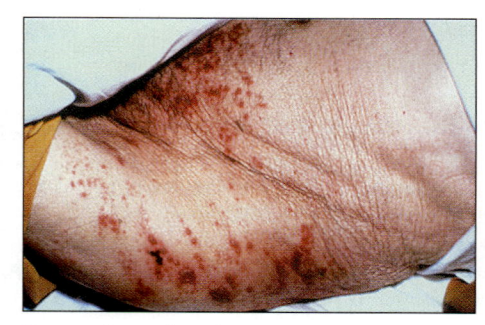

Purpura due to thrombocytopenia.

Investigations
- Initial investigations are used to identify primary platelet disorder and to exclude von Willebrand's disease in patients with a strong family history and lifelong bleeding disorder.

Full blood count: platelet count and mean platelet volume, to exclude other haematological disease and pseudothrombocytopenia due to clumping or EDTA (ethylenediaminetetraacetic acid)-induced aggregation.

Microscopic examination of film: for platelet morphology, to detect erythrocyte or leucocyte abnormality.

Coagulation screening: to exclude primary coagulopathy

Biochemistry profiles: to identify renal or hepatic disease.

Platelet function tests: bleeding time, if prolonged, suggests platelet function disorder or von Willebrand's disease (drugs that affect platelet function, e.g. aspirin, should be avoided for 10 days before testing); spontaneous in-vitro aggregation and response to ADP, collagen, and ristocetin should be recorded; if abnormal, response to other agonists (e.g. adrenaline, thrombin, arachidonate) should be assessed; release reaction of radiolabelled 5-HT; measurement of platelet adenine nucleotides; hereditary and some acquired platelet disorders have characteristic aggregation responses.

Bone-marrow aspiration and biopsy: in most patients with thrombocytopenia, to assess number and structure of megakaryocytes and bone-marrow function.

Platelet serology: in post-transfusion purpura and in neonates with alloimmune thrombocytopenia, to identify specific anti-platelet antigen antibodies.

Platelet-associated immunoglobulin measurement: nonspecific, often increases in immune thrombocytopenias.

Flow cytometry: to quantify platelet membrane glycoproteins, using monoclonal antibodies to detect hereditary disorders.

Complications
Iron-deficiency anaemia: caused by menorrhagia or recurrent epistaxis or gastrointestinal bleeding.

Neurological impairment or death: caused by intracranial bleeding.

Differential diagnosis

Bleeding disorders
Von Willebrand's disease.
Fibrinogen disorders.

Purpura
Vasculitis: e.g. Henoch–Schönlein syndrome.
Amyloid.
Senile purpura.
Scurvy.
Steroid treatment.
Collagen disorders (e.g. Ehlers–Danlos syndrome).
Hereditary haemorrhagic telangectasia (does not cause purpura but can lead to low platelet count in extreme forms).

Aetiology
- Causes include the following:

Decreased production
Bone-marrow failure: leukaemia, metastatic tumour, idiopathic aplasia, infiltration, abnormal production, myelodysplasia, aplastic anaemia, drugs (predictable, e.g. cytotoxic drugs, or idiosyncratic reactions).

Increased consumption
Immune: autoimmune (idiopathic, post-viral, HIV, associated with other autoimmune disorders), alloimmune against platelet-specific antigens, e.g. HPA-1.
Drugs: e.g. quinine, heparin, sulphonamides, rifampicin.
Coagulopathy: disseminated intravascular coagulation, thrombotic thrombocytopenic purpura.
Hypersplenism and splenomegaly.

Hereditary
Platelet membrane glycoprotein abnormalities, e.g. Bernard-Soulier and Glanzmann's syndromes.
Platelet storage pool abnormalities.
Other abnormalities, e.g. May–Hegglin anomaly.

Acquired
Platelet storage pool defects: e.g. aspirin, uraemia, ethanol, cirrhosis, myeloproliferative disorders.

Epidemiology
- Acquired disorders of platelet function are common and are associated with disorders such as chronic renal failure or the ingestion of aspirin.
- Chronic idiopathic thrombocytopenic purpura is relatively common (one group suggests that 0.18% of patients admitted to hospital in a 10-year period had the disease).

Treatment

Diet and lifestyle
- Patients should avoid trauma and contact sports.

Pharmacological treatment

For immune thrombocytopenia
- In children, the onset is usually acute and often follows a viral infection; spontaneous recovery is common, and treatment is given to those with severe or life-threatening bleeding to elevate the platelet count. In adults, the onset is more insidious, and it almost never remits spontaneously.

Standard dosage	*Children:* immunoglobulin 0.4 g/kg i.v. daily (in 4–6 h) for 5 days (sometimes 1.0 g/kg daily for 2 days); or prednisolone 1 mg/kg. *Adults:* prednisolone 1 mg/kg daily initially until maximum response, then tailed off.
Contraindications	*Prednisolone:* active infection, diabetes mellitus.
Main drug interactions	See drug data sheet.
Main side effects	*Immunoglobulin:* headache, hypertension tachycardia. *Prednisolone:* hypertension, diabetes mellitus, osteoporosis.

- Adults who do not respond or who relapse when steroids are reduced should be considered for splenectomy.
- Other treatments for adults failing steroids or splenectomy include i.v. immunoglobulin, azathioprine, vinca alkaloids, danazol, high-dose dexamethasone, or vitamin C.

For platelet functional defects
- The bleeding tendency is often mild, and specific treatment (platelet transfusion, arginine vasopressin [DDAVP]) is needed for major haemorrhage or to cover surgical procedures. Antifibrinolytic agents may be helpful to control minor bleeding; antiovulatory treatment may be needed for menorrhagia.

Standard dosage	One single donor platelet pack/10 kg body weight or one platelet pheresis pack should raise the platelet count by $20–40 \times 10^9$/L. DDAVP 0.4 µg/kg i.v. in 100ml 0.9% saline solution in 15–20 min. Tranexamic acid 0.5–1.0 g 3 times daily orally or i.v.
Contraindications	*DDAVP:* coronary artery disease. *Tranexamic acid:* history of thromboembolism.
Special points	*DDAVP:* ineffective in Glanzmann's thromboasthenia.
Main drug interactions	See drug data sheets.
Main side effects	*Platelet transfusion:* allergic reactions, HLA or alloimmunization in multitransfused patients; hepatitis B (rare) or C transmission. *DDAVP:* nausea, tremor, vomiting, angina, myocardial infarction. *Tranexamic acid:* nausea, vomiting, diarrhoea.

For bone-marrow disorders
- The risk of spontaneous haemorrhage increases when the platelet count is $<10 \times 10^9$/L. Prophylactic platelet transfusions are given to maintain the count above this level during the treatment of acute leukaemia or aplastic anaemia or during bone-marrow transplantation.
- In chronic thrombocytopenia due to bone-marrow failure, platelet transfusions are given for symptomatic bleeding.

For thrombotic thrombocytopenic purpura
Supportive therapy of medical complications, e.g. haemodialysis. Plasma exchange with fresh frozen plasma replacement (1.5 times plasma volume) for 7 days. Additional treatments include aspirin, dipyridamole, methylprednisolone, and vincristine.

For alloimmune thrombocytopenia, neonatal and post-transfusion
Antigen-negative platelet transfusion, i.v. immunoglobulin, prednisolone, or plasma exchange.

Treatment aims
To cure or alleviate symptoms, depending on underlying disease.

Other treatments
- Splenectomy is indicated for immune thrombocytopenia (not in children <6 years).
- Vaccination by Pneumovax and against *Haemophilus influenzae* type b and *Neisseria meningitidis* serogroups A and C should be given 1–2 weeks before surgery. Lifelong antipneumococcal prophylaxis (.e.g. penicillin V 250 mg twice a day) is recommended for splenectomy patients.

Prognosis
- Up to 90% of children with idiopathic thrombocytopenic purpura remit spontaneously, with 50% recovering in 1 month.
- 80% of adults with idiopathic thrombocytopenic purpura remit after treatment by steroids alone or after splenectomy.
- The bleeding tendency in patients with hereditary platelet defects varies.
- In patients with acquired platelet function defects, the prognosis is related to the underlying disease.
- Mortality in patients with untreated thrombotic thrombocytopenic purpura is up to 90%; 60–80% respond to treatment, reducing mortality to ~30%.
- Alloimmune thrombocytopenias are self-limiting but potentially fatal.

Follow-up and management
- The frequency of follow-up depends on the clinical severity and stability of the underlying disorder.

Key references
Bolan CD, Alving BM: Pharmacologic agents in the management of bleeding disorders. *Transfusion* 1990, **30**:541–551.

Caen JP (ed): Platelet disorders. *Baillières Clin Haematol* 1989, **2**:.

George JN, Shattil SJ: The clinical importance of acquired abnormalities of platelet function. *N Engl J Med* 1991, **324**:27–38.

Rock GA et al.: Comparison of plasma exchange with plasma infusion in the treatment of thrombotic thrombocytopenic purpura. *N Engl J Med* 1991, **325**:393–397.

Prothrombotic states — S.J. Machin

Diagnosis

Symptoms
Symptoms of venous or arterial thrombosis.

Signs
- Patients to investigate include those with the following:

Venous thromboembolism before the age of 40–45 years.
Recurrent venous thrombosis or thrombophlebitis.
Thrombosis in an unusual site: e.g. mesenteric vein, cerebral vein.
Unexplained neonatal thrombosis.
Skin necrosis.
Arterial thrombosis before the age of 30 years.
Relatives with a specific defect.
Unexplained prolonged coagulation screening tests.
Recurrent fetal loss, idiopathic thrombocytopenic purpura, SLE.

Investigations
- Functional and immunological assays are needed for a precise diagnosis.
- Screening tests and functional assays should be performed on fresh citrated blood samples collected with minimal venous stasis on all patients being investigated for a prothrombotic state.

Full blood count and film.
Measurement of prothrombin, activated partial thromboplastin, and thrombin time, fibrinogen, and euglobin lysis time (fibrinolytic activity).
Platelet aggregation studies.
Assays for antithrombin III, protein C, protein S, plasminogen, heparin cofactor II, anticardiolipin antibodies, lupus anticoagulant, factor XII, dysfibrinogenaemia, and homocystinuria.
Fibrinolytic tests: before and after stimulation (i.e. venous occlusion or DDAVP).
Fibrin plate, tissue-type plasminogen activator, and PA1-1 assays.
Platelet activation markers analysis: i.e. GMP-140 expression, plasma beta-thromboglobulin.

Complications
Arterial and venous thrombosis and embolism.

Differential diagnosis
Hyperviscosity.

Aetiology

Common acquired causes of thrombosis
Diabetes mellitus, hyperlipidaemia, malignancy, myeloproliferative disorders, chronic liver disease, SLE, paraproteinaemias, nephrotic syndrome.
- These disorders predispose to thrombosis in a multifactorial way; specific homeostatic assays are generally unhelpful in the investigation and management of individual patients.

Inherited defects with increased tendency to thrombosis
Antithrombin III, protein C, protein S, plasminogen, heparin co-factor II, factor XII, dysfibrinogenaemia, homocystinuria.
- Most of these disorders represent autosomal dominant traits with variable penetrance.
- Deficiency in the heterozygous state predisposes to thrombosis either spontaneously or in association with other high risk factors.

Pathophysiology
- The balance of the haemostatic mechanism can be shifted in favour of thrombosis in the following circumstances:

Increased coagulation system activity.
Increased platelet activity.
Decreased fibrinolytic activity.
Damaged vascular endothelial activity.

Epidemiology
- Epidemiological studies have shown an increased incidence of thrombotic events associated with raised concentrations particularly of fibrinogen, factor VII, and factor VIII:C, with a frequency of 1 in 2000–5000.

High risk factors for thrombosis
Surgical and nonsurgical trauma.
Age.
Immobilization.
Heart failure.
Prior venous thrombosis and varicose veins.
Paralysis of lower limbs.
Obesity.
Oestrogen treatment.
Pregnancy and puerperium.
Smoking.
Raised blood viscosity.

Treatment

Diet and lifestyle
- No special precautions are necessary.

Pharmacological treatment

Prophylaxis for venous thromboembolism
- The degree of risk must be assessed depending on the predisposing factors.

Low risk: early ambulation, graduated compression stocking.
Moderate risk: standard unfractionated heparin 5000 units s.c. every 8–12 h.
High risk: low molecular weight heparin s.c. every 12–24 h, dose depending on type of heparin.

- The degree of risk for surgical prophylaxis may be defined as follows:0

Low risk: <40 years, minor surgery lasting <1 h.
Moderate risk: >40 years, abdominal or thoracic surgery lasting >1 h.
High risk: >40 years, knee and hip orthopaedic surgery, obesity, and malignancy.

Heparin

Standard dosage	Unfractionated heparin 5000 units i.v. bolus, followed by 1000–2000 units/h i.v. for 5–7 days. Low molecular weight heparin s.c. once daily.
Contraindications	Rare hypersensitivity, risk of bleeding complications.
Special points	Activated partial thromboplastin time must be monitored 6 h after start of treatment, then at least every 24 h, with dose adjustment to maintain ratio at 1.5–2.5 times control.
Main drug interactions	Drugs that interfere with platelet aggregation or coagulation.
Main side effects	Bleeding, thrombocytopenia, rebound thrombosis, osteoporosis (if treatment lasts >3 months), rare alopecia, skin rash.

- Heparinization can be reversed by administering protamine sulphate 1 mg, which neutralizes ~100 units heparin; maximum dose, 40 mg i.v. in 10 min.

Warfarin

Standard dosage	Warfarin 10 mg orally on days 1 and 2, 5 mg orally on day 3, then adjusted daily according to prothrombin time, maintained at 1–20 mg daily.
Contraindications	Pregnancy.
Special points	Prothrombin time must be monitored, with results expressed as INR with therapeutic range of 2.0–4.5.
Main drug interactions	Many medications potentiate or antagonize effect; for any new medication, prothrombin time should be checked.
Main side effects	Bleeding, skin necrosis after first few days of treatment in the case of protein C or S deficiency.

- Anticoagulant effects can be reversed by an infusion of fresh frozen plasma or factor II, IX, and X concentrate if bleed is life-threatening; vitamin K_1 1–2 mg i.v. takes 6–24 h to reverse warfarin effect.

Antiplatelet agents
- These are indicated for prophylaxis and prevention of further arterial thrombotic events when platelet activation has been shown to be a primary pathological factor, particularly myocardial ischaemia and cerebrovascular thrombotic strokes including transient ischaemic attack, for secondary thrombocytosis (>800 × 10^9/L), and for essential thrombocythaemia.

Aspirin 75 mg orally daily or 300 mg twice weekly or dipyridamole up to 100 mg orally 3 times daily (dipyridamole may cause severe headaches).

Treatment aims
To prevent thrombosis.

Prognosis
- Prognosis depends on the underlying cause and the degree of risk of arterial or venous thrombosis or embolism.

Follow-up and management
- Lifelong expert management is needed.

Therapeutic ranges for oral anti-coagulation

INR 2.0–2.5: prophylaxis of deep-vein thrombosis.

INR 2.0–3.0: treatment of deep-vein thrombosis, pulmonary embolism, systemic embolism, prevention of venous thromboembolism in myocardial infarction, mitral stenosis with embolism, transient ischaemic attacks, atrial fibrillation.

INR 3.0–4.5: recurrent deep-vein thrombosis and pulmonary embolism, arterial disease including myocardial infarction, mechanical prosthetic heart valves (tissue prosthetic values can be controlled at 2.0–3.0).

Key references
Hirsh J: Low molecular weight heparin. *Thromb Haemost* 1993, **70**:204–207.

Lowe GDO: Risk of and prophylaxis for venous thromboembolism in hospital patients. *BMJ* 1992, **305**:567–574.

Poller L: Oral anticoagulation. *J Clin Pathol* 1990, **43**:177–183.

Sickle cell disease — S.C. Davies

Diagnosis

Symptoms

- Patients with SS and Sß° thalassemia are generally more severely affected than those with SC, Sß⁺ being the mildest disorder.

Acute painful vaso-occlusive crisis: causes >90% of hospital admissions affecting bones, joints, and muscles; initial presentation in one-third is the 'hand foot' syndrome from age of 4 months; limb pain in older children, more central pain distribution in adolescents and adults.

Chronic pain: in hip or shoulders, caused by avascular necrosis.

Signs

- Often patients present with no signs in mild crisis.

Constitutional upset mimicking septicaemia: in severe crisis (infection can precipitate crisis).

Localized swelling, tenderness, and redness of bone, joint, or muscle.

Abdominal pain mimicking more severe disease.

Limited range of hip or shoulder movement: with active avascular necrosis.

Investigations

For diagnosis

- Investigations should be made preferably when the patient is in a stable state.

Full blood count: to establish degree of anaemia.
Reticulocyte count: to establish degree of haemolysis.
Haemoglobin electrophoresis: to determine variant haemoglobins.
'Sickle test': to confirm presence of haemoglobin S.
Haemoglobin F estimation: high concentrations diminish severity.
Extended erythrocyte grouping: to ensure appropriate erythrocytes for transfusion.
Plasma U&E analysis: to monitor renal function.
Liver function tests: to monitor haemolysis and exclude hepatitis.
Hydroxybutyrate dehydrogenase analysis: to monitor haemolysis.

In crisis

- The results should be compared with those from the stable state.

Full blood count: haemoglobin raised with dehydration; falls in sequestration and aplasia.
U&E analysis: to detect dehydration.
Liver function tests: to measure dysfunction.
Cultures and viral screening: urine, blood, sputum, throat swab; to exclude infection (before antibiotic treatment); screening for parvovirus (not routine unless severely anaemic).
Reticulocyte count.
Viral screen, chest radiography, blood gas and arterial oxygen saturation measurement: if patient has chest pain or signs.

Complications

Stroke: in 8% of patients, median age 7 years.
Sequestration syndromes: common cause of death in UK; erythrocytes pooled in the organ, causing haemoglobin to fall by ≤2 g/dl, leading to dysfunction of the following organs: spleen (in infants; high risk of recurrence), liver (in children and adults), chest (a medical emergency, exchange transfusion if partial arterial oxygen pressure <60 mmHg), splanchnic circulation (in adults, clinical picture of paralytic ileus that resolves spontaneously).
Infection: common and serious or life-threatening because of auto-splenectomy, therefore susceptible to encapsulated bacteria, especially *Streptococcus pneumoniae* and *Salmonella* spp., aplastic crisis due to parvovirus B19.
Priapism, proliferative retinopathy, cholecystitis and cholelithiasis secondary to haemolysis.

Differential diagnosis

- It can be difficult to distinguish simple vasoocclusive crisis from that associated with infection.
- Other diseases may also manifest (e.g. appendicitis) or coexist.

Aetiology

- Sickle cell disease is inherited in a Mendelian recessive manner.
- Most UK patients are homozygous SS.
- Clinical problems also occur when haemoglobin S interacts with other variant haemoglobins (e.g. SC) and with a beta thalassaemia gene (ß° or ß⁺).

Epidemiology

- >5000 patients in the UK have sickle cell disease; they are predominantly of West Indian and Sub-Saharan origin, also Arabs, Italians, Greeks, and Asians.
- It is rarely manifest before the age of 4–6 months because of the continued production of fetal haemoglobin due to the late switching off of the fetal haemoglobin gene.

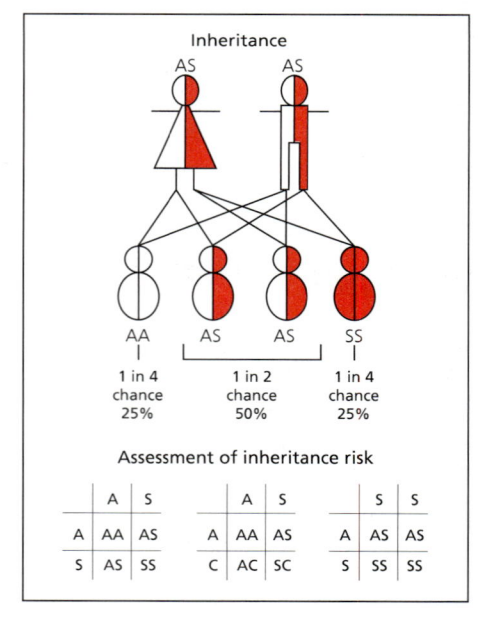

Assessment of inheritance risk.

Treatment

Diet and lifestyle
- Patients should avoid factors that precipitate painful crisis, e.g. infection, dehydration, exhaustion, cold, marked temperature changes, smoking, high altitude, and unpressurized aircraft; in some patients, stress is reported to be a precipitant.

Pharmacological treatment

Analgesia

Standard dosage	*For mild to moderate pain*: paracetamol 12–15 mg/kg 8-hourly, codeine phosphate 1–2 mg/kg 6-hourly (up to 3 mg/kg in 24 h), or diclofenac 1 mg/kg 8-hourly, all orally. *For severe pain*: morphine 0.1 mg/kg i.v. loading dose, then 1–2 mg/kg i.v. infusion over 24 h using patient-controlled analgesia system, or pethidine 50–150 mg i.m. every 1–4-h in adults.
Contraindications	*Oral drugs*: hepatic and renal impairment, peptic ulceration, asthma. *Parenteral drugs*: raised intracranial pressure.
Special points	*Pethidine*: respiratory rate must be monitored hourly.
Main drug interactions	*Codeine and morphine*: alcohol, anxiolytics and hypnotics, dompetidone and metoclopramide, cimetidine. *Diclofenac*: caution with other analgesics, anticoagulants, antihypertensives, beta-blockers, and cardiac glycosides.
Main side effects	*Oral drugs*: rashes, blood dyscrasias, acute pancreatitis, constipation, respiratory depression. *Morphine*: respiratory depression, nausea, bronchospasm, severe pruritus. *Pethidine*: fitting.

Antibiotics
- Antibiotics are indicated for patients in severe crisis or when infection is suspected.

Standard dosage	Amoxycillin 500 mg 3 times daily.
Contraindications	Penicillin allergy.
Special points	If pneumococcal infection is suspected, penicillin should be added.
Main drug interactions	Anticoagulants, antacids, oral contraceptives.
Main side effects	Nausea, diarrhoea, rashes, pseudomembranous colitis.

Non-pharmacological treatment

Rehydration
Oral fluids increased in patients with mild pain; i.v. clear fluids in patients with severe pain at 80 ml/kg/24 h.

Oxygen treatment
60% oxygen if partial arterial oxygen pressure on air is <60 mmHg; 35% if 60–70 mmHg; 28% if 70–80 mmHg.

Blood transfusion
See Transfusion medicine *for further details*.

Additive: when haemoglobin <5 g/dl and patient symptomatic from anaemia; for aplastic crisis, sequestration, bleeding (e.g. renal papillary necrosis).

Exchange: when haemoglobin >5 g/dl but improved oxygen transport needed. overall aim: haemoglobin S <20%, total haemoglobin 11–14.5 g/dl (possibly 3–4 procedures); for chest syndrome (if partial arterial oxygen pressure <60 mmHg), priapism (if >4 h), acute neurological deficit or splanchnic sequestration, severe or protracted crisis (occasionally), preoperatively in selected patients.

Long-term transfusion: to maintain haemoglobin at 11–14.5 g/dl, with haemoglobin S <25%; for neurological deficit, sickle chronic lung disease, prevention of pain (occasionally), pregnant women (selected).

Treatment aims
To provide early and effective relief of pain.
To treat infection.
To maintain hydration.
To maintain tissue oxygenation.

Prognosis
- All types of sickle cell disease are variable in clinical manifestations; no markers exist to predict severity for a particular patient.
- 87% of patients are alive at 20 years, 50% at 50 years.
- Deaths in childhood are most commonly due to infection.
- Deaths in adolescents and young adults are most commonly due to neurological and lung complications.
- Deaths in middle age are most commonly due to chronic organ failure.
- Successful outcome after bone-marrow transplantation has now been recorded and drugs that raise haemoglobin F levels look promising.

Follow-up and management
- Full education and counselling must be ensured, with family screening and genetic advice.
- Penicillin prophylaxis must be ensured for children, and anti-pneumococcal and haemophilus B vaccination should be considered.
- Children should be checked for upper airways obstruction.

Key references
Davies SC: Bone marrow transplant for sickle cell disease. *Blood Reviews* 1992, **7**:4–9.

Davies SC, Wonke B: The management of haemoglobinopathies. *Baillière's Clin Haematol* 1991, **4**:361–389.

Embury SH et al.: *Sickle Cell Disease: Basic Principles and Clinical Practice.* New York: Raven Press, 1994.

Pryle BJ et al.: Toxicity of norpethidine in sickle cell crisis. *BMJ* 1992, **304**:1478–1479.

Thalassaemia — B. Wonke

Diagnosis

Symptoms
- Beta thalassaemia is manifest during the first year of life in 90% of patients; a few present at 3–4 years (late-onset beta thalassaemia major).
- 10% of patients with beta thalassaemia major have a mild course (not dependent on transfusion).
- Patients may be asymptomatic; detection is from antenatal screening and diagnosis.

Poor weight gain.
Failure to thrive.
Fever.
Diarrhoea.
Increasing pallor.
Distended abdomen.

Signs
Pallor.
Heart failure.
Splenomegaly.
Jaundice.

Investigations
Blood tests: low haemoglobin, mean corpuscular haemoglobin, mean cell volume; absent or reduced haemoglobin A (β° or β^+ thalassaemia), variable haemoglobin F and A_2 (using electrophoresis).

Genetic analysis: defines specific mutations, may help to predict disease severity and prognosis and facilitate first-trimester diagnosis.

Complications
Splenomegaly leading to hypersplenism (neutropenia, thrombocytopenia, anaemia).
Anaemia causing severe bone changes, short stature, and heart failure.

Differential diagnosis
Iron-deficiency.

Aetiology
- Thalassaemia is caused by defective synthesis of the alpha or beta globin chain (alpha and beta thalassaemia, respectively).
- The disorder is inherited (Mendelian recessive).
- It occurs in Mediterranean, Asian, Arabic, and Chinese groups because of a selective advantage against *Plasmodium falciparum*.

Epidemiology
- Thalassaemia is one of the most common inherited disorders throughout the world
- In northwest Europe, >200 babies with beta thalassaemia are born each year, the number rising in migrant groups
- In southwest Europe, it is declining because of prevention programmes; in consanguineous marriages, the birth rate of beta thalassaemia increases by 30%

Treatment

Diet and lifestyle
- Patients must avoid red meat and liver, and they should be encouraged to lead a normal active lifestyle.

Pharmacological treatment

Treatment of transfusional iron overload
- Desferrioxamine is infused s.c. over 8–12 h from a portable syringe driver pump 5–6 nights/week.
- Chelation therapy is started when ferritin is 1000 μg/L (after 12–24 transfusions).
- Initial dose of 20 mg/kg desferrioxamine is diluted in 5–10 ml water for injection. Vitamin C 100–200 mg orally (increases urinary iron excretion) is added when the patient is on desferrioxamine.
- In iron-overloaded patients, the desferrioxamine dose is 50 mg/kg daily.
- For cardiomyopathy, continuous desferrioxamine is given through an i.v. delivery device (Hickman Line, Port-a-Cath).

Complications of treatment
Alloimmunization to blood group antigens (in 25% of patients), febrile and urticarial transfusion reactions (in 75% of patients), cytomegalovirus infection and immunosuppression, transfusion-transmitted hepatitis B and C viruses: due to chronic transfusion (risk of HIV, 1 in 65 000).

Cardiomyopathy (most common cause of death), reduced growth, hypoparathyroidism, diabetes, failure of puberty: due to inadequate chelation.

Short stature, bone changes (pseudo-rickets), visual disturbances, hypersensitivity, hearing problems, pulmonary oedema: due to desferrioxamine toxicity (overchelation).

Treatment aims
To provide good quality of life.
To provide a long life.

Other treatments
Bone-marrow transplantation: 94% success rate if patient compliant to desferrioxamine and has no liver fibrosis or enlargement; success rate affected by age and liver status.
Splenectomy for hypersplenism.

Prognosis
- Maintenance transfusion and regular iron chelation preserve excellent health, and the prognosis is now open-ended.
- Early death is generally the result of intractable heart failure secondary to iron overload and infections.

Follow-up and management
- The patient's ferritin, liver function, and bone metabolism must be monitored 3 times yearly, with annual anti-hepatitis C virus, anti-HIV, and hepatitis B surface antigen checks.
- Oral glucose tolerance tests must be done yearly from the age of 10 years in patients with a family history of diabetes or from the age of 16 years in those without.
- Other endocrine and cardiac investigations should be made if clinically indicated.
- Patients should have yearly audiometry and twice-yearly eye tests.
- Splenectomy patients have higher risk of infection and may need vaccinations.

Key references
Davies SC, Modell B, Wonke B: *Access to Healthcare for People from Black and Ethnic Minorities.* London: Royal College of Physicians, 1993, pp 147–168.

Davies SC, Wonke B: The management of haemoglobinopathies. *Baillières Clin Haematol* 1991, **4**:361–389.

World Health Organization: *The Haemoglobinopathies in Europe.* Geneva: World Health Organization, 1988.

Transfusion medicine — M. Brennan and M. Contreras

Indications

Erythrocytes
- A low haemoglobin level *per se* is not an indication for transfusion. Factors such as the patient's condition, the rate of fall of haemoglobin, and the cause of anaemia must be considered to determine the correct treatment.

Whole blood
For acute massive blood loss.

Erythrocyte concentrates
For chronic blood loss or anaemia.

For blood loss <1 blood volume in elective surgery (in additive solution).

Filtered blood
To prevent or delay non-haemolytic febrile transfusion reactions in patients who are erythrocyte-dependent.

For newly-diagnosed patients with aplastic anaemia who are potential bone-marrow transplant recipients.

When cytomegalovirus-antibody negative blood is indicated but not readily available.

For intrauterine transfusion.

Washed cells
For patients with proven hypersensitivity reactions to plasma proteins.

For neonates who have necrotizing enterocolitis.

Cryopreserved erythrocytes
For patients needing blood of rare phenotypes or blood compatible with multiple erythrocyte alloantibodies.

For patients with anti-IgA in the absence of IgA-negative blood.

Irradiated erythrocytes
For recipients at risk of graft-versus-host disease: in-utero transfusion, after bone-marrow transplantation.

For rare cases of transfusions from relatives.

Platelets
To prevent or treat bleeding in patients with thrombocytopenia and rarely to treat bleeding in patients with platelet function defects: the cause of thrombocytopenia and significance of haemorrhage influence the use of platelet transfusions.

For **acute bone-marrow failure (e.g. due to aplasia, chemotherapy)**: if platelet count $10-50 \times 10^9$/L, serious spontaneous bleeding is unlikely, although minor bleeding (purpura, epistaxis) may occur; prophylactic platelet transfusions to maintain count $>10 \times 10^9$/L reduces risk of haemorrhage as effectively as keeping count higher and reduces morbidity but not mortality; patients with fever, infection, coagulopathy, or rapid fall in platelet count should be transfused to maintain platelets $>20 \times 10^9$/L.

For **acute disseminated intravascular coagulation**: when thrombocytopenia is associated with bleeding (not indicated in chronic disseminated intravascular coagulation without bleeding).

For **massive blood loss**: to maintain platelets $>50 \times 10^9$/L.

Prophylaxis for surgery: to maintain platelets $>50 \times 10^9$/L or $>100 \times 10^9$/L for surgery in a critical site, e.g. brain or eye (not routinely with cardiopulmonary bypass).

For **autoimmune thrombocytopenia**: platelet transfusions rarely used.

Fresh frozen plasma
To replace single coagulation factor deficiencies when a specific or combined factor concentrate is unavailable.

For immediate reversal of warfarin effect.

For acute disseminated intravascular coagulation.

For thrombotic thrombocytopenic purpura.

For bleeding or disturbed coagulation associated with massive transfusion, liver disease, or cardiopulmonary bypass surgery.

Autologous transfusion

Advantages
- The possibilities of alloimmunization, immunosuppression, and transfusion-transmitted infection are avoided.

Disadvantages
- Not all patients are eligible.
- Predeposited blood may be unused, e.g. if surgery is cancelled, or may be insufficient to meet the patient's needs.
- Collecting predeposited autologous blood is more expensive than standard units.

Options
Autologous pre-deposit: up to 5 units of blood collected and stored during the weeks before surgery.

Acute normovolaemic haemodilution: blood drawn from patient under anaesthetic and replaced by crystalloid so that blood lost during surgery has a lower hematocrit; when blood loss starts or at end of procedure, patient's whole blood is returned.

Erythrocyte salvage: blood lost at operating site recovered and processed for transfusion.

Directed blood donations
- Blood donations from relatives or friends should be discouraged unless needed on medical grounds.
- Evidence suggests that 'directed' donations are generally less safe than blood supplied by the Transfusion Service.

Techniques

Erythrocytes

Whole blood: packed cell volume (PCV) 0.35–0.45, 1 unit = 510 ml ± 10%; if blood loss and replacement exceed twice the blood volume, thrombocytopenia and abnormalities of haemostasis may develop.

Fresh blood (<24 h): blood that has not been microbiologically tested must not be transfused.

Erythrocyte concentrates: PCV 0.55–0.75, 1 unit = 220–340 ml.

Erythrocyte concentrates in additive solution: PCV 0.5–0.7, 1 unit = 280–420 ml; not to be used for exchange or large-volume transfusion in neonates.

Filtered blood (leucodepleted $<5 \times 10^6$ leucocytes/unit): PCV and quantity variable; rigorous validation of blood processing and component preparation needed, quality assurance programme shows bedside filtration to be unreliable.

Washed cells (residual protein <0.5 g/unit): must be used within 24 h of preparation.

Cryopreserved erythrocytes (thawed and washed): volume usually <200 ml; must be used within 24 h of preparation.

Irradiated erythrocytes (minimum dose, 25 Gy): must be used within 1 day if for intrauterine transfusion because of increased potassium.

Platelets

Administration
- Platelets for transfusion should preferably be of the recipient ABO and RhD group.
- If RhD-positive platelets are transfused to a RhD-negative woman potentially capable of childbearing, 250 IU anti-D immunoglobulin should be given subcutaneously with each dose of platelets.

Dose and response
- A standard dose of 300×10^9 may be issued as pooled or single platelet concentrates derived from individual donations or as a single apheresis donation respectively to raise the platelet count (adult) by $\sim 40 \times 10^9$/L.
- Patient factors including sepsis, certain drugs, disseminated intravascular coagulation, splenomegaly, uraemia, and platelet antibodies can reduce the expected platelet increment.
- Patients who are repeatedly transfused with platelets may develop immunological refractoriness due to HLA alloimmunization and should receive platelets from HLA-matched donors.
- In some cases, platelet-specific alloantibodies develop, requiring type-specific platelet transfusions.

Fresh frozen plasma

Administration
- Fresh frozen plasma (FFP) should be ABO and RhD compatible, although compatibility testing is not required.
- Group O FFP should only be transfused to Group O recipients.
- If an RhD-negative woman potentially capable of childbearing is transfused with RhD-positive FFP, 50 IU anti-D immunoglobulin should be given per unit of FFP transfused.

Dose
- A generally accepted starting dose is 12–15 ml/kg.
- The clinical and laboratory responses should be monitored to assess response and plan further management.

Management of adverse effects of transfusion

Haemolytic transfusion reactions
(ABO incompatibility most severe)
Safe documentation and checking of systems for compatibility testing and blood administration; treatment for acute renal failure and disseminated intravascular coagulation may be needed.

Febrile non-haemolytic transfusion reactions
Treatment by antipyretics and use of leucodepleted cellular components if recurrent.

Allergic reactions to foreign proteins
Cessation of infusion; treatment of urticarial reactions by piriton; emergency treatment needed if anaphylaxis has developed; IgA-deficient patients who have anti-IgA should receive components from IgA-deficient donors.

Alloimmunization
Provision of antigen-negative units to transfusion-dependent patients.

Iron overload
Consideration of iron-chelation treatment in transfusion-dependent patients.

Transfusion-transmitted infection
Use of blood components from volunteer unpaid donors that have been screened by sensitive techniques for relevant viral markers; consideration of hepatitis A and B vaccination of transfusion-dependent patients.

Key references

Anonymous: *Leucocyte Depletion of Blood and Blood Components: Consensus Conference*. Edinburgh: Royal College of Physicians of Edinburgh, 1993.

Contreras M: *ABC of Transfusion* edn 2. London: British Medical Association, 1992.

Contreras M *et al.*: Guidelines for the use of fresh frozen plasma. *Transfusion Med* 1992, 2:57–63.

Mollision PL, Engelfriet CP, Contreras M: *Blood Transfusion in Clinical Medicine* edn 9. Oxford: Blackwell Scientific Publications, 1993.

Murphy MF *et al.*: Guidelines for platelet transfusion. *Transfusion Med* 1992, 2:311–318.

Strauss RG: Therapeutic granulocyte transfusions in 1993. *Blood* 1993, 81:1675–1678.

Waldenström's macroglobulinaemia — T.J. Hamblin

Diagnosis

Symptoms

Fatigue, weakness and weight loss: in >80% of patients.

Bleeding tendency: in 60%.

Sensorimotor peripheral neuropathy: in 15%.

Headache, dizziness, vertigo, confusion, stroke, drowsiness, breathlessness, dependent oedema: features of hyperviscosity syndrome in 20%.

Epistaxis, gastrointestinal haemorrhage, dependent purpura.

Signs

Lymphadenopathy: in 40%.

Splenomegaly: in 30%.

Hepatomegaly: in 30%.

Peripheral neuropathy: in 15%.

Ataxia, nystagmus, hemiplegia, dementia, coma, signs of congestive cardiac failure, dependent purpura, haemorrhage, dilated, tortuous retinal veins with 'sausage-like' segmentation, retinal haemorrhage, papilloedema: signs of hyperviscosity syndrome.

Investigations

Full blood count: shows normocytic, normochromic anaemia in 80% of patients; rouleaux, sometimes spuriously raised mean cell volume, neutropenia, thrombocytopenia; lymphocytes may be increased but seldom >5 × 10^9/L.

Cell marker analysis: surface immunoglobulin of single light chain class (κ or λ); CD19$^+$, CD20$^+$, CD37$^+$, CD38$^+$, CD5$^-$, CD10$^-$.

Bone-marrow aspiration: increase in small lymphocytes and plasmacytoid lymphocytes, sometimes in plasma cells.

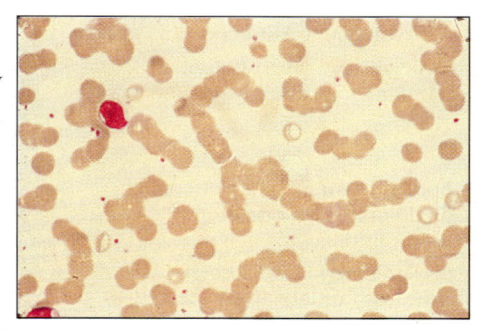

Rouleaux on Romanovsky-stained blood film.

Serum electrophoresis: monoclonal spike in beta or gamma globulins; identifiable as IgM by immunoelectrophoresis; serum IgG and IgA often reduced.

Plasma viscosity measurement: raised; hyperviscosity syndrome only if relative serum viscosity >4 times water.

Cryoglobulin analysis: proteins that precipitate at 4°C found in 15% of patients.

Cold agglutinin analysis: erythrocyte autoantibodies (anti-I or anti-i) agglutinate erythrocytes in the cold; idiopathic acquired variety monoclonal IgM.

• Clotting studies may indicate a pseudo von Willebrand's state with prolonged activated partial thromboplastin time, bleeding time, and abnormal platelet function.

Complications

Amyloid: in <10%.

IgM monoclonal protein autoantibody activity: occasionally.

Peripheral neuropathy, cold agglutination syndrome, acquired haemophilia: due, respectively, to anti-myelin, anti-erythrocyte, and anti-factor VIII.

Differential diagnosis

Diseases associated with IgM monoclonal proteins:

Essential (benign) monoclonal macroglobulinaemia (27%).

Cold agglutinin syndrome (3%).

Chronic lymphocyte leukaemia (10%).

Other B-cell lymphomas (30%).

IgM myeloma (3%).

Extramedullary plasmacytoma (2%).

Waldenström's macroglobulinaemia (25%).

Aetiology

• Presumably, a mutation event occurs in a susceptible clone.

• Proliferation of antibody-producing cells in response to antigenic stimulation may become autonomous when a mutation leads to a lack of control of the cell cycle.

Epidemiology

• Waldenström's macroglobulinaemia is predominantly a disease of the elderly; the median age at presentation being 65 years.

• The annual incidence is 1 in 200 000.

• It occurs more often in men than women.

• Familial incidence is slightly increased.

Bleeding abnormalities

• The IgM paraprotein interferes with the formation of the platelet plug.

• Platelet adhesiveness is reduced, as is the release of platelet factor 3.

• The paraprotein also interferes with the coagulation cascade and may be an antibody against factor VIII.

• Some paraproteins bind to fibrin and inhibit fibrin monomer aggregation, resulting in a bulky gelatinous clot with impaired clot retraction.

• Factor X deficiencies may be seen in patients who develop amyloidosis.

Treatment

Diet and lifestyle
- The patient should be encouraged to live as normal a life as possible.

Pharmacological treatment
- Chlorambucil, given under specialist supervision, is the mainstay of treatment, but only ~50% of patients respond.
- Other alkylating agents give similar responses and probably could be used interchangeably.
- Higher response rates have been reported using combination chemotherapy (e.g. BCNU, vincristine, cyclophosphamide, melphalan, and prednisolone), but such studies have been very small.
- Recent reports have suggested that fludarabine is a useful drug, but again, the number of patients treated has been small. Similarly, early reports indicate that alpha interferon may be of value.

Standard dosage	Chlorambucil orally daily for 2 weeks every 4 weeks.
Contraindications	No absolute contraindications.
Special points	Full blood count essential because chlorambucil may cause bone-marrow suppression.
Main drug interactions	No major interactions known.
Main side effects	Bone-marrow suppression, nausea and vomiting, diarrhoea, oral ulcers, hypersensitivity rashes, occasionally myelodysplasia, acute leukaemia.

Treatment aims
To relieve symptoms.
To prolong life.

Other treatments
- Plasma exchange should be instituted urgently for hyperviscosity syndrome; one plasma volume exchanged at regular intervals until relative viscosity <4 times that of water.
- Maintenance plasmapheresis alone may be sufficient to control the disease; viscosity need not be restored to normal.

Prognosis
- The disease is not curable.
- Median survival is 4 years in patients who respond to treatment, 2 years in non-responders; the peripheral neuropathy is frequently unresponsive.

Follow-up and management
- Patients should be followed up at regular intervals.
- Full blood count and IgM concentrations should be monitored.
- Plasma viscosity indicates whether plasmapheresis is indicated.
- No large controlled trials are available to guide the physician. By analogy with other low-grade lymphomas, it is reasonable to withhold treatment in asymptomatic patients.

Key references
Kantarjian HM *et al.*: Fludarabine therapy in macroglobulinaemic lymphoma. *Blood* 1990, **75**:1928–1931.

Index

A

ABCM chemotherapy for multiple myeloma 25
abdominal
    distension 16, 26, 36
    pain 24, 26, 34
ABVD chemotherapy for Hodgkin's disease 11
acyclovir for infections in haematological malignancy 13
adriamycin
    in ABCM for multiple myeloma 25
    in ABVD for Hodgkin's disease 11
    in CHOP
        for chronic lymphocytic leukaemia 21
        for non-Hodgkin's lymphoma 29
    in EVAP for Hodgkin's disease 11
    in PACEBOM for non-Hodgkin's lymphoma 29
    in VAD for multiple myeloma 25
agglutination syndrome, cold 40
ALG see antilymphocyte globulin
alkylating agents
    for chronic lymphocytic leukaemia 21
    for Waldenström's macroglobulinaemia 41
ALL see leukaemia, acute lymphoblastic
allergic reaction to foreign proteins 39
all-trans-retinoic-acid for acute myeloid leukaemia 19
allopurinol
    for acute lymphoblastic leukaemia 15
    for non-Hodgkin's lymphoma 29
aminoglycosides
    for acute myeloid leukaemia 19
    for pyrexia of unknown origin 13
amoxycillin for sickle cell disease 35
amphotericin B
    for acute myeloid leukaemia 19
    for infections in haematological malignancy 13
amyloidosis 24, 30, 40
anaemia 6, 14, 16, 18, 20, 24, 26, 34, 36, 38
    aplastic 2, 4, 14, 16, 30, 38
    Fanconi 2, 16
    haemolytic 4, 6, 20
    iron-deficiency 30
    megaloblastic 4
    normochromic normocytic 22, 40
    pernicious 4
anagrelide for essential thrombocythaemia 27
analgesia
    for multiple myeloma 25
    for sickle cell disease 35
angiitis see vasculitis
angiohaemophilia see von Willebrand's disease
anthracycline for leukaemia
    acute lymphoblastic 15
    acute myeloid 19
antibiotics see also antimicrobials
    for acute myeloid leukaemia 19
    for infections in haematological malignancy 13
    for multiple myeloma 25
    for sickle cell disease 35
anticoagulants
    for disseminated intravascular coagulation 7
    lupus 6, 32
antifibrinolytic agents for platelet disorders 31
antifungal agents for multiple myeloma 25
antilymphocyte globulin for aplastic anaemia 3
antimicrobials for acute lymphoblastic leukaemia 15, 17 see also antibiotics
antiovulatory treatment for platelet disorders 31
antiplatelet drugs for prothrombotic states 33
antipyretics for adverse effects of transfusion 39
antithymocyte globulin for aplastic anaemia 3
aplasia 30, 38
    post-hepatitic 2
    pure erythrocyte 2, 20
aplastic crisis 34
appendicitis 34
ARDS see respiratory distress, adult
arginine vasopressin for platelet functional defects 31
arteritis, temporal 24
arthritis 8
ascorbic acid see vitamin C
L-asparaginase for acute lymphoblastic leukaemia 15, 17
aspirin
    for essential thrombocythaemia 27
    for prothrombotic states 33
    for thrombotic thrombocytopenic purpura 31
    ingestion 30
ataxia 40
    telangiectasia 16
ATG see antithymocyte globulin
ATRA see all-trans-retinoic-acid
autosplenectomy 34
azathioprine for immune thrombocytopenia 31

B

BCNU
    for Waldenström's macroglobulinaemia 41
    in ABCM for multiple myeloma 25
    in BEAM for Hodgkin's disease 11
    in VBMCP for multiple myeloma 25
BEAM chemotherapy for Hodgkin's disease 11
bisphosphonates for multiple myeloma 25
bites
    insect 6
    snake 6
bleeding 6, 8, 14, 16, 18, 20, 22, 24, 26, 30, 38, 40
    capillary 30
    gastrointestinal 28
    gum 2
    intracranial 30
    mucosal 16, 30
    postpartum 8
    retinal 30
    vaginal 6
bleomycin
    in ABVD for Hodgkin's disease 11
    in PACEBOM for non-Hodgkin's lymphoma 29
blood
    donation, directed 38
    filtered 38
    pressure, high see hypertension
    product
        support
            for acute lymphoblastic leukaemia 15
            for multiple myeloma 25
        transfusion reaction 12
    viscosity, raised 32
    transfusion for sickle cell disease 35
    whole 38
bone-marrow
    failure 14, 16, 22, 28, 30, 38
    graft rejection 2
    transplantation
        for acute lymphoblastic leukaemia 15, 17
        for acute myeloid leukaemia 19
        for aplastic anaemia 3
        for chronic myeloid leukaemia 27
        for multiple myeloma 25
        for non-Hodgkin's lymphoma 29
        for thalassaemia 37
    tumour 16
bruising 2, 6, 8, 14, 16, 18, 20, 22, 26, 30
Burkitt's lymphoma 29
    virus 28 see also Epstein Barr virus
burns 6
busulphan for myeloproliferative disorders 27

C

carcinoma 2, 4, 6, 24
cardiac see heart
carmustine see BCNU
ceftazidime for pyrexia of unknown origin 13
cerebrovascular
    accident see stroke
    thrombotic stroke 33
chemical exposure 24
chlorambucil
    for non-Hodgkin's lymphoma 29
    for Waldenström's macroglobulinaemia 41
    in LOPP for Hodgkin's disease 11
2-chlorodeoxyadenosine
    for chronic lymphocytic leukaemia 21
    for hairy-cell leukaemia 23
    for non-Hodgkin's lymphoma 29
cholecystitis 34
cholelithiasis 34
CHOP chemotherapy

Index

for chronic lymphocytic leukaemia 21
for non-Hodgkin's lymphoma 29
Christmas disease *see* haemophilia
ciprofloxacin for infections in haematological malignancy 13
clodronate for multiple myeloma 25
clotting factor
  deficiency 8, 40
  preparations for haemophilia and von Willebrand's disease 9
coagulation
  disseminated intravascular 4, 6, 19, 30, 38
  factor deficiencies 38
coagulopathy 30, 38
  consumption *see* coagulation, disseminated intravascular
codeine phosphate for sickle cell disease 35
colistin for infections in haematological malignancy 13
collagen disease 24, 30
colony-stimulating factor, granulocyte–macrophage, for multiple myeloma 25
corticosteroids
  for acute lymphoblastic leukaemia 15, 17
  for immune thrombocytopenia 31
  for multiple myeloma 25
co-trimoxazole
  for acute lymphoblastic leukaemia 15, 17
  for infections in haematological malignancy 13
Crohn's disease 4
cryoprecipitate for disseminated intravascular coagulation 7
cutis hyperelastica *see* Ehlers–Danlos syndrome
cyclophosphamide
  for chronic lymphocytic leukaemia 21
  for multiple myeloma 25
  for Waldenström's macroglobulinaemia 41
  in ABCM for multiple myeloma 25
  in CHOP
    for chronic lymphocytic leukaemia 21
    for non-Hodgkin's lymphoma 29
  in VBMCP for multiple myeloma 25
cyclosporin
  for aplastic anaemia 3
  for multiple myeloma 25
cytarabine
  for acute lymphoblastic leukaemia 15, 17
  in BEAM for Hodgkin's disease 11
cytomegalovirus 2, 10, 12
cytopenia 14, 23
cytosine arabinoside for acute myeloid leukaemia 19

D

dacarbazine in ABVD for Hodgkin's disease 11
danazol for immune thrombocytopenia 31
daunorubicin for acute lymphoblastic leukaemia 15, 17
DDAVP
  for haemophilia 9
  for platelet functional defects 31
  for von Willebrand's disease 9
deafness 30
2'deoxycoformycin for hairy-cell leukaemia 23
desferrioxamine for thalassaemia 37
desmopressin *see* DDAVP
dexamethasone
  for immune thrombocytopenia 31
  for multiple myeloma 25
  in VAD for multiple myeloma 25
diabetes mellitus 32
dialysis
  for renal failure in multiple myeloma 25
  peritoneal 4
diet deficiency 4
diclofenac for sickle cell disease 35
dipyridamole
  for essential thrombocythaemia 27
  for prothrombotic states 33
  for thrombotic thrombocytopenic purpura 31
Down's syndrome 16
doxorubicin *see* adriamycin
dyskeratosis congenita 2

E

EBV *see* Epstein–Barr virus
ecchymoses 2, 26
ecthyma gangrenosum 12
effusion, pleural 28
Ehlers–Danlos syndrome 30
embolism
  amniotic fluid 6
  arterial 32
  pulmonary 33
  venous 32
enterocolitis, necrotizing 38
enteropathy, gluten-induced 4
eosinophilia 10
epipodophyllotoxin for acute lymphoblastic leukaemia 15, 17
epistaxis 8, 30, 38, 40
Epstein–Barr virus 2, 10, 28
erythrocyte
  aplasia, pure 2, 20
  transfusion
    concentrates 38
    cryopreserved 38
    irradiated 38
    packed
      for disseminated intravascular coagulation 7
      for megaloblastic anaemia 5
erythrocytosis *see* polycythaemia
erythroderma, Sezary *see* Sezary syndrome

etoposide
  for acute myeloid leukaemia 19
  for multiple myeloma 25
  in BEAM for Hodgkin's disease 11
  in EVAP for Hodgkin's disease 11
  in PACEBOM for non-Hodgkin's lymphoma 29
EVAP chemotherapy for Hodgkin's disease 11

F

factor
  VIII
    for haemophilia A 9
    for von Willebrand's disease 9
  IX
    deficiency *see* haemophilia
    for haemophilia B 9
  X deficiencies 40
  XI for haemophilia C 9
fetal loss, recurrent 32
fibrinolytic inhibitors for disseminated intravascular coagulation 7
fluconazole for infections in haematological malignancy 13
flucytosine for infections in haematological malignancy 13
fludarabine
  for chronic lymphocytic leukaemia 21
  for non-Hodgkin's lymphoma 29
  for Waldenström's macroglobulinaemia 41
folate deficiency 4
folic acid for megaloblastic anaemia 5
folinic acid for infections in haematological malignancy 13
foscarnet for infections in haematological malignancy 13
fracture, pathological 24
fresh frozen plasma 38
  for disseminated intravascular coagulation 7
  for platelet disorders 31
  for prothrombotic states 33

G

gammopathy, benign monoclonal 24
ganciclovir for infections in haematological malignancy 13
gangrene 6
gastric
  atrophy 4
  bypass 4
  carcinoma 4
  neoplasm 4
  polyp 4
gastritis, sclerosing 4
Gaucher's disease 26
Glanzmann's syndrome 30
glossitis 4
glycopeptides for infections in haematological malignancy 13

Index

gonadal failure 26
gout 26
graft-versus-host disease 12, 38
granulocyte–macrophage colony-stimulating factors for multiple myeloma 25
granuloma
  Hodgkin's see Hodgkin's disease
  malignant see Hodgkin's disease

H

haemarthrosis 8
haematemesis 6
haematological malignancy, infections in 12
haematoma 8
haematuria 26
haemodialysis for platelet disorders 31
haemoglobinuria, paroxysmal nocturnal 2
haemolysis 4, 7, 28, 34
haemophagocytosis 2
haemophilia 8, 40
haemoptysis 6
haemorrhage 6, 8, 38, 40 see also bleeding
  buccal 2
  fundal 16
  gastrointestinal 40
  retinal 2, 26, 30, 40
heart failure 4, 16, 24, 32, 36, 40
heparin
  for acute myeloid leukaemia 19
  for disseminated intravascular coagulation 7
  for prothrombotic states 33
hepatitis 2, 8, 34
hepatomegaly 20, 22, 26, 28, 40
hepatosplenomegaly 14, 16, 18, 24
herpes virus 10, 12
HIV 4, 8, 28, 30
Hodgkin's
  disease 10, 28
  granuloma see Hodgkin's disease
hydroxocobalamin for megaloblastic anaemia 5
hydroxyurea for myeloproliferative disorders 27
hypercalcaemia 24
hyperkalaemia 16
hyperleucostasis 21
hyperlipidaemia 32
hyperphosphataemia 16
hypersplenism 22, 30, 36
hypertension 26
hypertrophy, gum 18
hyperuricaemia 16
hyperviscosity syndrome 14, 24, 26, 32, 40
hypogammaglobulinaemia 20, 24
hypothyroidism 4

I

imipenem for pyrexia of unknown origin 13
immunoglobulin
  for chronic lymphocytic leukaemia 21
  for infections in haematological malignancy 13
  for platelet disorders 31
infarction
  pulmonary 12
  splenic 26
infection 2, 6, 10, 12, 14, 16, 18, 20, 22, 24, 26, 28, 34, 38
  in haematological malignancy 12
  of skin 24
  of respiratory tract 24
  of urinary tract 24
  transfusion-transmitted 39
interferon-α
  for hairy-cell leukaemia 23
  for multiple myeloma 25
  for myeloproliferative disorders 27
  for non-Hodgkin's lymphoma 29
  for Waldenström's macroglobulinaemia 41
iron
  chelation
    for adverse effects of transfusion 39
    for transfusional iron overload 37
  deficiency 36
  overload 37, 39
irradiation
  for acute lymphoblastic leukaemia
    cranial 15, 17
    craniospinal 17
  splenic for myelofibrosis 27
ischaemia, myocardial 33
ischaemic attack, transient 33
isoniazid for infections in haematological malignancy 13
itching see pruritus
itraconazole for infections in haematological malignancy 13

K

kala-azar see leishmaniasis, visceral

L

leishmaniasis 16
  visceral 16, 26
lesion
  bone 24
  small intestinal 4
  osteolytic 24
leucocytapheresis for chronic lymphocytic leukaemia 21
leucocytosis 26, 22
leucopenia 2, 14, 18
leukaemia 26, 30
  CNS 15
  hairy-cell 2, 20, 22
  intracranial 18
  lymphoblastic
    acute
      in adults 14
      in children 2, 16
    chronic see leukaemia, chronic lymphocytic
  lymphocytic
    chronic 20, 40
    T-cell see leukaemia, T-cell
  megakaryocytic see thrombocythaemia, essential
leukaemia cont.
  monocytic 18
  myeloblastic, acute see leukaemia, acute myeloid
  myelogenous, acute see leukaemia, acute myeloid
  myeloid 6
    acute 2, 4, 14, 18
    chronic 26
  prolymphocytic 20
  promyelocytic 6, 18
  T-cell 20
liver disease 4, 6, 32, 38
LOPP chemotherapy for Hodgkin's disease 11
lupus
  anticoagulant 6, 32
  erythematosus, systemic 2, 32
lymphadenopathy 10, 14, 16, 18, 20, 22, 24, 28, 40
lymphocytosis 20
lymphoglobuline for aplastic anaemia 3
lymphogranuloma see Hodgkin's disease
lymphoma 2, 16, 20, 26, 28
  B cell 22, 40
  follicle centre cell 20
  lymphoblastic 14, 29
  mantle cell 20
  non-Hodgkin's 10, 24, 28
  splenic 20, 22
  T cell 20
  virus, Burkitt's 28 see also Epstein–Barr virus
lymphopenia 10, 12

M

macroglobulinaemia
  monoclonal 40
  Waldenström's 24, 40
macroglossia 24
macrolides for infections in haematological malignancy 13
malaria 6, 12, 26
malignancy 32
  infections in haematological 12
May–Hegglin anomaly 30
melaena 6, 8
melphalan

Index

for multiple myeloma 25
for Waldenström's macroglobulinaemia 41
in ABCM for multiple myeloma 25
in BEAM for Hodgkin's disease 11
in VBMCP for multiple myeloma 25
menorrhagia 30
meperidine *see* pethidine
mercaptopurine for acute lymphoblastic leukaemia 15, 17
methotrexate
  for acute lymphoblastic leukaemia 15, 17
  in PACEBOM for non-Hodgkin's lymphoma 29
methylprednisolone
  for multiple myeloma 25
  for thrombotic thrombocytopenic purpura 31
monocytopenia 22
mononucleosis, infectious 16 *see also* Epstein–Barr virus
MOPP chemotherapy for Hodgkin's disease 11
morphine for sickle cell disease 35
mustine in MOPP for Hodgkin's disease 11
myelodysplasia 2, 4, 16, 18, 30
myelofibrosis 2, 4, 26
myeloma 4, 24, 25
  IgM 40
  multiple 24
  plasma cell *see* multiple myeloma
myeloproliferative disorders 18, 26, 30, 32
myelosclerosis *see* myelofibrosis
myopathy, peripheral 16

N

necrosis
  acute tubular 12
  avascular 34
  skin 32
  tissue 6
nephrotic syndrome 32
neuroblastoma 16
neuropathy 4
  peripheral 16, 24, 40
  vitamin B12 4
neutropenia 12, 18, 20, 22, 36, 40
neutrophilia 10
nucleoside analogues for chronic lymphocytic leukaemia 21
nystagmus 40

O

obesity 32
oedema 24, 40
  facial 16
  upper trunk 16
oestrogen treatment 32
osteoporosis 24
oxygen for sickle cell disease 35

oxymetholone for aplastic anaemia 3

P

PACEBOM chemotherapy for non-Hodgkin's lymphoma 29
pain
  abdominal 24, 26, 34
  back 24
  bone 16, 24
  hip 34
  limb 34
  shoulder 34
palsy, cranial nerve 16
pancytopenia 2, 16, 18
papilloedema 16, 40
paracetamol for sickle cell disease 35
paraesthesiae in feet 4
paralysis of lower limbs 32
paraproteinaemia 32
parvovirus B19 2, 34
penicillin
  for infections in haematological malignancy 13
  for sickle cell disease 35
pentamidine for infections in haematological malignancy 13
petechiae 2, 18, 30
pethidine for sickle cell disease 35
phlegmasia alba dolens *see* thrombophlebitis, thrombosis
phosphorus, radioactive for myeloproliferative disorders 27
piritron for urticarial reactions to transfusion 39
plasma
  exchange
    for multiple myeloma 25
    for platelet disorders 31
    for Waldenström's macroglobulinaemia 41
  fresh frozen 38
    for disseminated intravascular coagulation 7
    for platelet disorders 31
    for prothrombotic states 33
plasmacytoma 24, 40
plasmapheresis for Waldenström's macroglobulinaemia 41
platelet
  concentrates for disseminated intravascular coagulation 7
  disorders 30
  function defect 8, 30, 38
  transfusion 38
    for alloimmune thrombocytopenia 31
    for platelet disorders 31
pneumonia 2, 20
polyarteritis, microscopic 22
polycythaemia rubra vera 26
polymyalgia rheumatica 24

polyneuropathy 24
prednisolone
  for acute lymphoblastic leukaemia 15, 17
  for chronic lymphocytic leukaemia 21
  for platelet disorders 31
  for Waldenström's macroglobulinaemia 41
  in CHOP
    for chronic lymphocytic leukaemia 21
    for non-Hodgkin's lymphoma 29
  in EVAP for Hodgkin's disease 11
  in LOPP for Hodgkin's disease 11
  in MOPP for Hodgkin's disease 11
  in PACEBOM for non-Hodgkin's lymphoma 29
prednisone
  for multiple myeloma 25
  in VBMCP for multiple myeloma 25
priapism 26, 34
procarbazine
  in LOPP for Hodgkin's disease 11
  in MOPP for Hodgkin's disease 11
protamine sulphate for prothrombotic states 33
proteins, foreign, allergic reaction to 39
proteinuria 24
prothrombotic states 32
pruritus 10, 24, 26
pseudohaemophilia *see* von Willebrand's disease
pseudopolyarthritis, rhizomelic *see* polymyalgia rheumatica
pseudothrombocytopenia 30
purpura 14, 16, 20, 24, 30, 38, 40
  anaphylactoid *see* Henoch–Schönlein purpura
  fulminans 6
  Henoch–Schönlein 30
  non-thrombocytopenic *see* Henoch–Schönlein purpura
  post-transfusion 30
  rheumatoid *see* Henoch–Schönlein purpura
  thrombocytopenic
    idiopathic 30, 32
    thrombotic 6, 30, 38
pyrexia of unknown origin 13
pyrimethamine for infections in haematological malignancy 13

Q

quinolones for infections in haematological malignancy 13

R

radiation exposure 18, 24, 26
radiotherapy
  for Hodgkin's disease 11
  for multiple myeloma 25
  for non-Hodgkin's lymphoma 29
recombinant erythropoietin for multiple myeloma 25
rejection

Index

allograft 6
bone-marrow graft 2
renal
  dysfunction 16
  failure 24
    chronic 30
  occlusive disease 26
  tubular obstruction 26
respiratory distress, adult 6, 12
reticulocytopenia 2
reticulocytosis 4
reticuloendotheliosis, leukaemic *see* hairy-cell leukaemia
retinopathy, proliferative 34
runt disease *see* graft-versus-host disease

S

scurvy 30
sepsis 2
septicaemia 6, 12, 34
Sezary
  erythroderma *see* Sezary syndrome
  syndrome 20
shingles 20
shock 6
short stature 2, 36
sickle cell disease 34
SLE *see* lupus erythematosus, systemic
sodium clodronate for multiple myeloma 25
spinal cord compression 24
splenectomy
  for hairy-cell leukaemia 23
  for immune thrombocytopenia 31
  for myelofibrosis 27
  for thalassaemia 37
splenomegaly 2, 20, 22, 26, 28, 30, 36, 40
sprue, tropical 4
stagnant loop syndrome 4
stem cell
  autologous haematopoietic, for Hodgkin's disease 11
  peripheral blood, for multiple myeloma 25
stenosis, mitral 33
steroids *see* corticosteroids
stomach *see* gastric
stroke 34, 40
sulphadiazine for infections in haematological malignancy 13
sweats 26
  night 10, 20

T

teicoplanin for pyrexia of unknown origin in neutropenia 13
telangiectasia
  ataxia 16
  haemorrhagic 30
testicular enlargement 16
thalassaemia 26, 34, 36
thiabendazole for infections in haematological malignancy 13
thioguanine for leukaemia
  acute lymphoblastic 15, 17
  acute myeloid 19
thrombocythaemia
  essential 26, 33
  idiopathic *see* thrombocythaemia, essential
  haemorrhagic *see* thrombocythaemia, essential
  primary *see* thrombocythaemia, essential
thrombocytopenia 2, 6, 14, 18, 20, 22, 28, 30, 36, 38, 40
thrombocytosis 26, 33
thromboembolism, venous 32
thrombopenia *see* thrombocytopenia
thrombophlebitis, recurrent venous 32
thrombosis 30, 32
  arterial 32
  venous 32
thymoglobuline for aplastic anaemia 3
tranexamic acid
  for acute myeloid leukaemia 19
  for haemophilia 9
  for platelet functional defects 31
  for von Willebrand's disease 9
transcobalamin II deficiency 4
transfusion 6, 38
  blood, for sickle cell disease 35
  platelet
    for alloimmune thrombocytopenia 31
    for platelet disorders 31
  reaction 12
    febrile nonhaemolytic 38
    haemolytic 38
  transmitted disease 8
transplantation, bone-marrow
  for aplastic anaemia 3
  for leukaemia
    acute lymphoblastic 15, 17
    acute myeloid 19
    chronic myeloid 27
  for multiple myeloma 25
  for non-Hodgkin's lymphoma 29
  for thalassaemia 37
TTP *see* purpura, thrombotic thrombocytopenic
tuberculosis 2, 10, 16
tumour 16, 22, 30
  bone-marrow 16
  lysis syndrome 14, 16

U

ulcer
  gastroduodenal *see* peptic
  mouth 2
  peptic 26
  tongue 2
ureidopenicillin for acute myeloid leukaemia 19
urticarial reactions to transfusion 39

V

vaccination
  antipneumococcal for sickle cell disease 35
  haemophilus B for sickle cell disease 35
VAD chemotherapy for multiple myeloma 25
vancomycin
  for acute myeloid leukaemia 19
  for pyrexia of unknown origin 13
varicella–zoster virus 12
vasculitis 22, 30
  haemorrhagic *see* Henoch–Schönlein purpura
vaso-occlusive crisis 34
vasopressin for platelet functional defects 31
VBMCP chemotherapy for multiple myeloma 25
venesection for polycythaemia rubra vera 27
vinblastine in ABVD for Hodgkin's disease 11
vinca alkaloids for thrombocytopenia 31
vincristine
  for acute lymphoblastic leukaemia 15, 17
  for thrombotic thrombocytopenic purpura 31
  for Waldenström's macroglobulinaemia 41
  in CHOP
    for chronic lymphocytic leukaemia 21
    for non-Hodgkin's lymphoma 29
  in EVAP for Hodgkin's disease 11
  in LOPP for Hodgkin's disease 11
  in MOPP for Hodgkin's disease 11
  in PACEBOM for non-Hodgkin's lymphoma 29
  in VAD for multiple myeloma 25
  in VBMCP for multiple myeloma 25
visual disturbances 2, 26, 30
vitamin
  B_{12}
    deficiency 4
    neuropathy 4
  C
    for immune thrombocytopenia 31
    for thalassaemia 37
  K
    deficiency 6
    for acute myeloid leukaemia 19
    for prothrombotic states 33
von Willebrand's disease 8, 30

W

Waldenström's macroglobulinaemia 24, 40
warfarin
  effect 38
  for prothrombotic states 33
wasting disease, homologous *see* graft-versus-host disease
Willebrand's disease 8, 30

CURRENT DIAGNOSIS & TREATMENT

in

Hepatology

Edited by
Andrew Burroughs

Series editors
Roy Pounder
Mark Hamilton

A QUICK Reference for the Clinician

Contributors

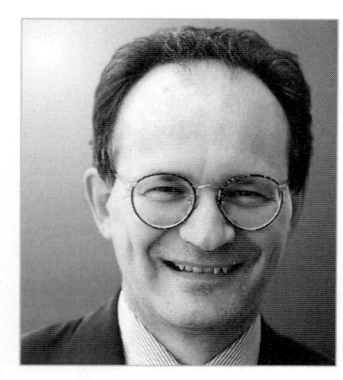

EDITOR

A K Burroughs

Dr Andrew Burroughs is Consultant Physician and Hepatologist at the Royal Free Hospital, London. He heads the medical side of the liver transplantation service. His special interests include portal hypertension, haemostasis in liver disease, primary biliary cirrhosis, and liver transplantation.

REFEREES

Professor Oliver F W James
Department of Medicine
University of Newcastle upon Tyne
Newcastle upon Tyne, UK

Dr E Elias
The Liver Unit
The Queen Elizabeth Hospital
Birmingham, UK

AUTHORS

ASCITES
Dr Alexander Gimson
Hepatobiliary and Liver Transplant Unit
Addenbrooke's Hospital
Cambridge, UK

CHOLANGITIS, PRIMARY SCLEROSING
Dr James S Dooley
Hepatobiliary and Liver Transplantation Unit
Royal Free Hospital
London, UK

CIRRHOSIS, PRIMARY BILIARY
Dr James M Neuberger
Liver Unit
Queen Elizabeth Hospital
Birmingham, UK

HEPATIC, ENCEPHALOPATHY
Dr Andrew K Burroughs
Department of Liver Transplantation and Hepatobiliary Medicine
Royal Free Hospital
London, UK

HEPATITIS, ACUTE
Dr Graeme Alexander
Department of Medicine
Clinical School of Medicine
Cambridge University
Cambridge, UK

HEPATITIS, CHRONIC
Dr JP Watson
Department of Haematology and Gastroenterology
Freeman Hospital
Newcastle upon Tyne, UK

Professor MF Bassendine
Department of Medicine
Freeman Hospital
Newcastle upon Tyne, UK

HEPATOCELLULAR CARCINOMA
Dr Geoffrey Dusheiko
University Department of Medicine
Royal Free Hospital
London, UK

LIVER FAILURE, FULMINANT
Dr John O'Grady
Liver Unit
St James' University Hospital
Leeds, UK

VARICEAL BLEEDING
Dr P Aidan McCormick
Liver Clinic
St Vincent's Hospital
Dublin, Ireland

Contents

2 **Ascites**
spontaneous bacterial peritonitis
uncomplicated ascites

4 **Cholangitis, primary sclerosing**

6 **Cirrhosis, primary biliary**

8 **Hepatic encephalopathy**
in chronic liver disease
in fulminant liver failure

10 **Hepatitis, acute**

12 **Hepatitis, chronic**

14 **Hepatocellular carcinoma**

16 **Liver failure, fulminant**
non-paracetamol-induced fulminant liver failure
paracetamol-induced fulminant liver failure

18 **Variceal bleeding**

20 **Index**

Ascites A. Gimson

Diagnosis

Symptoms

Uncomplicated ascites
Abdominal distension and discomfort.
Ankle oedema: rare.
Dyspnoea: due to splinting of diaphragm.

Spontaneous bacterial peritonitis
Deterioration in liver function, increasing jaundice, renal impairment, gastrointestinal haemorrhage, encephalopathy: often the only symptoms.
Pain, fever: in 15–20% of patients.

Signs

Uncomplicated ascites
Distension.
Shifting dullness on percussion of flanks.
Ballotable liver.

Spontaneous bacterial peritonitis
- Often no new clinical signs are manifest.
Fever.
Tenderness, rebound, rigidity: very uncommon.

Investigations

In all cases
Serum ascites–albumin gradient measurement: >11 g/dl indicates transudate.
Ascitic protein measurement: <30 g/L indicates transudate; >30 g/L indicates exudate.
Ascitic leucocyte and neutrophil or lymphocyte count: spontaneous bacterial peritonitis confirmed when ascitic leucocyte count >500 or neutrophil count >250 cells/high-power film.
Gram stain and culture of ascites: blood culture bottle inoculation.
Urine electrolytes analysis.

Specific tests
Ziehl–Neelson stain, adenine deaminase test: to detect tuberculous ascites.
Amylase measurement: concentration raised in pancreatic ascites.
Cholesterol or triglyceride measurement: concentration raised in chylous ascites.
Immunoglobulin analysis: for chylous ascites.
Cytology: for malignant ascites.
Laparoscopy and biopsy, abdominal ultrasonography, CT, lymphangiography: for tuberculosis and malignant peritonitis.

Complications

Spontaneous bacterial peritonitis: in 10% of patients who develop ascites.
Pleural effusion.
Inguinal, femoral, or umbilical herniae.
Mesenteric venous thrombosis.
Functional renal failure.

Differential diagnosis

Transudate
Cirrhosis, acute liver failure (rare), veno-occlusive disease, Budd–Chiari syndrome (protein may be high in 50% of patients).
Biventricular heart failure, constrictive pericarditis, tricuspid regurgitation.
Nephrotic syndrome, protein-losing enteropathy, malnutrition.
Meig's syndrome, recurrent polyserositis.

Exudate
Bacterial, fungal, or tuberculous infection, ruptured viscus, pancreatitis, biliary duct leak.
Primary or metastatic malignancy, myelo- or lymphoproliferative disease.
Hypothyroidism.

Chylous
Trauma and surgery, abdominal tuberculosis, lymphoma or other malignancy, filariasis.

Aetiology

- Common causes include the following:

General
Malignancy and cirrhosis.

Transudate
Overflow hypothesis: primary increase in renal sensitivity to aldosterone, causing sodium retention or volume expansion, ascites forming in abdomen because of portal hypertension and hypoalbuminaemia.
Underfill hypothesis: fluid sequestration in abdomen, causing renal hypoperfusion and secondary hyperaldosteronism, renal retention of sodium to maintain circulating volume.
Vasodilatation hypothesis: overflow factors initiating and underfill factors perpetuating ascites.

Exudate
Increased capillary permeability.

Chylous
Lymphatic leakage.

Epidemiology

- 80% of patients with chronic liver disease develop ascites during their course (spontaneous bacterial peritonitis in 10%).

Ascites

A. Gimson

Treatment

Diet and lifestyle
- Patients should have a low-salt diet (20–40 mmol daily).
- Bed-rest during mobilization of ascites lowers renin–angiotensin concentrations.

Pharmacological treatment

For uncomplicated ascites
- Initially, treatment should involve bed-rest and spironolactone.
- Frusemide can be added if no response is seen after 4 days and is more effective in patients with peripheral oedema.

Standard dosage	Spironolactone 100 mg daily or frusemide 40 mg daily; increased slowly depending on diuresis to maximum spironolactone 400 mg or frusemide 120 mg.
Contraindications	Renal failure.
Special points	Treatment must be stopped if creatinine >120 mmol/L or sodium <130 mmol/L; diuretics less effective if serum albumin <25 g/d; 5–20% albumin infusion should be given for 3 days; weight loss of 0.5–1.0 kg daily should be the aim.
Main drug interactions	Diuretics and aminoglycosides may have increased nephrotoxicity in this context.
Main side effects	Hyponatraemia, impaired renal function with raised creatinine. For patients with breast pain and enlargement from spironolactone, amiloride is an alternative (5–10 mg daily).

For functional renal failure
- Renal failure is often precipitated by infection, haemorrhage, hypotension, or over-aggressive diuretic treatment; it may reverse after orthotopic liver transplantation.
- Treatment involves central venous monitoring, volume expansion, and treatment of precipitating factors; renal vasodilators are of no proven benefit.

For spontaneous bacterial peritonitis
- 80% of organisms are aerobic Gram-negative bacilli; 20% are nonenteric organisms.
- Cefotaxime or ceftizoxime is effective in up to 85%; ciprofloxacin and amoxycillin may be as effective, but gentamycin and ampicillin are less effective and potentially more toxic.
- Treatment should last 5–7 days.
- Antibiotic treatment is influenced by hospital sensitivities.
- Clearance of ascitic leucocytes should be checked after 3 days, and renal function should be monitored daily.
- Long-term antibiotic prophylaxis with poorly absorbed antibiotics may prevent recurrence.

Treatment aims
To reduce ascitic volume.

Other treatments
For diuretic-resistant ascites: orthotopic liver transplantation or, if contraindicated for surgical or medical reasons, jugulo-peritoneal shunt, regular abdominal paracentesis with albumin infusion, or transhepatic intravascular portal systemic stent shunt.

Prognosis
- 1-year and 5-year survival rates after development of ascites without renal impairment are 50% and 20%, respectively.
- 80% of patients respond to medical treatment.
- 30% develop functional renal failure within 24 months.
- When urine sodium is <5 mmol/L or diuretic-resistant ascites has developed, 1-year survival is <50%.
- Spontaneous bacterial peritonitis has a hospital mortality of up to 50%.
- >50% of survivors have a recurrence in the following year.

Follow-up and management
- Patients with uncomplicated ascites must be monitored using weight and fluid input and output charts daily, and sodium, potassium, urea, and creatinine measurement 3 times weekly.
- If no response is seen at maximum tolerated dose of diuretic, the development of hepatoma, portal-vein thrombosis, or spontaneous bacterial peritonitis must be excluded.

Key references
Arroyo V et al.: Ascites, renal failure and electrolyte disorders in cirrhosis. Pathogenesis, diagnosis and treatment. In *Oxford Textbook of Clinical Hepatology.* Edited by McIntyre N et al. Oxford: Oxford Medical Publications, 1991, pp 429–470.

Bhuva M, Ganger D, Jensen D: Spontaneous bacterial peritonitis: an update on evaluation, management, and prevention. *Am J Med* 1994, 97:169–175.

Cholangitis, primary sclerosing — J.S. Dooley

Diagnosis

Symptoms

- 25% of patients are asymptomatic; diagnosis is made after discovery of abnormal liver function tests, particularly in patients with ulcerative colitis.

Itching, jaundice: intermittent.

Fatigue, weight loss, right upper-quadrant pain.

Fever: unusual unless previous intervention, e.g. endoscopic retrograde cholangio-pancreatography, surgery.

Bleeding oesophageal varices, oedema, ascites: late features.

Signs

- Signs are not always manifest.

Hepatomegaly.

Splenomegaly.

Jaundice.

Spider naevi, palmar erythema, ascites: late.

Investigations

Liver function tests: cholestatic pattern with raised alkaline phosphatase, gamma glutamyl transpeptidase, bilirubin (late); low albumin, prolonged prothrombin time (late); antinuclear and smooth-muscle antibodies variably positive; antimitochondrial antibody negative.

Cholangiography: the diagnostic test; endoscopic retrograde cholangiography first choice, percutaneous route only if endoscopic route fails; bile-duct stricturing interspersed with dilatation (beading); intra- and extrahepatic duct changes in most patients.

Liver biopsy: changes suggestive (portal oedema, fibrosis, duct proliferation) rather than diagnostic; biopsy staging: 1, portal changes; 2, periportal extension; 3, septum formation; 4, cirrhosis.

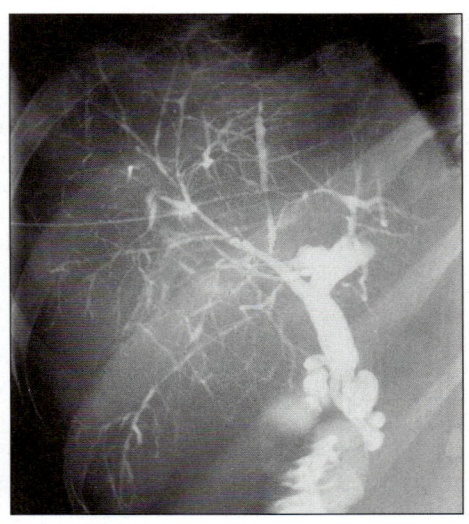

Classic intrahepatic changes of primary sclerosing cholangitis (bleeding and stricturing) on percutaneous cholangiography. The common bile duct is dilated because of involvement of the lower end by primary sclerosing cholangitis. Endoscopic cholangiography was unsuccessful.

Complications

Recurrent cholangitis.

Cholangiocarcinoma: in 10–15% of patients.

Metabolic bone disease.

Portal hypertension, variceal haemorrhage, oedema, ascites, encephalopathy: late.

Differential diagnosis

Bile duct stones.

Cholangiocarcinoma.

Drug-induced cholestasis.

Primary biliary cirrhosis.

Surgical stricture.

Secondary sclerosing cholangitis.

Metastatic tumour.

Granulomatous liver disease (e.g. sarcoid).

AIDS cholangiopathy.

- Distinction of benign primary sclerosing cholangitis stricture from cholangiocarcinoma is very difficult; brush or bile cytology is only 50–60% sensitive.

Aetiology

- Primary sclerosing cholangitis has a known strong association with inflammatory bowel disease (ulcerative colitis) and HLA B8 and DR3.
- The pathogenetic mechanism is unknown.
- The current hypothesis is that infection, or absorption of bacterial products or both occur in predisposed (HLA DR) individuals.

Epidemiology

- 70% of patients with primary sclerosing cholangitis have ulcerative colitis; 4% of patients with ulcerative colitis have primary sclerosing cholangitis.
- The prevalence of primary sclerosing cholangitis is 2–7 in 100 000.
- The male:female ratio is 2:1.
- The most common age of presentation is 25–45 years.

Treatment

Diet and lifestyle
- A healthy balanced diet is recommended.
- If steatorrhoea is problematic, fat intake may be reduced.

Pharmacological treatment

Symptomatic
- Drugs are indicated to relieve puritus.

Standard dosage	Cholestyramine 4–12 g daily.
Contraindications	Complete biliary obstruction.
Special points	May interfere with absorption of fat-soluble vitamins, so supplementation may be needed.
Main drug interactions	Delayed or reduced absorption of digitalis, tetracycline, chlorothiazide, warfarin, thyroxine.
Main side effects	Increased bleeding tendency, constipation, diarrhoea.

Prophylactic
- For proven fat-soluble vitamin deficiency or jaundice, the following are indicated:

Vitamin K 10 mg i.m. monthly.
Vitamin D 100 000 units i.m. monthly.
Vitamin A 100 000 units i.m. 3-monthly.

- Adequate calcium intake must be ensured.

Therapeutic
- No medical treatment has been known to delay progression or reverse changes of primary sclerosing cholangitis.
- Ursodeoxycholic acid 10–15 mg/kg orally daily improves liver function tests, but benefit for liver histology, cholangiography, or survival has not been established.
- The choice of antibiotics for cholangitis (when no remediable dominant stricture) depends on bile or blood culture; best choices without positive culture are trimethoprim, ciprofloxacin, ampicillin, and cephalosporin.

Treatment aims
To relieve symptoms.

Other treatments

Non-surgical
Endoscopic or radiographic palliation: for symptomatic dominant strictures (cholangitis, itching); endoscopic approach preferable to percutaneous; balloon dilatation possibly with stent.

Surgical
Surgical palliation: appropriate for dominant stricture only if transplantation is ruled out or endoscopic or percutaneous approach fails.
Orthotopic liver transplantation: for persistent jaundice, cholangitis, bleeding varices, fluid retention, encephalopathy, malnutrition; ~70% 1-year survival; unexpected cholangiocarcinoma often found (recurs).

Prognosis
- Prognosis varies greatly: patients may be asymptomatic for 25 years or need transplantation within a few years.
- Factors at presentation related to prognosis (Mayo model) include serum bilirubin concentration, histological stage on liver biopsy, age, and presence of splenomegaly.

Follow-up and management
- Follow-up depends on symptoms or complications.
- Patients should be reviewed monthly if they have symptomatic or biochemical deterioration and approaching transplantation.

Key references
Dickson ER et al.: Primary sclerosing cholangitis: refinement and validation of survival models. *Gastroenterology* 1992, **103**:1893–1901.

Lindor KD et al: Advances in primary sclerosing cholangitis. *Am J Med* 1990, **89**:73–80.

Wiesner RH et al.: Selection and timing of liver transplantation in primary biliary cirrhosis and primary sclerosing cholangitis. *Hepatology* 1992, **16**:1290–1299.

Cirrhosis, primary biliary — J. Neuberger

Diagnosis

Symptoms
- Disease may be an incidental finding (abnormal liver tests on routine screening for other conditions) or manifest in one of the following ways:

Lethargy and pruritus: in middle-aged women (classic).

Right-sided abdominal pain.

Ascites or variceal haemorrhage: indicating portal hypertension.

Associated symptoms: e.g. Raynaud's syndrome or thyroid disease.

Complications: e.g. end-stage liver disease, jaundice, or hepatocellular carcinoma, dry eyes and mouth (Sjögren's syndrome).

Signs
Jaundice: in later stages.
Pigmentation.
Xanthoma.
Hepatomegaly.
Splenomegaly.
Ascites: may be present in late stage.
Spider naevi: usually absent.

Investigations
Full blood count: usually normal, but mean cell volume possibly raised.

Liver tests: show cholestasis; in early stage, raised serum alkaline phosphatase, gamma GT, serum bilirubin concentrations; raised cholesterol concentration.

Immunological tests: raised serum IgM and IgG concentrations (IgG less marked); antimitochondrial antibodies (AMA M_2 subclass) almost diagnostic; other autoantibodies, e.g. antinuclear, occasionally manifest.

Liver histology: shows non-suppurative destructive cholangitis or hepatitis involving portal tracts, which may also contain granulomas.

Complications
- Complications are the same as for end-stage liver disease.

Variceal haemorrhage.
Ascites.
Osteoporosis: hepatic osteopenia.
Liver failure.
Hepatocellular carcinoma.

Differential diagnosis
Primary sclerosing cholangitis.
Autoimmune hepatitis.
Drug-induced jaundice.
Sarcoidosis.

Aetiology
- The cause is unknown, although the following may have a role:

Infectious agents: bacterial or viral.
Autoimmune disorders.
Drugs: benoxaprofen, chlorpromazine.

Epidemiology
- In the UK, estimates of point prevalence of primary biliary cirrhosis are 2.3–14.4 in 100 000 people.
- The disease is less common in Africa and India.

Associated syndromes
Common
Sicca syndrome.
Arthralgia.
Thyroid disease.
Sclerodactyly (CREST syndrome).
Raynaud's syndrome.

Rare
Glomerulonephritis.
Pulmonary fibrosis.
SLE.
Addison's disease.
Coeliac disease.

Histology
Stage 1
Florid duct lesions, septal duct damage surrounded by dense inflammatory infiltrate, lymphoid aggregates; granulomas.

Stage 2
Ductular proliferation, fibrosis, reduced duct numbers.

Stage 3
Scarring (less inflammation), fibrous septa expanding from portal tracts; periportal cholestatis.

Stage 4
True cirrhosis; paucity or absence of bile ducts.

Treatment

Diet and lifestyle
- Patients must avoid regular alcohol intake.

Pharmacological treatment

Symptomatic
- Drugs are indicated to relieve pruritus.

Standard dosage	Cholestyramine 4–16 g daily or colestipol.
Contraindications	Complete biliary obstruction.
Special points	May interfere with absorption of fat soluble vitamins, so supplementation may be needed.
Main drug interactions	Delayed or reduced absorption of digitalis, tetracycline, chlorothiazide, warfarin, thyroxine.
Main side effects	Increased bleeding tendency, constipation, diarrhoea.

- Treatment to prevent osteoporosis and supportive treatment for associated symptoms should also be provided.

Definitive
- Treatment should be done under specialist supervision.
- No drug has been shown to arrest disease; anti-inflammatories and antifibrotics (corticosteroids, azathioprine, cyclosporin A, colchicine, methotrexate, penicillamine) have been used with no major clinical benefit.
- Ursodeoxycholic acid may help; biochemistry is improved, but data on long-term survival are scanty and still debated.

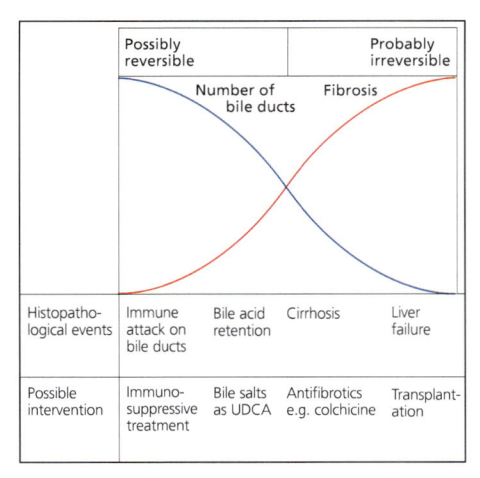

Progression of primary biliary cirrhosis and possible interventions. UDCA, ursodeoxycholic acid.

Treatment aims
To prevent progression.
To reverse symptoms.

Other treatments
Liver transplantation for end-stage disease or intractable symptoms.

Prognosis
- Prognosis depends on serum bilirubin concentration: >180 μmol/L implies an 18-month survival.
- The median time from diagnosis to death is 10 years.

Follow-up and management
- Progression must be monitored.
- Complications must be prevented or treated.

Key references

Coppel RI et al.: Primary structure of the human M_2 mitochondrial auto-antigen in PBC. *Proc Natl Acad Sci U S A* 1988, **85**:7317–7321.

Kaplan M: Primary biliary cirrhosis: a first step in prolonging survival. *N Engl J Med* 1994, **330**:1386–1387.

Mutchison HC, Bassendine MF: Auto-immune liver disease. *Aliment Pharmacol Ther* 1993, **7**:93–109.

Neuberger J et al.: Use of a prognostic index in evaluation of liver transplantation for primary biliary cirrhosis. *Transplantation* 1986, **41**:713–716.

Shapiro J, Smith H, Schaffner F: Serum bilirubin: a prognostic factor in PBC. *Gut* 1979, **20**:137–140.

Hepatic encephalopathy — A.K. Burroughs

Diagnosis

Definition
- Hepatic encephalopathy is a reversible neuropsychiatric syndrome that is a complication of fulminant or chronic liver disease.

Chronic liver disease: manifest as acute or chronic encephalopathy, usually in decompensated cirrhotic patients with precipitant cause, or as chronic encephalopathy due to spontaneous portal-systemic shunting with relatively good liver function.

Fulminant liver disease: associated with cerebral oedema and increasing intracranial pressure (see Liver failure, fulminant for further details).

- Hepatic encephalopathy may also be present in the rare cases of urea-cycle enzyme defects and portosystemic shunting in the absence of liver disease.
- Latent encephalopathy is a subclinical form occurring in chronic liver disease, only detected by psychometric testing.

Symptoms
- Wide differences are seen in presentation and evolution.

Inversion of normal sleep pattern.
Deterioration of intellectual function.
Slurred speech.
Tremor: absent at rest.
Personality changes: features of frontal-lobe syndrome.
Coma.
Symptoms of precipitating causes.

Signs
- Patients with impaired consciousness have intact pupillary reflexes.

Flapping tremor.
Hepatic foetor.
Constructional apraxia: Reitan trail test.
Brisk tendon reflexes: except in coma.
Increased muscle tone and rigidity.
Hyperventilation in deep coma.
Signs of precipitating causes.

Investigations
- No single parameter confirms the diagnosis.
- The underlying liver disease or its complications must be identified.
- A precipitant cause must always be sought.

Psychometric testing: essential to detect subclinical encephalopathy; number connection test (Reitan trail) and drawing a clock face easiest to perform.
EEG: slowing of normal frequency to severe slowing; characteristic triphasic waves; changes appearing first in frontal regions.
CT of head: to exclude subdural haematomas and other intracranial diseases; some atrophy of brain usually manifest, particularly in chronic encephalopathy.
Blood ammonia measurement: concentration usually raised.

Complications
Increase in intracranial pressure: in patients with fulminant liver failure; due to cerebral oedema, which can lead to coning and death.
Complications of coma: e.g. aspiration; in patients with encephalopathy.
Structural neuronal damage: with demyelination and a spastic paraplegia, in patients with chronic encephalopathy (rare); chronic cerebellar or basal ganglia signs may also be present with Parkinsonian features.
Focal fits: rare, other causes must be sought.

Differential diagnosis
Alcoholic brain damage.
Alcohol withdrawal syndrome.
Wernicke's encephalopathy.
Chronic subdural haematoma or other space-occupying lesion.
Other causes of metabolic coma.
Postictal state.
Meningitis, encephalitis.

Aetiology
- Precipitant causes include the following:

Constipation.
Gastrointestinal bleeding (occult or apparent).
Infection.
Overdiuresis.
Hypovolaemia.
Sedative and opiate drugs.
Diarrhoea and vomiting.
Dietary indiscretion.
Protein excess.
Acute worsening of chronic liver disease.
Urea and electrolyte abnormalities.
Uncontrolled diabetes.
Hypoglycaemia.
Surgery.

Epidemiology
- Chronic liver disease is usually progressive, so that most patients develop hepatic encephalopathy at some time, particularly secondary to a precipitant cause.
- Chronic encephalopathy is a rare syndrome.
- Subclinical or latent encephalopathy is present in most patients, but its clinical significance is unclear.
- Fulminant liver failure is a rare disorder that warrants immediate referral to a liver transplant centre.

Classification
Grade 1: confusion, altered behaviour, psychometric abnormalities.
Grade 2: drowsiness, altered behaviour.
Grade 3: stupor, obedience to simple commands, great confusion.
Grade 4: coma responsive to painful stimuli.
Grade 5: coma unresponsive to painful stimuli.

Treatment

Diet and lifestyle
- Patients must avoid dietary indiscretions (including alcoholic binges); a high-energy diet is indicated.
- Protein intake must be stopped for 24–48 h, then increased in 20 g/day aliquots from 20 g/day every 3 days to 60 g/day, if possible, to maintain adequate nutrition.
- The possible manifestations of encephalopathy must be explained to the patients so that early medical opinion can be obtained.

Pharmacological treatment
- The syndrome reverses when the precipitating causes are removed; hence, these must be treated.

For acute encephalopathy in chronic liver disease
Neutral or acid enemas twice daily to clear bowel.
Intravenous thiamine in alcoholics.
Oral antibiotics (metronidazole) in resistant cases for 5 days only.

Long-term treatment

Standard dosage	Lactulose or lactitol 20 ml twice daily or 1 sachet twice daily initially to produce two soft bowel motions daily; with dose adjustment by patient as needed.
Contraindications	Known hypersensitivity.
Special points	Protein intake should be reduced (minimum, 50 g/day) if patient is resistant; overall liver function should be improved, if possible; U&E monitored regularly if patient on diuretics; diabetes control optimized.
Main drug interactions	None known.
Main side effects	Bloatedness, flatulence.

Encephalopathy of fulminant liver failure
Correction of hypoglycaemia: 20% dextrose i.v.
Correction of electrolyte abnormalities.
Bowel decontamination: oral antibacterial and antifungal agents.
Early treatment of infection.
See Liver failure, fulminant *for further details*.

Other options
Oral bromocriptine: in some patients with chronic encephalopathy or rare spontaneous recurring acute or chronic encephalopathy; patients must be referred to a specialized centre.

Treatment aims
To correct or remove precipitating cause.
To prevent recurrence.

Other treatments
Refashioning, embolization, or ligation of surgical shunt.
Liver transplantation: for recurrent acute or chronic encephalopathy, some cases of chronic encephalopathy, and fulminant liver failure with adverse prognostic factors.

Prognosis
- Prognosis is determined by the underlying liver disease and avoidance of precipitating factors.

Follow-up and management
- Follow-up depends on the severity of the disease; patients usually should keep a 3-monthly diary and stool chart.

Key references
Butterworth RF: Pathogenesis and treatment of portal-systemic encephalopathy. *Dig Dis Sci* 1992, **37**:321–327.

Sherlock S, Dooley J (eds): Hepatic encephalopathy. In *Diseases of the Liver and Biliary System*. Oxford: Blackwell Scientific Publications, 1993, pp 86–101.

Hepatitis, acute G. Alexander

Diagnosis

Symptoms
- Symptoms range from absent or negligible to severe (rare), leading to occasionally life-threatening disease.

Headache, influenza, arthralgia, muscle pain, abdominal discomfort, nausea and vomiting: characterizing prodromal illness.

Hepatitic picture: may evolve into cholestatic disease, with pale stools, dark urine, and pruritis.

Virus infection: hepatitis C usually mild at onset; hepatitis A and B much milder illnesses in younger patients and probably not symptomatic before the age of 5 years; hepatitis E clinically more severe during pregnancy.

Signs
- Signs may be absent.

Jaundice.

Tender hepatomegaly.

Splenomegaly: in up to 25% of patients.

Stigmata of chronic liver disease: absent in uncomplicated acute hepatitis.

Hepatic fetor, hepatic encephalopathy or flap: signs of severe disease.

Investigations

Biochemical assays: should confirm hepatitic picture, with marked increase in serum transaminases, mild increase in alkaline phosphatase, variable increase in bilirubin; as disease progresses, cholestatic picture may evolve before recovery.

Full blood count or blood film: not usually helpful; features consistent with hypersplenism, however, suggest underlying chronic liver disease.

Prothrombin time: excellent prognostic value.

Virology tests: used with thought and precision on basis of probable cause, as follows:
Hepatitis A: to check for IgM antibody (present for 6–24 months; IgG antibody present for life).
Hepatitis B: to check for IgM anticore antibody (develops early in illness); hepatitis B surface antigen present in most symptomatic patients but may be eliminated quickly.
Hepatitis C: antibody may take several months to develop, although most patients become positive within 3 months.
Hepatitis D: sought by detection of total antibody; superinfection with hepatitis D virus in a chronic hepatitis B virus carrier (IgM anticore negative) must be differentiated from co-infection by hepatitis B (IgM anticore to hepatitis B positive).
Hepatitis E: can be sought by enzyme-linked immunosorbent assay.
Cytomegalovirus and Epstein–Barr virus: should be sought when viral cause suspected and other serological tests negative.

Liver biopsy: may be indicated in rare circumstances when diagnostic confusion exists or when underlying liver damage is suspected.

Screening for hepatitis B: source of infection may be carrier at risk of chronic liver disease, cirrhosis, and hepatocellular carcinoma; such a carrier must be screened and assessed because treatment may be beneficial.

Complications

Acute liver failure: rare.

Coma and death: rare.

Progression to chronic hepatitis.

Diagnosis of underlying chronic liver disease.

Differential diagnosis
Acute manifestation of chronic liver disease: e.g. acute onset of autoimmune disease with rapid progression.

Acute disease in a patient with underlying chronic liver disease: e.g. episode of acute alcoholic liver damage.

Aetiology
- Acute hepatitis is caused by the following:

Hepatitis A virus: transmitted by faecal–oral route; infection closely associated with foreign travel, consumption of shellfish, and some sexual practices; often, no source identified.

Hepatitis B virus: often transmitted sexually; vertical transmission also important; i.v. drug users at risk.

Hepatitis C virus: associated with i.v. drug use and transfusion; vertical transmission occurs; occasionally unexplained.

Hepatitis B and D virus: hepatitis D transmitted almost exclusively by i.v. drug use in UK, intrafamilial or other horizontal modes elsewhere.

Hepatitis E virus: transmitted by faecal–oral route.

Epstein–Barr virus.

Cytomegalovirus.

Epidemiology
- Local outbreaks of hepatitis A virus infection occur.
- Hepatitis E virus infection occurs in epidemics in developing countries (where people have little access to quality water).
- Carrier state for hepatitis B, C, and D may occur.

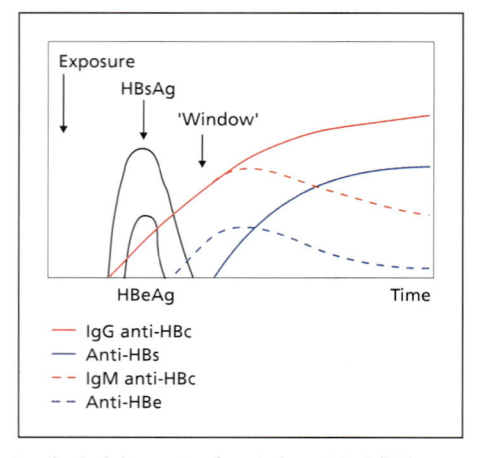

Serological diagnosis of acute hepatitis B (HB) infection. HBeAg, HBe antigen; HBsAg, HB surface antigen.

Treatment

Diet and lifestyle

- Avoidance of fat can be recommended in patients with acute hepatitis because fat intolerance is characteristic; ingestion does no harm but may cause discomfort.
- Abstinence from alcohol until recovery should be recommended; continued consumption may slow recovery and is associated with exacerbation of symptoms.
- Rest is recommended; many patients are unable to return to work for weeks or months and, even after return, may need time before normal function fully returns; academic performance may be suboptimal.
- Patients must understand the routes by which the hepatitis infection has been acquired and may therefore be transmitted; this may place certain restrictions on professional or sexual activities in the short term.

Pharmacological treatment

- The onset of jaundice is often associated with loss or significant reduction of infectivity in patients with hepatitis A and B; no specific treatment is available for acute viral hepatitis.
- Symptomatic improvement may be obtained in patients with prolonged cholestasis by ursodeoxycholic acid 600 mg at night, which is extremely safe, without significant drug interactions or side effects.
- For hepatitis A virus, an effective vaccine is available for protective immunization; immunoglobulin has a well defined role in short-term prophylaxis and for household contacts of patients with acute hepatitis.
- For hepatitis B virus, an effective vaccine is available; vaccination soon after exposure may still be effective; hepatitis B immunoglobulin no longer has a role in this setting but is given with vaccination to infants born of mothers who are hepatitis B surface antigen positive.

Treatment aims

To treat the symptoms.
To prevent infection.

Prognosis

- Acute hepatitis is often a debilitating illness, but recovery is usual, although patients may experience fatigue for several months before full recovery.
- Most patients infected by hepatitis C virus and some infected by hepatitis B become carriers; for the latter, chronic infection is rare after a severe, acute illness.
- The immediate prognosis for patients with hepatitis C who become carriers is excellent; chronic liver disease may develop but after a prolonged period.

Follow-up and management

- Patients with acute hepatitis A, B, or E should be followed until the liver function tests have clearly settled and the patient has made a full symptomatic recovery.
- Patients with hepatitis B should also be followed until hepatitis B surface antigen is eliminated; persistence of hepatitis Be antigen beyond 6 weeks suggests that a carrier state may be evolving.
- For hepatitis D, the prognosis depends ultimately on the outcome of the hepatitis B infection; a patient who remains hepatitis B surface antigen positive may well develop chronic liver disease; follow-up should therefore be for life.
- In the present state of uncertainty about the prognosis of patients with hepatitis C, they should be followed every 6–12 months unless evidence for persistent hepatitis C is lacking, i.e. disappearance of hepatitis C virus antibody or RNA.

Key references

Bradley DW: Virology, molecular biology and serology of hepatitis C virus. *Transfus Med Rev* 1992, **6**:93–102.

Brown JL *et al.*: The hepatitis B virus. *Baillières Clin Gastroenterol* 1990, **4**:721–747.

Krawczynski K: Hepatitis E. *Hepatology* 1993, **17**:932–941.

Ross BL *et al.*: Hepatitis A virus and hepatitis A infection. *Ad Virus Res* 1991, **39**:209–257.

Hepatitis, chronic
J.P. Watson and M.F. Bassendine

Diagnosis

Symptoms
- Often no symptoms are manifest.

Malaise, nausea, abdominal pain.

Arthralgia: in autoimmune disease.

Signs
- Often few clinical signs of chronic liver disease are manifest.

Palmar erythema and spider naevi: in some patients.

Gynaecomastia, abdominal striae, splenomegaly: possibly.

Jaundice: unusual in mild disease.

Hepatomegaly: unusual because liver is usually small or normal size.

Tattoos and needle track marks on arms: should be sought in viral hepatitis.

Investigations
Liver function tests: show chronic hepatocellular disease, with raised alanine transaminase (ALT), normal alkaline phosphatase, and normal or low albumin.

Coagulation screening: impaired hepatic synthetic function causes prolonged prothrombin time.

Full blood count: hypersplenism can cause leucopenia and thrombocytopenia.

Autoantibody analysis: antinuclear factor, double-stranded DNA, smooth-muscle antibody, and liver kidney microsomal antibody can all be positive in autoimmune disease.

Immunoglobulin measurement: IgG concentration raised in autoimmune disease.

Hepatitis B serology: interpreted as follows:
Immune, post-vaccination: surface antibody (sAb)+, surface antigen (sAg)–, c antibody (cAb)–, e antigen (eAg)–, e antibody (eAb)–, DNA–.
Immune, past exposure to hepatitis B virus: sAb+, sAg–, cAb+, eAg–, eAb+, DNA–.
Infected, low risk of transmission: sAb–, sAg+, cAb+, eAg–, eAb+, DNA–.
Infected, high risk of transmission: sAb–, sAg+, cAb+, eAg+, eAb–, DNA+.

Hepatitis C serology: interpreted as follows:
Positive, active disease: enzyme-linked immunosorbent assay (ELISA)+, recombinant immunoblot assay (RIBA)+ (2–4 bands), ALT increased, RNA+.
Positive, no active disease (perhaps immune): ELISA+, RIBA+ (2–4 bands), ALT normal, RNA–.
False-positive: ELISA+, RIBA– or indeterminate (1 band), ALT normal, RNA–.

Genetic marker analysis: HLA B8 and DRW 3 associated with autoimmune disease.

Copper, caeruloplasmin, alpha-1 antitrypsin measurement.

Liver ultrasonography or CT: often normal but may show small liver with splenomegaly.

Liver biopsy for histology: shows the following:
Hepatitis B/D virus: inflammatory cells spreading into parenchyma from enlarged portal tracts; hepatitis B surface antigen on immunohistochemistry; hepatitis D infection increases severity and can be detected by immunohistochemistry.
Hepatitis C virus: usually mild chronic hepatitis with lobular component, prominent lymphoid follicles in portal tracts, acidophil body formation, focal hepatocellular necrosis; no immunohistochemical staining currently available.
Autoimmune disease: periportal inflammatory infiltrate and piecemeal necrosis; negative to hepatitis B/D staining on immunohistochemistry.

Complications
Cirrhosis: in 20% of patients.

Variceal bleeding, portosystemic encephalopathy, ascites: due to portal hypertension.

Hepatocellular carcinoma: increased incidence in male patients with hepatitis B or C virus infection.

Differential diagnosis
Primary biliary cirrhosis: pruritus, common in middle-aged women, positive antimitochondrial antibody, bile-duct obliteration by lymphocytic infiltrate and granuloma formation (on liver biopsy).

Primary sclerosing cholangitis: associated with ulcerative colitis, strictured and beaded intrahepatic bile ducts (on endoscopic retrograde cholangiopancreatography).

Granulomatous hepatitis: multiple granulomata (on liver biopsy), sarcoid, tuberculosis, histoplasmosis, Q fever, brucella, lymphoma.

Alcoholic liver disease: inappropriately raised gamma glutamyl transferase (on liver function tests), raised mean cell volume (on full blood count), steatosis, Mallory's hyaline, necrosis of liver cells, and infiltration with polymorphonuclear leucocytes (on liver biopsy).

Aetiology
- Causes include the following:

Viral infection: hepatitis B, C, or D (B/D in 20% of patients, C in 40%).

Autoimmune disorder (in 25%).

Drugs: methyldopa, isoniazid, oxyphenisatin.

Genetic: Wilson's disease, alpha-1 antitrypsin deficiency.

Epidemiology
- Autoimmune hepatitis is more common in northern Europe.
- Viral hepatitis, particularly hepatitis C and D, is more common in southern Europe.

Treatment

Diet and lifestyle
- Alcohol must be avoided.
- Patients infected by hepatitis B virus must be advised on barrier methods of contraception unless the partner is vaccinated.

Pharmacological treatment
- Treatment should be given under specialist supervision.

For hepatitis B virus infection
- Treatment is indicated for patients with histological evidence of chronic hepatitis or who are positive for hepatitis B e antigen or virus DNA.

Standard dosage	Interferon-α s.c. 3 times weekly for 4–6 months.
Contraindications	Hypersensitivity.
Main drug interactions	None.
Main side effects	*Induction:* fever up to 39°C, malaise, arthralgia, myalgia, headache, anorexia, nausea, vomiting, diarrhoea. *Maintenance:* fatigue, anorexia, weight loss, alopecia, depression, neutropenia, thrombocytopenia, exacerbation of autoimmune disease, induction of thyroid disease (particularly in hepatitis C patients), myalgia.

- Steroid pretreatment may cause rebound immune stimulation; available data do not indicate that combination is superior to interferon alone.

For hepatitis C virus infection
- Treatment is indicated for patients with histological evidence of hepatitis or who are positive for recombinant immunoblot assay (2–4 bands) or virus RNA.
- Remission persists in only 25% of patients after treatment is stopped.

Standard dosage	Interferon-α s.c. 3 times weekly for 6–12 months. Ribavirin 1000–1200 mg orally daily for 6 months.
Contraindications	*Interferon-α:* hypersensitivity.
Special points	*Ribavirin:* currently being evaluated in clinical trials.
Main drug interactions	None.
Main side effects	*Interferon-α:* as above. *Ribavirin:* nausea, vomiting, haemolytic anaemia, insomnia, exacerbation of gout.

For hepatitis D virus infection
- Patients may respond to interferon-α, but remission does not usually persist after treatment is discontinued.

For autoimmune disease
- Treatment is indicated for patients with raised transaminase and IgG, histological evidence of chronic hepatitis, and positive ANF, SMA, LKM antibodies.

Standard dosage	Prednisolone 20–40 mg initially, reduced gradually (depending on clinical response); 5–10 mg daily maintenance dose often needed. Azathioprine 50–70 mg orally daily as adjunct.
Contraindications	Systemic infection.
Main drug interactions	None.
Main side effects	*Steroids:* osteoporosis, proximal myopathy, skin thinning, cataracts, diabetes mellitus, weight gain, amenorrhoea, depression, hypertension.

Vaccination
Hepatitis B: surface antigen suspension 20 μg i.m. injection at 0, 1, and 6 months; surface antibody must be >100 IU after third dose to ensure adequate seroconversion (if inadequate, a fourth dose should be given).
Hepatitis C: no vaccine available.
Hepatitis D: protection provided by adequate hepatitis B vaccination.

Treatment aims
To induce remission and thus prevent progression to cirrhosis.
To eliminate active replication of viruses.

Other treatments
- Orthotopic liver transplantation is the treatment of choice for end-stage liver disease in chronic hepatitis.
- The 5-year survival rate is 50–70%, depending on the cause.
- Pretreatment with antiviral therapy is recommended in patients with hepatitis B, C, or D virus infection to reduce or eliminate viral load before transplantation.

Prognosis
- Only a few patients with viral hepatitis respond to interferon-α in the long term (hepatitis B virus 35%, hepatitis C 25%).
- Maintenance immunosuppression is usually needed in autoimmune chronic hepatitis.

Follow-up and management
- During interferon-α treatment, patients must be monitored closely for leucopenia and thrombocytopenia, and autoantibodies and thyroid function must be checked because autoimmune disease can be exacerbated.
- Patients on long-term corticosteroid treatment should be monitored for diabetes mellitus and should have annual bone densitometry to check for osteoporosis.
- Patients who have progressed to cirrhosis should have alpha fetoprotein and liver ultrasound screening every 6 months because they are at risk of hepatocellular carcinoma.

Key references
Jacyna MR, Thomas HC: Antiviral therapy: hepatitis B. *Br Med Bull* 1990, **46**:368–382.

Lake JR, Wright TL: Liver transplantation for patients with hepatitis B: what have we learned from our results? *Hepatology* 1992, **13**:796–799.

Mitchison HC, Bassendine MF: Autoimmune liver disease. In *Recent Advances in Gastroenterology*. Edited by Pounder RE. Edinburgh: Churchill Livingstone, 1990, pp 225–243.

Scheuer PJ: Classification of chronic viral hepatitis: a need for reassessment. *J Hepatol* 1991, **13**:372–374.

Hepatocellular carcinoma — G.M. Dusheiko

Diagnosis

Symptoms
- Small hepatocellular carcinomas (<2 cm diameter) are asymptomatic; symptoms are usually manifest when the diameter is at least 10 cm.
- Onset is insidious.

Upper abdominal pain: right hypochondrial or epigastric.
Weight loss, weakness, anorexia.
Abdominal swelling: may be due to ascites or enlarged liver.
Low-grade pyrexia.
Features of cirrhosis.
Metastatic symptoms: e.g. bone pain.

Signs
Enlarged liver: hard and nodular surface.
Hepatic tenderness.
Arterial bruit: heard in 20% of patients.
Ascites.
Splenomegaly: in 20–30%.
Wasting: with more advanced disease.
Jaundice: in later stages of illness.
Pityriasis rotunda.

Investigations
Biochemistry: aspartate aminotransferase frequently higher than alanine aminotransferase; raised alkaline phosphatase concentration found in 60% of patients.
Haematology: may show evidence of pancytopenia (hypersplenism) or erythrocytosis.
Tumour marker analysis: combined with ultrasonography for early detection; alpha fetoprotein possibly normal in small hepatocellular carcinoma; fucosylated alpha fetoprotein may aid differentiation from rises seen in chronic hepatitis; des-gamma-carboxyprothrombin and carcinoembryonic antigen concentrations possibly raised; transcobalamin 1 and neurotensin concentrations raised in fibrolamellar variant.
Chest radiography: shows raised right hemidiaphragm or metastases.
CT: shows extent of tumour.
Ultrasonography: useful for screening patients with cirrhosis for small hepatocellular carcinoma; 1-cm lesions can be detected, often as hypoechoic lesions.
Coeliac axis angiography: tumours usually vascular and show features of malignant circulation.
Lipiodol CT: essential if surgery planned; most sensitive method for detecting small hepatocellular carcinoma; lipiodol, an oil contrast medium, cleared by hepatocytes but not by hepatocellular carcinoma; CT done 2 weeks after intra-arterial injection.
CT portography: frequently more sensitive than CT or MRI for small deposits.
MRI: diagnosis accuracy equal to CT.
Liver biopsy: aimed biopsy usually indicated; thin needle preferable to prevent seeding; aspiration biopsy can be used but less diagnostic.

Complications
Acute intraperitoneal haemorrhage: may be terminal.
Intravascular and intraductal growth.
Portal vein, inferior vena cava, and right atrial involvement.
Metastases: lung, bone, skin, brain, adrenal, and lymphogenous.
Hypoglycaemia, hypercalcaemia, polycythaemia, hyperlipidaemia, porphyria cutanea tarda, dysfibrinogenaemia.
Hepatic failure.
Variceal bleeding.

Differential diagnosis
Cystic lesions, hepatic metastatic carcinoma from other sites, abscess, adenoma, focal nodular hyperplasia.
Benign haemangioma.

Aetiology
- Most cases of hepatocellular carcinoma coexist with cirrhosis, including disease caused by the following:

Chronic hepatitis B or C virus infection.
Alcohol abuse.
Autoimmune hepatitis or primary biliary cirrhosis.
Haemochromatosis.
Other inherited disorders of metabolism.
Tyrosinosis, alpha-1-antitrypsin deficiency.
Environmental carcinogens: aflatoxin is a potent chemical carcinogen, produced by *Aspergillus flavus*, which contaminates food in high-incidence areas; genetic changes have been documented.
Membranous inferior vena cava obstruction.
Androgenic anabolic steroids.
Contraceptives (uncertain).

Epidemiology
- Areas of high, intermediate, and low incidence correspond crudely to prevalence of hepatitis B and C infection; low-incidence areas include northern Europe and North America.
- Hepatocellular carcinoma is more frequent in immigrants from high- and intermediate-prevalence countries (sub-Saharan Africa, China, southern and eastern Europe, Middle East).

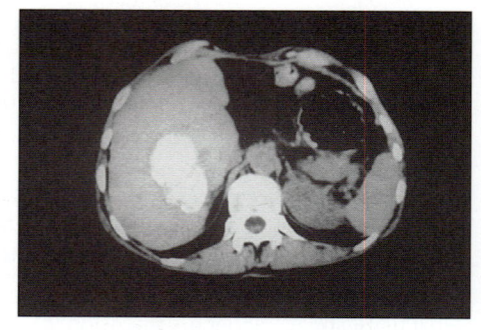

Retention of lipiodol within a hepatocellular carcinoma.

Treatment

Diet and lifestyle
- No special precautions are necessary.

Pharmacological treatment

Targeted therapies
- Alcohol is generally used in patients with 1–3 nodules <3 cm.
- Lipiodol-targeted chemotherapy, given under specialist supervision, is indicated for non-resectable carcinoma in patients with Child's A or B cirrhosis.

Standard dosage	Alcohol 10–20 ml intratumoural injection 3 times weekly for up to 12 treatments.
	Injected chemotherapy (including doxorubicin, mitomycin, and cisplatin) linked to lipiodol by emulsification, repeated every 2–3 months if necessary.
Contraindications	*Alcohol:* large (>3 cm) or multiple (>3) tumours.
Special points	*Alcohol:* causes immediate coagulative necrosis; cheap and widely available; trials needed to establish whether this is an alternative to surgery or should be reserved for small tumours not suitable for resection.
	Lipiodol-targeted chemotherapy: activity of cytotoxic agents may be prolonged by retention of lipiodol within tumour; tumour necrosis has been shown, but no definitive evidence shows that prognosis is changed.
Main drug interactions	None of importance.
Main side effects	*Alcohol:* pain, fever, intrahepatic or intraperitoneal bleeding.
	Lipiodol-targeted chemotherapy: abdominal pain, nausea, fever, abnormal aminotransferases (common); leucopenia, alopecia, pancreatitis, gastric mucosal lesions, jaundice, cholecystitis (rare); fatal hepatocellular failure may occur in patients with Child's C cirrhosis.

Chemotherapy for palliation
- Treatment should be given under specialist supervision.

Standard dosage	Doxorubicin, epirubicin, cisplatin, mitozantrone every 3–4 weeks.
Contraindications	*All:* hypersensitivity.
	Doxorubicin: bone-marrow suppression, buccal ulcerations (after first dose).
	Cisplatin: pre-existing renal impairment, hearing disorders, bone-marrow suppression.
Special points	Other adjunctive agents, e.g. tamoxifen, interferon, and interleukin 2 may be used.
	Doxorubicin: ECG, ejection fraction, and echocardiogram must be monitored.
	Cisplatin: hydration must be maintained; blood count, serum creatinine, and blood-urea-nitrogen must be monitored; audiometry needed.
Main drug interactions	*Cisplatin:* use with aminoglycoside or cephalosporins may cause increased ototoxicity or nephrotoxicity.
Main side effects	*Doxorubicin:* mucositis, bone-marrow suppression, alopecia, nausea, vomiting, diarrhoea, cardiotoxicity.
	Cisplatin: nephrotoxicity, myelosuppression, neurotoxicity, ototoxicity, immunosuppression, nausea, vomiting.
	Mitozantrone: leucopenia, thrombocytopenia, anaemia, nausea, vomiting, alopecia, diarrhoea, mucositis, cardiovascular effects (rare), blue-green discoloration of urine.

Lipiodol ^{131}I radiotherapy
- By replacing part of the iodine component of lipiodol with radioactive ^{131}I, tumourocidal radiotherapy can be selectively delivered to hepatocellular carcinoma; retention of the isotope results in sustained irradiation and necrosis of tumour foci.

Treatment aims
To cure disease or prolong survival without recurrence.
To alleviate symptoms.

Other treatments
Transcatheter arterial embolization: for unresectable carcinoma, not for portal-vein thrombosis or Child's C cirrhosis; side effects include abdominal pain and fever; can be used with lipiodol-targeted chemotherapy.

Local resection or segmentectomy: potential cure but high recurrence rates in patients with cirrhosis; for selected patients with small tumours involving one lobe of liver; preoperative lipiodol-targeted chemotherapy or transcatheter arterial embolization can be added.

Hepatic transplantation: for patients with ≤3 small lesions (<3 cm) after exclusion of extrahepatic spread; side effects include recurrence of hepatitis B and C.

Prognosis
- <25% of patients have partial responses to current chemotherapeutic regimens.
- 60% 5-year survival rates have been reported after intratumoural injection of alcohol for small tumours.
- The 5-year survival rate of lipiodol combined with surgical resection for small tumours is 70%.
- 1-year survival rates of 78% after transcatheter arterial embolization are reported.
- Perioperative mortality is 10%; the 5-year survival rate after surgery is 25%; patients with encapsulated tumours, negative resection margins, no intracapsular or intravascular invasion of tumour cells, and Child's class A have better prognosis.

Follow-up and management
- Imaging of the liver, lung, and bones is needed every 2 months to detect recurrence.
- Serial alpha-fetoprotein concentrations should be measured if initially high.

Key references
Dusheiko GM *et al.*: Treatment of small hepatocellular carcinomas. *Lancet* 1992, **340**:285–288.

Okuda K: Hepatocellular carcinoma: Recent progress. *Hepatology* 1992, **15**: 948–963.

Liver failure, fulminant — J. O'Grady

Diagnosis

Symptoms

Lethargy, nausea, vomiting: prodromal symptoms of viral hepatitis.
Abdominal pain, haematemesis: common after paracetamol overdose.
Drowsiness or confusion: in grades 1 and 2 encephalopathy.
Restlessness, agitation: possibly aggressive; in grade 3.
Unresponsiveness: in grade 4.

Signs

Jaundice: usual but not always manifest at presentation.
Encephalopathy of varying severity: although foetor and asterixis are not prominent features.
Normal or reduced liver size: although hepatomegaly suggests malignancy or Budd–Chiari syndrome.
Ascites: late finding.
Systemic hypertension, decerebrate posturing, hyperventilation: indicating cerebral oedema.

Investigations

- Extensive investigations are needed, but the following are particularly important:

Prothrombin time or INR measurement: prognostic significance in all cases.
Haemoglobin measurement: haemolytic anaemia suggests Wilson's disease.
Platelet count: thrombocytopenia may occur in paracetamol-induced cases.
Serum bilirubin measurement: prognostic significance in non-paracetamol-induced cases.
Serum creatinine measurement: urea underestimates renal impairment; prognostic significance in paracetamol-induced cases.
Arterial pH and electrolytes measurement: pH has prognostic significance in paracetamol-induced cases.
Glucose measurement: regularly to detect hypoglycaemia.
Amylase measurement: especially in paracetamol-induced cases.
Paracetamol measurement.
Hepatitis A serology: to detect IgM anti-hepatitis A virus.
Hepatitis B and D serology: to detect IgM anti-core, hepatitis B surface antigen, anti-hepatitis D virus.
Ultrasonography: to assess liver size and texture.

Complications

- All of the following are late complications, mainly occurring in patients with advanced encephalopathy.

Hypoglycaemia.
Renal failure: in 75% of paracetamol-induced cases and 30% of other cases.
Cerebral oedema: in 40–70%.
Bleeding, infection: bacterial in 80–90%, fungal in 30%.
Respiratory failure.
Hypotension.

Differential diagnosis

Acute decompensation of chronic liver disease.
Reye's syndrome.
Other metabolic encephalopathy.

Aetiology

- Causes include the following:

Paracetamol ingestion: in >50% of patients in the UK.
Hepatitis A, B, B/D, or E virus infection, seronegative hepatitis (non-A, non-B, non-C), halothane hepatitis, idiosyncratic drug reactions.
Pregnancy-related, Budd–Chiari syndrome, autoimmune liver disease, malignancy, mushroom poisoning.

Epidemiology

- Fulminant liver failure complicates 0.1–4.7% of hospitalized patients with viral hepatitis, depending on the cause.

Classification

Hyperacute liver failure
Encephalopathy within 7 days of onset of jaundice, characterized by high incidence of cerebral oedema; despite this, many patients survive with medical management.

Acute liver failure
Encephalopathy within 8–28 days of onset of jaundice, high incidence of cerebral oedema, but poorer prognosis without liver transplantation.

Subacute liver failure
Encephalopathy 5–12 weeks after onset of jaundice, low incidence of cerebral oedema and less severe prolongation of prothrombin times, but poor prognosis.

Treatment

Diet and lifestyle
- Parenteral or enteral nutritional support is usually needed.
- Survivors return to a normal diet and lifestyle, unless they are recipients of liver grafts, in which case they need lifelong follow-up and immunosuppressive treatment.

Pharmacological treatment

N-acetylcysteine
- Indications have been extended after paracetamol ingestion; administration >16 h after overdose is beneficial.
- It also improves haemodynamics in patients with oxygen debt, irrespective of cause.

Standard dosage	N-acetylcysteine 150 mg/kg loading dose, followed by 6.2 mg/kg/h.
Contraindications	Hypersensitivity.
Special points	Lower threshold for starting treatment in patients on enzyme-inducing drugs and chronic alcohol consumers.
Main drug interactions	None.
Main side effects	Occasional hypersensitivity reactions.

Gastric protection
- H_2 antagonists or sucralfate reduce the incidence of gastrointestinal bleeding.

Standard dosage	Ranitidine 50 mg i.v. 8-hourly. Sucralfate 1 g 6-hourly.
Contraindications	Hypersensitivity.
Main drug interactions	None relevant.
Main side effects	*Ranitidine:* thrombocytopenia.

Selective bowel decontamination
- Treatment reduces the incidence of sepsis if started early.

Standard dosage	Colistin 100 mg, tobramycin 80 mg, or amphotericin B 500 mg, all 6-hourly.
Contraindications	Hypersensitivity.
Main drug interactions	None.
Main side effects	None.

Lactulose or lactitol
- This is usually ineffective and recommended only in patients with grade 1 or 2 encephalopathy.

Standard dosage	Lactulose 30 ml or lactitol 200 mg/kg, each 8-hourly; doses titrated to two bowel movements daily.
Contraindications	Gastrointestinal obstruction, galactosaemia, lactose intolerance.
Main drug interactions	*Lactitol:* antacids, neomycin.
Main side effects	Nausea, flatulence, abdominal discomfort.

Treatment aims
To anticipate and treat complications.

Other treatments
- Liver transplantation is indicated for the following:

Paracetamol-induced cases
Metabolic acidosis >24 h after overdose (pH <7.3, or <7.25 if treated by N-acetylcysteine). Coexistent advanced encephalopathy, renal failure (serum creatinine concentration >300 µmol/L) and prothrombin time >100 s.

Non-paracetamol-induced cases
Prothrombin time >100 s or three of the following:
Seronegative or drug induced hepatitis.
Age <10 years or >40 years.
Acute or subacute liver failure.
Prothrombin time >50 s.
Serum bilirubin concentration >300 µmol/L.

Prognosis
- Survival rates are 40–80% for patients progressing to grade 4 encephalopathy, depending on the underlying cause.
- Most patients who do not progress beyond grade 2 encephalopathy survive.
- Survivors make complete recoveries; progression to chronic liver disease is unusual.

Follow-up and management
- Long-term medical follow-up is rarely needed, except in liver-graft recipients.
- Psychiatric and social support is important in overdose cases.

Key references
Blei AT et al.: Complications of intracranial pressure monitoring in fulminant hepatic failure. *Lancet* 1993, **341**:157–158.

Harrison PM et al.: Improvement by N-acetylcysteine of hemodynamics and oxygen transport in fulminant hepatic failure. *N Engl J Med* 1991, **324**:1853–1857.

O'Grady JG, Portmann BC, Williams R: Fulminant hepatic failure. In *Fulminant Hepatic Failure.* Edited by Schiff E, Schiff L. Philadelphia, JB Lippincott, 1993, pp 1077–1090.

O'Grady JG, Schalm SW, Williams R: Acute liver failure: redefining the syndromes. *Lancet* 1993, **342**:273–275.

Ronaldo N et al.: Prospective study of bacterial infection in liver failure: an analysis of fifty patients. *Hepatology* 1990, **11**:49–53.

Variceal bleeding
P.A. McCormick

Diagnosis

Symptoms and signs
Major haematemesis or melaena.
Chronic blood loss, with iron-deficiency anaemia: indicating portal-hypertensive gastropathy.
- Sites of bleeding in patients with portal hypertension are oesophageal (most frequent); fundal, lesser curve, antral, in hiatus hernia (gastric varices); ileostomy, colostomy, colonic, and rectal (ectopic varices). These may give massive rectal bleeding.

Investigations
Gastroscopy, barium swallow and meal: to identify varices.
Doppler ultrasonography, angiography: to establish patency of portal vein.
Blood tests, CT, liver biopsy: to identify underlying liver disease.
Measurement of portal venous, wedged hepatic venous, splenic pulp, and intra-variceal pressure: endoscopic needle, endoscopic pressure gauge; special investigations, mainly for research use.
Measurement of azygos blood flow: to estimate variceal blood flow (research use).

Complications
Infection: in ~30% of patients during admission.
Renal failure: acute tubular necrosis, hepatorenal syndrome.
Delirium tremens, Wernicke–Korsakoff syndrome: related to alcohol withdrawal.
Ascites: precipitated by fluid overload.
Portal systemic encephalopathy: precipitated by blood in gut and liver hypoxia.

Differential diagnosis
Bleeding caused by the following:
Peptic ulcer.
Mallory–Weiss tear.
Gastric erosions.
Gastric carcinoma.
Portal-hypertensive gastropathy.
Gastric vascular malformations.
Other sources of gastrointestinal bleeding.

Aetiology
- Precipitants of variceal bleeding include the following:
Infection.
Drugs: e.g. aspirin, NSAIDs.
Development of hepatocellular carcinoma or portal-vein thrombosis in cirrhotic patients.
Heavy alcohol binges in cirrhotic patients.

Epidemiology
- ~10% of UK patients presenting with upper gastrointestinal bleeding have varices.
- Varices develop in 90% of patients with cirrhosis; the risk of haemorrhage is highest in the first 2 years after identification.
- The risk of bleeding is highest in patients with large oesophageal varices (>5 mm diameter), red signs on varices, and poor liver function.

Conditions complicated by variceal bleeding
Precirrhotic severe alcoholic hepatitis/fatty liver.
Cirrhosis.
Schistosomiasis.
Portal-vein thrombosis.
Splenic-vein thrombosis: usually causes gastric fundal varices, with no oesophageal varices.
Budd–Chiari syndrome.
Congenital hepatic fibrosis.
Idiopathic portal hypertension.
Nodular regenerative hyperplasia of liver.
Partial nodular transformation of liver.

Pugh's modified grading of the severity of liver disease

Points	1	2	3
Encephalopathy	None	Grade 1–2	Grade 3–4
Ascites	Absent	Slight	Moderate
Bilirubin (µmol/L)	<34	34–51	>51
Albumin (g/L)	>35	28–35	<28
Prothrombin (secs, prolonged)	1–3	4–10	>10

Pugh's grade A, 5–6; B, 7–9; C, 10–15 points.

Treatment

Diet and lifestyle
- Patients must avoid NSAIDs or aspirin.
- Alcohol should be avoided if the liver disease is alcoholic cirrhosis.
- Patients should be cautioned about travelling to underdeveloped areas with poor medical services.

Pharmacological treatment

Emergency drug treatment
- Drugs are useful when emergency endoscopy is not available or is delayed.
- Somatostatin and octreotide are as effective as terlipressin and have fewer side effects.

Terlipressin 2 mg i.v. bolus and 1 mg 4–6-hourly i.v. for 24 h, possible with transdermal nitroglycerin 10 mg/12 h.

Octreotide 25–50 µg/h i.v. for 5 days.

Somatostatin 250 µg i.v. bolus and 250 µg/h i.v. for 5 days.

Vasopressin: now obsolete.

Prophylaxis: primary and secondary
- Propranolol or nadolol reduces the risk of first haemorrhage; the resting pulse rate should be reduced to 60 beats/min or by 25%. Treatment is recommended in cirrhotic patients with large varices and red signs.
- For prevention of recurrent haemorrhage, drugs are cheaper than endoscopic sclerotherapy or banding, but many patients cannot tolerate beta blockade.

Non-pharmacological treatment

Resuscitation
Airway protection to prevent aspiration.

Insertion of large i.v. line (cross-matching of at least 6 units blood).

Crystalloid and colloid infusion to maintain circulation while cross-matched blood awaited.

Vasoconstriction.

Possible use of filters and blood warmers after transfusion of 4 units of blood.

Insertion of central venous line to guide further replacement therapy when systolic blood pressure >100 mmHg.

Fresh frozen plasma to correct clotting abnormalities.

Platelet transfusion occasionally.

Emergency treatment
Emergency endoscopy to confirm variceal bleeding.

Emergency endoscopic sclerotherapy or banding: treatment of choice; complications include fever, aspiration, oesophageal perforation, and mediastinitis; gastric fundal varices respond poorly to sclerotherapy.

Balloon tamponade for temporary control of torrential bleeding; many complications.

Other options
Transjugular intrahepatic portal-systemic stent shunt: if emergency endoscopic treatment fails; also under evaluation for prevention of recurrent haemorrhages, but high rate of shunt occlusion (30% at 1 year).

Emergency shunt surgery.

Emergency oesophageal transection.

Liver transplantation: can be considered for prevention of recurrent haemorrhage in patients with liver failure.

Treatment aims
- The aims of treatment, in order of importance, are as follows:
To resuscitate.
To control bleeding quickly.
To maintain liver function.
To identify and treat complications.
To prevent rebleeding.

Prognosis
- Sclerotherapy has high success rates, with bleeding controlled in 90% of patients after 2–3 sessions.
- 70% of patients rebleed after balloon tamponade, so definitive treatment must be arranged.
- Mortality is 30–40% with the first variceal bleed, 15–20% with subsequent bleeds.
- Prognosis depends on the underlying liver function.
- Approximately one-third of deaths in cirrhotic patients are related to bleeding.

Follow-up and management
- Patients should be followed-up every 3 months for the first year after the varices have been obliterated by sclerotherapy, then 6-monthly, or again 3-monthly if a stent is inserted and then yearly.

Key references
Burroughs A, Bosch J: Clinical manifestations and management of bleeding episodes in cirrhotics. In *Oxford Textbook of Clinical Hepatology*. Edited by McIntyre N et al. Oxford: Oxford University Press, 1991, pp 408–425.

Rossle M et al.: The transjugular intrahepatic portosystemic stent-shunt procedure for variceal bleeding. *N Engl J Med* 1994, **330**:165–171.

Stiegman GV et al: Endoscopic sclerotherapy as compared with endoscopic ligation for bleeding oesophageal varices. *N Engl J Med* 1992, **326**:1527–1532.

Index

A

abdominal
   pain 2, 6, 10, 12
   striae 12
abscess, hepatic 14
acetaminophen *see* paracetamol
acetylcysteine for fulminant liver failure 17
adenoma, hepatic 14
alcohol
   abuse 14
   for hepatocellular carcinoma 15
   withdrawal 8, 18
amoxycillin for spontaneous bacterial peritonitis 3
amphotericin B for fulminant liver failure 17
ampicillin for primary sclerosing cholangitis 5
anaemia
   haemolytic 16
   iron-deficiency 18
antibiotics
   for hepatic encephalopathy 9
   for primary sclerosing cholangitis 5
   for spontaneous bacterial peritonitis 3
ascites 2, 4, 6, 12, 14, 16, 18
aspiration 8, 19
azathioprine for chronic hepatitis 13

B

balloon
   dilatation for primary sclerosing cholangitis 5
   tamponade for variceal bleeding 19
Besnier–Boeck disease *see* sarcoidosis
beta blockade for variceal bleeding 19
bile-duct
   obstruction, common *see* cholestasis
   stone 4
biliary
   cirrhosis, primary 4, 6, 12
   duct leak 2
bleeding 16 *see also* haemorrhage
   antral 18
   colonic 18
   fundal 18
   gastrointestinal 8, 18
   oesophageal 18
   rectal 18
   variceal 12, 14, 18
blood
   loss, chronic 18
   pressure, high *see* hypertension
bowel
   decontamination
      for fulminant liver failure 17
      for hepatic encephalopathy 9
   disease, inflammatory 4
brain
   atrophy 8
   damage, alcoholic 8
bromocriptine for hepatic encephalopathy 9
bromocrytin *see* bromocriptine
bruising *see* haematoma
Budd–Chiari syndrome 2, 16, 18
Burkitt's lymphoma *see* Epstein–Barr virus

C

cancer *see* malignancy
carcinoma
   gastric 18
   hepatocellular 6, 10, 12, 14, 18
cefotaxime for spontaneous bacterial peritonitis 3
ceftizoxime for spontaneous bacterial peritonitis 3
cephalosporins for primary sclerosing cholangitis 5
Chiari's disease *see* Budd–Chiari syndrome
cholangiocarcinoma 4
cholangiopathy, AIDS 4
cholangitis 6
   primary sclerosing 4, 6, 12
cholestasis 4, 6, 11
cholestyramine
   for primary biliary cirrhosis 7
   for primary sclerosing cholangitis 5
ciprofloxacin
   for primary sclerosing cholangitis 5
   for spontaneous bacterial peritonitis 3
cirrhosis 2, 4, 10, 12, 14, 18
   primary biliary 4, 6, 12
cisplatin for hepatocellular carcinoma 15
coeliac disease 6
colestipol for primary biliary cirrhosis 7
colistin for fulminant liver failure 17
colitis, ulcerative 4, 12
confusion 16
constipation 8
CREST syndrome 6
cytomegalovirus 10

D

delirium tremens 18
demyelination 8
dextrose for hepatic encephalopathy 9
diabetes mellitus 8, 13
doxorubicin for hepatocellular carcinoma 15
dysfibrinogenaemia 14

E

embolization, transcatheter arterial, for hepatocellular carcinoma 15
encephalitis 8
encephalopathy 2, 4, 16
   acute 8
   chronic 8
   hepatic 8, 10 *see also* liver failure, fulminant
   latent 8
   portal systemic 12, 18 *see also* liver failure, fulminant
   subclinical 8
   Wernicke's 8
enema for acute encephalopathy in chronic liver disease 9
enteropathy, protein-losing 2
epirubicin for hepatocellular carcinoma 15
Epstein–Barr virus 10
erythema, palmar 4, 12
erythrocytosis 14

F

fibrosis 4
   congenital hepatic 18
   pulmonary 6
fits, focal 8
foetor, hepatic 8, 10, 16
frusemide for ascites 3

G

gastric
   carcinoma 18
   erosion 18
   varices 18
   vascular malformation 18
gastropathy, portal hypertensive 18
glomerulonephritis 6
granuloma 6

Index

granulomata 12
gynaecomastia 12

H

H₂ antagonists for fulminant liver failure 17
haemangioma 14
haematemesis 16, 18
haematoma, subdural 8
haemochromatosis 14
haemorrhage *see also* bleeding
    gastrointestinal 2
    intraperitoneal 14
    variceal 4, 6
hepatic *see also* liver
    abscess 14
    adenoma 14
    carcinoma, metastatic 14
    encephalopathy 8, 10 *see also* liver failure, fulminant
    failure 14
    fibrosis, congenital 18
    foetor 8, 10
    osteopenia 6
hepatitis 6
    A 10, 16
    acute 10
    autoimmune 6, 14
    B 10, 12, 14, 16
    C 10, 12, 14
    chronic 10, 12, 14
    D 10, 12, 16
    E 10, 16
    viral 16
hepatocellular carcinoma 6, 10, 12, 14, 18
hepatolenticular degeneration *see* Wilson's disease
hepatomegaly 4, 6, 10, 12, 16
hernia
    femoral 2
    hiatus 18
    inguinal 2
    umbilical 2
histoplasmosis 12
hypercalcaemia 14
hyperlipidaemia 14
hypersplenism 10, 14
hypertension 16
    portal 4, 6, 12, 18
hyperventilation 16
    in deep coma 8
hypoglycaemia 8, 14, 16
hypoplasia, focal nodular 14
hypotension 16
hypothyroidism 2
hypovolaemia 8

I

immunoglobulin
    for hepatitis A 11
    for hepatitis B 11
infection 8, 16, 18
    bacterial 2, 6, 16
    fungal 2, 16
    viral 6, 10
intellectual function, deterioration of 8
interferon-α
    for hepatitis 13
    for hepatocellular carcinoma 15
interleukin 2 for hepatocellular carcinoma 15
itching 4 *see also* pruritus

L

lactitol
    for fulminant liver failure 17
    for hepatic encephalopathy 9
lactulose
    for fulminant liver failure 17
    for hepatic encephalopathy 9
lesion
    cystic 14
    space-occupying 8
lipiodol for hepatocellular carcinoma 15
liver *see also* hepatic
    disease
        alcoholic 10, 12
        autoimmune 16
        chronic 8, 10, 16
        end-stage 6
        granulomatous 4
    enlarged 14
    failure 2, 6, 10
        acute 16
        fulminant 8, 16
        hyperacute 16
        subacute 16
    function, deterioration in 2
    hyperplasia 18
    transplantation
        for fulminant liver failure 17
        for hepatic encephalopathy 9
        for hepatocellular carcinoma 15
        for primary biliary cirrhosis 7
        for variceal bleeding 19
        orthotopic
            for ascites 3
        for chronic hepatitis 13
        for primary sclerosing cholangitis 5
lupus erythematosus, systemic 6
lymphoma 2, 12
lymphoproliferative disease 2

M

malignancy 2, 16
Mallory–Weiss tear 18
malnutrition 2
Meig's syndrome 2
melaena 18
meningitis 8
metronidazole for acute encephalopathy in chronic liver disease 9
mitomycin for hepatocellular carcinoma 15
mitozantrone for hepatocellular carcinoma 15
muscle tone, increased 8
mushroom poisoning 16
myeloproliferative disease 2

N

nadolol for variceal bleeding 19
naevi, spider 4, 6, 10
necrosis
    acute tubular 18
    of liver cells 12
nephrotic syndrome 2

O

octreotide for variceal bleeding 19
oedema 4
    ankle 2
    cerebral 8, 16
    portal 4
oesophageal transection for variceal bleeding 19
osteopenia, hepatic 6
osteoporosis 6, 13
overdiuresis 8

P

pancreatitis 2
pancytopenia 14
paracentesis, abdominal, for ascites 3

Index

paracetamol overdose 16
paraplegia, spastic 8
peritonitis, spontaneous bacterial 2
personality changes 8
pigmentation 6
pityriasis rotunda 14
plasma, fresh frozen, for variceal bleeding 19
platelet transfusion for variceal bleeding 19
polycythaemia 14
polyserositis 2
porphyria cutanea tarda 14
prednisolone for chronic hepatitis 13
propranolol for variceal bleeding 19
protein excess 8
pruritus 6, 10, 12 *see also* itching
pseudotuberculosis *see* sarcoidosis

Q

Q fever 12

R

ranitidine for fulminant liver failure 17
Raynaud's syndrome 6
reflex, brisk tendon 8
regurgitation, tricuspid 2
renal
    failure 2, 16, 18
    impairment 2
respiratory failure 16
restlessness 16
retinol *see* vitamin A
Reye's syndrome 16
ribavirin for hepatitis C infection 13

S

sarcoid 4, 12
sarcoidosis 6
schistosomiasis 18
sclerodactyly 6
sclerotherapy for variceal bleeding 19
segmentectomy for hepatocellular carcinoma 15
shunt
    jugular peritoneal, for ascites 3
    transhepatic intravascular portal-systemic stent, for ascites 3
    transjugular intrahepatic portal-systemic stent, for variceal bleeding 19
Sicca's syndrome 6
Sjögren's syndrome 6
SLE *see* lupus erythematosus, systemic
sleep pattern, inversion of normal 8
somatostatin for bleeding varices 19
speech, slurred 8
spironolactone for ascites 3
splenomegaly 4, 6, 10, 12, 14
steatosis 12
stomach *see* gastric
stones, bile duct 4
sucralfate for fulminant liver failure 17

T

tamoxifen for hepatocellular carcinoma 15
tamponade, balloon, for variceal bleeding 19
terlipressin for variceal bleeding 19
thiamine for hepatic encephalopathy 9
thrombocytopenia 12, 16
thrombosis 170
    mesenteric venous 2
    portal-vein 18
    splenic-vein 18
thyroid disease 6
tobramycin for fulminant liver failure 17
transplantation, liver
    for fulminant liver failure 17
    for hepatic encephalopathy 9
    for hepatocellular carcinoma 15
    for primary biliary cirrhosis 7
    for variceal bleeding 19
    orthotopic
        for ascites 3
        for chronic hepatitis 13
        for primary sclerosing cholangitis 5
tremor 8
trimethoprim for primary sclerosing cholangitis 5
tuberculosis 2, 12
tyrosinosis 14

U

UDCA *see* ursodeoxycholic acid
ulcer
    gastroduodenal *see* ulcer, peptic
    peptic 18
unresponsiveness 16
ursodeoxycholic acid
    for acute hepatitis 11
    for primary biliary cirrhosis 7
    for primary sclerosing cholangitis 5

V

vaccination
    for hepatitis A 11
    for hepatitis B 11, 13
variceal
    bleeding 12, 14, 18
    haemorrhage 4, 6
varices
    bleeding oesophageal 4
    ectopic 18
    gastric 18
varicose veins *see* varices
vasoconstriction for variceal bleeding 19
veno-occlusive disease 2
viscus, ruptured 2
vitamin
    A for primary sclerosing cholangitis 5
    D for primary sclerosing cholangitis 5
    K for primary sclerosing cholangitis 5

W

Wernicke's encephalopathy 8
Wernicke–Korsakoff syndrome 18
Wilson's disease 12, 16

X

xanthoma 6

CURRENT DIAGNOSIS & TREATMENT

in

Infectious diseases

Edited by
Glyn Williams

Series editors
Roy Pounder
Mark Hamilton

A QUICK Reference for the Clinician

Contributors

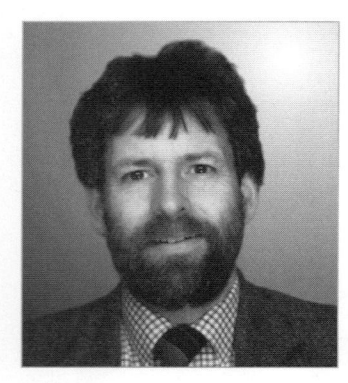

EDITOR

G R Williams

Dr Glyn Williams is consultant physician in infectious diseases at Ayrshire Central Hospital, Irvine. He is interested in the clinical presentation of infection and its reaching (especially in relation to travel-related illness, salmonellosis, and toxic shock syndrome) and the safe management of infected patients within the district general hospital.

REFEREES

Professor Roger Finch
Department of Microbiology
City Hospital
Nottingham, UK

Dr C Christopher Smith
Infection and Tropical Diseases Unit
City Hospital
Aberdeen, UK

AUTHORS

CHRONIC FATIGUE SYNDROME
Dr Darrell O Ho-Yen
Microbiology Department
Raigmore Hospital
Inverness, UK

ERYTHEMA MULTIFORME AND STEVENS-JOHNSON SYNDROME
Dr WTA Todd
Infectious Diseases Unit
Monklands and Bellshill Hospitals
Airdrie, UK

ERYTHEMA NODOSUM
Dr WTA Todd
Infectious Diseases Unit
Monklands and Bellshill Hospitals
Airdrie, UK

FUNGAL INFECTIONS, INVASIVE
Dr KT Khoo
Department of Respiratory Medicine
City General Hospital
Stoke-on-Trent, UK

Dr David W Denning
Department of Infectious Diseases and Tropical Medicine
North Manchester General Hospital
Manchester, UK

GRAM-NEGATIVE SEPTICAEMIA
Dr William A Lynn
Infectious Diseases and Bacteriology Unit
Hammersmith Hospital
London, UK

HENOCH-SCHÖNLEIN PURPURA
Dr WTA Todd
Infectious Diseases Unit
Monklands and Bellshill Hospitals
Airdrie, UK

HERPES SIMPLEX INFECTION
Dr Karl Nicholson
Department of Microbiology and Immunology
Leicester Royal Infirmary
Leicester, UK

HERPES ZOSTER AND VARICELLA
Dr Fred J Nye
Infectious Diseases Unit
Fazakerley Hospital
Liverpool, UK

LEPTOSPIROSIS
Dr Ian Ferguson
Former Director of Public Health Laboratory
County Hospital
Hereford, UK

LYME DISEASE
Dr Darrell O Ho-Yen
Microbiology Department
Raigmore Hospital
Inverness, UK

MALARIA
Professor Malcolm Molyneux
School of Tropical Medicine
University of Liverpool
Liverpool, UK

MEASLES
Dr Philip D Welsby
Department of Communicable Diseases
City Hospital
Edinburgh, UK

PARVOVIRUS B19 INFECTION
Dr Philip D Welsby
Department of Communicable Diseases
City Hospital
Edinburgh, UK

PHARYNGITIS
Dr Glyn R Williams
Department of Infectious Diseases
Ayrshire Central Hospital
Irvine, UK

RHEUMATIC FEVER, ACUTE
Dr WTA Todd
Infectious Diseases Unit
Monklands and Bellshill Hospitals
Airdrie, UK

RUBELLA (GERMAN MEASLES)
Dr Philip D Welsby
Department of Communicable Diseases
City Hospital
Edinburgh, UK

SKIN INFECTIONS
Dr Philip D Welsby
Department of Communicable Diseases
City Hospital
Edinburgh, UK

TOXIC SHOCK SYNDROME
Dr Glyn R Williams
Department of Infectious Diseases
Ayrshire Central Hospital
Irvine, UK

TUBERCULOSIS, EXTRAPULMONARY
Dr Dermot H Kennedy
Department of Infection and Tropical Medicine
Ruchill Hospital
Glasgow, UK

TYPHOID AND PARATYPHOID FEVERS
Dr Bibhat K Mandal
Department of Infectious Diseases and Tropical Medicine
Monsall Hospital
Manchester, UK

Contents

2 Chronic fatigue syndrome

4 Erythema multiforme and Stevens-Johnson syndrome

6 Erythema nodosum

8 Fungal infections, invasive
  Aspergillus infection
  Candida infection
  cryptococcal infection
  histoplasmosis
  mucormycosis (zygomycosis)

10 Gram-negative septicaemia

12 Henoch-Schönlein purpura

14 Herpes simplex infection
  cutaneous herpes
  eczema herpeticum
  genital herpes
  herpes encephalitis
  herpes meningitis
  ocular herpes
  orolabial herpes (cold sores)
  primary gingivostomatitis

16 Herpes zoster and varicella
  chickenpox
  shingles

18 Leptospirosis
  anicteric leptospirosis
  icteric leptospirosis (Weil's syndrome)

20 Lyme disease

22 Malaria
  complicated falciparum malaria
  uncomplicated malaria

24 Measles

26 Parvovirus B19 infection

28 Pharyngitis
  diphtheria
  follicular tonsilitis
  hand, foot, and mouth disease
  infectious mononucleosis
  streptococcal infection (scarlet fever)

30 Rheumatic fever, acute

32 Rubella (German measles)

34 Skin infection
  abscesses
  boils
  carbuncles
  cellulitis
  erysipelas
  impetigo
  methicillin-resistant *Staphylococcus aureus* (MRSA)

36 Toxic shock syndrome
  menstrual toxic shock syndrome
  non-menstrual toxic shock syndrome

38 Tuberculosis, extrapulmonary

40 Typhoid and paratyphoid fevers

42 Index

Chronic fatigue syndrome — D.O. Ho-Yen

Diagnosis

Symptoms

Major

Fatigue: lasting >3–6 months, with 50% reduction in activity; worsened by physical or mental stress; relapsing, with good and bad days.

Prominent disturbance of concentration or short-term memory.

Minor

Initiating viral-like illness, with pyrexia and malaise, common.

Myalgia: especially limb and chest pain; worse after activity.

Joint pain: especially in large joints.

Abdominal pain or bloatedness, nausea, alternating constipation and diarrhoea.

Headaches, dizziness, tinnitus, paraesthesiae.

Sleep disturbance: initially more sleep, followed by disturbed sleep or vivid dreams.

Sensitivity to heat or cold, inappropriate sweating.

Adverse effects of alcohol.

Signs

- Most patients have been previously well; few clinical signs are manifest.

Localized areas of tender muscle: about 1 cm diameter in affected muscle groups.

Enlarged lymph nodes, glands, or inflamed throat: in periods of relapse.

Muscle weakness: in patients who have been ill for many years.

Investigations

- Diagnosis must not be made on the presence of fatigue alone; the two major symptoms and at least four minor items from symptoms, clinical signs, or positive laboratory investigations must be present.
- No diagnostic test exists; investigations are designed to exclude other causes of a similar clinical syndrome.

Initial investigations

- All of the results should be normal, if other illness are to be excluded.

Haemoglobin measurement: to exclude anaemia.

Leucocyte count: to identify infection or a haematological condition.

Thyroid function tests: to exclude thyroid disease.

Plasma viscosity or ESR and CRP measurement: nonspecific indicator of an underlying disorder.

Further investigations

T-helper, T-suppressor, and natural killer cell count: abnormalities often found.

- Other conditions suggested by the patient's history or examination must be excluded, especially infection, e.g. tick bites (Lyme disease) or consumption of raw meat (toxoplasmosis).

Complications

Psychiatric disorder: especially depression and anxiety.

Irritable bowel syndrome.

Severe disability: patient may become bedridden.

Differential diagnosis

Infections, especially Epstein–Barr virus, Lyme disease, toxoplasmosis, hepatitis A, brucellosis.

Endocrine disease, especially hypothyroidism.

Psychiatric disease, especially if patient has been ill for many years.

Malignancy.

Autoimmune disease, sarcoidosis.

Drugs or toxins.

Aetiology

- The cause is unknown; probably several conditions are involved, including continuing infection and immune response to infection.

Epidemiology

- Chronic fatigue syndrome occurs throughout the world.
- ~1.3 in 1000 population are affected.
- Both sexes and all ages are affected; women are more likely to have prolonged illness.

Nomenclature

- Chronic fatigue syndrome is also known as the following:

Post viral fatigue syndrome.

Myalgic encephalomyelitis (ME).

Royal Free disease.

Neurasthenia.

Effort syndrome.

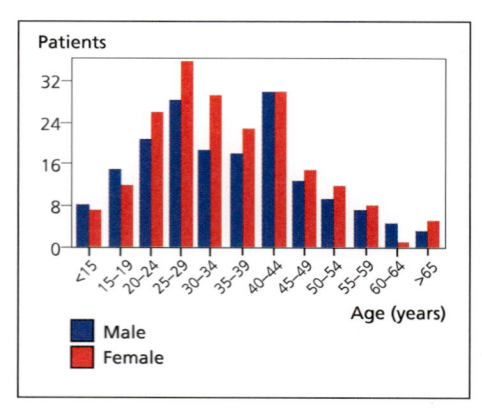

Patients affected by chronic fatigue syndrome, according to age and sex (204 females, 177 males; raio, 1.2:1.

Treatment

Diet and lifestyle
- If patients have a normal diet, vitamins or mineral supplements are unnecessary.
- Patients should remain within their energy limits; sleep should not be resisted (at least 10 h/day); sleep and relaxation techniques increase energy levels; energy is lost through physical activities and mental exertion (such as concern about jobs, finances, and relationships).

Pharmacological treatment
- Although moderating activity is the best method of controlling symptoms, many patients need additional supportive treatment.
- Several drugs may have to be tried before the most appropriate is found.

Analgesics
- Mild analgesics, e.g. paracetamol or aspirin should be tried initially; if they are unsuccessful, dihydrocodeine or ibuprofen may help.

Benzodiazepines
- Because of their hypnotic, sedative, anxiolytic, and muscle-relaxant actions, these drugs are useful in patients with difficulty sleeping.
- Intermediate-acting compounds are best (temazepam, lormetazepam).

Standard dosage	Temazepam 10 mg orally at night for 3–4 weeks.
Contraindications	Respiratory depression, phobic or obsessional states.
Main drug interactions	Alcohol.
Main side effects	Drowsiness, dizziness.

Antidepressants
- The most useful agents are amitriptyline, doxepin, dothiepin, and fluoxetine.

Standard dosage	Amitriptyline 10 mg orally at night.
Contraindications	Heart disease.
Special points	Patients should be given low doses initially, with gradual increase if necessary.
Main drug interactions	Alcohol.
Main side effects	Dry mouth, blurred vision, nausea, constipation.

Treatment aims
To reduce fatigue and prevent relapses.
To relieve other symptoms.
To allow patient to resume normal activity, e.g. to return to work or school.

Prognosis
- Patients may recover after a fluctuating illness, usually in the first 4 years, achieve stability at a lower energy level, or deteriorate and become chronically disabled.

Follow-up and management
- Patients should keep a daily diary, monitoring activities and energy levels.
- Activities may be increased and a return to work or school encouraged when energy levels are 70–80% of normal.

Causes of treatment failure
Overoptimistic reassurance of recovery.
Patient's inability to change lifestyle.
Too much energy being spent pursuing alternative cures.

Key references
Ho-Yen DO: *Better Recovery from Viral Illnesses* edn 3. Inverness: Dodona Books, 1993.

Thomas PK: The chronic fatigue syndrome: what do we know? *BMJ* 1993, **306**:1557–1558.

Tirelli U *et al.*: Clinical and immunologic study of 205 patients with chronic fatigue syndrome. *Arch Intern Med* 1993, **153**:116–120.

Wessely S: Chronic fatigue syndrome: current issues. *Rev Med Micro* 1992, **3**:211–216.

Erythema multiforme and Stevens–Johnson syndrome
W.T.A Todd

Diagnosis

Symptoms
- These conditions form a spectrum from the relatively mild erythema multiforme syndrome to the severe and potentially life-threatening Stevens–Johnson syndrome.

Nonspecific upper respiratory tract infection: prodromal syndrome.

Intensely itchy skin rash.

Painful, bullous lesions: involving two or more mucous membranes in Stevens-Johnson syndrome; shallow ulcers result if the bulla ruptures.

Fever, malaise, cough, sore throat, chest pain, vomiting, diarrhoea, myalgia, arthralgia: severe systemic reaction in Stevens–Johnson syndrome.

Signs

Erythema multiforme
Classic 'target' lesions: develop abruptly and symmetrically, heaviest peripherally; often involve palms and soles.

Urticarial plaques: may develop but do not evolve rapidly as with a true urticaria.

Vesicles and bullae: may develop in pre-existing lesions, usually heralding a more severe form of disease; severe disease with mucosal involvement and constitutional upset indicates Stevens–Johnson syndrome.

Stevens–Johnson syndrome
Bullous lesions on mucous membranes: abrupt appearance 1–14 days after other symptoms; often on oral mucosa, lips, and conjunctivae, often with variable involvement of other mucous surfaces; urethral, vulvo-vaginal, and balanitic involvement may lead to urinary retention.

Pain from oral lesions: possibly severe enough to compromise fluid intake and breathing.

Patchy pulmonary disease, pneumonia, renal failure, diarrhoea, paronychia, nail loss, polyarthritis, otitis media, and coma.

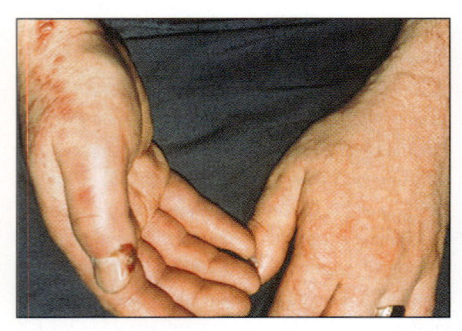

Typical 'target' lesions on hands.

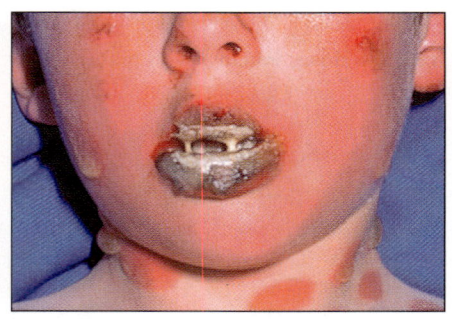

Buccal mucous membrane involvement.

Investigations
History of drug ingestion: very important.

Throat swab: to detect coxsackie viruses, herpes simplex virus, adenoviruses.

Serology: for *Mycoplasma pneumoniae*, coxsackie, herpes simplex virus, adenovirus.

Autoimmune serology: to detect collagen diseases.

Full blood count and ESR measurement: total leucocyte count often raised and may show excess of eosinophils; ESR and CRP usually raised.

U&E and albumin measurement: urea raised because of catabolic state and fluid loss if skin lesions extensive; exudation from lesions may cause hypoalbuminaemia.

Skin biopsy: shows characteristic range of changes from mild dermal inflammation to full epidermal necrosis.

Complications
Blindness: caused by corneal involvement.

Recurrence: especially of disease caused by herpes simplex virus or drugs.

Differential diagnosis
- Classic cases with target lesions should prove no problem; atypical cases may resemble any of the following:

Chronic urticaria.
Toxic erythema (drugs or infection).
Collagen diseases.
Secondary syphilis.
Acute HIV seroconversion.
Haemorrhagic fevers.
Kawasaki syndrome.
Toxic epidermal necrolysis.
Chronic meningococcaemia.

Aetiology
- The condition is produced by a hypersensitivity reaction mediated by immune complexes in dermal blood vessels.
- In ~50% of patients, no cause is identified.
- Common antigenic triggers involve the following:

Infection by virus (especially herpes simplex, enteroviruses), *Mycoplasma pneumoniae*, chlamydiae, histoplasmosis.

Drugs: antibiotics (e.g. penicillins, sulphonamides), anticonvulsants (especially phenytoin), aspirin, corticosteroids, cimetidine.

Neoplasia: leukaemia, lymphoma, multiple myeloma, internal (cryptic) malignancy.

Collagen diseases: lupus erythematosis, polyarteritis, rheumatoid arthritis.

Others: sarcoidosis, foods (e.g. emulsifiers in margarine).

Epidemiology
- Erythema multiforme and Stevens–Johnson syndrome account for up to 1% of dermatology outpatient consultations.
- Children <3 years and adults >50 years are rarely affected.
- The incidence peaks in the second and third decades, with 50% of patients <20 years.
- The male:female ratio is 1.5:1.
- The illness is most severe in young adults and children, especially boys.
- Seasonal epidemics occur, related to the common provoking agents, e.g. *Mycoplasma* spp., herpes virus, and adenoviral infections.

Treatment

Diet and lifestyle

- In rare cases of a dietary 'trigger', e.g. emulsifiers in margarine, this must be avoided.
- If the oral contraceptive is implicated, obvious lifestyle changes must follow.

Pharmacological treatment

For the underlying 'trigger' condition

- Possible drug precipitants should be withdrawn.
- Acyclovir is indicated for herpes simplex virus, and the appropriate antibiotic for *Mycoplasma* infection (macrolide or tetracycline).

Standard dosage	Acyclovir applied directly every 4 h (ointment) or 200 mg 5 times daily.
	Erythromycin 500 mg 4 times daily.
Contraindications	*Acyclovir*: renal impairment, severe dehydration.
	Erythromycin: hypersensitivity.
Main drug interactions	*Acyclovir*: other antivirals, e.g. zidovudine (produces lethargy).
	Erythromycin: increase in theophylline concentrations.
Main side effects	*Acyclovir*: rashes, gastrointestinal disturbances.
	Erythromycin: gastrointestinal disturbances, nausea, vomiting, pain, diarrhoea.

For skin lesions

- Antihistamines are indicated for pruritus, salicylates or NSAIDs for symptomatic relief (salicylates have been implicated as causative agents), and steroids or icthammol soaks for broken lesions.

Standard dosage	Chlorpheniramine 4 mg orally every 6–8 h.
	Naproxen 250 mg every 6–8 h.
Contraindications	*Naproxen*: active peptic ulceration; to be avoided in children (paracetamol analgesia instead).
Special points	*Chlorpheniramine*: patients must not drive if drowsiness ensues.
Main drug interactions	*Chlorpheniramine*: alcohol or sedatives.
	Naproxen: oral anticoagulants.
Main side effects	*Chlorpheniramine*: drowsiness, headache, gastrointestinal disturbances.
	Naproxen: gastrointestinal disturbances.

For severe cases (Stevens–Johnson syndrome)

- Withdrawal of any drug precipitant and treatment of infective causes is vital.
- No data from well controlled trials are available, but the dermatological manifestations respond to a short course of high-dose steroids.
- Because of mouth involvement, enteric or parenteral feeding may be needed and should be considered during the first week.
- Intravenous fluid replacement should be instituted early.

Standard dosage	Prednisolone 80–100 mg daily.
Contraindications	Active peptic ulceration.
Special points	Possible adrenal suppression on withdrawal.
Main drug interactions	NSAIDs, oral anticoagulants.
Main side effects	Cushing's syndrome, growth retardation in children.

Treatment aims

To remove or treat underlying 'triggers'.

To provide adequate pain relief for mucosal involvement.

To provide symptomatic relief for generalized skin involvement.

To maintain nutrition and fluid replacement in this hypercatabolic state.

Other treatments

- Urethral or renal tract involvement may necessitate catheterization, especially in children.
- Management in a unit used to burns care may be needed for severely ill patients.
- Careful skin nursing is essential to prevent secondary infection.

Prognosis

- The rash heals completely if the precipitant causes are removed or treated.
- Complete recovery is normal, but corneal scarring may occur after *Mycoplasma* infection.
- Untreated Stevens–Johnson syndrome has a 5–15% mortality.
- Typical erythema multiforme runs a mild course, subsiding to normal after 2–3 weeks.
- Cases related to herpes simplex usually follow a simple course but may recur with further reactivation of herpes simplex; prophylactic acyclovir is then indicated.
- Cases related to *Mycoplasma* infection or drugs often subside more slowly and will more probably progress to Stevens–Johnson syndrome.

Follow-up and management

- Prophylaxis against herpes simplex virus (topical or occasionally systemic acyclovir) is important if the virus precipitates erythema multiforme; this should reduce the incidence of further attacks.

Key references

Hurwitz S: Erythema multiforme: a review of its characteristics, diagnostic criteria, and management. *Pediatr Rev* 1990, **11**:217–222.

Renfro L *et al.*: Controversy: are systemic steroids indicated in the treatment of erythema multiforme? *Pediatr Dermatol* 1989, **6**:43–50.

Erythema nodosum W.T.A. Todd

Diagnosis

Symptoms

Painful red nodules: on lower legs and occasionally on thighs and forearms; pain worse on weight-bearing; gradual appearance; can become almost confluent; gradual healing (3–6 weeks), with bruising but no scarring.

'Crops' of lesions: occurring at different times, so that lesions manifest at different stages of evolution.

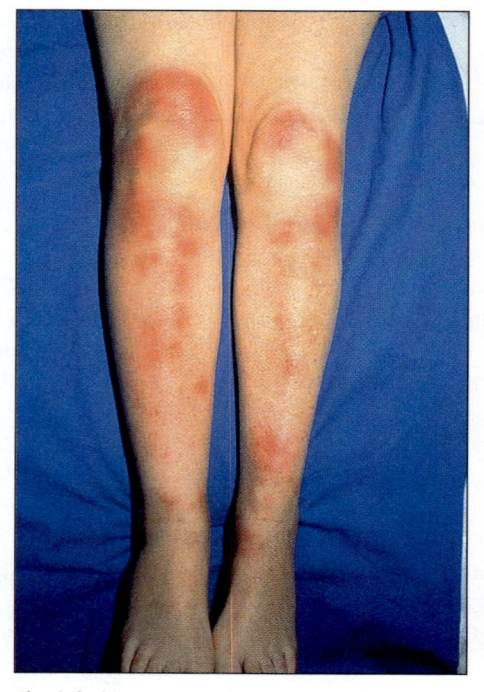

Classic lesions over pretibial region.

Signs

Tender erythematous nodules: 1–5 cm diameter; usually bilateral over pretibial areas; no ulceration or blistering; involution over 3–6 weeks, with yellow–purple bruising.

Fever and systemic reaction: variable but may precede lesions by 1–7 days.

Investigations

- Discovering the cause is important because treatment of this prevents recurrences.

History: for drugs (e.g. oral contraceptive), pregnancy, contact with tuberculosis, bowel upset (inflammatory bowel disease, yersiniosis).

Full blood count, ESR analysis: acute-phase reactants always raised.

Chest radiography: to detect features of sarcoidosis, tuberculosis, disseminated fungal infection.

Bacteriology: sputum or early morning urine for acid/alcohol-fast bacilli; throat swab or antistreptolysin O titre for evidence of streptococcal infection.

Mantoux test: strongly positive in tuberculosis, negative in sarcoidosis.

Kveim test: positive granuloma formation indicates sarcoidosis, but negative reaction does not exclude diagnosis.

Serum angiotensin-converting enzyme measurement.

Complications

- The skin lesions have no complications.
- Any complications relate to the underlying condition; if this is not controlled, the skin lesion may continue to be manifest (lasting up to 4–5 months).

Differential diagnosis

Erythema nodosum leprosum: in multi-bacillary leprosy, unrelated acute reactional state to the release of mycobacterial protein during treatment.

Erythematous skin lesions of pretibial area: e.g. pretibial myxoedema.

Rheumatoid nodules (usually on elbows, wrists, or palms).

Aetiology

- Erythema nodosum is a septal panniculitis in subcutaneous fat due to a hypersensitivity reaction to antigenic or other stimulus.
- Causes include the following:

Drugs: e.g. penicillin, sulphonamides, oral contraceptive pill in 25% of patients.

Infections: e.g. tuberculosis, streptococci, *Yersinia*, *Salmonella*, *Campylobacter* spp., deep fungal infection, leprosy.

Inflammatory conditions: e.g. sarcoidosis, inflammatory bowel disease, Behçet's syndrome, pregnancy, thyroid disease.

- 20–40% of cases are idiopathic.

Epidemiology

- The peak age is 20–30 years, but erythema nodosum can occur at any age.
- The female:male ratio is 3:1.
- Patients with tuberculosis-related disease are usually <20 years.
- Patients with disease caused by pregnancy or inflammatory bowel disorders are usually 15–40 years.
- Patients with disease caused by Behçet's syndrome or sarcoidosis are usually 20–40 years.
- Fever and systemic reactions occur more often and for longer in older patients.

Treatment

Diet and lifestyle
- During the acute phase of the inflammation, prolonged weight-bearing should be avoided.
- Bed-rest is advised during the first 3–5 days.

Pharmacological treatment
- Treatment of skin lesions is primarily symptomatic.
- Management of the underlying condition prevents further erythema nodosum.

For pain relief
- NSAIDs should be sufficient.

Standard dosage	Naproxen 250 mg every 6–8 h.
Contraindications	Hypersensitivity, active peptic ulceration; caution with concomitant anticoagulation and asthma.
Main drug interactions	Warfarin.
Main side effects	Gastrointestinal disturbances, discomfort, nausea, ulceration.

Systemic steroids
- Steroids are effective, but extreme caution must be observed; they should be used only if the underlying conditions, e.g. tuberculosis, have been adequately treated.

Standard dosage	Prednisolone 20–40 mg initially, reduced rapidly over 10 days to nil.
Contraindications	Active peptic ulceration.
Special points	Possible adrenal suppression on sudden withdrawal.
Main drug interactions	NSAIDs, oral anticoagulants.
Main side effects	Cushing's syndrome, growth retardation in children, glucose intolerance, osteoporosis.

Treatment aims
To provide symptomatic relief of lesion-related pain or discomfort.
To remove or treat underlying cause.

Other treatments
Potassium iodide.
Wet dressings to the lesions for symptomatic relief.

Prognosis
- Lesions usually clear in 3–6 weeks.
- Spontaneous resolution is usual.

Follow-up and management
- The most important aspect of erythema nodosum management is diagnosis of any underlying precipitant.

Key references
Fox MD, Schwartz RA: Erythema nodosum. *Am Fam Physic* 1992, **46**:818–822.

Hannuksela M: Erythema nodosum. *Clin Dermatol* 1986, **4**:88–95.

Fungal infections, invasive
S.H. Khoo and D.W. Denning

Diagnosis

Symptoms and signs

Candida infections
White plaques in mouth or tongue, angular cheilitis.
Vulvovaginal discharge, pruritus.
Cutaneous candidiasis, intertrigo, folliculitis, balanitis, perianal or interdigital infection, nappy rash.
Paronychia or onychomycosis.
Cystitis, urethritis, passage of fungal balls.
Disseminated candidiasis involving several organs, intravascular infection, endocarditis, peri- or myocarditis, meningitis, cerebral microabscesses.
Pneumonia, allergic wheeze, breathlessness.
Peritonitis, oesophagitis, gastritis, small and large bowel plaques, and ulceration.

Aspergillus infections
Wheeze, breathlessness: indicating allergic bronchopulmonary aspergillosis.
Fever, cough, hypoxia, chest discomfort or pleuritic pain, haemoptysis, pneumonia: indicating invasive aspergillosis.
Blocked nose, facial pain, nasal discharge, chronic headache: indicating allergic or saprophytic sinus infection.
Chronic otitis media or externa, meningitis or cerebral microabscesses, endocarditis, endophthalmitis, osteoarticular disorders.

Cryptococcal infections
- Onset is insidious.

Fever, headache, nausea, vomiting, neck stiffness, photophobia: indicating meningitis.

Histoplasmosis
Breathlessness, lung infiltrates: indicating pulmonary histoplasmosis.
Pancytopenia, pneumonia, lymphadenopathy, hepatosplenomegaly, oral or gastrointestinal ulcers, adrenal masses: indicating disseminated histoplasmosis.

Agents of mucormycosis (zygomycosis)
Headache, facial pain, orbital cellulitis, lower cranial nerve palsies: indicating rhinocerebral infection.
Pneumonia, disseminated disease.

Investigations
Biopsy of tissue and bone marrow with culture and histology (histoplasmosis only), culture of blood, sputum, fluid (including CSF), and sinuses.
Antigen tests: for cryptococcal infections, candidaemia, *Aspergillus* infection.
CT for *Aspergillus* infections: of thorax for aspergilloma and invasive infections; of sinuses for allergy, saprophytic, acute invasion; of brain for brain abscess.
Endoscopy, colonoscopy, barium meal, swallow, follow-through: for oesophagitis, gastritis, small and large bowel plaques, and ulceration.
Radiography of chest, thorax, and sinuses.
Bronchoscopy: lavage, biopsy, for airways disease and diagnosis.

Complications

Candida infections
Oesophageal candidiasis, azole-resistant thrush, endometritis, ascending renal infection in intensive care or surgical patients, prostatitis, multiple organ involvement, hepatosplenic candidiasis in leukaemic patients.

Other infections
Pulmonary fibrosis: after 5–10 years; complication of allergic bronchopulmonary aspergillosis.
Haemoptysis: in *Aspergillus* infections and zygomycosis.
Hydrocephalus, impaired mental function, blindness: complications of cryptococcal infections; hydrocephalus usually communicating.

Differential diagnosis
Other infections.
Lymphoma.
Tuberculosis.

Aetiology
- Predisposing causes include the following:

Superficial *Candida* infections
Antibiotics, steroids, diabetes mellitus, AIDS immunocompromise, pregnancy, oral contraceptives, macerated skin, wet nappies, occupation, frequent wetting of hands, abnormal T-cell response to *Candida* antigens.

Systemic *Candida* infections
Urinary catheterization, immunosuppression, surgery, burns, premature birth, endocarditis, valvular heart disease, prosthetic valves, peritoneal dialysis, abdominal surgery, bowel perforation, haematological malignancies, CSF shunts.

Aspergillus infections
Asthma, cystic fibrosis, neutropenia, organ transplantation, AIDS, steroids, chronic granulomatous disease, previous pulmonary tuberculosis, sarcoidosis, bronchiectasis, chronic lung disease, diabetes mellitus, alcoholism, previous ear disease, i.v. drug abuse, valve replacement.

Cryptococcal infections
AIDS, lymphoma, steroids, sarcoidosis.

Histoplasmosis
History of exposure, e.g. endemic area, bat caves (acute), emphysema (chronic), AIDS, immunocompromise (disseminated).

Mucormycosis
Acidosis, diabetes mellitus, neutropenia, bone-marrow transplantation, i.v. drug abuse, desferrioxamine treatment.

Epidemiology
- Vaginal candidiasis affects 70% of all women, and 5% have frequent recurrences.
- Oral thrush affects 90% of AIDS patients and 15–30% of leukaemia patients.
- Invasive aspergillosis affects 5–40% of immunocompromised patients.
- Cryptococcal meningitis affects 4–35% of AIDS patients, depending on country.

Treatment

Diet and lifestyle
- No special precautions are necessary.

Pharmacological treatment

Amphotericin B
- Amphotericin B is indicated for the following:

Candida infections (oropharyngeal, urogenital tract, candidaemia, endocarditis, pneumonia, visceral, CNS).
Aspergillus infections (invasive or chronic necrotizing aspergillosis, acute invasive sinus, or paranasal granuloma).
Cryptococcal infections (meningitis).
Histoplasmosis (chronic pulmonary, disseminated).
Agents of mucormycosis (rhinocerebral).

Standard dosage	Amphotericin B 0.5–1.5 mg/kg i.v.
Contraindications	Hypersensitivity.
Special points	Resistant strains include *Candida lusitaniae*, *Fusarium* spp., *Pseudallescheria boydii*, *Trichosporon beigellei*, Mucorales (limited activity).
Main drug interactions	Increased nephrotoxicity with aminoglycosides or cyclosporin.
Main side effects	Infusion-related fever or rigors, nausea, phlebitis, renal toxicity, anaemia, electrolyte disturbances.

Azoles
- Fluconazole is indicated for *Candida* infections (oropharyngeal, vulvovaginal, nail infections, chronic mucocutaneous candidiasis, urogenital tract, visceral candidiasis) and for cryptococcal infections (meningitis in AIDS).
- Itraconazole is indicated for *Aspergillus* infections (pulmonary, acute invasive sinus, paranasal granuloma) and for histoplasmosis (severe acute, chronic pulmonary, less seriously ill, disseminated; maintenance in AIDS).

Standard dosage	Fluconazole 50–400 mg orally or i.v. daily. Itraconazole 100–200 mg orally daily; 200 mg loading doses 3 times daily initially in severe or life-threatening disease. Ketoconazole 200–400 mg orally daily.
Contraindications	Azole hypersensitivity.
Special points	*Fluconazole*: resistant strains include *Histoplasma capsulatum*, Mucorales, *Candida krusei* and *glabrata*, *Aspergillus* and *Fusarium* spp. *Itraconazole*: resistant strains include *C. glabrata*, *Fusarium*, Mucorales. *Ketoconazole*: resistant strains include *C. glabrata*, *Cryptococcus neoformans*, *Aspergillus* and *Fusarium* spp.
Main drug interactions	Altered azole or drug concentrations with phenytoin, cyclosporin, rifampicin, phenobarbitone, carbamazepine, warfarin, terfenadine, astemizole, digoxin.
Main side effects	*Fluconazole*: nausea, rash, liver dysfunction (rare). *Itraconazole*: gynaecomastia, peripheral oedema, hypokalaemia, liver dysfunction (rare). *Ketoconazole*: liver dysfunction, nausea, reduced libido, menstrual irregularities, gynaecomastia.

Other drugs
Flucytosine 50–100 mg/kg orally or i.v. daily only in combination with amphotericin B: for *Candida* infections (candidaemia, endocarditis, CNS infections), *Aspergillus* infections (invasive aspergillosis), and cryptococcal infections (meningitis).
Topical nystatin: for mucosal *Candida* infection.
Topical antifungals: for cutaneous *Candida* and dermatophyte infections.
Inhaled steroids, bronchodilators: for allergic pneumonitis.
Oral steroids: for exacerbations of allergic bronchopulmonary aspergillosis.

Treatment aims
To eradicate infection.
To prevent recurrence of infection.
To remove underlying cause.

Other treatments
Removal or replacement of catheter or shunt.
Surgery: for invasive aspergillosis, aspergilloma, allergic sinus infection, fungus ball, paranasal granuloma, rhinocerebral infection (radical clearance).
Removal of CSF in cryptococcal meningitis.

Prognosis
- In patients with candidaemia, overall mortality is 55%; in surgical patients with candida peritonitis, mortality is 37%.
- In patients with invasive aspergillosis, mortality is 30–90%, depending on the host group: poor prognosis in patients with late-diagnosis and persistent neutropenia, 85–90% in bone-marrow transplant recipients, 95% in patients with disseminated disease or cerebral aspergillosis.
- In patients with haemoptysis resulting from aspergilloma, mortality is 10%; spontaneous resolution is 10%.
- 50% of leukaemia patients with acute invasive *Aspergillus* sinus infection relapse.
- In patients with meningitis, acute mortality is 15–20%, lower if intracranial hypertension is treated aggressively.
- More than one-third of patients who have had meningitis relapse without prophylaxis.

Follow-up and management
- Patients with life-threatening invasive fungal infections should have specialist treatment and prolonged follow-up.

Key references
British Society for Antimicrobial Chemotherapy Working Party: Antifungal chemotherapy in patients with acquired immunodeficiency syndrome. *Lancet* 1992, **340**:648–651.

Denning DW, Stevens DA: Antifungal and surgical treatment of invasive aspergillosis: review of 2121 published cases. *Rev Infect Dis* 1990, **12**:1147–1201.

Warnock DW, Richardson MD (eds): *Fungal Infection in the Immunocompromised Patient*. Chichester: Wiley & Sons, 1991.

Gram-negative septicaemia — W.A. Lynn

Diagnosis

Symptoms
Sweats, chills, or rigors.
Cough, possibly with sputum, pleuritic chest pain, breathlessness.
Dysuria, urinary frequency.
Abdominal pain, nausea, vomiting, diarrhoea.
Headache, neck stiffness, confusion.

Signs
- Focal clinical signs, if present, may help to localize the site of infection.

Tachycardia: >90 beats/min.
Tachypnoea: >20 breaths/min.
Temperature >38°C or <35.6°C: hypothermia associated with worse prognosis.
Hypotension: systolic blood pressure <90 mmHg or fall of 40 mmHg from baseline.
Oliguria: <20 ml/h.
Petechial or purpuric skin rash: suggesting meningococcal septicaemia; ecthyma gangrenosum associated with *Pseudomonas* infection in neutropenic patients.

Investigations
- Investigations are directed towards ascertaining the microbiology, site of infection, severity, and complications of Gram-negative sepsis.
- Ideally, culture specimens should be taken before antimicrobial treatment, but treatment should not be unduly delayed in seriously ill patients.

Blood cultures: at least two, preferably three.
Urine and sputum microscopy and culture.
Gram-stain and culture of available pus or body fluids: may provide rapid diagnosis.
Chest radiography, further radiography directed by clinical picture.
Haemoglobin count: to detect severe anaemia (may need to be corrected).
Leucocyte count: to detect neutrophil leucocytosis or toxic granulation; leucopenia associated with poor prognosis.
Platelet count and coagulation studies: for evidence of disseminated intravascular coagulation.
Arterial blood gas analysis: shows respiratory alkalosis early and metabolic acidosis later; possibly hypoxia.
Liver function tests: abnormal results in 40–60% of patients.

Complications
Renal failure: acute tubular necrosis, usually reversible.
Disseminated intravascular coagulation.
Adult respiratory distress syndrome: in 15–40% of patients.
Hepatic failure.

Differential diagnosis
- More than one factor may contribute to shock in an individual patient.

Other causes of shock: cardiogenic, hypovolaemic, redistribution of fluid (e.g. burns, pancreatitis, anaphylaxis), toxins.
Other infections: e.g. Gram-positive bacteria, fungi, malaria, or viral infections, staphylococcal or streptococcal toxic shock syndrome.

Aetiology
- Gram-negative septicaemia is usually associated with *Escherichia coli*, *Klebsiella*, *Enterobacter*, *Serratia*, *Proteus*, and *Pseudomonas* spp., and *Neisseria meningitidis*; enteric Gram-negative bacteria account for most cases.
- The most common sources are intra-abdominal or urinary tract infections and pneumonia.
- Host risk factors include the following:

Surgery (especially gastrointestinal, genitourinary, hepatobiliary).
Abnormalities of genitourinary tract.
Intravenous lines.
Hospitalization.
Cancer.
Neutropenia.
Immunosuppression.

Epidemiology
- Gram-negative septicaemia and shock have been increasing over the past 30 years.
- Bacteraemia is found in ~7 in 1000 hospital admissions.
- Septic shock complicates 20% of bacteraemias.
- ~30 000 to 50 000 patients are affected annually in the UK.

Pathogenesis of Gram-negative shock
- Bacterial endotoxin (lipopolysaccharide) and other bacterial products initiate the release of inflammatory mediators from monocyte/macrophages, endothelial cells and polymorphonuclear leukocytes.
- The interaction of these mediators leads to an 'inflammatory cascade' of reactions, leading to widespread endothelial damage, hypotension, refractory shock, multiorgan failure, and death.

Treatment

Diet and lifestyle
- No special precautions are necessary.

Pharmacological treatment

Indications
- Antibiotic treatment depends on the site of the infection and host and environmental factors.

Urinary tract (community-acquired): co-amoxiclav or cefotaxime.

Urinary tract or pneumonia (hospital-acquired): ceftazidime, or piperacillin with gentamicin.

Intra-abdominal: cefotaxime with metronidazole, or piperacillin with gentamicin.

Biliary tract: piperacillin with gentamicin.

Cefotaxime or ceftazidime
Standard dosage	Cefotaxime or ceftazidime 1–2 g 8-hourly.
Contraindications	Previous cephalosporin hypersensitivity.
Special points	Dose adjusted in moderate to severe renal failure.
Main drug interactions	None.
Main side effects	Rashes, diarrhoea, haemolysis, or raised transaminases (rare).

Co-amoxiclav (Augmentin)
Standard dosage	Augmentin 1.2 g 8-hourly.
Contraindications	Penicillin hypersensitivity.
Special points	Dose adjusted in moderate to severe renal failure.
Main drug interactions	None.
Main side effects	Pseudomembranous colitis, hypersensitivity.

Gentamicin
Standard dosage	Gentamicin 2.5 mg/kg 12-hourly (normal renal function).
Contraindications	Myasthenia gravis.
Special points	Concentrations must be monitored before and after dose.
Main drug interactions	Loop diuretics, curare-type anaesthetic agents.
Main side effects	Nephrotoxicity, ototoxicity.

Metronidazole
Standard dosage	Metronidazole 500 mg 8-hourly i.v. or 1 g every 8–12 h *per rectum*.
Contraindications	Hypersensitivity.
Special points	To be used in pregnancy only if essential; accumulation in liver disease.
Main drug interactions	Alcohol, warfarin, phenobarbitone, lithium.
Main side effects	Leucopenia, peripheral neuropathy (long-term use).

Piperacillin
Standard dosage	Piperacillin 2 g 6-hourly.
Contraindications	Penicillin hypersensitivity.
Special points	Dose adjusted in moderate to severe renal failure.
Main drug interactions	Inactivates aminoglycosides if mixed in solution.
Main side effects	Hypersensitivity, hepatotoxicity in 3% of patients, platelet dysfunction.

Treatment aims
To control infection.
To maintain organ perfusion and tissue oxygen delivery.
To minimize complications

Other treatments
Drainage of infected collections of pus.
Surgical debridement of dead or infected material.

Prognosis
- Mortality is 10–20% in patients with bacteraemia, 40–60% in those with shock, and >90% in those with multiorgan failure.

Follow-up and management
- Patients need careful management in the convalescent stage, which may be prolonged after acute septic shock; they may relapse if the predisposing condition remains.

Management of Gram-negative bacterial shock
- Monitoring of the following is needed:
Systolic blood pressure (must be kept >90 mmHg or high enough to maintain renal perfusion).
Central venous pressure or post-capillary wedge pressure (to exclude hypovolaemia).
Cardiac output.
Systemic vascular resistance (normal, >1000; in septic shock, generally <1000).
Catheterization (for urine measurement).
Oxygen saturation (arterial pressure falls, venous pressure rises because of failure in tissue oxygenation).
- Treatment includes the following:
Colloid to restore intravascular volume (blood for severe anaemia).
Pressor or inotropic agents, if necessary.
Renal dopamine 2–4 µg/min to maintain renal perfusion.
Inspired oxygen at minimum to maintain arterial oxygenation.
Nutritional support.

Key references
Edwards JD: Management of septic shock. *BMJ* 1993, **306**:1661–1664.
Parillo JE: Pathogenetic mechanisms of septic shock. *N Engl J Med* 1993, **328**:1471–1477.
Rietschel ET, Brade H: Bacterial endotoxins. *Sci Am* 1992, **267**:26–31.

Henoch–Schönlein purpura W.T.A. Todd

Diagnosis

Symptoms
- In most patients, symptoms occur 24–48 h after infection (usually upper respiratory tract infection) or drug ingestion (antibiotics).
- ~50% of adults develop only the characteristic rash and malaise.

Florid palpable purpuric skin rash: predominantly on lower legs but also on buttocks and arms (cardinal symptom).

Cramping abdominal pains: in 60–70% of patients

Joint pains: in 60–70%.

Blood in urine or stool: in 20–30%.

Symptoms of intestinal obstruction: due to intussusception, in young children.

Fever and toxicity: if severe.

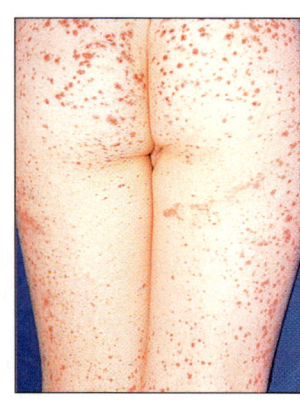

Typical purpuric lesions on buttocks (left) and pretibial areas and lower legs (right).

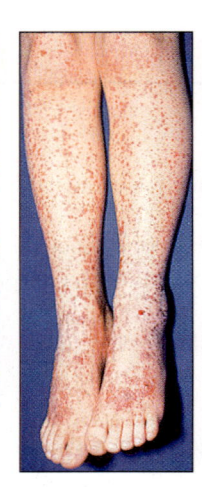

Signs
Rash: 'papular purpura' lesions that do not blanch on pressure, some forming a necrotic centre that may vesiculate, usually on buttocks, natal cleft, and extremities; usually painless; in adults, may persist or recur for up to 2 months.

Joint involvement: mild to moderate symmetrical arthropathy in 60–70%; some periarticular swelling; a few patients also have angioedema of hands and feet.

Gut involvement: cramping abdominal pain, and some rebound tenderness in 25%; frank blood in stool in 10–20%; obstructive symptoms (intussusception) or perforation.

Renal involvement: ~30% of patients develop nephritis.

Investigations
Skin biopsy: may show cutaneous necrotizing venulitis but does not indicate cause.

History: may be positive for recent infective episodes or drug ingestion (antibiotic).

Full blood count: may show mild polymorphonuclear leucocytosis.

Serology: for recent viral or streptococcal infection.

Stool and urine analysis: regularly during and after rash, with formal microscopy if positive; 30% of patients show evidence of erythrocytes, raised protein concentration, and casts on urinalysis.

Formal renal investigations, including biopsy: if findings indicate renal disease.

Complications
- In children, this condition is often thought of as 'harmless'.

Secondary infection of vasculitic lesions.

Glomerulonephritis, IgA nephropathy: in ~30% of patients; 15–20% of these progress to renal failure in 6 months (adults).

Renal failure: in 5–10% of all patients.

Gastrointestinal or surgical problems: e.g. intussusception or perforation in young children; of the 60–70% of patients with gastrointestinal complications, a few develop intramural haematomata, associated with intussusception, infarction, or gut perforation; protein-losing enteropathy.

Renal problems: e.g. immunoglobulin nephropathy in older children and adults.

Differential diagnosis
Other forms of vasculitic or purpuric rash (e.g. meningococcal septicaemia).
Embolic phenomena from acute or subacute bacterial endocarditis.
Systemic Gram-negative sepsis.
Collagen vascular disease, especially polyarteritis nodosa.

Aetiology
- Henoch–Schönlein purpura is essentially idiopathic.
- Triggers include the following:

Nonspecific upper respiratory infection (in ~33% of patients).
Sulphonamide or penicillin treatment.
Streptococcal infection.
Streptokinase treatment for myocardial infarction.

Epidemiology
- Henoch–Schönlein purpura can occur at any age, but it predominantly affects children.
- It has a seasonal variation, occurring most often in winter months in temperate climates.

Treatment

Diet and lifestyle
- Other than bed-rest during the acute phase, no special precautions are necessary.

Pharmacological treatment
- Treatment is symptomatic and does not alter the course or outcome of the condition or its complications.
- Local treatment of the rash, if needed, should be designed to prevent secondary infection, e.g. potassium permanganate soaks.
- Steroids have no effect on renal abnormalities and are associated with a significant incidence of gastrointestinal side effects.

For pain relief
Standard dosage	NSAIDs, e.g. naproxen 250 mg every 6–8 h (adults).
Contraindications	Active peptic ulceration.
Special points	Asthma may be exacerbated.
Main drug interactions	Oral anticoagulants.
Main side effects	Gastrointestinal disturbances, discomfort, nausea, or ulceration.

For joint abnormalities
Standard dosage	Corticosteroids, e.g. prednisolone 40–60 mg daily.
Contraindications	Active peptic ulceration.
Special points	Possible adrenal suppression on sudden withdrawal.
Main drug interactions	NSAIDs, oral anticoagulants.
Main side effects	Cushing's syndrome, growth retardation in children, osteoporosis.

Treatment aims
To prevent secondary infection in vasculitic skin lesions.
To relieve symptoms of joint or abdominal pain.

Other treatments
- Renal replacement therapy may be needed in the 5–10% of patients who develop renal failure or nephrotic syndrome.

Prognosis
- The prognosis of the rash alone is good.
- Crops of lesions may recur within 4–8 weeks, especially in adults.
- Spontaneous remission is the norm.
- Relapses of the rash alone often occur in adults.
- 15–20% of adults with IgA nephropathy progress to renal failure in 6 months.
- Generally, 5–10% of patients develop renal failure; this is most probable in adults or adolescents.

Follow-up and management
- Renal function or urinary sediment must be monitored for evidence of renal involvement.
- If renal involvement is detected, full renal investigation, including biopsy is needed.

Key references
Fogazzi GB *et al.*: Long term outcome of Schönlein Henoch nephritis in the adult. *Clin Nephrol* 1989, **31**:60–66.

Ford EG, Jennings LM, Andrassay RJ: Management of Henoch–Schönlein purpura and polyarteritis nodosum. *Tex Med* 1987, **83**:54–58.

Schreiner DT: Purpura. *Dermatol Clin* 1989, **7**:481–490.

Herpes simplex infection — K.G. Nicholson

Diagnosis

Symptoms

Pain, burning, itching, tingling lasting 6–12 h, vesicles (generally ulcerating or crusting within 48 h): recurrent orolabial herpes (cold sores).
Fever, malaise, headache, altered personality, confusion, convulsions, paresis, paralysis, or coma: herpes encephalitis.
Fever, malaise, headache, nausea, vomiting, photophobia, neck stiffness: herpes meningitis.
Pain, photophobia, oedema of the eyelid, lacrimation, blurring of vision: ocular herpes (spectrum ranges from superficial infections to stromal keratitis and iridocyclitis affecting inner eye).
Fever, sore mouth, swelling of gums, vesicles, ulceration in anterior half of mouth, tender anterior cervical lymph nodes: primary gingivostomatitis (frequently asymptomatic).
Pain, burning, itching, tingling, vesicles followed by ulcers and crusts in perineum, vaginal discharge, dyspareunia: genital herpes; symptoms vary in severity, extent, and duration, depending on whether the infection is primary (usually most severe) or recurrent; may be asymptomatic.
Vesicles, ulcers, crusts, malaise, fever, lymphadenopathy: eczema herpeticum.
Pruritis, severe localized pain, vesicles, ulcers, crusts, fever, lymphadenopathy: other cutaneous herpes infections (herpes whitlow or gladiatorum, herpetic nipple).

Signs

Erythema progressing to vesicles, ulcers, and crusts: cutaneous lesions.
Altered personality, fluctuating levels of consciousness, focal or generalized convulsions, focal neurological findings, drowsiness, stupor, coma: herpes encephalitis.
Neck stiffness, positive Kernig's test: herpes meningitis.
Small blister or predendritic ulcers on cornea: ocular herpes; dendritic ulcers have serpentine branching appearance on fluoroscopy after fluorescein instillation.

Investigations

Cutaneous lesions

- Laboratory tests are usually not needed because symptoms and signs are diagnostic.

Electron microscopy: may show herpes virus in newly formed vesicle fluid.
Immunofluorescence: can show viral antigens in cell smears.
Virus culture: from vesicle fluid or ulcers.
Serology: of most practical value in primary infection.

Herpes encephalitis

CT, MRI, EEG: show temporal lobe localization; EEG shows temporal spike and slow wave activity in 80% of patients.
CSF analysis: shows pleocytosis, usually 50–500 cells/mm^3, with lymphocyte predominance; erythrocytes often present, specimen may be xanthochromic; protein or red erythrocyte count may be raised, sugar usually normal; csf can be examined for virus DNA (polymerase chain reaction) or viral antigens (immunology), but treatment should not await results.
Brain biopsy: may show presence of virus and Lipschütz inclusions.

Herpes meningitis

Lumbar puncture: to show CSF abnormalities of aseptic meningitis; herpes meningitis assumed when findings accompany mucocutaneous herpes, usually primary genital.

Ocular herpes

Ophthalmic examination and fluorescein: show presence of dendritic ulceration.
Abrasion of corneal cells: shows viral antigens; can be used for virus isolation.

Complications

Erythema multiforme, aseptic meningitis, urethritis, urinary retention, myelitis: due to mucocutaneous herpes.
Death, severe neurological sequelae: due to herpes encephalitis.
Visual loss, rupture of the globe (rare): due to recurrent ocular herpes.

Differential diagnosis

Mucocutaneous lesions
Causes of gingivitis and stomatitis.
Aphthous ulceration.
Coxsackie virus infection (hand, foot, and mouth).
Behçets syndrome.
Inflammatory bowel disease.
Varicella–zoster virus.
Sexually transmitted disease.

Herpes encephalitis
Other encephalitides.
Space-occupying lesions (e.g. abscess, tumour, tuberculoma).

Herpes meningitis
Other causes of meningitis (e.g. viruses, bacteria, fungi).

Ocular herpes
Ocular infections.

Aetiology

Herpes simplex virus types 1 and 2: enveloped DNA viruses.

Exposure to strong sunlight, ultraviolet light, pneumonia, meningitis and malaria: cause reactivation (cold sores).

Fever, stressful events, depression, menstruation, sexual activity: causes of recurrences of genital herpes.

Immunosuppression: cause of mucocutaneous herpes.

Inoculation of virus into a finger or direct contact: cause of herpetic whitlow and gladiatorum.

Bites and other traumatic forms of viral inoculation (e.g. from needles, razors, contaminated finger nails): causes of herpetic nipple.

Epidemiology

- Seroepidemiological studies show that 30–50% of patients in higher socio-economic groups and 100% of those in lower groups are infected with herpes simplex virus 1 by puberty.
- The prevalence of antibodies to herpes simplex virus 2 varies from 3% in nuns to ~70% in prostitutes.
- ~50 000 new cases of genital herpes occur in the UK each year.
- ~50 000 people are affected by ocular herpes in the UK each year.
- The prevalence of herpes encephalitis is 0.1–0.4 in 100 000 people, with ~50–100 cases in the UK each year.

Treatment

Diet and lifestyle
- Parents or grandparents with cold sores should not kiss young children.
- Laboratory tests have shown latex condoms to be effective mechanical barriers to herpes simplex virus.

Pharmacological treatment
- Acyclovir is of proven clinical value in some infections.
- It is not recommended for orolabial herpes or treatment of recurrent genital herpes.
- No other licensed compound has the combined safety and efficacy of acyclovir.
- Famcyclovir is now available and quite effective.

Standard dosage	*For initial genital herpes:* acyclovir 200 mg 5 times daily for 10 days. *For recurrent genital herpes (prophylaxis):* acyclovir 400–800 mg daily in 2–4 divided doses (continuous suppressive therapy). *For mucutaneous herpes in immunocompromised patients:* acyclovir i.v. or oral. *For herpes encephalitis:* acyclovir 10 mg/kg i.v. 3 times daily for 10 days. *For ocular herpes simplex:* acyclovir 400 mg 5 times daily more effective than 3% ointment.
Contraindications	Hypersensitivity.
Special points	Limited experience in pregnancy and lactation so should be used only when potential benefits outweigh risks. Bioavailability of drug possibly reduced in patients being treated for malignancy so i.v. route advised.
Main drug interactions	Probenecid increases acyclovir half-life. No detrimental interactions recognized.
Main side effects	Raised urea and creatinine concentrations due to deposition of acyclovir crystals in tubules after rapid bolus doses, occasional nausea and vomiting, inflammation and ulceration at site of infusion if extravasation of drug occurs.

Treatment aims
To accelerate healing.
To reduce virus replication and dissemination.
To prevent recurrence, death and neurological complications, and blindness.

Prognosis
- Treatment of mucocutaneous herpes results in accelerated healing and reduced viral shedding.
- Treatment of herpes encephalitis results in reduced mortality and morbidity, especially in young patients with high Glasgow Coma Scale scores who are treated early.
- Treatment of ocular herpes has varying outcomes, depending on previous inflammation and scarring.
- Prophylactic treatment reduces the incidence and severity of recurrences in patients with recurrent genital herpes and viral shedding in immunocompromised patients.

Follow-up and management
- Pregnant women should inform their obstetrician of a past history of genital herpes.

Key references
Prober CG *et al.*: The management of pregnancies complicated by genital infections with herpes simplex virus. *Clin Infect Dis* 1992, **15**:1031–1038.

Herpes zoster and varicella — F.J. Nye

Diagnosis

Symptoms

Chickenpox (varicella)
Fever and malaise: in prodromal phase, variable.

Headache, myalgia.

Vesicular rash: frequently itchy.

Shingles (herpes zoster)
Pain in affected dermatome: may precede rash by a few days.

Mental confusion, depression: common in elderly patients.

- Symptoms often continue for weeks or months.

Signs

Chickenpox
Vesicular rash: maximal on face and trunk; rapidly evolving from macules and papules to vesicles and crusts; crops of new vesicles continuing to appear for 3–4 days; drying up in 7–10 days; possibly involving conjunctivae, oropharynx, vulva, vagina; larger lesions and slow evolution suggest underlying immune deficiency.

Shingles
Unilateral, segmental skin rash: lesions similar to chickenpox but often confluent; possibly ulcerating; often a few scattered lesions elsewhere; severe multiple dermatome or recurrent disease suggests underlying immune deficiency, including HIV infection.

Investigations

- Virological investigations are needed only when the clinical diagnosis is uncertain.

Electron microscopy: of material from vesicular skin lesions for rapid confirmation of herpes virus infection.

Tissue culture: to distinguish varicella–zoster virus from herpes simplex virus.

Serology: examination of acute and convalescent sera by standard methods, e.g. complement fixation.

Complications

Chickenpox
Secondary bacterial infection of skin: usually *Staphylococcus aureus* or *Streptococcus pyogenes*.

Chickenpox pneumonia: particularly in adults, smokers, and pregnant women.

Systemic spread: in immunocompromised patients.

Haemorrhagic rash: in immunocompromised patients.

Encephalitis, polyneuritis, transverse myelitis: rare.

Reye's syndrome: in children, rare.

Haemolytic anaemia, coagulopathy with haemorrhagic rash: rare.

Shingles
Uveitis, keratitis: in patients with ophthalmic herpes zoster.

Lower motor neurone paralysis.

Ramsey–Hunt syndrome: herpes zoster of geniculate ganglion, with facial palsy, loss of taste, ipsilateral oral ulcers and skin lesions in pinna of ear.

Bowel and bladder dysfunction: in patients with sacral herpes zoster infection.

Encephalitis: rare.

Cerebral vasculopathy: trigeminal herpes zoster virus infection, with delayed cerebral infarction and hemiplegia; rare.

Differential diagnosis
Herpes simplex virus.
Other vesicular rashes, especially erythema multiforme.

Aetiology
- Chickenpox is caused by direct contact or airborne transmission of varicella–zoster virus from either chickenpox or shingles.
- After primary infection, the virus probably incorporates its DNA into the satellite cells of dorsal-root or cranial-nerve ganglion cells.
- Later reactivation causes shingles.

Epidemiology
- Chickenpox affects 1 in 200 people annually in the UK, mostly children.
- 2% of cases of chickenpox but 25% of deaths due to the disease occur in people aged >20 years.
- The prevalence of shingles rises steadily with age, 1 in 100 people >80 years being affected.
- Shingles in infants and young children probably is caused by a reactivation of intra-uterine infection.
- Both chickenpox and shingles are cross-infection hazards in hospitals.

Infection in pregnancy
- Chickenpox in pregnant women may be severe and complicated by varicella pneumonia; patients should be monitored closely.
- Intra-uterine infection may damage the fetus and cause limb scarring and hypoplasia, microcephaly or hydrocephalus, and eye abnormalities.
- This fetal varicella syndrome has an incidence of 1–3% in the first trimester (much lower risk in subsequent trimesters).
- Termination of pregnancy on the grounds of maternal chickenpox is not indicated, because the risk to the fetus is small and unpredictable.
- Maternal herpes zoster infection is not a risk to the fetus.

Infectivity
Incubation period (chickenpox): 17 days.
Infectivity: from 2 days before onset of rash until lesions have dried.
Increased infectivity and susceptibility with immunodeficiency or immunosuppression.

Treatment

Diet and lifestyle
- Patients should avoid contact with susceptible individuals (e.g. immunocompromised) until their skin lesions have dried.

Pharmacological treatment

Acyclovir
- Acyclovir is a highly selective antiviral agent that inhibits viral DNA polymerase and causes premature DNA chain termination.

Standard dosage	*For chickenpox and shingles in immunocompromised patients, chickenpox pneumonia:* acyclovir 10 mg/kg i.v. 8-hourly. *For cutaneous shingles:* acyclovir 800 mg orally 5 times daily for 7 days (started within 72 h of rash onset). *For ophthalmic shingles:* acyclovir orally as above for 10 days. *For severe maternal or neonatal chickenpox:* acyclovir i.v. *Alternatively for herpes zoster infection:* famciclovir 250 mg 3 times daily for 7 days (started within 72 h of rash onset); valaciclovir 1000 mg 3 times daily for 7 days.
Contraindications	Hypersensitivity.
Special points	High cost; no effect on latency or recurrence; not licensed for uncomplicated chickenpox.
Main drug interactions	Extreme lethargy has been reported on administration of zidovudine with i.v. acyclovir.
Main side effects	Rashes and gastrointestinal disturbances (occasionally), alterations in biochemical and haematological indices (more rarely), headaches and neurological reactions, particularly with i.v. administration, some risk of crystalluria and renal impairment at high dose (maximum oral dose in renal failure, 800 mg 3 times daily).

Varicella–zoster immune globulin
- This is distributed by the Public Health Laboratory Service (in short supply).
- It is used for highly susceptible contacts of chickenpox or shingles, including the following:

Bone-marrow transplant recipients (despite history of previous chickenpox).
Patients with debilitating disease (despite history of previous chickenpox).
HIV-positive patients with symptoms but no known varicella–zoster virus antibody.
Pregnant women without antibody (patients without a definite history of previous chickenpox must be screened for antibody).
Immunosuppressed patients who have been treated by high-dose steroids within the 3 months before contact (screened first).
Neonates up to 4 weeks old whose mothers develop chickenpox between 1 week before and 1 month after delivery or those in contact with chickenpox or shingles whose mothers have no history of previous varicella–zoster infection or no antibody.
Premature babies <30 weeks gestation or weighing <1 kg at birth in contact with chickenpox.

Standard dosage	Varicella–zoster immune globulin, depending on age: *0–5 years,* 250 mg; *6–10 years,* 500 mg; *11–14 years,* 750 mg; *≥15 years,* 1000 mg.
Contraindications	Hypersensitivity to human immunoglobulin.
Special points	Must be given as soon as possible and not more than 10 days after exposure.
Main drug interactions	None.
Main side effects	Hypersensitivity reactions (rare).

- Live attenuated varicella vaccine is available, on a named-patient basis, for immunocompromised patients, especially children with leukaemia.

Treatment aims

Chickenpox
To relieve symptoms in previously healthy patients.
To contain infection and reduce morbidity and mortality in immunocompromised patients or those with chickenpox pneumonia or maternal or neonatal infection.

Shingles
To accelerate healing and curtail pain.
To prevent complications in patients with ophthalmic herpes zoster.
To prevent progressive disease in immunocompromised patients.

Prognosis
- Mortality from chickenpox is increased in patients aged >20 years.
- Morbidity and mortality are reduced by acyclovir treatment in immunocompromised patients.

Follow-up and management
- Patients must be monitored for the development of complications.
- Pain continuing at the site of herpes zoster 30 days or more after an acute attack indicates postherpetic neuralgia, which should be treated by amitriptyline or sodium valproate. *See* Neuralgia, postherpetic *for details.*

Key references
Anonymous: Acyclovir in general practice. *Drug Ther Bull* 1992, **30**:101–104.

Anonymous: Varicella/herpes zoster. In *Immunisation Against Infectious Diseases.* London: HMSO, 1992.

Bowsher D: Neurogenic pain syndromes and their management. *Br Med Bull* 1991, **47**:644–666.

Gilbert GL: Chickenpox during pregnancy. *BMJ* 1993, **306**:1079–1080.

Wallace MR *et al.*: Treatment of adult varicella with oral acyclovir. A randomised, placebo-controlled trial. *Ann Intern Med* 1992, **117**:358–363.

Leptospirosis — I.R. Ferguson

Diagnosis

Symptoms and signs
- Any organ or tissue can be infected, so the clinical picture can vary enormously.
- The disease follows a biphasic course: the incubation period lasting 7–12 days (range, 2–20 days) is followed by the septicaemic phase lasting 4–7 days, which precedes the immune phase lasting 4–30 days.

Anicteric leptospirosis
- This occurs in 90% of patients.
- Onset is abrupt.

Fever, headache, myalgia, malaise, prostration.

Abdominal pain, nausea, vomiting, occasionally diarrhoea.

Excruciating headache: usually heralds meningitis in immune stage.

Joint pains, myalgia, conjunctival suffusion: common findings.

Sore throat, cough, bronchitis, pneumonitis, rashes, adenopathy, hepatosplenomegaly: less frequent (in UK at least).

Lymphocytic meningitis: usually lasting a few days, never fatal.

Icteric leptospirosis (Weil's syndrome)
- This form occurs in 10% of patients.

Impaired renal and hepatic function: with anuria and deepening jaundice.

Hepatosplenomegaly, severe haemorrhages into skin, pleura, peritoneum, or gastrointestinal tract.

Vascular collapse and alterations in consciousness.

Myocarditis, haemorrhage, adult respiratory distress syndrome, multiorgan failure: causing death in 10–20% of icteric patients.

Investigations
- Diagnosis is confirmed by isolation of the organism or detection of a rise in antibody titres.

Isolation: special media needed; organisms isolated from blood or CSF during septicaemic phase and from urine during third week in untreated patients.

Serology: slide agglutination tests unreliable; antibodies appear in 6–12 days, reach maximum in 4 weeks, can be suppressed by antibiotic treatment; enzyme-linked immunosorbent assay IgM test detects antibodies from day 5 of illness; microagglutination test is specific and identifies infecting serovar.

Full blood count and coagulation screen: to identify bleeding disorder and thrombocytopenia.

Liver function tests: usually normal except for raised bilirubin.

Serum creatinine measurement: to identify degree of renal impairment.

CSF analysis: to confirm lymphocytic meningitis.

Complications
Uveitis 6–12 weeks after original illness and chronic persistent leptospiruria: extremely rare.

Transplacental transmission, with fetal death and abortion: has occurred.

Differential diagnosis
Influenza-like illness, viral infections, aseptic meningitis, encephalitis.

Enteric-fever-like illness.

Infective hepatitis, other causes of jaundice.

Atypical pneumonia, rickettsioses.

Septicaemia, nephritis.

Leukaemia, thrombocytopenic purpura, meningococcal disease.

Aetiology
- In the UK, prevalent serovars of pathogenic leptospires, Leptospira interrogans, are hardjo, icterohaemorrhagiae, saxkoebing, ballum, australis, autumnalis, hebdomadis, and canicola (the first three are the most common in humans).
- Wild and domestic animals, especially rats (icterohaemorrhagiae) and cattle (hardjo) are infection reservoirs.
- Contact of mucous membranes or abraded skin with infected animal tissue or urine or contaminated water or soil can lead to transmission.

Epidemiology
- People at risk include farmers, dairyworkers, abattoir workers, veterinarians, and those working or engaged in recreational pursuits on or in natural inland waters.
- On average, 63 cases and three deaths are diagnosed annually in the UK: 90% in working men, 75% in summer and autumn, peaking in October.

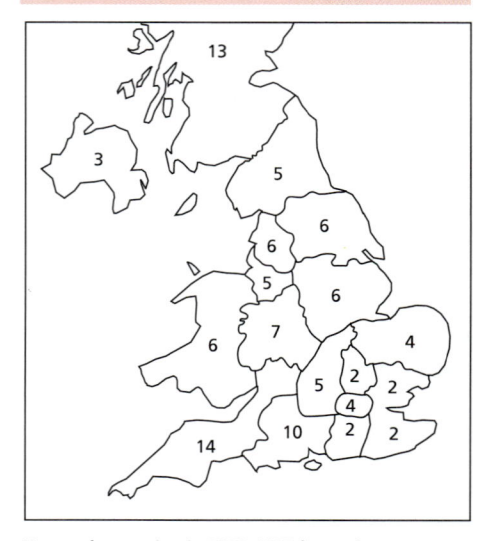

Human leptospirosis 1968-1992 by region.

Treatment

Diet and lifestyle

- Rodents must be controlled in and around human habitations.
- Contamination of living, working, and recreational areas by infected urine should be prevented.
- Cuts should be covered by waterproof dressings, and protective clothing be worn.
- Immersion in natural inland waters should be avoided.
- Participants should shower after swimming, canoeing, windsurfing, or waterskiing.
- Safety cards should be issued to people at risk to show medical staff if illness occurs.
- Patients should be educated on modes of transmission and preventive measures.
- Domestic animals, especially cattle and dogs, should be immunized.

Pharmacological treatment

Antibiotics

- Antibiotics can only influence the course of the disease if given in the first week.
- Intensive treatment is needed for severe infections.

Standard dosage	Benzylpenicillin 900 mg, ampicillin 1 g, or erythromycin 500 mg all parenterally 4 times daily for 1 week. Amoxycillin 500 mg orally 3 times daily or doxycycline 100 mg twice daily for 1 week.
Contraindications	Hypersensitivity; oral agents should be avoided in pregnancy, infancy, and childhood.
Special points	*Penicillin:* can induce a short-lived exacerbation with pyrexia and hypotension: this 'MacKay–Dick' reaction is regarded as a sign of leptospiral lysis.
Main drug interactions	*Penicillins:* inactivate aminoglycoside in syringe. *Erythromycin:* potentiates digoxin, warfarin, and carbamazepine. *Doxycycline:* affects anticoagulant treatment.
Main side effects	*Parenteral agents:* anaphylactic reaction, gastrointestinal reactions (rare). *Doxycycline:* photosensitivity (rare), permanent teeth discoloration.

For symptoms

Prompt correction of electrolyte imbalance.

Fresh blood, platelets, or clotting factors for haemorrhage.

Pethidine or morphine for severe pain.

Diazepam and phenytoin for seizures.

Steroids for thrombocytopenia.

Haemodialysis for renal failure.

Treatment aims

To alleviate symptoms.

Prognosis

- Most cases are mild and often undiagnosed; patients recover spontaneously.
- In Weil's syndrome with hepatorenal involvement, mortality is 10–20%.
- No ill effects are seen after renal or hepatic involvement in surviving patients.
- Death without jaundice is extremely rare.
- Reinfection by a different serovar is possible.

Follow-up and management

- Supportive treatment includes analgesics, sedation, and antiemetics.
- Renal and cardiac function must be monitored daily.

Key references

Ferguson IR: Leptospirosis surveillance: 1990–1992. *Commun Dis Rep* 1993, 3:R47–R48.

Ferguson IR: Leptospirosis update. *BMJ* 1991, 302:128–129.

Lyme disease
D.O. Ho-Yen

Diagnosis

Symptoms
- Patients may be asymptomatic.

Acute disease
- Symptoms occur 3–32 days after tick bite.

Influenza-like illness: malaise, pyrexia, myalgia, arthralgia, sore throat.

Rash.

Stiff neck.

Photophobia.

Chronic disease
- Symptoms occur weeks or months later.

Headache, stiff neck, photophobia, confusion, concentration and memory impairment.

Chest pain.

Joint pain and swelling.

Abdominal pain, tenderness, diarrhoea.

Rashes.

Signs

Acute disease
Pyrexia, tender muscles or joints, inflamed throat.

Erythema chronicum migrans: characteristic rash, red macule or papule at site of tick bite, enlarges peripherally with central clearing over several weeks; metastatic lesions may develop; can last months.

Lymphadenopathy.

Meningism.

Erythema chronicum migrans.

Chronic disease
Meningitis, encephalitis, cranial neuritis (especially Bell's palsy), radiculoneuritis, peripheral neuropathies.

Atrioventricular block, myopericarditis.

Arthritis.

Hepatomegaly, splenomegaly.

Acrodermatitis chronica atrophicans: vivid red lesions becoming sclerotic or atrophic.

Lymphadenosis benigna cutis: especially in earlobes or nipples.

Investigations

Microscopy, histopathology, and culture: lack sensitivity and not widely available but may be diagnostic.

Serological tests: widely available but not diagnostic (support clinical diagnosis); IgM tests positive 3–6 weeks after infection, may persist for many months, but may not be reproducible; IgG tests positive 6–8 weeks after infection, may remain positive for years, but more reproducible so are mainstay of diagnosis; immunofluorescence tests and enzyme linked immunosorbent assays most widely available.

- False-negative antibody results may occur early in illness, with antibiotic treatment or due to immune complexes; a negative antibody test does not exclude the diagnosis. False-positive results are due to other spirochaete infections, other infections, or the test; Western blotting may distinguish true- from false-positive results.

Complications
CNS abnormalities.

Cardiac conduction disturbances.

Oligoarthitis.

Differential diagnosis

Erythema chronicum migrans
Erythema marginatum.
Erythema multiforme.
Granuloma annulare.

Lymphadenopathy
Infectious mononucleosis.
Cytomegalovirus.
Toxoplasmosis.

Neurological symptoms
Infectious diseases.
Toxoplasmosis.
Guillain–Barré syndrome.
Multiple sclerosis.

Cardiac symptoms
Infectious diseases.
Chronic heart disease.
Digitalis use.

Arthritis
Rheumatoid arthritis.
Reactive arthritis.

Other dermatological symptoms
Erythema nodosum.
Circulatory insufficiencies.
Lymphoma.

Aetiology
- Infection is transmitted by tick bites, usually *Ixodes ricinus* in the UK.
- The causative organism is *Borrelia burgdorferi*, a spirochaete.

Epidemiology
- Lyme disease is found in the USA, Europe, Russia, China, Japan, and Australia.
- Occurrence parallels distribution and infection in ticks (0–25%).
- In forested areas, 5–10% of the population have antibodies.
- Infection peaks in June and July.
- It is found in patients of all ages but especially in the most active and those exposed to ticks.

Treatment

Diet and lifestyle
- No special precautions are necessary.

Pharmacological treatment

Criteria for treatment
- The risk depends on infected tick attachment: <24 h, little risk; 48 h, 50% risk; 72 h, almost certain infection.
- Infection occurs in ~10% of people bitten by infected ticks, so empirical treatment is not justified in areas where infected ticks are rare.
- Erythema chronicum migrans must be treated; acute disease with positive serology and chronic disease when other causes are excluded warrant treatment.
- Treatment should be considered in anxious patients with possible infection but without high expectation of success.
- Asymptomatic individuals with positive serology probably should not be treated.

For acute disease

Standard dosage	Doxycycline 200 mg orally daily for 14 days. Amoxycillin 500 mg 3 times daily for 14 days. Ceftriaxone 2 g i.v. or i.m. daily for 14–21 days.
Contraindications	*Doxycycline:* pregnancy, lactation, children <12 years, SLE, porphyria. *Amoxycillin:* penicillin hypersensitivity. *Ceftriaxone:* cephalosporin hypersensitivity, pregnancy, lactation.
Main drug interactions	*Doxycycline:* anticoagulants, antiepileptics, oral contraceptives. *Amoxycillin:* anticoagulants, oral contraceptives.
Main side effects	*Doxycycline:* nausea, vomiting, diarrhoea, headache. *Amoxycillin:* nausea, diarrhoea, rashes. *Ceftriaxone:* gastrointestinal complaints, allergic reactions, rashes, haematological disturbance, liver dysfunction.

- Erythromycin and clarithromycin are less effective but can be used in penicillin-sensitive children.
- Azithromycin has great promise but is not yet licensed in the UK.

For chronic disease

Standard dosage	Ceftriaxone 2 g i.v. or i.m. daily for 14–21 days. Cefotaxime 12 g i.v. or i.m. twice daily for 14–21 days. Penicillin G 3 g i.v. 4 times daily for 14–21 days.
Contraindications	*Cefotaxime:* cephalosporin hypersensitivity, porphyria. *Penicillin:* hypersensitivity.
Main drug interactions	*Cefotaxime:* anticoagulants, probenecid. *Penicillin:* anticoagulants, oral contraceptives.
Main side effects	*Cefotaxime:* gastrointestinal complaints, allergic reactions, rashes, haematological disturbance, liver dysfunction. *Penicillin:* sensitivity reactions, especially urticaria, angioedema, anaphylaxis.

Treatment aims
To kill organism.
To prevent disease progression.
To alleviate symptoms.

Prognosis
- Despite antibiotic treatment, symptoms recur in 50% of patients, although severity and duration are greatly reduced; occasionally, recurrent symptoms may last several years.
- Acute Lyme disease and carditis have good prognosis.
- Cranial nerve palsies and meningitis have good prognosis; radiculoneuritis, peripheral neuropathy, encephalitis, and encephalomyelitis usually have a favourable outcome, but a tendency toward chronic or recurrent disease is seen.
- Arthritis often resolves, but response may be slow, often needing further treatment.
- In chronic disease, recurrence is not usual.

Follow-up and management
- Patients may need careful monitoring for months or years, depending on the severity of the symptoms.

Key references
Guy EC: The laboratory diagnosis of Lyme borreliosis. *Rev Med Microbiol* 1993, **4**:89–96.

Magid D *et al.*: Prevention of Lyme disease after tick bites. *N Engl J Med* 1992, **327**:534–541.

Rahn DW, Malawista SE: Recommendations for diagnosis and treatment. *Ann Intern Med* 1991, **114**:472–481.

Weber K, Pfister H: Clinical management of Lyme borreliosis. *Lancet* 1994, **343**:1017–1020.

Malaria
M.E. Molyneux

Diagnosis

Symptoms
- The diagnosis may be disastrously overlooked, especially if a travel history is not obtained. A brief stop-over in an endemic area is sufficient to allow inoculation with the parasite.
- Illness usually occurs 1–4 weeks after mosquito bite but may be delayed for weeks or even years.

Uncomplicated malaria
Fever: usually rapid onset; rigors, malaise, headache, and myalgia followed by profuse sweating; fever paroxysms every 2–3 days develop in some patients.

Nausea, vomiting, anorexia, diarrhoea, cough: possible early symptoms.

Complicated falciparum malaria
Altered consciousness, convulsions, oliguria, jaundice, respiratory distress, haemorrhage.

Signs
- Fever is usual; it may, however, be intermittent, so some patients are afebrile when first seen. Occasionally, patients remain afebrile throughout the illness.

Uncomplicated malaria
Fever: either continuous or episodic.

Rigors.

Moderately enlarged liver or spleen.

Complicated falciparum malaria
Confusion.
Delirium.
Coma.
Abnormal posturing.
Opisthotonos.
Acidosis.
Pallor.
Jaundice.
Shock syndrome.

Investigations

Urgent
Blood films: thick and thin, stained with Giemsa for malaria parasites, to identify species of malaria and density of parasitaemia; a single blood film may be negative in malaria; repeat films may reveal parasites.

Blood glucose profile: repeated at intervals.

Haemoglobin and full blood count: regularly, because haemoglobin may fall rapidly.

In severe falciparum malaria
Urine output, plasma urea, creatinine, electrolytes, and arterial blood gas analysis: to identify renal failure and respiratory distress syndrome.

Platelet count: if $<50 \times 10^9$/L, bleeding time, serum fibrinogen, and fibrin degradation products should be checked to identify disseminated intravascular coagulation.

Chest radiography: peripheral shadows indicate pulmonary oedema or adult respiratory distress syndrome.

Blood culture: for bacterial pathogens in patients with shock.

Complications
- Complications occur only with *Plasmodium falciparum* malaria; they are more likely if treatment is delayed.

Cerebral malaria: altered consciousness with or without convulsions.

Extreme prostration.
Shock.
Hypoglycaemia.
Lactic acidosis.
Intravascular haemolysis.
Jaundice.
Severe anaemia.
Disseminated intravascular coagulation.
Respiratory distress syndrome.
Acute renal failure.

Differential diagnosis

Uncomplicated malaria
Any fever.
Influenza or upper respiratory tract infection.
Hepatitis, gastroenteritis.

Complicated falciparum malaria
Fulminant hepatitis.
Meningitis, encephalitis, rabies.
Leptospirosis, heat stroke, ketoacidosis.
Septicaemia or septic shock.
Pneumonia or pulmonary oedema.
Acute tubular necrosis.

Aetiology
- Malaria is a protozoal infection transmitted by mosquitoes.
- Four parasite species infect humans: *Plasmodium falciparum*, *P. vivax*, *P. malariae*, and *P. ovale*.
- Only *P. falciparum* malaria progresses to complicated disease, which may be fatal.

Epidemiology
- 1–3 million children die of malaria annually throughout the world.
- ~2000 cases are diagnosed in the UK annually, with an average of 10 deaths each year.
- In the UK, imported malaria is increasing as more people travel to endemic areas and parasites develop resistance to drugs.

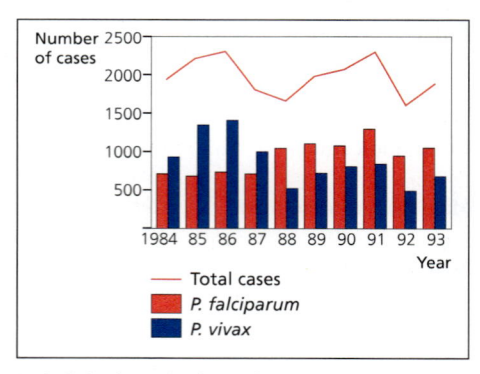

Malaria in the United Kingdom: reports to the Malaria Reference Laboratory 1984–1993. © PHLS.

M.E. Molyneux **Malaria**

Treatment

Diet and lifestyle

- Travellers to endemic areas should remember the following points:
- Mosquito bites can be prevented by using permethrin-impregnated bed-net or sleeping in well screened buildings, wearing long sleeves and trousers in evenings or after dark, and applying insect repellent containing diethyl toluamide (DEET) for journeys into swamp or jungle (Mosigard is an alternative).
- Antimalarial prophylactic drugs appropriate to the area to be visited should be taken.
- Immediate diagnosis and treatment should be sought for any fever developing during or after travel.
- A supply of antimalarial drugs suitable for immediate treatment of possible malaria should be taken on any journey far from medical services.

Pharmacological treatment

For malaria due to *Plasmodium vivax, P. malariae,* or *P. ovale*

- Oral treatment should be given when possible. Doses are for chloroquine base.

Standard dosage	Chloroquine phosphate or sulphate 600 mg (child, 10 mg/kg) on days 1 and 2; 300 mg (child, 5 mg/kg) on day 3.
Contraindications	Rare hypersensitivity.
Special points	*P. vivax* acquired in southeast Asia may be resistant to chloroquine: alternative treatment is Fansidar 3 tablets once daily (adults).
Main drug interactions	None of importance.
Main side effects	Rare hypotension, pruritus in blacks.

For malaria due to *P. vivax* or *P. ovale*

Chloroquine as above and primaquine 15 mg (child, 0.25 mg/kg) daily for 15 days to eliminate dormant hepatic parasites: contraindicated in glucose-6-phosphate dehydrogenase deficiency; status must be checked before primaquines prescribed.

For uncomplicated malaria due to *P. falciparum*

- Treatment is needed urgently because complications may develop quickly; in non-endemic countries (e.g. UK), hospital admission is advised, at least for initiation of treatment. Oral treatment is recommended when possible.

Standard dosage	Quinine sulphate salt 600 mg (child, 10 mg/kg) 3 times daily for 7 days, with Fansidar 3 tablets (child, *see drug data sheet*). Alternatively, mefloquine 500 mg orally, repeated after 6 h.
Contraindications	*Quinine*: caution in cardiac disease. *Fansidar*: sulphonamide hypersensitivity. *Mefloquine*: pregnancy, beta blocker treatment, history of epilepsy or chronic neurological disease.
Main drug interactions	*Quinine*: may potentiate cardiotoxic effect of other cardiac drugs.
Main side effects	*Quinine*: hypoglycaemia (especially in pregnancy), hypotension, tinnitus (always).

For *P. falciparum* malaria with complications

- This is a medical emergency: immediate hospital admission is vital, preferably with intensive care facilities.

Standard dosage	Quinine dihydrochloride salt 20 mg/kg (up to 1400 mg) i.v. infusion in saline solution over 4 h, then 10 mg/kg over 4 h for each dose every 12 h; changed to oral treatment as soon as possible. Alternatively, quinidine gluconate.
Contraindications	Caution in elderly patients or those with cardiac disease.
Special points	First dose 10 mg/kg if quinine, mefloquine, or halofantrine taken in preceding 24 h. When condition satisfactory, Fansidar can be added.
Main drug interactions	None of importance.
Main side effects	None of importance.

Treatment aims

To support patients with complicated disease while drugs eliminate parasites.

To clear blood of parasites.

To eliminate liver-stage dormant parasites (*Plasmodium vivax, P. ovale*).

Prognosis

- Full recovery is expected for patients with non-falciparum infection.
- Prompt correct treatment of *Plasmodium falciparum* malaria should result in cure.
- After complications have developed, the mortality in falciparum malaria is 10–40%, determined by the extent and severity of the complications and the quality of intensive care offered.
- Recovery from renal failure or coma is usually complete; a few patients have neurological sequelae after cerebral malaria.

Follow-up and management

- Patients must be told to report promptly with any fever because recrudescence or relapse may occur.
- Organ complications must be followed up in their own right.
- Haemoglobin concentrations must be adequately restored and maintained; this must be monitored.

Useful addresses

- Centres in the UK where advice on malaria may be obtained include the following:
Liverpool School of Tropical Medicine, Pembroke Place, Liverpool L3 5QA, tel 0151 708 9393.

Hospital for Tropical Diseases, 4 St Pancras Way, London NW1 0PE, tel. 0171 387 4411.

Key references

Bradley D *et al.*: Prophylaxis against malaria for travellers from the United Kingdom. *BMJ* 1993, **306**:1247–1252.

Molyneux ME, Fox R: Diagnosis and treatment of malaria in Britain. *BMJ* 1993, **306**:1175–1180.

World Health Organization: Severe and complicated malaria. *Trans R Soc Trop Med Hyg* 1990, **84 (suppl 2)**:1–65.

Measles
P.D. Welsby

Diagnosis

Symptoms
Fever: for 3–4 days.
Rash.
Systemic upset; 'misery'.
Unproductive cough.
Catarrh.
Conjunctivitis.

Signs

Prodromal period before rash
Fever.
Enanthem, Koplik's spots: pathognomic small greyish-white spots on reddened mucous membranes, notably the buccal mucosa.
Rash: maculopapular, blotchy, not itchy; starts on face and behind ears; spreads downwards over a few days; lasts ~5 days; almost invariably stains (persisting discoloration that does not blanch on pressure) from erythrocyte leakage during active rash.

Associated with development of rash
Reddened throat.
'Muffled' bronchitic cough.
Conjunctivitis.
Lymph-node enlargement.

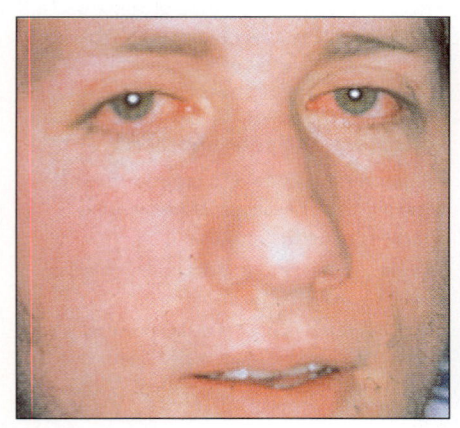

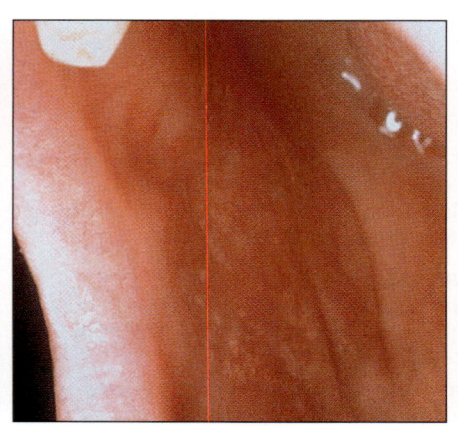

Blotchy rash of measles, misery, and conjunctivitis.　　Koplik's spots in measles.

Investigations
- The clinical picture is usually diagnostic.

Throat swab or nasopharyngeal aspirate: measles virus may be grown (technically difficult).
Immunofluorescent staining of throat secretions: may identify measles virus.
Serology: measles-specific IgM may be present in blood early in illness.
Paired sera examination: may show diagnostic rises in antibody (about fourfold).

Complications
- Complications are more severe in old or very young patients.

Measles bronchiolitis: when rash heaviest on trunk.
Secondary bacterial pneumonia and otitis media: in ~15%, especially children.
Febrile convulsions: in children, especially during prodrome.
Post-acute measles encephalitis: immune-mediated, at about day 6 of illness.
Subacute sclerosing pancephalitis: caused by persisting measles virus infection in nervous system, usually fatal; develops several years after acute infection.
Gastroenteritis: in malnourished children can lead to kwashiorkor and acute vitamin A deficiency.
Thrombocytopenia.
Giant-cell pneumonia or measles encephalitis: progressive in immunocompromised patient.

Differential diagnosis
Drug rashes: do not usually evolve from above downwards, may be itchy, only occasionally stain, often not associated with fever.
Rubella: patients not usually systemically unwell, rash not usually blotchy.
Adenovirus or enterovirus infection.
- Koplik's spots are not a feature in any of the above.

Aetiology
- Measles is caused by Measles virus, an RNA virus.
- Transmission is by respiratory droplets.

Epidemiology
- Measles occurs worldwide.
- Marked reduction in incidence can be expected after the schools' MR campaign at the end of 1994; this mass immunization programme is one of the strategies recommended by the World Health Organization to achieve global eradication.

Infectivity
- Measles is highly infectious: patients are infectious for about 4 days before the rash and until the rash has stained.
- Active infection without illness and a rash is extremely rare.
- Immunity after an attack is for life.
- Maternally derived antibodies protect babies for about the first 6 months of life.
- There is no infective carrier state.

Mean incubation period
To febrile illness: 10 days.
To rash: 14 days.

Treatment

Diet and lifestyle
- Patients should be isolated during the period of infectivity, which usually lasts from the onset of symptoms until the rash has stained.

Pharmacological treatment

Symptomatic
Analgesics, e.g. paracetamol.

Antibacterial drugs for bacterial complications.

- Ribavin may be of benefit for giant-cell pneumonia.

Prophylactic
Vaccination by live virus preparation in second year of life as MMR: may cause mild measles-like illness.

Pooled human immunoglobulin: protective if given shortly after exposure.

- Vaccination and pooled human immunoglobulin can be given together if vaccination of vulnerable patients (e.g. those with cystic fibrosis) is desired.
- Vitamin A deficiency (clinical or subclinical) increases the severity, complications, and risk of death from measles.
- In countries where the measles fatality rate is 1% or more, vitamin A should be given in all cases; elsewhere, it should be given in severe cases.

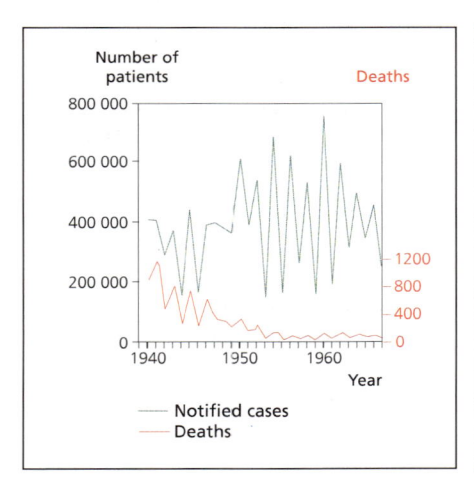

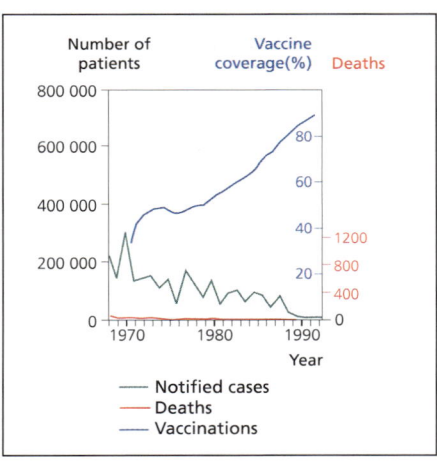

Measles notifications: cases and deaths in England and Wales 1940–1968 (left), when mass immunization was introduced, and 1968–1993 (right); vaccine coverage 1970–1993. © PHLS.

Treatment aims
To relieve symptoms.
To treat complications promptly.

Prognosis
- Most patients make a full recovery and are immune thereafter.

Follow-up and management
- No follow-up is necessary.

Key references
Anonymous: Measles surveillance. *Commun Dis Rep CDR Wkly* 1993, **3**:21.

Dales LG et al.: Measles epidemic from failure to immunize. *West J Med* 1993, **159**:455–464.

Makhene MK, Diaz PS: Clinical presentations and complications of suspected measles in hospitalized children. *Pediatr Infect Dis J* 1993, **12**:836–840.

Tohani VK, Kennedy FD: Vaccine efficacy in a measles immunisation programme. *Commun Dis Rep CDR Rev* 1992, **2**:R59–R60.

Parvovirus B19 infection — P.D. Welsby

Diagnosis

Symptoms
- Often no symptoms are manifest.

Mild feverish illness: in children.

Mild feverish illness with arthralgia or arthritis: in adults.

Symptoms of an aplastic crisis: in patients with haemolytic anaemias or occasionally normal people; onset usually acute but self-limiting.

Symptoms of persistent severe anaemia: in immunosuppressed patients.

Signs
- The illness, when accompanied by a rash, is known as erythema infectiosum, fifth disease, or slapped cheek syndrome.

Rash: usually seen in children; appears on cheeks, giving slapped-cheek appearance; lasts 1 week; recurs for several months on exposure to sun or wind; variable but often reticular maculopapular rash may also develop on arms and legs but rarely affects palms or soles.

Lymph-node enlargement: in adults.

Arthralgia or arthritis: often involving wrists and knees in adults; can occur without rash; usually last 2–4 weeks, occasionally longer.

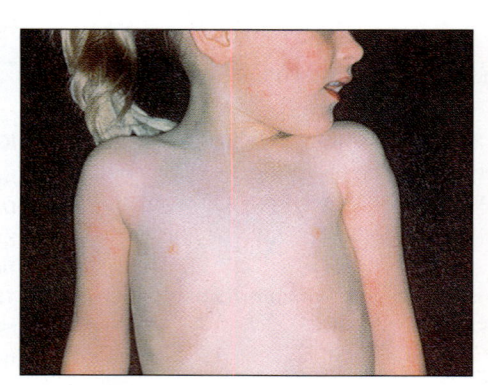

Slapped-cheek appearance of parvovirus B19 infection and reticular rash on arms.

Investigations
Serology: IgM specific to parvovirus B19 manifest in early illness; parvovirus B19 IgG antibody develops early in illness and falls within 1–2 months.

Complications
Aplastic crisis.

Fetal anaemia, hydrops fetalis, and death: especially during second trimester, although effect on pregnancy uncertain; about one-third of pregnant women with primary infection transmit it to fetus.

Differential diagnosis
Scarlet fever: parvovirus has no oral stigmata.

Measles: no Koplik's spots or marked syndrome in parvovirus infection.

Rubella, enteroviral infections, cytomegalovirus, Epstein–Barr virus, toxoplasmosis.

Aetiology
- Infection is by parvovirus B19, a DNA virus.
- Transmission is by respiratory droplets.

Epidemiology
- Infection occurs worldwide.
- Most infections are in spring or early summer.
- In England, antibody prevalence rises from 45% in 10-year-olds to 60–70% in adults.

Infectivity
- In England, primary infection is estimated to develop in 1 in 400 pregnancies; only ~10% of these are recognised.
- Parvovirus B19 is moderately infective.
- Immunity is apparently for life after an acute episode.

Mean incubation period
To the mild febrile illness: 6–8 days.
To the rash: 17–18 days.

Treatment

Diet and lifestyle
- People known to be infected should avoid contact with pregnant women.

Pharmacological treatment
Analgesics, e.g. paracetamol.
NSAIDs for reactive arthralgia.

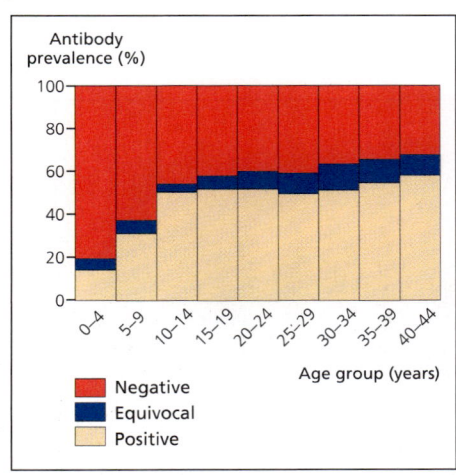

Antibody prevalance to parvovirus B19 by age (England). © PHLS.

Treatment aims
To relieve symptoms (if any).

Prognosis
- Prognosis is good in acquired illness.
- Mortality is 9% in recognised fetal infections.

Follow-up and management
- Follow-up is not needed.

Key references
Gay NJ et al. Age specific antibody prevalence to parvovirus B19: how many women are infected in pregnancy? *Comm Dis Rep* 1994, **4**:R104–R107.

Pattison JR: Human parvovirus B19. *BMJ* 1994, **308**:149–150.

Pharyngitis G.R. Williams

Diagnosis

Symptoms
Sore throat: with difficulty swallowing.
Concurrent coryza, laryngitis, productive cough: suggesting viral cause.
Malaise, fever, headache: common.

Signs

General
Injected mucous membranes of pharynx, tonsils, conjunctivae, and tympanic membranes.
Enlarged tonsils: sometimes with exudates.
Enlarged cervical lymph nodes.

Streptococcal infection
Grey exudates in tonsillar follicles.
Enlarged injected tonsillar and peri-tonsillar area.
Coated tongue with foetor.
Enlarged, tender jugulodigastric nodes.
Occasional meningism.
Diffuse punctate erythema, flushed cheeks, circumoral pallor, reddened mucous membrane, white then red strawberry tongue, desquamation of hands and feet (after 7–10 days): signs of scarlet fever.

Infectious mononucleosis
Prolonged fever: often for 10–14 days.
Nasal voice/'fish mouth' breathing.
Enlarged lymph nodes and splenomegaly.
Palatal petechiae and clean tongue.
Enlarged tonsils: sometimes almost meeting in middle, with confluent white exudates.
'Ampicillin or amoxycillin rash': in 95% of patients.

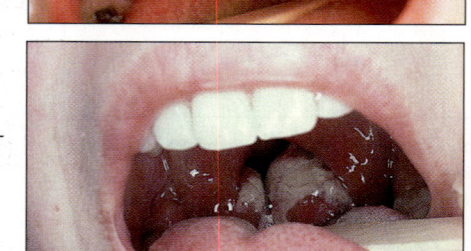

Hand, foot, and mouth disease
5–10 small aphthoid ulcers: scattered over oral cavity.
Firm vesicular lesions: along sides of fingers and on feet (usually few).
Papular lesions: especially on feet and lower legs, occasionally up to buttocks.

Herpangina
Posterior pharyngeal and soft-palate ulcers: often not painful, enlarging for 7–10 days.

Diphtheria
Toxic, listless, tachycardia due to myocarditis: fever usually low-grade or nonexistent.
Adherent whitish membrane: spreading from tonsils to oropharynx or oral cavity.
Enlarged anterior cervical lymph nodes: with surrounding oedema.

Streptococcal follicular tonsillar exudates (top) and confluent exudates (bottom) in infectious mononucleosis.

Investigations
Throat swab: to check for streptococcal infection and diphtheria.
Throat and faeces swab in viral transport medium or direct immunofluorescence: to check for enteroviruses, adenoviruses, influenza, parainfluenza.
Differential leucocyte count: elevated neutrophil leucocytosis indicates streptococcal infection; elevated, many atypical mononuclear cells indicate infectious mononucleosis.
Serology: for Epstein–Barr virus, adenovirus, mycoplasma, influenza, and parainfluenza.

Complications
Peritonsillar abscess, reactive phenomena (rheumatic fever, glomerulonephritis, erythema nosodum, Henoch–Schönlein purpura): with streptococcal infection.
Respiratory obstruction, hepatitis, splenic rupture: with infectious mononucleosis.
Nerve palsies, myocarditis: with diphtheria.
Erythema multiforme: with *Mycoplasma pneumoniae* infection.

Differential diagnosis
- Differential diagnosis depends on the underlying cause.

Aetiology
- Causes include the following:

Pharyngitis with nonspecific features
Viral infection, especially adenoviruses, enteroviruses, influenza or parainfluenza virus, Epstein–Barr virus.
Beta-haemolytic *streptococcus pyogenes* group A, C, or G.
Mycoplasma pneumoniae, Corynebacterium diphtheriae, Neisseria gonorrhoeae.

Pharyngitis with clinically recognisable features
Streptococcus pyogenes infection: cause of follicular tonsillitis, scarlet fever.
Epstein–Barr virus infection: cause of infectious mononucleosis.
Coxsackie virus infection: cause of hand, foot, and mouth disease (A16), herpangina (A).
Corynebacterium diphtheriae infection: cause of diphtheria.

Epidemiology
- Up to six episodes of pharyngitis occur per person each year.
- Adenoviral infection is the most common viral type identified in children with respiratory illnesses, which are more prevalent in crowded conditions.
- Enteroviral infection usually occurs in late summer or early autumn, with one or two types dominating (out of >70).
- Some influenza virus activity is usual each winter, with some larger outbreaks.
- Epstein–Barr virus circulates throughout childhood but is usually only manifest as anginose variety in teenagers and young adults.
- Streptococcal infection occurs in late winter and early spring, especially in school children.
- Very few cases of diphtheria occur in the UK each year; the bacteria are usually transmitted from healthy carriers from developing countries.

Treatment

Diet and lifestyle
- Infants should be breast-fed and subsequently provided with adequate nutrition throughout childhood.
- Respiratory secretions must be disposed of hygienically.

Pharmacological treatment
- Immunization should be given as nationally recommended: e.g. against diphtheria, influenza A; the combined tetanus and low-dose diphtheria booster was introduced for UK school leavers in 1994. It can be used for travellers to developing countries and Eastern Europe without previous Schick testing.
- Symptomatic treatment is indicated for presumed viral infections: e.g. throat lozenges, paracetamol.

Antibiotics
- Penicillins are effective against streptococcal and diphtherial infections.

Standard dosage	Benzylpenicillin 300–600 mg i.v. 6-hourly. Phenoxymethylpenicillin 500 mg orally 6-hourly.
Contraindications	Hypersensitivity.
Special points	Erythromycin or new macrolides are other options.
Main drug interactions	None.
Main side effects	Sensitivity reactions, diarrhoea.

Antitoxin
- Antitoxin should be given immediately on clinical suspicion of diphtheria.

Standard dosage	Antitoxin 10 000–100 000 units i.m. (most of larger doses may be given i.v. after 0.5–2 h).
Contraindications	Hypersensitivity.
Special points	Test dose is needed before full dose because of equine origin of antitoxin.
Main drug interactions	None.
Main side effects	Sensitivity reactions, including serum sickness.

Treatment aims
To provide symptomatic relief.
To reduce infectivity.
To prevent rheumatic fever (in streptococcal infections).
To neutralize circulating toxins of diphtheria promptly.

Other treatments
Drainage of peritonsillar abscess, indicated by marked inferior and posterior displacement of tonsil.
Intubation or tracheostomy for respiratory obstruction in infectious mononucleosis that does not respond to i.v. hydrocortisone.
Tonsillectomy in children with recurrent tonsillitis that disrupts schooling.

Prognosis
- Full rapid recovery is usual.
- Occasionally, patients suffer from post-viral fatigue, especially after influenza, Epstein–Barr, or enteroviral infections.
- Mortality from diphtheria is 5–10%; survivors usually recover completely.

Follow-up and management
- Patients who have apparently recovered from streptococcal tonsillitis may continue to have enlarged and tender jugulodigastric nodes that subsequently spread infection as cellulitis or septicaemia.
- Patients with diphtheria should be followed up after 2–6 weeks for late nerve palsies and myocarditis.

Notification
- Diphtheria and scarlet fever are legally notifiable diseases in the UK.
- Suspected diphtheria should be notified promptly by telephone to enable the source to be traced and contacts to be identified, assessed, and treated or immunized.

Key references
Dittmann S, Roure C: *Plan of Action for the Prevention and Control of Diphtheria in the European Region (1994–1995)*. Copenhagen: WHO Europe, 1994.
Schulman ST: Streptococcal pharyngitis: clinical and epidemiological factors. *Pediatr Infect Dis J* 1989, **8**:816–819.

Rheumatic fever, acute
W.T.A. Todd

Diagnosis

Symptoms
- Acute rheumatic fever is a multisystem disorder occurring 1–5 weeks after group A streptococcal infection.
- Its manifestation is variable, involving any of the following:

Joint pain (migratory polyarthropathy): ranging from simple pain to disabling arthritis; classically involves large joints in succession, with 'overlapping' involvement.

Breathlessness and chest pain (pancarditis): cardiac failure with occasional clinical pericardial involvement.

Rapid purposeless involuntary movements (Sydenham's chorea): including slurred speech, jerky movements, facial tics and grimacing, emotional lability; manifest only during wakefulness; may occur as late isolated feature of disease.

Subcutaneous nodules: painless firm lesions (up to 2 cm diameter) over bony prominences and tendons; tend to appear late and last 1–2 weeks.

Erythema marginatum: red rash extending circumferentially on trunk and proximal limbs; changes rapidly over minutes.

Signs
Joint involvement: joints may be exquisitely tender, red, swollen; refusal to bear weight (especially in children).

Signs of cardiac failure, tachycardia, cardiomegaly, pericardial rub, mitral regurgitation, Carey–Coombs aortic regurgitation, first-, second-, or third-degree atrioventricular block.

Chorea: 'bag of worms' tongue of chorea (fasciculation on protrusion), 'Milkmaid's grip' (squeezing and relaxing motion on gripping the hand), pendular knee jerks.

Skin rash and nodules.

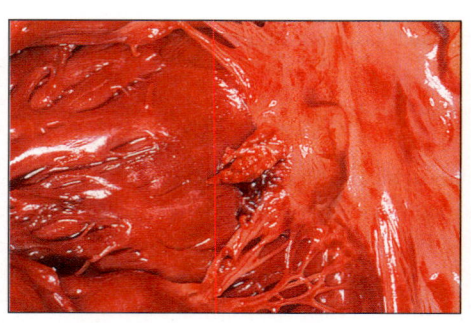

Vegetation on mitral valve, the major reason for continued prophylaxis after rheumatic heart disease.

Investigations
- No single test is diagnostic; the diagnosis is simplified by application of the Duckett-Jones criteria.
- The most important laboratory contribution is evidence of antecedent streptococcal infection.
- No significant laboratory abnormality may be seen in pure chorea.

Throat swab: usually negative, but positive result indicates increased disease activity.

Antistreptolysin O, anti-DNAse B, antihyaluronidase titres: if all three done, 95% chance of positive result.

Full blood count: leucocytosis common; moderate normochromic, normocytic anaemia often seen.

ESR, CRP measurement: usually raised.

Liver function tests: aspartate transaminase possibly raised.

Urinalysis: sediment positive for leucocytes and erythrocytes (not pathognomonic of glomerulonephritis).

ECG: shows tachycardia and first-, second-, or, rarely, third-degree heart block.

Echocardiography: shows myocardial thickening and dysfunction, pericardial effusion, and valvular dysfunction.

Complications
Recurrent episodes: with continuing evidence of inflammatory activity.
Rheumatic heart disease: major long-term sequela.

Differential diagnosis
Other causes of polyarthropathy, fever, and cardiac involvement.
Viral arthritides, e.g. rubella, hepatitis B.
Septic arthritis e.g. *Neisseria* spp. infection.
Infective endocarditis.
Acute rheumatoid arthritis.
Stills' disease.
Serum sickness, e.g. after penicillin.
SLE.
Pre-purpuric phase Henoch–Schönlein purpura.

Aetiology
- Acute rheumatic fever is an exudative, proliferative inflammation of connective tissues, especially heart, joints, and subcutaneous tissues.
- It only occurs after group A streptococcal infection of the upper respiratory tract.
- Particular serotypes, e.g. types 5 and 18, are often implicated, whereas others, e.g. type 12, are not.

Epidemiology
- The incidence of acute rheumatic fever mirrors that of acute streptococcal pharyngitis in a population.
- The peak incidence is at 5–15 years; it is rare in children <4 years but well described in adults.
- The overall male : female ratio is equal; women, however, are more likely to develop Sydenham's chorea and mitral stenosis.

Duckett-Jones criteria for diagnosing acute rheumatic fever
Modified by the American Heart Association.
- Acute rheumatic fever is indicated by two major or one major and two minor criteria if supported by evidence of preceding streptococcal infection.

Major manifestations
Carditis.
Polyarthritis.
Chorea.
Erythema marginatum.
Subcutaneous nodules.

Minor manifestations
Previous rheumatic fever or rheumatic heart disease.
Arthralgia.
Fever.
Raised ESR and CRP concentration, leukocytosis, prolonged PR interval.

Rheumatic fever, acute

W.T.A. Todd

Treatment

Diet and lifestyle
- Strict bed- or chair-rest is advised for the first 4 weeks of illness (if carditis), with gradual mobilization according to clinical status thereafter.

Pharmacological treatment

Antibiotics
- Antibiotics do not modify an acute attack or influence the development of carditis.
- They are used to eradicate streptococci from the pharynx and tonsils to prevent recurrence and further valve damage, as prophylaxis for all rheumatic carditis patients, or to cover dental extractions and other surgical interventions (long-term benzathine penicillin i.m. 4-weekly).

Standard dosage	Phenoxymethylpenicillin 500 mg 4 times daily for 10 days (adult; *see drug data sheets for children*). Erythromycin 250 mg 4 times daily for 10 days (adults; *see drug data sheets for children*).
Contraindications	Hypersensitivity.
Special points	Shorter courses may not eradicate streptococci from pharynx.
Main drug interactions	Oral anticoagulants, theophylline preparations (erythromycin).
Main side effects	Hypersensitivity and rash (penicillin), gastrointestinal intolerance.

Anti-inflammatory agents
- These do not cure or prevent subsequent development of rheumatic disease.
- Early indiscriminate use may obscure diagnosis in mild cases.

Standard dosage	Aspirin 80–100 mg/kg daily (children), 6–8 g daily (adults); reduced after 2 weeks and continued for 6–8 weeks. *For more severe carditis or patients intolerant of high-dose salicylates:* prednisolone 40–60 mg daily for 2 weeks, reduced over next 3–4 weeks, followed by aspirin.
Contraindications	*Aspirin:* breast feeding, gastrointestinal ulceration, haemophilia. *Prednisolone:* current acute gastrointestinal blood loss.
Special points	*Aspirin:* one of the few indications for aspirin treatment in childhood. *Prednisolone:* possible adrenal suppression on sudden withdrawal.
Main drug interactions	*Aspirin:* anticoagulants. *Prednisolone:* danger of gastrointestinal haemorrhage if combined with NSAIDs.
Main side effects	*Aspirin:* hypersensitivity, gastrointestinal bleeding. *Prednisolone:* glucose intolerance, Cushing's syndrome, growth retardation.

Other options
Diuretics, possibly with angiotensin-converting enzyme inhibitors.
Digoxin.
Anticoagulants.
- Use is determined by the degree of carditis or cardiac failure and the stage of illness.

Treatment aims
To eradicate current streptococcal infection and prevent reinfection.
To prevent further episodes of acute disease.
To relieve acute arthritic symptoms.
To prevent infective endocarditis on valves already damaged by carditis.

Prognosis
- Untreated acute rheumatic fever usually lasts up to 3 months.
- Severe carditis extends acute illness to 6 months.
- Most patients with valvular disease develop cardiological complications needing intervention by middle age.
- 6% of patients free of carditis during an acute attack have rheumatic heart disease at 10 years.
- 30% of patients with mild carditis and no pre-existing disease have murmurs at 10 years.
- 40% of patients with apical or basal murmurs in an acute attack have residual disease at 10 years.
- 70% of patients with cardiac failure or pericarditis in an acute attack have residual disease at 10 years.
- Exceptions are patients with 'pure' chorea, who frequently develop rheumatic heart disease despite absence of signs of carditis at outset.

Follow-up and management
- Patients must be kept under strict supervision until signs of acute inflammation have subsided.
- Penicillin or alternative prophylaxis is needed at least until the age of 18 years (some clinicians advocate life-long prophylaxis).
- Adequate prophylaxis is needed for minor surgical interventions, e.g. dental treatment.

Key references
Homer C et al.: Clinical aspects of acute rheumatic fever. *J Rheumatol* 1991, **18** (suppl 29):2–12.

Simmons NA: Recommendations for endocarditis prophylaxis. *J Antimicrob Chemother* 1993, **31**:437–438.

Rubella (German measles) — P.D. Welsby

Diagnosis

Symptoms
- Symptoms are mostly trivial; patients are systemically well.

Mild fever.

Rash: in ~50% of infected patients.

Signs
Rash: fine, erythematous pink macules, almost confluent on trunk on second day, rarely lasts >3 days.

Reddened throat: sometimes with tonsillar exudates.

Enlarged lymph nodes: notably occipital, sometimes splenomegaly.

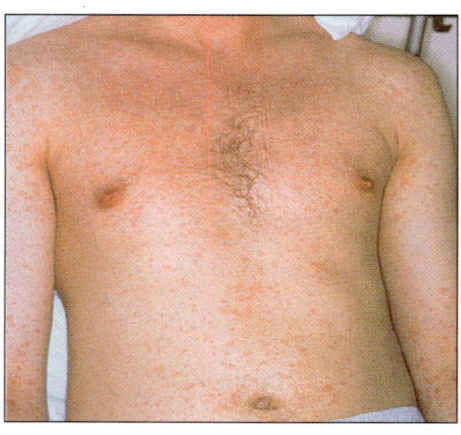

Fine non-blotchy rash of Rubella.

Investigations
- The clinical diagnosis of rubella is wrong in ~50% of patients.
- Only serological proof is acceptable evidence of (relative) immunity.
- A patient's unconfirmed history of rubella should be discounted.

Serology: IgM detectable in serum within 1–2 days of rash; haemagglutination-inhibiting antibodies rise within 1–2 days of rash, peak in 6–12 days, and thereafter fade but remain detectable at lower levels.

Complications

General
Arthralgia or arthritis of fingers, wrists, and knees: usually in young women.

Encephalitis.

Thrombocytopenia.

Neuritis.

Congenital rubella
Cataract, retinopathy, microphthalmia, glaucoma.

Patent ductus arteriosus, ventricular septal defect, pulmonary stenosis.

Deafness.

Thrombocytopenic purpura, hepatosplenomegaly, hepatitis, CNS defects, bone lesions.

Differential diagnosis
- Patients with rubella are usually well and the rash is not blotchy.

Measles: marked prodrome, malaise, dusky-red maculopapular erythematous rash that travels down body over 3 days.

Adenovirus or enterovirus infections, mild scarlet fever, cytomegalovirus or Epstein–Barr virus infection, toxoplasmosis.

Aetiology
- Infection is by rubella virus, an RNA virus.
- Transmission is by respiratory droplets.
- Fetal infection occurs secondary to maternal viraemia; the incidence and type of defect are related to the age of the fetus at the time of infection.
- Significant defects are found with early infection.

Epidemiology
- Rubella occurs worldwide.
- Since the introduction of MMR in 1988, the incidence of congenital rubella syndrome in the UK has declined markedly.
- The provisional total for 1991 to mid-1994 is 14 babies, including one set of triplets.
- The circulation of wild virus will have declined further after the schools' MR programme in late 1994.

Infectivity
- ~16% of affected infants have major defects at birth after maternal rubella in the first trimester.
- Rubella is moderately infectious: patients are infectious during the rash and probably for ~7 days before and up to 5 days after illness, although the virus is detectable in throat secretions up to 10 days before and until 16 days after the rash.
- Babies with congenital rubella excrete the virus in throat and urine for prolonged periods.

Mean incubation period
~18 days.

P.D. Welsby **Rubella (German measles)**

Treatment

Diet and lifestyle
- No special diet is necessary.
- Affected patients should keep away from pregnant women.

Pharmacological treatment

Symptomatic
Analgesics, e.g. paracetamol.

Prophylactic
- Vaccination is by live attenuated virus: this may produce a mild rubella-like illness; women should not be pregnant or become so within 8–12 weeks of vaccination.
- It is routinely recommended in the second year of life as part of MMR, for 10–14-year-old girls at present, and any identified susceptible adult women of child-bearing potential.
- Prompt serological testing of pregnant contacts of a patient with rubella is essential to assess susceptibility.
- The use of hyperimmune globulin should be considered if the risk is significant and if therapeutic abortion would not be considered should rubella develop later.

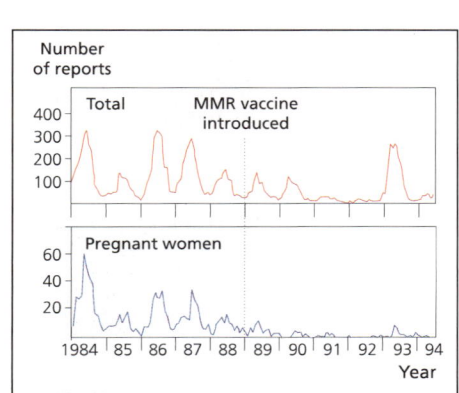

Laboratory reports of rubella: England and Wales, 1984 to June 1994. Incidence has declined since 1988, although outbreaks still occur. © PHLS.

Treatment aims
To relieve symptoms.
To prevent congenital rubella.

Prognosis
- The prognosis in rubella is excellent.
- Deaths are rare and usually associated with encephalitis.

Follow-up and management
- Follow-up and management is not needed except in pregnancy, when risks and discussion of termination should be considered.

Key references
Anonymous: *Immunization against Infectious Diseases.* London: HMSO, 1992

Miller E et al.: Rubella surveillance to June 1994. *Comm Dis Rep* 1994, **4**:R146–R152.

Morgan-Capner P. Diagnosing rubella. *BMJ* 1989; **229**:338–339.

Skin infections
P.D. Welsby

Diagnosis

Symptoms and signs

Impetigo
Isolated lesions or multiple small areas of golden yellow crusts, weeping areas, blisters: ruptured lesions leave raw areas.

Erysipelas
Inflammation substantially limited to skin, erythema with well defined and palpable margins, swelling, local heat, mild superficial pain, fever and malaise.

Deep infections
More swelling, deeper pain, less well defined edges than in erysipelas, perhaps crepitus on palpation, and overlying skin necrosis: indicating cellulitis.

Boils or abscesses: focal areas of pus formation, often painful, abscesses may be enlarged and pointing.

Severe boil with central necrosis and multiple discharging sinuses: carbuncle.

Methicillin-resistant *Staphylococcus aureus* infections
- Patients are usually asymptomatic, i.e. colonized, but some may have local or generalized life-threatening sepsis.

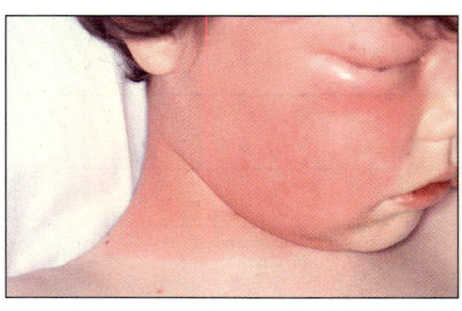

Erysipelas.

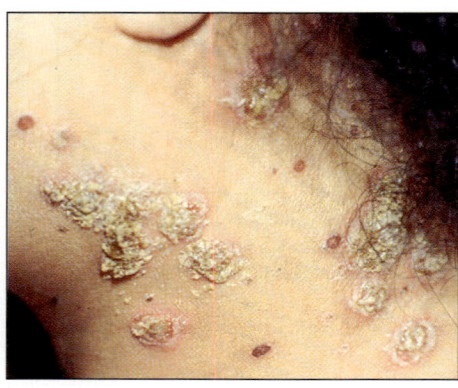

Impetigo.

Investigations

Microbiology: areas of impetigo should be swabbed; methicillin-resistant *Staphylococcus aureus* infection cannot be diagnosed clinically; swabs should be taken from nose, throat, perineum, eczematous areas, axillae, sputum, urine (if catheter present), any site of possible infection (including surgical wounds), intravenous access points;

often not needed for classic erysipelas; if confirmation of causative organism of erysipelas or cellulitis desired, a few millilitres of saline solution can be injected into involved area and immediately aspirated (using same needle, which should not be withdrawn); site of entry of infection should be swabbed; abscess pus should be sent for microscopy and culture.

Blood culture: if skin is intact over areas of cellulitis.

Complications

Lymphangitis, scarlet fever, septicaemia, post-streptococcal rheumatic fever: rare complications of erysipelas.

Spread of infection to contiguous tissue, septicaemia: complications of cellulitis.

Rupture, septicaemia: complications of boils.

Differential diagnosis
Not applicable.

Aetiology
- Impetigo is usually caused by *Staphylococcus aureus*, especially when bullous, occasionally by *Streptococcus pyogenes*.
- Erysipelas is caused by *Strep. pyogenes*.
- Cellulitis is usually caused by *Strep. pyogenes* but also by a wide range of anaerobes, e.g. *Clostridium perfringens*, and facultative anaerobes; often several pathogens are isolated.
- Boils and carbuncles are caused by *Staph. aureus*.

Epidemiology
- Up to 40% of the population are nasal carriers of *Staphylococcus aureus*.
- Where antibiotic use is intense, e.g. hospitals, most staphylococci are resistant to penicillin but retain sensitivity to methicillin, cloxacillin, and flucloxacillin.
- Outbreaks of methicillin-resistant *S. aureus*, usually in hospitals, have been reported since 1960; some strains are virulent, whereas others are harmless unless they infect vulnerable patients.
- Most strains of methicillin-resistant *S. aureus* are resistant to other frequently used antibiotics, and some strains are highly transmissible ('epidemic strains').
- Pharyngeal carriage of *Streptococcus pyogenes* is more common in younger age groups and can reach 15–20% in crowded conditions, especially in winter.
- Impetigo is most common in children aged 2–5 years in warm climates and with poor hygiene; the incidence increases in summer.
- The frequency and severity of invasive streptococcal disease has been increasing in the USA and Europe since the late 1980s.

P.D. Welsby **Skin infections**

Treatment

Diet and lifestyle
- No special precautions are necessary.

Pharmacological treatment

For erysipelas
- Erysipelas usually responds to penicillin parenterally if the illness is severe.

Standard dosage	Benzylpenicillin 300–600 mg i.v. 6-hourly Phenoxymethylpenicillin 500 mg orally 6-hourly.
Contraindications	Hypersensitivity.
Special points	Erythromycin or new macrolides are other options.
Main drug interactions	None.
Main side effects	Gastrointestinal disturbances, sensitivity reactions.

For cellulitis

Standard dosage	Flucloxacillin 0.5–1 g i.v. 6-hourly
Contraindications	Hypersensitivity.
Special points	Erythromycin is an alternative.
Main drug interactions	None.
Main side effects	Gastrointestinal disturbances, sensitivity reactions.

For boils and abscesses
- No antibiotics are needed in the case of free drainage, with no surrounding inflammation.
- Otherwise, flucloxacillin or erythromycin should be used.

For methicillin-resistant *Staphylococcus aureus* (MRSA) infection
- If the patient is widely colonized, topical antiseptics can be tried (including tridosan, hexachlorophane, chlorhedixine, povidone iodine), although success is uncertain.
- If the carriage is limited, particularly to the nose, topical mupirocin can be used.
- If the patient has an invasive infection or if eradication of MRSA is necessary to allow more appropriate treatment for underlying conditions, treatment with antibiotics under specialist supervision may be appropriate.
- MRSA strains are often sensitive to vancomycin or teicoplanin; fusidic acid, rifampicin, or ciprofloxacin may also have a role.

Standard dosage	Hexachlorophane applied sparingly every 4–6 h after washing. Mupirocin applied to nares 3 times daily for up to 10 days. Vancomycin 500 mg i.v. over 60 min every 6 h
Contraindications	*Hexachlorophane:* damaged skin, pregnancy, breast-feeding, children <2 years. *Mupirocin, vancomycin:* hypersensitivity.
Main drug interactions	*Vancomycin:* cholestyramine, aminoglycosides, loop diuretics.
Main side effects	*Hexachlorophane:* redness (overgenerous application). *Mupirocin:* minor burning, stinging, itching. *Vancomycin:* hypotension, nephrotoxicity, ototoxicity, bone-marrow suppression, sensitivity reactions, phlebitis, muscle spasm.

- Clearance is accepted if weekly sets of screening swabs are negative over 3 weeks.
- Patients must initially be isolated on further admission, and continued carriage must be assessed.

Treatment aims
To eradicate infection.
To avoid spread of methicillin-resistant *Staphylococcus aureus* infection.

Other treatments
Surgical exploration to define the extent and nature of anaerobic cellulitis and to treat it. Incision of pointing abscesses.

Prognosis
- Further attacks of erysipelas are common at the same site; patients should report promptly for antibiotic treatment.

Follow-up and management
- No follow-up is needed.

Prevention of spread of methicillin-resistant *Staphylococcus aureus* (MRSA)
- The patient must be isolated.
- The Infection Control Team must be contacted immediately.
- The source of the MRSA must be sought.
- The risk to other patients must be assessed.
- The patient's notes must be marked 'MRSA infected'.
- Infected staff must be identified and controlled.
- Hands must be washed after any patient contact.
- Gloves must be worn when infected tissue or dressings are being handled.
- Facemasks must be worn if exposure to infected aerosols is possible.
- 'Infection Control' disposal of soiled material is vital.
- Rooms must be terminally disinfected.
- The patient can be discharged unless contacts are vulnerable; if discharge is not possible, infected individuals must be isolated (even if asymptomatic).
- Unnecessary staff–patient contact must be minimized (barrier nursing).
- The use of staff not familiar with the involved ward must be minimized.

Key references
Duckworth DJ: Diagnosis and management of methicillin resistant *Staphylococcus aureus* infection. *BMJ* 1993, **307**:1049–1052.

Toxic shock syndrome — G.R. Williams

Diagnosis

Definition
- Definition criteria require fever, rash, hypotension, clinical or test evidence of involvement of three systems, negative results from blood (except in the case of *Staphylococcus aureus*), CSF, and throat culture, and exclusion of measles, leptospirosis, and, in the Americas, Rocky Mountain spotted fever.
- Mild or near-miss toxic shock syndrome that does not reach the clinical severity of the full definition is almost certainly more prevalent and poorly recognised. It may resolve because of general antibiotic use or end of menstruation.

Symptoms
High temperature: often to 40°C.
Vomiting and diarrhoea: usually watery.
Faintness: especially on standing.
Aching muscles.
Rash.

Signs
Hypotension: systolic blood pressure <90 mmHg or postural drop of >15 mmHg; below fifth percentile for age in children <16 years.
Rash: patchy erythema, likened to sunburn, especially on trunk, thighs, palms, soles.
Tender muscles.
Reddened mucosal surfaces: conjunctival, oral, vaginal.
'Red strawberry' tongue.
Confusion: without focal neurological signs.
Puffy hands and feet.

Investigations
Haematology: thrombocytopenia usual.
Biochemistry: to assess renal function and liver inflammation; creatine kinase concentration often high.
Bacteriology: cultures of blood, stool, urine, vagina, cervix, wounds; *Staphylococcus aureus* isolates to be forwarded for toxin production and phage typing.

Complications
Renal failure, coma, peripheral gangrene, adult respiratory distress: in varying combinations due to hypotension.
Marked desquamation: especially of palms, soles, and digits, 1–2 weeks after onset.
Hair loss, occasional nail loss: after 2–3 months.

Differential diagnosis
Infective gastroenteritis.
Septicaemia, especially Gram-negative.
Scarlatina.
Kawasaki disease.

Aetiology
- Toxins are produced by *Staphylococcus aureus*, mostly toxic shock syndrome toxin-1, but also enterotoxin A, B, or C. (Streptococcal toxins can produce a similar illness.)
- They are absorbed into the body during menstruation (especially with tampons) or at sites of infection (wound or burn, sinusitis, empyema, post-influenzal bronchopneumonia, conjunctivitis).

Epidemiology
- In the USA, where illness fulfilling diagnostic criteria is notified, for the past 7 years, only 50% of the notifications have been menstrually related.
- Menstrual toxic shock syndrome occurs most often in high-absorbency tampon users aged 15–25 years.
- The incidence of menstrual toxic shock syndrome has declined since the early 1980s in the USA, probably as a result of increased health education, reduced tampon absorbency, and removal of acrylate fibres from tampons.
- Toxic shock syndrome has also been associated with the use of contraceptive diaphragms and sponges.
- Non-menstrual toxic shock syndrome develops in both sexes and at any age.
- ~80% of adults have toxic shock syndrome toxin-1 antibodies, suggesting that mild or subclinical immunizing events happen frequently.
- In the UK, ~20 cases are validated each year by the reference laboratory; this inevitably understates the true incidence.

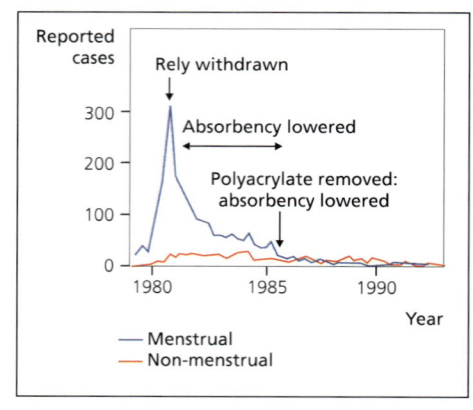

Incidence of toxic shock syndrome in the USA 1979–1993.

Treatment

Diet and lifestyle

- To reduce the likelihood of menstrually related toxic shock syndrome, women must wash hands before and after inserting tampons, use the lowest absorbency tampons that cope with their needs, change tampons regularly (at least every 4–6 h), use pads overnight, remove and stop using tampons if acute symptoms develop during menstruation, and inform their GPs of symptoms and remind of current menstruation. Details of toxic shock syndrome are given on leaflets within tampon cartons, and a health warning is printed on the outside.

Pharmacological treatment

General resuscitation

- Severely ill patients need management and monitoring in intensive care units.
- Crystalloid solutions should be used, initially with inotropic support.
- Other modalities, e.g. dialysis, ventilation, should be used when indicated.

Antibiotics

- Although flucloxacillin does not appear to speed resolution of toxic shock syndrome, it is used empirically in case of septicaemia and for localized infections at other sites.

Standard dosage	Flucloxacillin 0.5–1 g i.v. 6-hourly.
Contraindications	Hypersensitivity, porphyria.
Special points	Reduces recurrence rate in future menstrual periods. Third-generation cephalosporin can be used instead.
Main drug interactions	None.
Main side effects	Sensitivity reactions, jaundice.

Antitoxin

- The therapeutic usefulness of toxic shock syndrome toxin-1 antibodies (found in normal immunoglobulin or plasma) has not been determined.

Treatment aims

To limit hypoxic damage (prompt resuscitation).

To stop further toxin production and absorption (removal of tampons, drainage of pus, i.v. flucloxacillin).

To prevent subsequent relapses (flucloxacillin, advice on future tampon use).

Prognosis

- Mortality is 3%.
- Chronic morbidity varies and is related to acute ischaemic damage to vital organs.
- The risk of recurrence during the next menstrual period is small, and symptoms tend to be milder.
- Recurrences may also follow non-menstrual toxic shock syndrome, especially if anti-staphylococcal antibiotics are not used, and often follow subsequent skin or mucous membrane infection.

Follow-up and management

- Women should be advised against using tampons for the first few periods but can then reintroduce low-absorbency tampons, with frequent changing, and gradual return to advised standard routine thereafter.
- If further menstrual symptoms develop, tampon use must be stopped, and the patient should be given flucloxacillin and resuscitative measures in relation to symptoms.

Key references

Centers for Disease Control: Reduced incidence of menstrual toxic shock syndrome – United States 1980–1990. *MMWR Morb Mortal Wkly Rep* 1990, **39**:421–423.

Communicable Diseases Surveillance Centre: Toxic shock syndrome and related conditions in the United Kingdom: 1992 and 1993. *Commun Dis Rep CDR Rev* 1994, **4**:65.

Kain KC, Schulzer M, Chow AW: Clinical spectrum of nonmenstrual toxic shock syndrome. *Clin Infect Dis* 1993, **16**:100–106.

Tuberculosis, extrapulmonary — D.H. Kennedy

Diagnosis

Symptoms
- Disease may be focal, disseminated, or multifocal. Proportion by site: lymphatic ~35%; genitourinary, bone, joint ~15% each; disseminated, abdominal, cerebral <10% each; cutaneous, other sites <5% each.
- Systemic symptoms usually imply more wide-spread disease; focal disease may be acute or insidious (more usual).

Fever, malaise, fatigue, weight loss, night sweats.
Pain: in bone or joint, abdomen, gastrointestinal tract, or meninges.
Tissue swelling: in lymph node, joint, or peritoneum.
Frequency, dysuria, loin pain: in renal disease.
Cough, fever: in disseminated disease.
Headache, vomiting, confusion: in CNS disease.

Signs
Fever, wasting: due to tuberculous toxicity.
Erythema nodosum: a hypersensitivity reaction.
Choroidal tubercles: in miliary disease.
Non-tender, fluctuant lymph node: perhaps discharging.
Frank haematuria, loin tenderness.
Bone or joint deformity, cold abscess, spinal-cord signs.
Chest signs, hepatosplenomegaly: in dissemination.
Ascites, abdominal distension, bowel obstruction.
Nuchal rigidity, obtundation, focal signs: indicating meningitis.

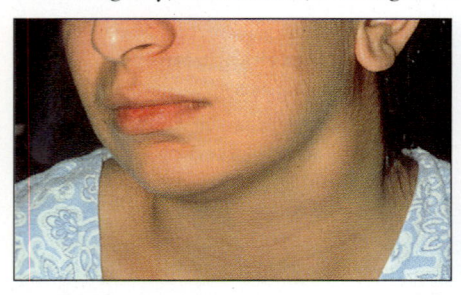

Asian woman with multiple tuberculous lymph nodes (most typical manifestation of extrapulmonary tuberculosis in Asian patients).

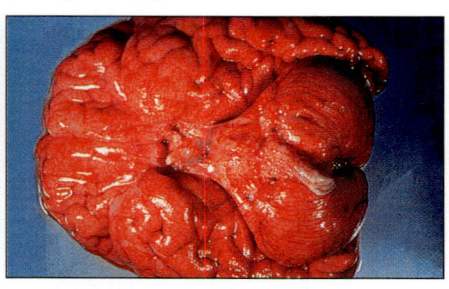

Massive cerebral oedema typical of advanced tuberculous meningitis.

Investigations
- Tests may suggest the diagnosis (ESR, skin test, radiography), identify the site (CT or ^{67}Ga scanning, specialized radiography, intravenous pyelography, isotope renography), or confirm the diagnosis (culture in ~50%, microscopy in ~35%, histology in ~35%).

Chest radiography: to check for new or old changes.
Blood analysis: may show anaemia, high ESR, pancytopenia, or leukaemoid reaction.
Tuberculin skin test: possibly negative (especially in disseminated infection).
Sputum or urine culture.
Biopsy of bone marrow, liver, lymph node, joint, or bowel.

Complications
Cryptic disseminated tuberculosis, acute miliary disease, or meningitis: due to dissemination from a focal lesion.
Focal damage: from vasculitis, fibrosis, abscess, sinus formation, or caseation.
Hydrocephalus, spinal block, cerebral vasculitis.
Adult respiratory distress syndrome: in miliary disease.
Ureteric obstruction or renal destruction by caseation.
Spinal-cord involvement: in 20% of patients with vertebral disease.
Bone or joint deformity.
Gastrointestinal stenosis, adhesions, obstruction.

Differential diagnosis
Lymphoma, toxoplasmosis, atypical mycobacterioses.
Infection: e.g. endocarditis, brucellosis, pneumocystosis.
Noninfective disease: e.g. lymphoma, collagenoses.
Chronic pyelonephritis.
Other arthritides, osteomyelitis, neoplasm.
Crohn's disease, starch or sarcoid peritonitis.
Viral or fungal infections or CNS neoplasm.

Aetiology
- Tuberculosis is caused by infection by *Mycobacterium tuberculosis* (now rarely *M. bovis*).
- Extrapulmonary disease may be due to lymphohaematogenous, contiguous, or 'down-stream' mucosal spread.
- Predisposing factors include genetics and race (rate in ethnic groups from Indian subcontinent 50 times European rate), immunocompromise (due to disease, drugs, alcohol), extremes of age, and HIV infection.

Epidemiology
- Extrapulmonary tuberculosis develops in ~25% of patients; pulmonary infection may coexist.
- The annual notification rate is ~4 people in 100 000, or ~1500 cases in the UK.

Tuberculosis and HIV infection
- ~3.5 million people world wide are co-infected.
- The infections may be mutually synergistic.
- Dissemination is much more probable.
- Many patients have extrapulmonary disease.
- Patients are more likely to be anergic on skin testing.
- Response to standard triple or quadruple treatment is usually good.

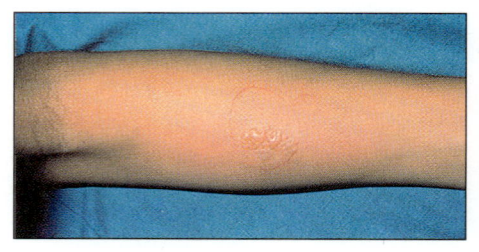

Strongly positive Mantoux reaction.

Tuberculosis, extrapulmonary

D.H. Kennedy

Treatment

Diet and lifestyle
- Weight loss and malnutrition must be reversed.
- Alcohol or drug addiction should be treated.
- Social circumstances, e.g. homelessness, should be improved.

Pharmacological treatment
- The advice of a tuberculosis specialist must be sought and the case notified.
- In a seriously ill patient, empirical treatment is justified even when the diagnosis is unconfirmed; treatment is invariably instituted before sensitivities are available.
- Efforts should be made to establish diagnosis, but procrastination may be dangerous.
- Patients must comply with the drug regimen for the duration of treatment.

Standard chemotherapy

Standard dosage	*Initial phase (2 months):* three or more drugs, usually isoniazid, with pyridoxine, rifampicin, pyrazinamide. *Continuation phase (4 months):* two drugs, usually isoniazid and rifampicin.
Contraindications	*Isoniazid:* drug-induced liver disease, porphyria. *Rifampicin:* jaundice, porphyria. *Pyrazinamide:* liver damage, porphyria.
Special points	For suspected resistance: addition of ethambutol. For documented resistance: drugs as indicated by sensitivities. For cerebral, bone and joint, and drug-resistant infections: longer treatment (9 months). For unreliable compliance: intermittent, supervised treatment 2–3 times weekly.
Main drug interactions	*Rifampicin:* oral contraceptive.
Main side effects	*Isoniazid:* neuropathy (pyridoxine prophylaxis), hepatitis, hypersensitivity reactions. *Rifampicin:* hepatitis, gastrointestinal upset, influenza symptoms, purpura. *Pyrazinamide:* hepatitis, gastrointestinal upset.

Steroids
- Steroids should be considered when the host's inflammatory response contributes significantly to the disease process; they are indicated for the following:

Severely ill patients who are moribund due to overwhelming infection or who have miliary disease with alveolar-capillary block or cerebral disease.

Patients with peritonitis, pericarditis, spinal block, renal infection (to reduce adhesions, effusions, and fibrosis).

Patients with lymph-node or cerebral infection (to reduce swelling).

Patients with drug hypersensitivity reactions.

Treatment aims
To secure survival (especially in disseminated and cerebral disease).
To preserve organ function and prevent deformity.
To relieve symptoms.
To prevent relapse by eradicating infection.
To prevent drug resistance by ensuring compliance.

Other treatments
- Surgery is often done both before and after the diagnosis is confirmed.
- It is indicated for the following forms of tuberculosis:

All: for biopsy diagnosis (>35% of patients), relief of obstruction due to inflammatory response, and correction of deformity.
Lymphatic: for chronic sinus and unresponsive or marked node enlargement.
Renal: ureteric obstruction or stricture, obstinate symptoms (e.g. pain).
CNS: for hydrocephalus, cerebral oedema.
Spinal: for cord pressure, bone graft.
Joint: to minimize deformity.
Gut: for obstruction, adhesions, strictures.
Pericardial: to relieve constriction.
Female genital: for stricture, infertility.

Prognosis
- Prognosis is related to the precariousness of the organ involved, the stage of disease progression, and the vulnerability of host.
- Mortality is significant in cerebral disease (10–30%) and disseminated disease (10–25%).
- Survival can be expected in other forms, although chronic sequelae may develop.
- The prognosis in lymph-node and dermatological tuberculosis is excellent.

Follow-up and management
- Drug toxicities that may affect compliance must be identified.
- The patient must be monitored for complications and long-term sequelae.

Key references
Langdale LA *et al.*: Tuberculosis and the surgeon. *Am J Surg* 1992, **163**:505–509.
Shafer RW *et al.*: Extrapulmonary tuberculosis in patients with human immunodeficiency virus infection. *Medicine* 1991, **70**:384–397.

Typhoid and paratyphoid fevers — B.K. Mandal

Diagnosis

Symptoms

Persistent fever: developing after recent visit to endemic country.

Mounting fever, headache, malaise, anorexia, dry cough, constipation: in first week of illness.

Continuing fever, mental apathy: in second week.

Abdominal distension, 'pea-soup' diarrhoea: in third week.

Signs

Pyrexia: in first week.

Rose spots: 2–4 mm erythematous maculopapules in crops on lower chest and upper abdomen in 30% of patients in second week.

Vagueness and withdrawal, splenomegaly, relative bradycardia: in second week.

Delirium or stupor, distended tender abdomen, dehydration, poor-volume rapid pulse, signs of complications: in third week.

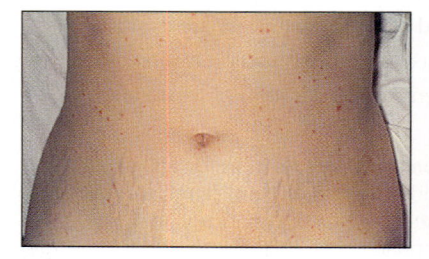

Rose spots in a patient with typhoid fever.

Investigations

- Definitive diagnosis needs positive blood or bone-marrow culture.

Blood culture: highest positivity during first week (80%), declining thereafter; often negative if patient has already been given antibiotic.

Bone-marrow culture: often remains positive despite antibiotic administration.

Stool and urine culture: often positive from third week onwards; diagnostic only if clinical picture is compatible.

Widal test: unreliable and difficult to interpret, so rarely performed.

Full blood count: leucocyte count decreased, with relative lymphocytosis after first week.

Liver function tests: often mildly raised aspartate and alanine transaminase concentrations.

Complications

- Complications occur only in untreated patients after the second week.

Intestinal haemorrhage: indicated by sudden drop in temperature, rise in pulse rate, and rectal bleeding.

Intestinal perforation: signs of peritonitis may be difficult to detect in an already tender and distended abdomen; presence of gas under diaphragm and ascites may be the only signs.

Myocarditis: indicated by rapid, thready pulse and ECG abnormalities.

Jaundice: may be due to cholangitis, hepatitis, or haemolysis.

Typhoid abscesses: in different organs (rare).

Differential diagnosis

- Fever in a traveller returning from endemic areas may also be due to the following:

Malaria (most important).
Tropical viral infections.
Typhus.
Amoebic liver abscess.
Trypanosomiasis and leishmaniasis.
Other causes of fever that are common world wide.

Aetiology

- Causes include the following:

Infection by *Salmonella typhi* or *paratyphi* A, B, or C.
Prolonged bacteraemia.
Gallbladder infection.
Inflamed Peyer's patches in small intestine (may ulcerate during third week, leading to bleeding or perforation).

Epidemiology

- The disease is endemic in the Indian subcontinent, southeast Asia, the Middle East, Africa, and Central and South America; paratyphoid B also occurs in southern and eastern Europe.

- Transmission is through food or water contaminated by faeces or urine of a sufferer or carrier.

- About 200 patients with typhoid and 100 patients with paratyphoid infection are seen in the UK annually, mostly contracted abroad.

Treatment

Diet and lifestyle
- Adequate nutrition and fluid replacement must be ensured.
- Chronic carriers, especially those handling foods, must practice strict hygiene because of the faecal–oral transmission of the disease; in such patients, attempts should be made to clear carriage.

Pharmacological treatment

General and supportive care
- Patients should be barrier-nursed in a single room, and the relevant authorities must be notified.
- Nutritional and fluid-electrolyte deficiencies should be corrected in patients presenting late.

Specific treatment
- 4-quinolones are currently the drug of choice in adults.
- Defervescence occurs in 3–5 days.
- Treatment failure, relapse, and chronic carriage are rare.
- Other drugs include third-generation cephalosporins and corticosteroids (in severe toxaemia).

Standard dosage	Ciprofloxacin 500 mg orally twice daily for 14 days (200 mg i.v. with vomiting or diarrhoea). *In children (but see below):* 10 mg/kg orally or i.v. daily in 2 divided doses. Ceftriaxone 3–4 g i.v. daily as single dose or 75–100 mg/kg i.v. daily in 2 divided doses for 7–10 days (shorter duration may be equally effective). Adjunctive dexamethasone 3 mg/kg i.v. initially, then 1 mg/kg 6-hourly for 48 h.
Contraindications	Hypersensitivity. *Dexamethasone:* caution in pregnancy, renal insufficiency, hypertension, and diabetes.
Special points	*Ciprofloxacin:* currently not recommended in pregnant women and children because of arthropathy in growing animals; this has not, however, been observed in children, and ciprofloxacin should not be withheld if benefits outweigh risks. *Ceftriaxone:* can be used in children and pregnant women but must be given intravenously.
Main drug interactions	*Ciprofloxacin:* NSAIDs, oral iron, anticoagulants. *Ceftriaxone:* probenecid. *Dexamethasone:* phenytoin, barbiturates, ephedrine or rifampicin may increase the metabolic clearance of corticosteroids.
Main side effects	*Ciprofloxacin:* nausea, abdominal pain, diarrhoea (all unusual). *Ceftriaxone:* headache, nausea, rash. *Dexamethasone:* fluid and electrolyte disturbances.

Treatment of chronic carriers
- Ciprofloxacin 750 mg or norfloxacin 400 mg twice daily for 28 days is highly effective.

Drug resistance
- Chloramphenicol, co-trimoxazole, and amoxycillin are highly effective if the infecting strains are sensitive to the above drugs.
- *Salmonella typhi* strains simultaneously resistant to all three drugs, however, are now widely prevalent in the Indian subcontinent, where most infections seen in the UK originate.

Treatment aims
To achieve clinical cure.
To prevent complications and relapse.
To prevent chronic faecal carriage after recovery.

Other treatments
- Surgery is needed for intestinal perforation (haemorrhage managed conservatively).
- Cholecystectomy should be reserved for carriers with symptomatic gallbladder disease.

Prognosis
- Untreated, typhoid and paratyphoid fevers have a mortality of up to 20%, mostly from myocarditis and intestinal haemorrhage or perforation; these complications are rarely seen in the UK.
- Recovery begins in the fourth week in the absence of complications.

Follow-up and management
- ~10% of patients relapse, and 3% become chronic faecal carriers after treatment with chloramphenicol, co-trimoxazole, or amoxycillin, but rarely after ciprofloxacin treatment.
- After clinical recovery, six consecutive negative stool and urine cultures should be obtained over 3 weeks.

Key references
Lassere R, Sangalang RP, Santiago L: Three day treatment of typhoid fever with two different doses of ceftriaxone, compared to 14 day therapy with chloramphenicol: a randomised trial. *J Antimicrob Chemother* 1991, **28**:765–772.

Mandal BK: Modern treatment of typhoid fever. *J Infect* 1991, **22**:1–4.

Index

A

abscess 14
  brain 8
  amoebic liver 40
  cold 38
  typhoid 40
ACE inhibitors *see* angiotensin-converting enzyme inhibitors
acetaminophen *see* paracetamol
acidosis 8, 22
  lactic 22
  metabolic 8
acrodermatitis chronica atrophicans 20
acyclovir
  for herpes simplex infection 5, 15
  for herpes zoster and varicella infection 17
adenomyosis *see* endometriosis
adenopathy 18
adenovirus 4, 24, 32
AIDS 8
alcohol, adverse effects of 2
alcoholism 8
alkalosis, respiratory 10
allergy 8 *see also* hypersensitivity reaction
alveolitis, fibrosing *see* fibrosis, pulmonary
amaurosis fugax *see* blindness
amitriptyline
  for chronic fatigue syndrome 3
  for postherpetic neuralgia 17
amoxycillin
  for acute Lyme disease 21
  for leptospirosis 19
  for paratyphoid fever 41
  for typhoid fever 41
amphotericin B for fungal infections 9
ampicillin for leptospirosis 19
anaemia 2, 10
  fetal 26
  haemolytic 16, 26
  microangiopathic *see* anaemia, haemolytic
analgesics
  for chronic fatigue syndrome 3
  for leptospirosis 18
  for measles 25
  for parvovirus B19 infection 27
anaphylaxis 10 *see also* hypersensitivity reaction
angioedema 12
angiotensin-converting enzyme inhibitors
  for acute rheumatic fever 31
anodynes *see* analgesics
antibacterial drugs for measles 25
antibiotics
  for diphtherial infections 29
  for Gram-negative septicaemia 11
  for leptospirosis 18
  for *Mycoplasma* infection 5
  for streptococcal infections 29
  for toxic shock syndrome 37

anticoagulants for acute rheumatic fever 31
antidepressants for chronic fatigue syndrome 3
antiemetics for leptospirosis 18
antifungal agents for fungal infections 9
antihistamines for erythema multiforme and Stevens–Johnson syndrome 5
anti-infective agents *see* antiseptics
anti-inflammatory drugs, nonsteroidal *see* NSAIDs
antimicrobial agents *see* antibiotics
antinociceptive agents *see* analgesics
antirheumatic agents *see* NSAIDs
antiseptics for MRSA infection 35
antitoxin
  for diphtheria 29
  for toxic shock syndrome 37
anuria 18
anxiety 2
aortic
  incompetence *see* aortic regurgitation
  regurgitation, Carey–Coombs 30
  valve
    incompetence *see* aortic regurgitation
    insufficiency *see* aortic regurgitation
aplastic crisis 26
ARDS *see* respiratory distress, adult
arthralgia 4, 20, 26, 32
arthritide
  hepatitis B 30
  rubella 30
arthritis 20, 26, 32 *see also* polyarthritis
  bacterial *see* arthritis, septic
  infectious *see* arthritis, septic
  Neisseria 30
  reactive 20
  rheumatic *see* rheumatic fever
  rheumatoid 4, 20, 30
  septic 30
arthropathy 12
aspergilloma 8
aspergillosis
  allergic bronchopulmonary 8
  invasive 8
aspirin
  for acute rheumatic fever 31
  for chronic fatigue syndrome 3
asthma 8
atelectasis, congestive *see* respiratory distress, adult
atrioventricular block 20
Augmentin *see* co-amoxyclav
azithromycin for acute Lyme disease 21
azoles for fungal infections 9

B

bacteraemia 10
balanitis 8

Behçet's syndrome 6, 14
benzathine penicillin for rheumatic fever 31
benzodiazepines for chronic fatigue syndrome 3
benzylpenicillin
  for diphtherial infections 29
  for leptospirosis 19
  for streptococcal infections 29
Berger's disease *see* glomerulonephritis
Besnier–Boeck disease *see* sarcoidosis
bladder dysfunction 16
bleeding *see* haemorrhage
blindness 4, 8
blister, corneal 14
blood
  in stool 12
  in urine 12
  poisoning *see* septicaemia
Boeck's disease *see* sarcoidosis
boils 34
Bouillaud's disease *see* heart disease, rheumatic
bowel
  disease, inflammatory 6, 14
  dysfunction 16
  syndrome, irritable 2
bradyarrhythmia *see* bradycardia
bradycardia, relative 40
breathlessness 8, 10
Bright's disease *see* glomerulonephritis
bronchiectasis 8
bronchitis 18
bronchodilators for fungal infections 9
brucellosis 2
bullae 4
burns 8, 10

C

cancer 10 *see also* malignancy
candidaemia 8
candidiasis
  cutaneous 8
  hepatosplenic 8
  oesophageal 8
  vaginal 8
carbuncle 34
cardiac *see also* heart
  conduction disturbance 20
  failure 30
cataracts 32
cefotaxime
  for chronic Lyme disease 21
  for Gram-negative septicaemia 11
ceftazidime for Gram-negative septicaemia 11
ceftriaxone
  for Lyme disease 21
  for paratyphoid fever 41
  for typhoid fever 41

Index

cellulitis 34
  orbital 8
cephalosporins
  for paratyphoid fever 41
  for typhoid fever 41
cheilitis, angular 8
chickenpox 16
chills 10
chloramphenicol
  for paratyphoid fever 41
  for typhoid fever 41
chlorhexidine for MRSA infection 35
chloroquine for Plasmodium malaria 23
chlorpheniramine for erythema multiforme and Stevens–Johnson syndrome 5
chorea 30
  Sydenham's 30
chronic fatigue syndrome 2
ciprofloxacin
  for MRSA infection 35
  for paratyphoid fever 41
  for typhoid fever 41
clarithromycin for acute Lyme disease 21
coagulation, disseminated intravascular 10, 22
coagulopathy 16
  consumption see disseminated intravascular coagulation
co-amoxyclav for Gram-negative septicaemia 11
cold sensitivity 2
coma 4, 14, 22, 36
concentration disturbance 2, 20
confusion 10, 14, 16, 20
conjunctivitis 24
consciousness, altered 14, 18
constipation 2, 40
convulsions 14, 22
  febrile 24
corticosteroids
  for erythema nodosum 7
  for extrapulmonary tuberculosis 39
  for fungal infections 9
  for Henoch–Schönlein purpura 13
  for thrombocytopenia 19
  for paratyphoid fever 41
  for Stevens–Johnson syndrome 5
  for typhoid fever 41
co-trimoxazole
  for paratyphoid fever 41
  for typhoid fever 41
cough 4, 8, 10, 18
  dry 40
cystitis 8
cytomegalovirus 20, 26, 32

D

deafness 32
dehydration 40
delirium 22, 40
depression 2, 14, 16
dexamethasone
  for paratyphoid fever 41
  for typhoid fever 41
diabetes mellitus 8
diarrhoea 2, 4, 10, 18, 20, 22
  'pea soup' 40
diazepam for seizures 19
digoxin for acute rheumatic fever 31
dihydrocodeine for chronic fatigue syndrome 3
diphtheria 28
disability, severe 2
disorientation see confusion
distension, abdominal 40
diuretics for acute rheumatic fever 31
dopamine for Gram-negative septic shock 11
dosulepin see dothiepin
dothiepin for chronic fatigue syndrome 3
doxepin for chronic fatigue syndrome 3
doxycycline
  for acute Lyme disease 21
  for leptospirosis 19
drug abuse 8
ductus arteriosus, patent 32
dyspareunia 14
dysuria 10

E

ear disease 8
EBV see Epstein–Barr virus
ecthyma gangrenosum 10
eczema herpeticum 14
effort syndrome see chronic fatigue syndrome
emphysema 8
encephalitides 14
encephalitis 16, 18, 20, 22, 32
  acute measles 24
  herpes 14
encephalomyelitis 21
  myalgic see chronic fatigue syndrome
endocarditis 8
  bacterial 12
    subacute 12, 30
  infective 30
  lenta see endocarditis, subacute bacterial
endometritis 8
endophthalmitis 8
enteropathy, protein-losing 12
Epstein–Barr virus 2, 28
  syndrome, chronic see chronic fatigue syndrome
erysipelas 34
erythema 14
  annulare centrifugum see erythema multiforme
  chronicum migrans 20

marginatum 20, 30
multiforme 4, 14, 16, 20
nodosum 6, 20
  leprosum 6
toxic 4
erythromycin
  for abscesses 35
  for acute Lyme disease 21
  for acute rheumatic fever 31
  for boils 35
  for erysipelas 35
  for erythema multiforme and Stevens–Johnson syndrome 5
  for leptospirosis 19

F

famcyclovir for herpes simplex infection 15
Fansidar for *Plasmodium falciparum* malaria 23
fatigue syndrome
  chronic 2
  postviral see chronic fatigue syndrome
fever
  enteric see typhoid fever
  haemorrhagic 4
  paratyphoid 40
  rheumatic
    acute 30
    post-streptococcal 34
  scarlet 26, 28, 32, 34
  typhoid 40
fibrosis
  cystic 8
  pulmonary 8
flucloxacillin
  for abscesses 35
  for boils 35
  for toxic shock syndrome 37
fluconazole for fungal infections 9
flucytosine for fungal infections 9
fluoxetine for chronic fatigue syndrome 3
folliculitis 8

G

gangrene 36
gastritis 8
gastroenteritis 24
  infective 36
gentamicin for Gram-negative septicaemia 11
German measles 32 see also rubella
gingivitis 14
gingivostomatitis 14
gland, enlarged 2
glaucoma 32
glomerulonephritis 12
granulation, toxic 10
granuloma
  annulare 20
  paranasal 8

Index

Guillain–Barré syndrome 20

H

haematomata, intramural 12
haemolysis, intravascular 22
haemoptysis 8
haemorrhage 18, 22, 40
hand, foot, and mouth disease 28
hearing loss *see* deafness
heart *see also* cardiac
    block *see* atrioventricular block
    disease
        chronic 20
        rheumatic 30
        valvular 8
heat
    sensitivity 2
    stroke 22
hemiplegia 16
hepatic
    failure 10
    function, impaired 18
hepatitis
    A 2
    infective 18
hepatomegaly 20
hepatosplenomegaly 8, 18
herpangina 28
herpes
    simplex 4, 14, 16
        encephalitis 14
        genital 14
        gladiatorum 14
        meningitis 14
        mucocutaneous 14
        ocular 14
        orolabial 14
        whitlow 14
    virus, Burkitt *see* Epstein–Barr virus
    zoster 16
        ophthalmic 16
        sacral 16
        trigeminal 16
herpetic nipple 14
histoplasmosis 4, 8
    pulmonary 8
HIV 16
hydrocephalus 8
    fetal 16
hydrophobia *see* rabies
hypersensitivity reaction 4 *see also* allergy, anaphylaxis
hypoalbuminaemia 4
hypoglycaemia 22
hypotension 10
hypothermia 10
hypothyroidism 2
hypoxia 8, 10

I

ibuprofen for chronic fatigue syndrome 3
icthammol soak for erythema multiforme and Stevens–Johnson syndrome 5
immunization, active *see* vaccination
immunoblastoma *see* lymphoma
immunoglobulin
    pooled human, for measles 25
    varicella–zoster, for herpes zoster and varicella infection 17
impetigo 34
inclusion disease *see* cytomegalovirus
infarction, cerebral 16
infection 2
    adenovirus 4, 24, 32
    Aspergillus 8
    bacterial
        Gram-positive 10
        of skin 16
    Borrelia burgdorferi 20
    Campylobacter 6
    Candida 8
    chlamydiae 4
    Corynebacterium diphtheriae 28
    coxsackie virus 4, 14, 28
    cryptococcal 8
    enteroviral 4, 24, 26, 32
    Escherichia coli 10
    fungal 6, 8, 10
    interdigital 8
    intra-abdominal 10
    intravascular 8
    Klebsiella 10
    mycoplasma 4
    Neisseria 10
    ocular 14
    parvovirus B19 26
    perianal 8
    plasmodium *see* malaria
    Proteus 10
    Pseudomonas 10
    renal 8
    rhinocerebral 8
    Salmonella 6
    Serratia 10
    sinus
        allergic 8
        saprophytic 8
    Staphylococcus aureus, methicillin-resistant 34
    streptococcal 6, 12, 28
    upper respiratory tract 4, 12
    urinary tract 10
    viral 4, 10, 12, 14, 18, 38
    Yersinia 6
influenza 22
intertrigo 8
intussusception 12
iridocyclitis 14
irritable bowel syndrome 2
itraconazole for fungal infections 9

J

jaundice 22
    haemolytic *see* anaemia, haemolytic
joint disorders *see* arthritis, polyarthritis

K

Kawasaki syndrome 4, 36
keratitis 16
    stromal 14
    ulcerative *see* ulcer, corneal
ketoacidosis 22
ketoconazole for fungal infections 8
kinase II inhibitors *see* angiotensin-converting enzyme inhibitors
Koplik's spots 24

L

lacrimation 14
leishmaniasis 40
lens opacities *see* cataracts
leprosy 6
leptospirosis 18, 22
    anicteric 18
    icteric 18
leptospiruria 18
lesions 6
    bullous 4
    cutaneous 14
    in pinna of ear 16
    oral 4
    space-occupying 14
    vasculitic 12
leucocytosis
    neutrophil 10
    polymorphonuclear 12
leucopenia 10
leukaemia 4, 18
lormetazepam for chronic fatigue syndrome 3
lung disease
    chronic 8
    interstitial *see* fibrosis, pulmonary
lupus erythematosus 4
Lyell's syndrome *see* necrolysis, toxic epidermal
Lyme
    disease 2, 20
lymph node
    cervical 14, 28
    enlarged 2
lymphadenopathy 8, 14, 20
lymphadenosis benigna cutis 20
lymphangitis 34
lymphoma 4, 8, 20
    virus, Burkitt's *see* Epstein–Barr virus

Index

M

macrolide for Mycoplasma infection 5
malaria 10, 14, 22, 40
   falciparum 22
malignancy 2, 4 see also cancer
   haematological 8
ME see chronic fatigue syndrome
measles 24, 26
   encephalitis, acute 24
   German 32 see also rubella
mefloquine for uncomplicated *Plasmodium falciparum* malaria 23
memory disturbance 2, 20
meningism 20, 28
meningitis 8, 14, 18, 20, 22
   aseptic 14, 18
   cryptococcal 8
   herpes 14
   lymphocytic 18
meningococcaemia 4
mental function, impaired 8
meperidine see pethidine
metronidazole for Gram-negative septicaemia 11
microabscess, cerebral 8
microcephaly, fetal 16
microphthalmia 32
mitral
   regurgitation 30
   valve, floppy 256
mononucleosis, infectious 20, 28
   like syndrome, chronic see chronic fatigue syndrome
   virus see Epstein–Barr virus
morphine for leptospirosis 19
MRSA see infection, *Staphylococcus aureus*
mucormycosis 8
mucoviscidosis see fibrosis, cystic
muscle
   tender 2
   weakness 2
myalgia 2, 4, 16, 18, 20
mycoplasma 4
myelitis 14
   transverse 16
myeloma, multiple 4
myocarditis 8, 18, 40
myopericarditis 20
myxoedema, pretibial 6

N

nail loss 4
naproxen
   for erythema nodosum 7
   for Henoch–Schönlein purpura 13
   for erythema multiforme and Stevens–Johnson syndrome 5

nasal discharge 8
neck stiffness 8, 10, 14, 20
necrolysis, toxic epidermal 4
necrosis
   acute tubular 10, 22
   epidermal 4
   skin 34
nephritis 12, 18
   Heymann see glomerulonephritis
nephropathy, immunoglobulin 12
neuralgia, postherpetic 17
neurasthenia see chronic fatigue syndrome
neuritis 32
   cranial 20
neuropathy, peripheral 20
neutropenia 8, 10
nodules
   erythematous 6
   rheumatoid 6
nonsteroidal anti-inflammatory drugs see NSAIDs
nose, blocked 8
NSAIDs
   for erythema nodosum 7
   for Henoch–Schönlein purpura 13
   for erythema multiforme and Stevens–Johnson syndrome 5
nystatin for fungal infections 9

O

obstruction, intestinal 12
oedema
   eyelid 14
   pulmonary 22
oesophagitis 8
oligoarthritis 20
oliguria 10, 22
onychomycosis 8
opisthotonos 22
osteoarticular disorders 8
otitis
   externa 8
   media 4, 8, 24
oxygen for Gram-negative bacterial shock 11

P

pain
   abdominal 2, 10, 12, 18, 20
   chest 2, 4, 10, 20, 30
   facial 8
   from oral lesion 4
   joint 2, 12, 18, 20
   pleuritic 8
palsy
   Bell's 20
   cranial nerve 8
   facial 16
pancarditis 30

pancreas, fibrosing disease of see fibrosis, cystic
pancreatitis 10
pancytopenia 8
panencephalitis, subacute sclerosing 24
paracetamol
   for chronic fatigue syndrome 3
   for measles 25
   for parvovirus B19 infection 27
   for rubella 33
paraesthesia 2
paralysis 14
   lower motor neurone 16
paratyphoid fever 40
paresis 14
paronychia 4, 8
penicillin
   for chronic Lyme disease 21
   for erysipelas 35
perforation
   gastrointestinal 12
   intestinal 40
periadenitis mucosa necrotica recurrens see ulcer, aphthoid
pericarditis 8
peritonitis 8
   sarcoid 38
   starch 38
personality, altered 14
pethidine for leptospirosis 19
pharyngitis 28
   streptococcal 28
phenoxymethylpenicillin
   for acute rheumatic fever 31
   for diphtherial infections 29
   for streptococcal infections 29
phlegmon see cellulitis
photophobia 8, 14, 20
piperacillin for Gram-negative septicaemia 11
plaque
   bowel 8
   urticarial 4
   white, in mouth 8
pleuropneumonia-like organisms see mycoplasma
pneumonia 4, 8, 10, 14, 18, 22, 24
   chickenpox 16
pneumonitis 18
polyarteritis 4
   nodosa 12
polyarthritis 4 see also arthritis
polyarthropathy, migratory 30
polyneuritis 16
polyradiculoneuritis see Guillain–Barré syndrome
potassium
   iodide for erythema nodosum 7
   permanganate soaks for Henoch–Schönlein purpura 13

Index

povidone iodine for MRSA infection 35
PPLO see mycoplasma
prednisolone
   for acute rheumatic fever 31
   for erythema nodosum 7
   for Henoch–Schönlein purpura 13
   for Stevens–Johnson syndrome 5
prostatitis 8
pruritus 8, 14
pseudotuberculosis see sarcoidosis
psychiatric disorder 2
purpura
   allergic see purpura, Henoch–Schönlein
   anaphylactoid see purpura, Henoch–Schönlein
   Henoch–Schönlein 12, 30
   non-thrombocytopenic see purpura, Henoch–Schönlein
   rheumatoid see purpura, Henoch–Schönlein
   thrombocytopenic 18, 32
   thrombopenic see purpura, thrombocytopenic
pyrazinamide for extrapulmonary tuberculosis 39
pyrimethamine/sulphadoxine see Fansidar

Q

quinidine for complicated *Plasmodium falciparum* malaria 23
quinine for malaria 23
quinolones
   for paratyphoid fevers 41
   for typhoid fevers 41

R

rabies 22
radiculoneuritis 20
Ramsey–Hunt syndrome 16
rash 4, 12, 18, 20
   ampicillin 28
   drug 24
   haemorrhagic 16
   nappy 8
   skin 10, 12, 16
   slapped cheek 26
   vesicular 16
regurgitation
   Carey–Coombs aortic 30
   mitral 30
renal
   failure 4, 10, 12, 22, 36
   function, impaired 18
respiratory distress 22
   adult 10, 18, 36, 38
retinopathy 32
Reye's syndrome 16
rheumatism, acute articular see fever, rheumatic
rickettsioses 18
rifampicin for extrapulmonary tuberculosis 39

rigors 10, 22
Royal Free disease see chronic fatigue syndrome
rubella 24, 26, 32
   arthritide 30
rubeola see measles

S

salicylates for erythema multiforme and Stevens–Johnson syndrome 5
salivary gland disease see cytomegalovirus
sarcoidosis 2, 4, 6, 8
scalded skin syndrome, nonstaphylococcal see necrolysis, toxic epidermal
scarlet fever 26, 28, 32, 34
Schaumann's disease see sarcoidosis
sclerosis
   disseminated see sclerosis, multiple
   multiple 20
sepsis, Gram-negative 12
septal defect, ventricular 32
septicaemia 18, 22, 36
   Gram-negative 10
   meningococcal 10, 12
Septrin see co-trimoxazole
sexually transmitted disease 14
shock
   cardiogenic 10
   endotoxic see septic shock, toxic shock
   hypovolaemic 10
   lung see respiratory distress, adult
   septic 10, 22 see also toxic shock
   toxic see also septic shock
      syndrome 10, 36
         toxin-1 antibodies for toxic shock syndrome 37
sleep disturbance 2
sodium valproate for postherpetic neuralgia 17
sore
   canker see ulcer, aphthoid
   cold 14
splenomegaly 20, 40
stenosis
   gastrointestinal 38
   pulmonary 32
      valve see stenosis, pulmonary
steroids see corticosteroids
Stevens–Johnson syndrome 4
Still's disease 30
stomatitis 14
   aphthous see ulcer, aphthoid
stroke, heat 22
stupor 14, 40
suffusion, conjunctival 18
sulphadoxine/pyrimethamine see Fansidar
sweating 10
   inappropriate 2
   night 38

swelling
   joint 20
   of gums 14
   periarticular 12
syphilis 4

T

tachycardia 10
tachypnoea 10
taste, loss of 16
teicoplanin for MRSA infection 35
temazepam for chronic fatigue syndrome 3
tetracycline for Mycoplasma infection 5
throat
   inflamed 2
   sore 4, 18, 20, 28
thrombocytopenia 18, 24, 32
thrombopenia see thrombocytopenia
thrush
   azole-resistant 8
   oral 8
thymoanaleptics see antidepressants
thymoleptics see antidepressants
thyroid disease 2, 6
tick bites 2, 20
tinnitus 2
toxoplasmosis 2, 20, 26, 32, 38
transplantation, organ 8
triple symptom complex see Behçet's syndrome
trypanosomiasis 40
tuberculoma 14
tuberculosis 6, 8
   cryptic disseminated 38
   extrapulmonary 38
   miliary 38
   pulmonary 8
tumour 14
typhoid fever 40
typhus 40

U

ulcer 4
   aphthoid, small 28
   aphthous 14
   bowel 8
   corneal 14
   gastrointestinal 8
   oral 8, 14, 16
   posterior 28
   soft-palate 28
urethritis 8, 14
urinary
   frequency 10
   retention 14
urticaria 4
uveitis 16, 18

Index

V

vaccination
  against rubella 33
  for measles 25
  for varicella 17
vaginal discharge 14
vancomycin for MRSA infection 35
varicella–zoster 14, 16
  immune globulin for varicella–zoster infection 17
vasculitis, haemorrhagic *see* purpura, Henoch–Schönlein
vasculopathy, cerebral 16
venereal disease *see* sexually transmitted disease
ventricular septal defect 32
venulitis, cutaneous necrotizing 12
vesicles 4, 14
vision
  blurring of 14
  loss of 14
vulvovaginal discharge 8

W

weakness 2
Weil's syndrome 18
wheeze 8
  allergic 8

Z

zygomycosis 8

CURRENT DIAGNOSIS & TREATMENT

in

Nephrology

Edited by
Paul Sweny

Series editors
Roy Pounder
Mark Hamilton

A **QUICK** Reference for the Clinician

Contributors

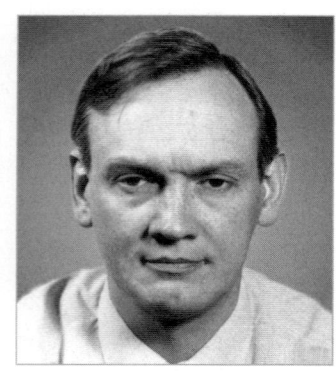

EDITOR

P Sweny

Dr Paul Sweny is a NHS Consultant at the Royal Free Hospital, London. Special interests include immunological renal disease and the medical management of renal transplantation. He has published three books and many review articles and original papers on a wide range of renal issues.

REFEREES

Nephrology

Dr Steve Nelson
Department of Nephrology
King's College Hospital
London, UK

Professor Charles D Pusey
Renal Unit
Hammersmith Hospital
London, UK

AUTHORS

DIALYSIS

Dr James Tattersall
Renal Unit
Lister Hospital
Stevenage, UK

GLOMERULONEPHRITIS

Dr Paul Sweny
Renal Unit
Royal Free Hospital
London, UK

HAEMOLYTIC URAEMIC SYNDROME

Professor Guy Neild
Institute of Urology and Nephrology
University College Hospital
London, UK

HYPERKALAEMIA AND HYPOKALAEMIA

Dr Paul Sweny
Renal Unit
Royal Free Hospital
London, UK

HYPERNATRAEMIA AND HYPONATRAEMIA

Dr Paul Sweny
Renal Unit
Royal Free Hospital
London, UK

NEPHROPATHIES, TUBULOINTERESTITIAL

Dr Ken Farrington
Renal Unit
Lister Hospital
Stevenage, UK

POLYCYSTIC KIDNEY DISEASE, AUTOSOMAL-DOMINANT

Dr Áine Burns
Renal Unit
Royal Free Hospital
London, UK

RENAL ARTERY STENOSIS

Dr John E Scoble
Renal Unit
Dulwich Hospital
London, UK

RENAL FAILURE, ACUTE

Dr Paul Sweny
Renal Unit
Royal Free Hospital
London, UK

RENAL FAILURE, CHRONIC

Dr Áine Burns
Renal Unit
Royal Free Hospital
London, UK

RENAL TRANSPLANTATION

Ms Rozanne Lord
Transplant Unit
Cardiff Royal Infirmary
Cardiff, UK

RENAL TUBULAR ACIDOSIS

Dr John E Scoble
Renal Unit
Dulwich Hospital
London, UK

URINARY TRACT INFECTION

Dr Ken Farrington
Renal Unit
Lister Hospital
Stevenage, UK

Contents

2 **Dialysis**
continuous ambulatory peritoneal dialysis
haemodialysis
haemofiltration
home haemodialysis

4 **Glomerulonephritis**
non-proliferative glomerulonephritis (minimal change, membranous)
proliferative glomerulonephritis (endocapillary: diffuse proliferative, focal segmental proliferative, mesangial IgA disease, mesangiocapillary, focal, necrotizing; extracapillary: crescentic)

6 **Haemolytic uraemic syndrome**
haemolytic uraemic syndrome
thrombotic thrombocytopenic purpura

8 **Hyperkalaemia and hypokalaemia**

10 **Hypernatraemia and hyponatraemia**

12 **Nephropathies, tubulointerstitial**
acute interstitial nephritis
acute tubular necrosis
analgesic nephropathy
chronic interstitial nephritis
papillary necrosis
reflux nephropathy

14 **Polycystic kidney disease, autosomal-dominant**

16 **Renal artery stenosis**
atherosclerotic disease
fibromuscular dysplasia

18 **Renal failure, acute**
postrenal acute renal failure
prerenal acute renal failure
renal acute renal failure (acute interstitial nephritis, acute tubular necrosis, focal necrotizing and crescentic glomerulonephritis, haemolytic uraemic syndrome, pigment nephropathy and kidney myeloma, renal infection, thrombotic thrombocytopenic purpura)

20 **Renal failure, chronic**

22 **Renal transplantation**
immunosuppression
rejection

24 **Renal tubular acidosis**
distal renal tubular acidosis
hyporeninaemic hypoaldosteronism
proximal renal tubular acidosis

26 **Urinary tract infection**
lower urinary tract infection (cystitis, prostatitis)
upper urinary tract infection (pyelonephritis, renal abscess)

28 Index

Dialysis J.E. Tattersall

Diagnosis

Indications for dialysis

Acute renal failure: usually part of a multisystem disease, especially with hypovolaemia or shock; if the renal failure cannot be reversed rapidly, recovery from the underlying disease is delayed or prevented, possibly resulting in death; early dialysis is needed to reverse acidosis, hyperkalaemia, and uraemia and to remove fluid from an oliguric patient to allow i.v. treatment and to relieve pulmonary oedema.

Chronic renal failure: irreversible, progressive failure is eventually fatal without dialysis; ideally, dialysis should be started before symptoms or signs develop; early dialysis is needed to prevent acidosis, hyperkalaemia, uraemia, and fluid overload.

Severe heart failure, certain poisonings: rare.

- Treatable causes of renal failure should be excluded before starting dialysis, especially when rapid deterioration in renal function has occurred; these include the following:

Hypovolaemia: central venous pressure and lying and standing blood pressure must be checked (postural drop of systolic blood pressure >10 mmHg suggests up to 10% hypovolaemia).

Outflow obstruction: patient must be checked for palpable bladder.

Investigations

Bicarbonate measurement: dialysis indicated in renal metabolic acidosis except when renal tubular acidosis occurs (rare); dialysis indicated if concentration <18 mmol/L.

Potassium measurement: dialysis indicated if concentration >6.5 mmol/L, especially in acute renal failure and if ECG changes are present.

Urea measurement: difficult to interpret because influenced by generation rate (from protein catabolism); dialysis indicated if concentration >30 mmol/L in well nourished patients or >20 mmol/L in malnourished patients.

Creatinine measurement: generated from muscle protein; dialysis indicated if concentration >1.0 mmol/L in patients with normal build or >0.5 mmol/L in patients with low muscle mass (e.g. elderly).

Creatinine clearance tests: most helpful, especially if normalized to patient's surface area; dialysis indicated if clearance rate <10 ml/min/1.75 m^2.

Hepatitis serology: precautions must be taken when dialysing hepatitis B or C antigen-positive patients; most dialysis units do not dialyse patient unless antigen status known.

HIV status: if positive, dialysis not contraindicated, but special precautions are needed.

Complications of dialysis

Acute

Peritonitis: in continuous peritoneal dialysis; usually follows contamination of catheter connections; occurs on average every 2 years; occasionally fatal; treated by intraperitoneal antibiotics and catheter removal if severe.

Bleeding: due to excessive anticoagulation.

Hypotension: due to excessive fluid removal.

Fever: due to contamination of blood circuit or dialyser with pyrogens or bacteria.

Disequilibrium: rare; cerebral oedema caused by osmotic effects when patient with very high urea concentration is dialysed excessively rapidly.

Chronic

Amyloidosis: beta-2 microglobulin is poorly cleared by dialysis and accumulates as amyloid; causes a disabling arthropathy and the carpal tunnel syndrome.

Malnutrition: uraemia causes anorexia and protein malnutrition unless adequate dialysis is provided; in continuous ambulatory peritoneal dialysis, this is exacerbated by protein losses from the peritoneum and may be masked by obesity caused by excessive uptake of glucose from the dialysis fluid.

Neuropathy: may result from inadequate dialysis or aluminium overload.

Acquired cystic disease: in native kidneys (malignant potential).

- Hypertension, anaemia, cardiovascular disease, hyperparathyroidism, and osteomalacia are common in dialysis patients as a result of the uraemic state.

Epidemiology

- 600 patients in one million population are on dialysis or have a functioning transplant.
- 100 new patients in one million population annually are treated by dialysis.
- The mean age of dialysis patients is 55 years.
- Dialysis costs £20 000 per patient per year.

Patients suitable for dialysis

- Any patient is suitable except those unlikely to survive more than a few months even with normal renal function.
- Dialysis units prefer to decide for themselves if a patient is suitable.
- Many patients on dialysis are elderly or have diabetes, myeloma, or other multisystem disease.
- Patients with severe heart failure need not be refused dialysis; this often improves on dialysis.

Procedures to avoid

Contrast radiography

- Radiography will probably not be helpful and may worsen renal failure.

Cannulation of forearm veins

- Cannulation may destroy the veins needed for dialysis access; hand or antecubital veins should be used.

Urethral catheterization

- In oliguria, catheterization causes urinary tract infection and septicaemia and may worsen renal failure.

Blood transfusion

- Transfusion causes fluid overload and hyperkalaemia and should be avoided unless performed at the same time as dialysis.
- HLA sensitization may make transplantation difficult.

Treatment

Diet and lifestyle
- Dialysis patients tend to have protein malnutrition and usually need an increased-protein diet or protein supplements; low-protein diets should be avoided.
- Most patients need moderate fluid, potassium, and sodium restriction.
- Supplements of iron and water-soluble vitamins are needed.

Dialysis techniques

Haemodialysis
- The patient's blood is pumped through a dialyser at 200–500 ml/min.
- Uraemic toxins diffuse from the blood through a permeable membrane in the dialyser into a dialysis fluid.
- Bicarbonate diffuses in the opposite direction to correct the acidosis.
- Up to 140 litres of dialysis fluid per treatment is produced by the dialysis machine from purified water and an electrolyte concentrate.
- Excess fluid is removed from the patient by ultrafiltration of the blood in the dialyser, driven by a controlled pressure gradient across the membrane.
- The patient is usually heparinized during treatment.

Haemofiltration
- Haemofiltration is similar to haemodialysis but without the dialysate.
- Uraemic toxins and excess fluids are removed by ultrafiltration rates up to 150 ml/min across a permeable membrane.
- The ultrafiltrate is then replaced by an i.v. infusion of up to 30 litres of sterile solution.
- Haemofiltration is more efficient then haemodialysis at removing high-molecular-weight toxins but is more expensive.
- Both haemodialysis and haemofiltration are performed 3 times weekly in chronic renal failure and take 3–5 h per session. The treatments may also be performed slowly and continuously for acute renal failure in the intensive care unit. 30 litres of dialysate or infusate are needed each day and are available ready-prepared in bags, avoiding the need for a dialysis machine.

Continuous ambulatory peritoneal dialysis
- 60% of dialysis patients are now treated by this method.
- . The treatment is done by the patient at home and allows considerable independence.
- Uraemic toxins diffuse into 2–3 litres of dialysate within the peritoneum.
- Excess fluid is removed by osmosis; the dialysate contains a variable glucose concentration to achieve this.
- The patient aseptically exchanges the dialysate with fresh fluid 4 times daily via a peritoneal catheter.

Home haemodialysis
- Home haemodialysis is suitable for well motivated patients who will probably remain on dialysis for many years.
- It is gradually being replaced by continuous ambulatory peritoneal dialysis in the UK.

Treatment aims
To restore quality of life and prolong life expectancy.

Prognosis
- A typical 60-year-old dialysis patient with coexisting cardiovascular disease has an expected survival of 4–5 years.
- Younger patients with no other disease have a near-normal life expectancy.

Follow-up and management
- Dialysis patients are usually followed up at least 3-monthly in the dialysis unit.
- Blood pressure, fluid balance and nutritional status, haemoglobin, calcium, and bicarbonate should be maintained within the normal range.
- Parathyroid hormone should be maintained at about twice the normal upper limit, and phosphate at 1–2 mmol/L.
- The amount of dialysis delivered is monitored to ensure adequate dialysis delivery.

Access
Cimino fistula: created surgically between artery and vein (usually radial).

Tenckhoff catheter: cuffed, tunnelled, silicone catheter implanted into peritoneal cavity for continuous ambulatory peritoneal dialysis.

Long-bore central venous catheter: can be inserted into right atrium or femoral vein.

Scribner shunt: surgically implanted catheters in both artery and vein for haemodialysis.

Key references
Ota K et al.: The Dialysis Patient. In *The Oxford Textbook of Clinical Nephrology*. Edited by Cameron S et al. Oxford: Oxford University Press, 1992, pp 405–415.

Greenwood RN: High-reflux short-duration haemodialysis: a new approach. In *Advanced Renal Medicine*. Edited by Raine AEG. Oxford: Oxford University Press, 1992, pp ???

Michael J: Continuous ambulatory peritoneal dialysis: current role and future prospects. In *Advanced Renal Medicine*. Edited by Raine AEG. Oxford: Oxford University Press, 1992, pp 405–424.

Glomerulonephritis
P. Sweny

Diagnosis

Definition
- Glomerulonephritis is immunologically mediated glomerular inflammation, often with associated tubulointerstitial lesions and sometimes part of a multisystem vasculitis.
- In different patients, the same cause can produce different histological lesions; similarly, different histological appearances can be caused by similar insults in different patients.
- The following classification is based on that of the World Health Organization (terms are purely descriptive and are not necessarily specific disease entities):

Non-proliferative
Minimal-change glomerulonephritis: normal on light microscopy.
Membranous glomerulonephritis: thick-basement membranes, subepithelial immune complexes.
Focal segmental glomerulosclerosis: mesangial and capillary loop scarring.

Proliferative: endocapillary
Diffuse proliferative glomerulonephritis: overcellular glomeruli.
Focal segmental proliferative glomerulonephritis: overcellular glomeruli.
Mesangial IgA disease: large deposits of IgA in mesangium.
Mesangiocapillary glomerulonephritis: thick capillary loops with expanded overcellular mesangium; also called membranoproliferative glomerulonephritis.
Focal necrotizing glomerulonephritis: segment of necrosis in peripheral capillary loop.

Proliferative: extracapillary
Crescentic glomerulonephritis: sheaves of macrophages and other cells filling all or part of Bowman's space with variable underlying glomerular lesions.

Symptoms and signs
- Glomerulonephritis is often silent, manifesting as chronic renal failure after insidious deterioration in renal function.

Proteinuria: asymptomatic (usually <2 g/24 h); nephrotic (>3 g/24 h).
Haematuria: microscopic (detected by stick test); macroscopic (smoky urine).
Acute nephritic illness.
Acute renal failure.
Chronic renal failure.

Investigations
Urine microscopy (phase contrast): dysmorphic erythrocytes and casts imply glomerular inflammation.
24-h urinalysis: for creatinine clearance and urine protein.
U&E and creatinine measurement.
Albumin and lipid measurement.
Tests for vasculitides: e.g. anti-double-stranded DNA antibody, anti-neutrophil cytoplasmic antibody (ANCA).
Antiglomerular basement membrane antibody measurement.
Investigation for appropriate associated infections.
Complement studies: CH50, C3, C4, C3 nephritic factor.
Plain abdominal radiography and ultrasonography or intravenous pyelography.
Renal biopsy: light, electron, and immunofluorescent microscopy all needed.

Complications
Hypertension: can be severe.
Acute or chronic renal failure.
Nephrotic syndrome: venous and arterial thromboses, pleural effusions, ascites, intravascular volume depletion, infection, accelerated atherosclerosis.

Differential diagnosis

Nephritic syndrome
Severe hypertension.
Scleroderma renal crisis.
Thrombotic microangiopathies (e.g. haemolytic uraemic syndrome).
Acute interstitial nephritis.

Nephrotic syndrome
Preeclampsia.
Amyloidosis.
Diabetes mellitus.
Congestive cardiac failure.
Cirrhosis with oedema and ascites.
NSAID use.

Other
Orthostatic proteinuria.
Other causes of hypertension or acute or chronic renal failure.

Aetiology

Immunopathogenesis
Immune complex: in-situ formation (built up within glomerulus) or, less commonly, deposition of preformed immune complexes from circulation.
Direct antibody-mediated injury: antiglomerular basement membrane antibody (Goodpasture's disease); this is rare.
Unknown, but possibly cell-mediated; probably important in many forms of glomerulonephritis.

Associated diseases
Primary: no known association (idiopathic).
Secondary: postinfectious, e.g. viruses, (hepatitis B, HIV), bacterial (post streptococcal), protozoal (malarial);
drug-induced, e.g. gold or penicillamine;
associated with vasculitis;
associated with neoplasia.

Epidemiology
- Glomerulonephritis is the most common cause of chronic renal failure (~20–25%).
- Minimal-change glomerulonephritis is the most common cause of nephrotic syndrome in children.
- Mesangial IgA disease is the most common cause of recurrent episodes of macroscopic haematuria in young adults.

Treatment

Diet and lifestyle

- Patients must not have added salt if they have oedema or hypertension.
- Nephrotic patients should have a normal protein intake.
- Renal failure patients should have a low protein intake (0.5 g/kg daily).
- Oral intake of fluids should be restricted if the patient is oedematous.
- Pregnant patients are at increased risk of preeclampsia (high risk if creatinine raised).
- Occasionally, pregnant patients experience deterioration of renal function.

Pharmacological treatment

Immunosuppression

- Patients are chosen on the basis of clinical syndrome and histology.
- Aggressive treatment is indicated for heavy proteinuria or falling glomerular filtration rate.
- Histology is most helpful for choosing treatment.

For minimal-change glomerulonephritis:
remission induction: high-dose steroids, cyclosporin A;
maintenance: low-dose steroids or cyclosporin A;
prevention of relapse: cyclophosphamide.

For membranous glomerulonephritis: trial of steroids, possibly with chlorambucil in selected patients.

For focal segmental glomerulosclerosis: high-dose steroids or cyclosporin A, or both (prolonged treatment needed).

For mesangial IgA disease: fish oil (eicosapentaenoic acid).

For postinfectious diffuse proliferative glomerulonephritis: observation.

For mesangiocapillary glomerulonephritis: no treatment effective; trial of immunosuppression in selected patients.

For focal necrotizing or crescentic glomerulonephritis: steroids with cyclophosphamide (pulse i.v. methylprednisolone for 3 days may help); additional plasma exchange in selected patients (immediate plasma exchange mandatory in Goodpasture's disease).

Supportive

Control of fluid balance: diuretics (combinations may be needed).

Protection of intravascular volume: nephrotic patients may need volume expansion with human albumin solutions.

Control of blood pressure: angiotensin-converting enzyme inhibitors if possible; calcium antagonists should be avoided (oedema).

Aggressive treatment of intercurrent infections (cellulitis, pneumonia, spontaneous bacterial peritonitis).

Anticoagulation: should be considered for nephrotic patients, especially if they are immobile.

Treatment aims

To suppress glomerular inflammation.
To prevent progressive glomerular scarring and progression to chronic renal failure.
To minimize proteinuria.
To control hypertension and fluid balance.
To avoid overimmunosuppression, particularly of burnt-out glomerulonephritis with intrarenal scarring.

Prognosis

- A bad prognosis is associated with severe hypertension, heavy persistent proteinuria, and raised creatinine when first seen.
- Prognosis is closely related to histology:
Minimal-change glomerulonephritis: excellent, eventually resolves despite relapses.
Focal segmental proliferative glomerulonephritis: <10% of patients progress to chronic renal failure (CRF).
Membranous glomerulonephritis: 30% resolve, 30% remain static, 30% progress to CRF
Mesangial IgA disease: 25% progress to CRF.
Postinfectious diffuse proliferative glomerulonephritis: >90% resolve.
Mesangiocapillary glomerulonephritis: >75% progress to CRF.
Focal necrotizing and crescentic glomerulonephritis: <30% progress to CRF if given early aggressive treatment.

Follow-up and management

- Follow-up should be for life if the patient has raised creatinine, persistent haematuria, proteinuria, or hypertension.
- Obsessional control of blood pressure is needed, using angiotensin-converting enzyme inhibitors whenever possible because this class of drug reduces glomerular blood pressure and proteinuria and may protect the kidney.
- Immunosuppressive drugs must be titrated to disease activity.
- Lipids must be controlled.

Key references

D'Amico G: Influence of clinical and histological features on actuarial renal survival in adult patients with idiopathic IgA nephropathy, membranous nephropathy and membranoproliferative glomerulonephritis. *Am J Kidney Dis* 1992, **20**:315–323.

Mason PD, Pusey CD: Glomerulonephritis: diagnosis and treatment. *BMJ* 1994, **309**:15571563.

Haemolytic uraemic syndrome
G.H. Neild

Diagnosis

Definition
- Haemolytic uraemic syndrome (HUS) is a syndrome, not a disease; it is defined by the following:

Acute renal insufficiency.

Microangiopathic haemolytic anaemia.

Thrombocytopenia.

- Thrombotic thrombocytopenic purpura (TTP) is closely related and often indistinguishable from HUS; the term should be reserved for the following:

A relapsing form of HUS.

Associated fever and fluctuating CNS signs.

- Both HUS and TTP are associated with normal clotting times. Thrombocytopenia and a microangiopathic haemolytic anaemia with prolonged clotting times indicate septicaemia and disseminated intravascular coagulation.

Symptoms
Malaise, nausea, tiredness: nonspecific symptoms of renal insufficiency.

Oliguria, discoloured urine, difficulty concentrating, other subtle CNS changes.

Abdominal cramps, watery diarrhoea, then bloody diarrhoea, fever <38°C: indicating infection by *Escherichia coli*.

Signs
Pallor: from anaemia.

Yellow tinge: occasionally, from the haemolysis.

Bruising or prolonged bleeding: if thrombocytopenia is severe.

Investigations
Full blood count: shows thrombocytopenia; fragmented erythrocytes seen on film.

Clotting times: prothrombin time and partial thromboplastin time should be normal.

Biochemistry: shows raised urea, creatinine, and urate concentrations, hyponatraemia, hypoalbuminaemia in severely ill patients, raised lactate dehydrogenase (an index of erythrocyte haemolysis).

Renal biopsy: usually not needed in children; contraindicated during severe thrombocytopenia; typically shows glomerular and arteriolar thrombosis and acute tubular necrosis in patients with diarrhoea, and severe intimal proliferation of preglomerular arterioles and small arteries, with varying degrees of glomerular endothelial injury, in patients without diarrhoea.

Stool culture for *Escherichia coli* 0157:H7 and isolation of verocytotoxin: can confirm diagnosis in patients with associated diarrhoea.

Serology: for neutralizing antibodies to *E. coli* 0157:H7.

Complications
Bloody diarrhoea, gut infarction, rectal prolapse: in patients with associated diarrhoea.

Severe malignant hypertension, cardiomyopathy: in patients without diarrhoea.

Irritability, restlessness, twitching, generalized or focal seizures, transient visual disturbance, drowsiness, cerebellar ataxia, reduced level of consciousness, decerebrate spasms, coma.

Skin petechiae or purpura: rare unless platelets are $\leq 20 \times 10^9$/L.

Differential diagnosis

Septicaemia associated with disseminated intravascular coagulation
Gram-negative bacilli.
Infection by *Staphylococcus aureus*, *Pneumococcus* spp., or *Meningococcus* spp.
Psittacosis.
Mycoplasma.

Viral and other diseases: thrombocytopenia without haemolysis
Hantavirus.
Dengue haemorrhagic fever.
Malaria.
Leptospirosis.
Snake bite.

Associated with pregnancy (associated with disseminated intravascular coagulation)
Septic abortion.
Amniotic fluid embolus.
Prolonged intrauterine fetal death.
Antepartum haemorrhage.

Aetiology

Infectious causes
Escherichia coli associated with diarrhoea (in most patients): infection acquired from contaminated beef or dairy products.
Shigella spp.
HIV.

Sporadic, noninfectious causes
Idiopathic or familial disorders, drugs (mitomycin, cyclosporin A), tumours, pregnancy, SLE, transplantation, scleroderma, malignant or accelerated hypertension.
Superimposed on glomerulonephritis.

Epidemiology
- Patients with diarrhoea-associated haemolytic uraemic syndrome are usually aged <5 years or >65 years.

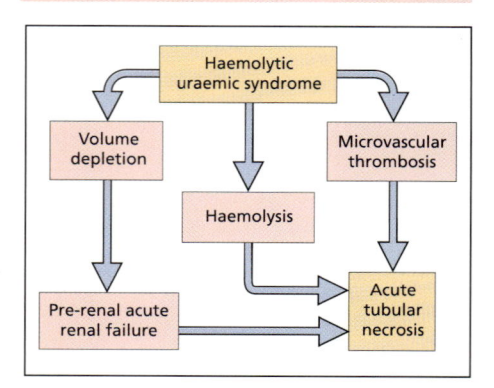

Pathogenesis of acute tubular necrosis from haemolytic uraemic syndrome.

Treatment

Diet and lifestyle
- No special precautions are necessary.

Pharmacological treatment
Intravenous saline solution and frusemide: to correct circulating volume and reverse prerenal failure and to establish diuresis.

Antiplatelet drugs (e.g. aspirin, dipyridamole): have a logic but no proven benefit.

Prostacyclin infusions: of theoretical value and useful to control hypertension.

Non-pharmacological treatment
Erythrocyte transfusion: for anaemia.

Platelet transfusion: if count $<50 \times 10^9$/L and some surgical intervention needed.

Haemodialysis: when indicated, i.e. for volume overload, hyperkalaemia, 'uraemia', acidosis.

Infusions of fresh frozen plasma: may induce remission; amount necessary not known but probably 1–2 litres daily; mechanism of benefit not known but may include neutralizing toxins, restoring antioxidant activity, and inducing prostacyclin synthesis; infusions should be continued until erythrocyte fragmentation ceases and platelet count rises $\sim 100 \times 10^9$/L.

Plasma exchange: may be needed to create intravascular space for repeated infusions of fresh frozen plasma.

Treatment aims
To establish diuresis if possible.
To provide dialysis if necessary.
To control blood pressure.
To try to induce haematological remission.
To prevent fits.

Prognosis
- The natural history of haemolytic uraemic syndrome, when preceded by a diarrhoeal illness and associated with glomerular thrombi, is one of spontaneous recovery, although patients may have some residual injury; most children are in this category.
- Idiopathic patients, particularly adults, often have major preglomerular vascular disease and irreversible renal failure.
- 3–10% of patients die during the acute illness (usually from CNS involvement); 10–20% remain dependent on dialysis; 10% have long-term neurological sequelae; 70% recover with no residual evidence of renal disease.

Follow-up and management
- Recovery of renal function and disappearance of proteinuria must be established.
- If this is not possible, long-term follow-up is needed.
- Blood pressure should be controlled by angiotensin-converting enzyme inhibitors, which may help to limit occlusive arteriopathy.

Key references
Milford DV, Taylor CM: New insights into the haemolytic uraemic syndromes. *Arch Dis Child* 1990, **65**:713–715.

Neild GH: Haemolytic uraemic syndrome: clinical practice. *Lancet* 1994, **343**:398–401.

Neild GH: Haemolytic uraemic syndrome (including disseminated intravascular coagulation and thrombotic purpura). In *Oxford Textbook of Clinical Nephrology*. Edited by Cameron JS et al. Oxford: Oxford University Press, 1992, pp 1041–1060.

Rock GA et al.: Comparison of plasma exchange with plasma infusion in the treatment of thrombotic thrombocytopenic purpura. *N Engl J Med* 1991, **325**:393–397.

Hyperkalaemia and hypokalaemia — P. Sweny

Diagnosis

Symptoms
- Often no symptoms are manifest.

Hyperkalaemia
Skeletal muscle weakness: causing collapse, paralysis.
Formication. — a prickling sensation said to resemble feeling of ants crawling over skin.

Hypokalaemia
Muscle weakness and fatigue.
Polyuria and polydipsia.
Palpitations.

Signs

Hyperkalaemia
Skeletal muscle weakness.
Irregular pulse.
Ileus.
Ventricular arrythmias, cardiac arrest (asystolic).

Hypokalaemia
Postural hypotension: indicating autonomic neuropathy.
Ileus. — intestinal obstruction usually of the small intestine.
Skeletal muscle weakness: quadriplegia, respiratory distress.
Cardiac arrhythmias: atrial and ventricular premature beats, atrial or ventricular tachycardia.

Investigations
- Estimation must be repeated urgently with optimal venepuncture technique and rapid transfer to laboratory.

Renal function tests: urea, creatinine.
ECG.
Acid–base analysis.
Urinary potassium and pH measurement.
Plasma magnesium measurement.
Creatine kinase measurement.
Plasma phosphate measurement.
Plasma glucose measurement.

Complications

Hyperkalaemia
Sudden death: asystole.

Hypokalaemia
Rhabdomyolysis on vigorous exertion (acute).
Growth retardation in children.
Nephrogenic diabetes insipidus.
Negative nitrogen balance.
Interstitial nephritis: renal impairment.
Glucose intolerance.
Myocardial fibrosis.

Differential diagnosis
Artefact of sampling technique (hyperkalaemia).

Aetiology

Hyperkalaemia
- The most common cause is a combination of renal impairment with the following:

Excessive potassium intake: due to diet, salt substitutes, potassium penicillins, transfusion of stored blood.
Redistribution: due to acidosis, exercise, hyperkalaemic familial periodic paralysis, hormonal deficiencies (insulin, aldosterone, cortisol), drugs (beta blockers, alpha antagonists), release from damaged tissues, hyperosmolality.
Impaired renal excretion: due to acute or chronic renal failure, potassium-conserving diuretics, inadequate mineralocorticosteroid hormones, angiotensin-converting enzyme inhibitors, NSAIDs, cyclosporin A, pentamidine, type IV renal tubular acidosis.
Impaired gut excretion: due to colectomy in patients with pre-existing renal failure.

Hypokalaemia
- The most common cause is a combination of gut loss with the following:

Inadequate intake: due to diet.
Redistribution: due to anabolic states, correction of severe anaemia, transfusion of washed or frozen erythrocytes, metabolic alkalosis, some myeloproliferative disorders, beta agonists, correction of hyperglycaemia, hypokalaemic periodic paralysis, barium intoxication.
Gut losses: due to vomiting or nasogastric aspiration, diarrhoea, purgative abuse.
Urinary losses: due to diuretics, hyperaldosteronism, Bartter's syndrome, Cushing's syndrome, liquorice abuse, excess adrenocorticotrophic hormone, renal tubular acidosis, tubular toxins (e.g. cisplatin, amphotericin, aminoglycosides), urinary diversion into gut, magnesium depletion.

Epidemiology
- Hyperkalaemia rarely occurs without renal impairment.
- Hypokalaemia is more common, being associated with the use of common drugs (diuretics and purgatives) and as a common complication of diarrhoeal states.

Treatment

Diet and lifestyle
- Hyperkalaemic patients with underlying chronic renal failure need dietary advice to restrict the daily potassium intake to 40–60 mmol/day; high-potassium foods include fruits, chocolate, nuts, and instant coffee.
- Hypokalaemia can rarely be corrected by dietary means.

Pharmacological treatment

For hyperkalaemia: moderate
- For moderate hyperkalaemia with an acute rise in potassium to <6.5 mmol/L and a normal ECG, the following measures should be taken:

Intake of potassium decreased.
Offending drug removed.
Good urinary output ensured.
Plasma potassium concentration measured every 6 h to ensure falling values.

For hyperkalaemia: severe
- An acute rise in potassium to >6.5 mmol/L and abnormal ECG or chronically raised potassium >8 mmol/L is a medical emergency.
- ECG monitoring is needed.
- Rapid correction is vital.
- Emergency dialysis is needed if the patient is oliguric and volume overloaded.

Standard dosage	10% calcium gluconate solution 10 ml i.v. slowly. 50% glucose solution 50 ml, containing insulin 10 units i.v. 4-hourly. 8.4% sodium bicarbonate solution 50 ml i.v. if acidotic. Calcium resonium 15 g and lactulose 10 ml orally 6-hourly or calcium resonium by rectal retention enema. Frusemide or bumetanide i.v. every 4–6 h to achieve urine flow rate >50 ml/h, e.g. bumetanide 1 mg initially, increased to 5 mg. Salbutamol infusion 5–20 µg/min can be given.
Contraindications	None.
Special points	Patient must be checked for hypoglycaemia after i.v. glucose and insulin. *Calcium gluconate:* a cardioprotective agent, does not lower plasma potassium concentration.
Main drug interactions	None.
Main side effects	*Sodium bicarbonate:* volume overload. *Frusemide:* deafness (i.v. doses >120 mg).

For hypokalaemia

Standard dosage	Effervescent potassium chloride 80–200 mmol orally daily. Potassium chloride 60–120 mmol i.v. over 24 h.
Contraindications	None.
Special points	Potassium as chloride must be used with alkalosis to avoid continued urinary losses. Oral supplements should be used whenever possible. Intravenous repletion is potentially dangerous: 10 mmol/h is usually safe; higher rates may be used, but ECG monitoring is essential.
Main drug interactions	Hypokalaemia exacerbates digoxin toxicity.
Main side effects	Late hyperkalaemia due to delayed gastrointestinal absorption after oral potassium supplements.

Treatment aims
To restore acid–base balance and plasma potassium slowly over 24–72 h.

Prognosis
- Prognosis depends on the underlying condition.

Follow-up and management
- If deviations are gross, frequent and repeated measurements of plasma potassium are essential for several days.

Key references
Androgue HJ, Wesson DE: Potassium. In *Blackwell's Basics of Medicine.* Oxford, Blackwell Scientific Publications, 1994.

Jacobsen HR, Rector FC (eds): Renal regulation of extracellular fluid composition. *Kidney Int* 1990, **38**:569–743.

Schrier RW (ed): *Renal and Electrolyte Disorders* edn 4. Boston: Little Brown & Co, 1992.

Tannen RL: Potassium metabolism. In *Current Nephrology* vol 15. Edited by Gonick HC. St Louis: Mosby Year Books, 1992, pp 109–148.

Hypernatraemia and hyponatraemia
P. Sweny

Diagnosis

Symptoms

Hypernatraemia
Restlessness.
Irritability.
Lethargy.
Muscle twitches.

Hyponatraemia
Lethargy.
Confusion and disorientation.
Agitation.
Anorexia.
Nausea.
Muscle cramps.

Signs

Hypernatraemia
Increased reflexes.
Increased muscle tone.
Depressed consciousness.
Fits.
Coma.

Hyponatraemia
Decreased reflexes.
Hypothermia.
Pseudobulbar palsy.
Fits.
Cheyne–Stokes respiration.
Coma.
Altered consciousness.

Investigations

- Most sodium is extracellular, so changes in sodium balance are reflected in changes in extracellular fluid volume (ECFV).
- Changes in serum sodium concentration reflect alterations in the sodium : water ratio in the extracellular fluid and can occur with increased, normal, or decreased ECFV (increased, normal, or reduced total body sodium).

Detection of oedema, estimation of jugular venous pressure, tissue turgor, erect and supine pulse and blood pressure, peripheral perfusion, auscultation of lung bases, and patient weighing: vital for accurate documentation of state of ECFV; oedema always indicates raised total body sodium (water, being freely diffusable, does not accumulate as oedema).

Renal function tests, chest radiography, ECG, liver function tests, albumin and glucose measurement, urine and plasma osmolality, U&E analysis, endocrine tests (thyroid and adrenal), echocardiography if cardiac disease suspected.

Complications

Hypernatraemia
Shrinkage of brain cells.
Rupture of cerebral veins.
Cerebral venous (sinus) thrombosis.
Intracranial haemorrhage.

Hyponatraemia
Cerebral oedema.
Raised intracranial pressure.
Coning: herniation.
Central pontine myelinolysis: related to over-rapid correction; causes permanent residual neurological deficits.

Differential diagnosis

Hyperlipidaemia or hyperproteinaemia: may cause pseudohyponatraemia; reduced water volume of plasma reduces apparent sodium concentration/ml whole plasma.

Aetiology

Causes of hypernatraemia
Normal (slightly reduced) extracellular fluid volume (ECFV): diabetes insipidus, dry ventilation, hypodipsia, sweating.
Increased ECFV (oedema): excessive sodium intake, excessive adrenocortical hormones.
Decreased ECFV (without free access to water): excessive loss of sodium in urine, excessive loss of gastrointestinal secretions, burns, sweating.

Causes of hyponatraemia
Normal (slightly expanded) ECFV: excessive water intake, syndrome of inappropriate antidiuretic hormone secretion (drug-induced).
Increased ECFV (oedema): acute or chronic renal failure, cardiac failure, cirrhosis with ascites, nephrotic syndrome, pregnancy.
Decreased ECFV (with free access to water): excessive loss of sodium in urine, excessive loss of gastrointestinal secretions, burns, sweating.

Epidemiology

- Hypernatraemia is common in elderly patients (hypodipsia) and in immobile or unconscious patients.
- Hyponatraemia is common in hospitals because of inappropriate fluid replacement, usually with dextrose saline solution or over-diuresis of patients with cardiac failure.

Treatment

Diet and lifestyle
- Hypernatraemia and hyponatraemia usually develop in hospitals; the primary underlying disease dominates the clinical picture.
- Alterations in sodium intake are needed for patients with changes in their extracellular fluid volume, e.g. sodium restriction for those with oedema.
- Compulsive water drinkers and drug abusers may need psychiatric counselling.

Pharmacological treatment

Hypernatraemia
- Extracellular fluid volume must first be defined and corrected; a decrease should be corrected by normal saline solution, an increase by diuretics or dialysis.
- Then the hypernatraemia can be corrected *slowly* by .5% dextrose or dextrose saline or N saline solution infused at a rate that reduces the hypernatraemia by 1 mmol/L/h – over-rapid correction may cause brain damage.
- Central venous pressure monitoring and urethral catheterization for monitoring urine output may be needed.

Hyponatraemia
- For mild to moderate chronic dilutional hyponatraemia, restriction of water intake alone may be sufficient.
- For oedematous states, diuretics should be given, with human albumin if the patient is nephrotic or cirrhotic.
- Patients with true sodium depletion should be given N saline or 5% hypertonic saline solution infused slowly, with diuretics to correct serum sodium concentrations – over-rapid correction may cause brain damage (hyponatraemia should be corrected by 1.5–2 mmol/h if acute onset or ≤ 1 mmol/h if chronic).
- Administration of sodium to oedematous patients may precipitate cardiac failure; diuretics may be needed to normalize intravascular volume.
- Restoring plasma oncotic pressure with albumin solutions may be needed, but their sodium content can be high (160 mmol/L); serum sodium must be measured every 4–6 h, with treatment adjusted to achieve desired correction rate.
- In severe cases, central venous pressure monitoring and urethral catheterization to monitor urine output are needed.

Treatment aims
To correct extracellular fluid volume.
To correct serum sodium concentration.

Prognosis
- Prognosis depends on the underlying condition.
- Acute changes in onset or correction are more dangerous than slow changes.
- Very old or very young patients are most vulnerable.
- Permanent neurological deficits are common, especially if correction is over-rapid.

Follow-up and management
- Follow-up depends on the underlying condition.

Key references

Adrogue HJ, Wesson DE: Salt and water. In *Blackwell's Basics of Medicine*. Oxford: Blackwell Scientific Publications, 1994.

Buckalen VM, Kramer HJ: Natriuretic hormones and sodium homeostasis: roles of digitalis-like factors and atrial natriuretic peptides. In *Current Nephrology* vol 15. Edited by Gonick HC. St Louis: Mosby Year Books, 1992, pp 207–244.

Richardson RMA: Water metabolism. In *Current Nephrology* vol 15. Edited by Gonick HC. St Louis: Mosby Year Books, 1992, pp 149–206.

Schrier RW: Body fluid volume regulation in health and disease: a unifying hypothesis. *Ann Intern Med* 1990, **113**:155–159.

Sterns RH: Central nervous system complications of hyponatraemia. In *International Year Book of Nephrology*. Edited by Andreucci VE, Fine LG. Berlin: Springer-Verlag, 1992, pp 55–74.

Nephropathies, tubulointerstitial — K. Farrington

Diagnosis

Symptoms and signs

Acute interstitial nephritis
- This is usually manifest as acute (potentially reversible) non-oliguric renal failure, less often as acute on chronic renal failure.
- The clinical picture may be dominated by the disease process for which an offending drug was administered or by features of extrarenal infection.

Fever, skin rash, and eosinophilia: in 30% of cases associated with drug allergy; NSAID-associated cases may be complicated by nephrotic syndrome.

Arthralgias and lymphadenopathy.

Anterior uveitis and granulomatous infiltration of other organs: in a small group of patients with idiopathic disease.

Chronic interstitial nephritis
- This usually manifests insidiously as chronic (irreversible) renal failure.
- The clinical picture may be dominated by features of an underlying disease process or by the condition for which analgesics were taken.
- No specific features allow differentiation from other causes of chronic renal failure.

Investigations

Full blood count: with differential for eosinophilia in acute interstitial nephritis.

U&E, creatinine clearance, 24-h urinary protein excretion measurement: to quantify renal function.

Blood cultures and other specific serological tests: if systemic infection, connective tissue disease, or vasculitis suspected (casts, eosinophiluria).

Microscopy and culture of midstream urine.

Urinary Bence-Jones protein and serum protein electrophoresis: to screen for myeloma.

Ultrasonography of urinary tract and plain abdominal radiography: in all patients.

Intravenous urography: in patients with adequate renal function (serum creatinine <250 µmol/L) in whom papillary necrosis or reflux nephropathy is suspected, except in diabetic patients with significant renal impairment (serum creatinine >150 µmol/L) and myeloma.

Renal biopsy: in all patients with renal impairment and normal sized, non-hydronephrotic kidneys on ultrasonography, except those in whom diagnosis is apparent from clinical features (e.g. prerenal cause of acute tubular necrosis) or previous investigations (e.g. intravenous urographic diagnosis of reflux nephropathy or papillary necrosis); renal biopsy is dangerous in patients with small kidneys – a careful history provides more reliable diagnostic clues in these.

Radiographic features and progression of analgesic nephropathy.
(Labels: Forniceal extension: calyceal 'horn'; 'Egg in cup' focal necrosis; Normal calyx; Lobster claw; Sloughed papilla: calculus; Sloughing of papilla; Late scarring overlying papilla; Ring shadow, isolation and calcification of papilla; Hypertrophy of cortical columns of Bertin.)

Complications

Acute interstitial nephritis
- The major complications are those of acute renal failure.

Chronic interstitial nephritis
- The major complications are those of chronic renal failure.

Salt wasting, renal tubular acidosis, occasionally Fanconi's syndrome.

Symptomatic anaemia inappropriate to level of renal function: in patients with analgesic nephropathy.

Differential diagnosis

Acute interstitial nephritis
Other causes of acute renal impairment, especially rapidly progressive glomerulonephritis (either idiopathic or associated with systemic vasculitis).

Chronic interstitial nephritis
All other causes of chronic renal failure.

Aetiology

Causes of acute interstitial nephritis
Drug hypersensitivity: beta lactam antibiotics (e.g. methicillin, ampicillin), other antibiotics (e.g. sulphonamides, rifampicin), NSAIDs (e.g. fenoprofen, indomethacin), diuretics (e.g. thiazides, frusemide), and other miscellaneous drugs (e.g. phenindione, phenytoin, allopurinol).

Infections: complicating urinary tract infection (especially in diabetic patients) or complicating extrarenal infection (e.g. with streptococci, legionella, brucella, leptospira, mycoplasma, toxoplasma, infectious mononucleosis, hantavirus).

Immunological disorders: interstitial lesions sometimes overshadow glomerular.

Idiopathic.

Causes of chronic interstitial nephritis
Toxic and metabolic: analgesics, lithium, cis-platinum, lead, cadmium, hypercalcaemia.

Granulomatous: sarcoidosis, tuberculosis, drugs.

Immunological: associated with primary glomerular disease, Sjögren's syndrome, transplant rejection.

Miscellaneous: reflux nephropathy, post-obstructive, myeloma, sickle cell disease, radiation nephritis, Balkan nephropathy, hereditary.

Causes of papillary necrosis
Analgesic nephropathy, sickle cell disease, diabetes mellitus, obstruction with infection, tuberculosis, cryoglobulinaemia.

Epidemiology

- The true incidence of acute interstitial nephritis is unknown.
- Renal biopsy studies suggest that it accounts for up to 8% of cases of acute renal failure; this is almost certainly an underestimate.
- 20–40% of patients being treated for end-stage renal failure have primary tubulointerstitial disease.

Treatment

Diet and lifestyle
- Patients who habitually abuse analgesics may benefit from psychological support and counselling.
- Occupational health measures have helped to limit industrial exposure to heavy metals.
- Patients with chronic renal failure have accelerated atherogenesis; smoking should be discouraged, and a diet low in saturated fat recommended.
- Patients with drug-related interstitial nephritis should be advised never to take the same or a related drug in the future.

Pharmacological treatment
- Patients may present with features of severe uraemia and need stabilization by urgent dialysis before definitive investigation and treatment can safely be carried out.

For acute interstitial nephritis
Drug-associated: withdrawal of offending drug; prednisolone 40 mg daily, with rapid tapering according to response, may hasten resolution.

Infection-associated: antibiotic treatment tailored to causative organism; steroids not indicated at least until infection is controlled.

Idiopathic disease associated with uveitis: steroids as for drug-associated disease dramatically improve renal and ocular lesions.

For chronic interstitial nephritis
Toxin-induced: withdrawal of causative agents.

Reflux nephropathy: childhood urinary tract infection must be eradicated by appropriate antibiotics; this should be followed by long-term low-dose chemoprophylaxis until reflux is resolved or renal growth complete.

Sarcoidosis: long-term steroid treatment, using minimum dose to maintain stable renal function. *See* Sarcoidosis *for details*.

Tuberculosis: antituberculous chemotherapy; concurrent use of low-dose steroids may limit renal scarring. *See* Tuberculosis, extrapulmonary *for details*.

Myeloma: referral to haematologist or oncologist recommended for institution of appropriate treatment regimen; hypovolaemia must be avoided; allopurinol to prevent acute urate nephropathy. *See* Multiple myeloma *for details*.

For analgesic nephropathy
Withdrawal of offending drugs.

Provision of psychological support.

Monitoring and treatment of the following:
Hypertension: antihypertensive agents (diuretics often inappropriate).
Salt wasting: oral slow sodium may improve glomerular filtration rate.
Renal tubular acidosis: oral sodium bicarbonate.
Inappropriate anaemia (gastrointestinal blood loss): misoprostol, iron supplements.
Early renal osteodystrophy: alpha calcidol and calcium carbonate.
Frequent urinary tract infection: prolonged treatment for upper tract infections.
Obstruction due to sloughed papillae: nephrostomy or double-J stents.
Increased incidence of urothelial tumours: regular urine cytology.
Increased atheromatous renovascular disease.

Treatment aims

Acute interstitial nephritis
To provide dialysis support if needed, pending restoration of normal renal function.

Chronic interstitial nephritis
To stabilize renal function.
To reduce rate of progression and complications of chronic renal failure.
To institute renal replacement therapy when necessary.

Prognosis

Acute interstitial nephritis
- Normal renal function is recovered in many patients by prompt treatment.

Chronic interstitial nephritis
- Withdrawal of offending toxins or specific treatment (when possible) may stabilize or improve renal function (occasionally).
- When renal damage has been severe (serum creatinine, >300 µmol/L), progression to end-stage renal disease is probable; even in chronic glomerular disease, the degree of interstitial damage is the major correlate of progression.

Follow-up and management

Acute interstitial nephritis
- When recovery of renal function is incomplete, long-term follow-up is needed.

Chronic interstitial nephritis
- Long-term follow-up is needed.
- Control of hypertension slows progression.
- Salt wasters (5–10%) need supplements of sodium chloride or bicarbonate.
- Phosphate binders (e.g. calcium carbonate) help prevent secondary hyperparathyroidism; hypercalcaemia must be avoided.
- Preparations for renal replacement therapy should be made in good time.

Key references

Cameron JS: Allergic interstitial nephritis: clinical features and pathogenesis. *QJM* 1988, **66**:97–115.

Nath KA: Tubulointerstitial changes as a major determinant in the progression of renal damage. *Am J Kidney Dis* 1992, **20**:1–17.

Stewart JH (ed): Analgesic and NSAID-induced kidney disease. In *Oxford Monographs on Clinical Nephrology* vol 2. Oxford: Oxford Medical Publications, 1993.

Polycystic kidney disease, autosomal-dominant
A. Burns

Diagnosis

Definition
- Autosomal-dominant polycystic kidney disease is a subset of renal cystic disorders in which cysts are distributed throughout the cortex and medulla of both kidneys.

Symptoms and signs
- Although the process is usually not clinically apparent until the third or fourth decade, it has been found in infants and aborted fetuses, and all carriers show evidence of disease by the eighth or ninth decade.

Abdominal pain.
Haematuria.
Polyuria or nocturia.
Hypertension.
Abdominal distension.
Nephromegaly.

Investigations
Palpation: very enlarged cystic livers and kidneys are easily palpable.
CT: most sensitive; shows multiple cysts in kidneys and occasionally liver, pancreas, and spleen.
Ultrasonography: only cysts >1 cm are detectable.
Intravenous urography: shows stretched calyces.
Radioisotope scanning: shows multiple cystic defects in isotope image.

Complications
Chronic renal failure.
Hypertension: in 50% of patients.
Cyst rupture: pain, haematuria, and intrarenal haemorrhage.
Nephrolithiasis and nephrocalcinosis: in 10–18% of patients.
Infection: within renal cysts or above obstructed ureter (gallium scan useful).
Malignant tumours: have been found.
Obstruction: clot or stone (acute on chronic renal failure).
Polycythaemia.
Distal renal tubular acidosis.

Differential diagnosis
Autosomal-recessive polycystic kidney disease.
Tuberous sclerosis.
Cystic dysplasia of kidneys.
Benign noninherited cysts.

Aetiology
Genetics
- The disease is autosomal dominant, with almost complete penetrance and variable expression.
- The spontaneous mutation rate is relatively high (20% no family history).
- 85% of cases are linked to abnormal gene on chromosome 16 (ADPKD1 locus).

Pathogenesis
- The disease probably begins *in utero*.
- Cysts are formed from proximal or distal tubules, only 1% of which are affected.
- Renal damage is caused by compression of normal kidney tissue.

Epidemiology
- The autosomal-dominant form is the most common polycystic kidney disease.
- It affects 1 in 1000 world wide.
- The male:female ratio is equal.
- 10% of patients on dialysis suffer from the disease.

Associated extrarenal conditions
Aneurysms: berry, intracranial, abdominal aortic, dissecting thoracic, aortic root, and annulus aneurysms; 6% of patients with subarachnoid haemorrhage have autosomal dominant polycystic kidney disease; 10–36% of patients with autosomal dominant polycystic kidney disease have intracranial aneurysms.
Liver cysts (in 20–50% of patients): can cause obstructive jaundice and portal hypertension (rare); not communication with biliary tree; occasionally origin of cholangiocarcinoma.
Pancreatic cysts (in 5–10%).
Cysts in other organs: ovary, uterus, spleen, thyroid, seminal vesicles, epididymis.
Valvular heart lesions: mitral incompetence, mitral valve prolapse (in 30%), tricuspid incompetence, pulmonary valve incompetence.
Diverticulosis (in 80%).
Herniae.

Treatment

Diet and lifestyle
- No special precautions are necessary in most patients; some are unusually susceptible to physical trauma.
- Genetic counselling should be offered.

Pharmacological treatment
- No specific treatment is available for the disorder, but the following can be considered:

Bed-rest and analgesia for pain.

Blood pressure control.

Treatment of acidosis if present.

Treatment of renal failure when needed.

Prolonged antibiotic treatment for upper urinary tract infection.

Non-pharmacological treatment
- Haemodialysis and peritoneal dialysis are both suitable in patients with autosomal-dominant polycystic kidney disease.
- Polycythaemia and repeated clotting of fistulae can be a problem in the haemodialysis group.
- Survival rate for these patients on dialysis is better than for patients with other renal diseases.
- Infection after renal transplantation is common; patients may require nephrectomy.

See Dialysis and Renal transplantation for details.

Treatment aims
To treat complications as they arise.
To control blood pressure.
To prepare patient for renal replacement therapy.

Prognosis
- 50% of patients progress to end-stage renal failure by the age of 75 years.

Follow-up and management
- Annual monitoring of blood pressure and renal function is needed (more frequently in patients with impaired renal function) because when or whether renal failure will develop in an individual patient generally cannot be predicted.

Key references
Chapman AB, Rubinstein D, Hughes R: Intracranial aneurysms in autosomal dominant polycystic kidney disease. *N Engl J Med* 1992, **327**:916–920.

Gabow PA: Autosomal dominant kidney polycystic kidney disease – more than a renal disease. *Am J Kidney Dis* 1990, **16**:403–413.

Gabow PA: Autosomal dominant polycystic kidney disease. *N Engl J Med* 1993, **329**:322–342.

Gabow PA: Polycystic kidney disease: clues to pathogenesis. *Kidney Int* 1991, **40**:989–996.

Milutinovic J, Rust PF, Fialkow PJ: Intra-familial phenotypic expression of autosomal dominant polycystic kidney disease. *Am J Kidney Dis* 1992, **19**:465–472.

Renal artery stenosis — J.E. Scoble

Diagnosis

Symptoms
Symptoms of hypertension.

Symptoms of associated coronary, cerebral, and peripheral vascular disease: in atherosclerotic disease.

Acute dyspnoea: in 'flash' pulmonary oedema.

Signs
Hypertension.

Epigastric or renal angle bruits.

Femoral bruits and absent leg pulses: in atherosclerotic disease.

Investigations
Plasma creatinine measurement.

Renal ultrasonography: to measure kidney size (kidneys <8 cm long seldom worth revascularization.

DTPA (diethylenetriaminepentaacetic acid) nuclear medicine scanning: paired pre- and post-captopril scans may increase sensitivity and specificity.

Renal angiography.

- Other examinations are those for atherosclerotic disease elsewhere.

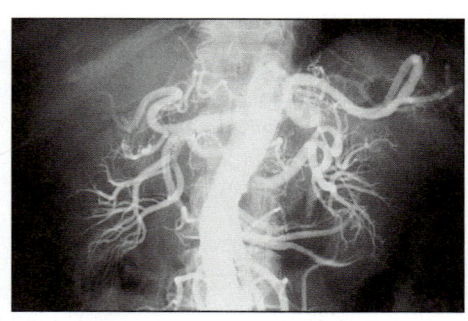

Widespread atherosclerotic disease in presence of renovascular disease, shown on angiography.

Complications
Hypertension, renal failure: in both fibromuscular and atherosclerotic forms (rare in fibromuscular dysplasia).

Differential diagnosis
Other causes of hypertension.
Other causes of renal failure.
Left ventricular dysfunction.

Aetiology
- Causes include the following:

Fibromuscular disease: medial muscular hyperplasia.

Atherosclerotic disease: as for atherosclerosis elsewhere.

Large-vessel vasculitis, e.g. Takayasu's arteritis.

Epidemiology
- Fibromuscular disease is rare (more common in younger female patients).
- Atherosclerotic disease occurrs in 30% of patients with abnormal coronary angiograms and 42% with abnormal peripheral angiograms.

Treatment

Diet and lifestyle
- Patients should take measures to alleviate atherosclerotic disease, e.g. stopping smoking, losing weight, and reducing lipids.

Pharmacological treatment
- Hypertension is treated by the usual agents (*see* Hypertension *for details*), except in the following cases:

Fibromuscular dysplasia: angiotensin-converting enzyme (ACE) inhibitors should be avoided because they may reduce renal function in kidneys with renal artery stenosis.

Atherosclerotic disease: ACE inhibitors and beta blockers should be avoided because most patients have peripheral vascular disease.

Treatment aims

To control hypertension.
To preserve renal function.
To prevent 'flash' pulmonary oedema.

Other treatments

Percutaneous angioplasty: for fibromuscular disease, with surgery if not successful.
Angioplasty or surgery: for atherosclerotic disease, depending on patient (ostial lesions usually need surgical treatment).

Prognosis

- The 5-year survival rate is 92% for fibromuscular disease and 67% for atherosclerotic disease.
- Renal artery stenosis may recur, especially after angioplasty.

Follow-up and management

- Blood pressure and plasma creatinine measurement and DTPA scans should be repeated, with re-angiography, if restenosis is possible.

Key references

Conolly JO *et al.*: Presentation, clinical features and outcome in different patterns of atherosclerotic renovascular disease. *Am J Med* 1994, **87**:413–421.

Stansby G, Hamilton G, Scoble JE: Atherosclerotic renal artery stenosis. Br J Hosp Med 1993, **49**:388–395.

Renal failure, acute
P. Sweny

Diagnosis

Symptoms
- The clinical features are usually dominated by those of the primary condition.

Nausea, vomiting, pruritus, malaise, lethargy, fits, coma: features of uraemia; develop if diagnosis unduly delayed.

Signs
Oliguria: <400 ml urine daily; classic but not universal sign.
Oedema.

Investigations
- Priorities are the detection and documentation of possibly life-threatening complications, exclusion of prerenal and postrenal factors, diagnosis of intrinsic renal disease, distinction of acute from chronic renal failure, and monitoring of response to treatment.

Central venous pressure monitoring and pulmonary capillary wedge pressure measurement: using Swan–Ganz catheter, if in any doubt about prerenal factors.
Chest radiography: for fluid overload.
Cardiac output and systemic vascular resistance measurement: can be helpful in infected patients.
ECG, echocardiography: to exclude prerenal factors.
Ultrasonography, plain abdominal radiography: to exclude postrenal factors.
Urine sodium and osmolality: can identify prerenal acute renal failure.
Urine microscopy: using a phase contrast microscope, for dysmorphic erythrocytes, erythrocyte casts, other casts to diagnose intrinsic renal disease.
Serology: for glomerulonephritis and vasculitis.
Creatine kinase and hydroxybutyrate dehydrogenase measurement: for rhabdomyolysis and haemolysis.
Calcium measurement: for metastatic bone deposits, iatrogenic, hypercalcaemia.
Blood film: for fragments and platelet count, to detect microangiopathic haemolytic anaemia.
Blood cultures: for sepsis.
Coagulation tests, fibrinogen and fibrin degradation products analysis: for disseminated intravascular coagulation.
Liver function tests: for hepato–renal syndrome.
Renal biopsy: possibly indicated in patients with renal acute renal failure when the insult is not sufficient to have caused acute tubular necrosis.
Ultrasonography, alkaline phosphatase measurement, bone radiography: for kidney size, evidence of metabolic bone disease, and anaemia, respectively, to distinguish acute from chronic renal failure.
Immunoglobulin and protein electrophoresis: for myeloma in elderly patients.

Complications
Sepsis, adult respiratory distress syndrome (non-cardiogenic pulmonary oedema): usually seen in patients with multiple organ failure.
Gastrointestinal haemorrhage: caused by gastric stress ulceration.
Bleeding: uraemic platelet–endothelial dysfunction and sepsis lead to a bleeding diathesis.
Superadded infections, poor wound healing, muscle wasting: due to hypercatabolic state associated with uraemia and infection.
Hypertension: often related to fluid overload, sometimes to primary renal disease.
Hypotension: often related to sepsis, occasionally to occult myocardial ischaemia.
Hyperkalaemia: especially in presence of acidosis and tissue breakdown.

Differential diagnosis
Prerenal: inadequate perfusion of otherwise normal kidneys.
Intrinsic renal disease: process within kidney substance.
Postrenal: blockage to flow of urine from otherwise normal kidneys.

Aetiology
- Aetiology is often complex, with more than one mechanism at play. Causes include the following:

Prerenal
Shock (hypovolaemia, inadequate cardiac output, lack of peripheral resistance – sepsis, anaphylaxis).
Hepatorenal syndrome.
Angiotensin-converting enzyme inhibitors.

Renal
Acute tubular necrosis: ischaemia, toxins (e.g. aminoglycosides, paracetamol, calcium).
Acute glomerulonephritis.
Acute interstitial nephritis: e.g. NSAIDs, antibiotics (sulphonamides, penicillins), infection (leptospirosis, Legionnaires disease).
Thrombotic microangiopathies: e.g. haemolytic uraemic syndrome, thrombotic thrombocytopenic purpura, related conditions (e.g. scleroderma renal crisis, accelerated-phase hypertension, pre-eclampsia, acute fatty liver of pregnancy, postpartum acute renal failure).
Vascular catastrophes: renal-vein thrombosis, renal-artery embolus or thrombosis, dissection of aorta, cholesterol emboli.
Pigment nephropathy: rhabdomyolysis, intravascular haemolysis.
Multiple myeloma: light-chain nephropathy.
Infection: bilateral pyelonephritis.

Postrenal
Intrarenal obstruction: urate, drugs, haemoglobin, myoglobin, light chains.
Extrarenal obstruction: stones, tumours, blood clots, bladder outflow, retroperitoneal fibrosis.

Epidemiology
- ~50 people in one million annually develop acute renal failure needing dialysis.
- Most acute renal failure develops in the context of other acute illnesses.

Treatment

Diet and lifestyle
- Acute renal failure is a medical emergency, usually occurring in hospital; diet is modified to supply sufficient energy while minimizing accumulation of toxins (protein 40–60 g, sodium 40–60 mmol, potassium 40–60 mmol daily).

Pharmacological treatment

For acute tubular necrosis
Resuscitation.

Maximization of perfusion of vital organs and exclusion of obstruction.

Diuretics only after restoration of euvolaemia and maximization of cardiac output: escalating doses of a loop diuretic (bumetanide 2–5 mg i.v. every 4–6 h depending on urine flow rate) and dopamine (2.5–5 μg/kg/min) may restore urine flow; contraindicated in presence of obstruction, before hypovolaemia is corrected, or if risk of cardiac arrhythmia.

Prompt identification and vigorous treatment of infection: culture of available body fluids, repeated frequently; regular change of venous lines; CRP monitoring and leucocyte count.

Control of acidosis and hyperkalaemia.

Enteral feeding, total parenteral nutrition if necessary; fluid balance must be controlled before feeding.

Haematological support: haemoglobin should be kept at ~10 g/dl and albumin maintained by i.v. human albumin solutions.

H_2 blockers to prevent gastric stress ulceration.

For focal necrotizing and crescentic glomerulonephritis
Steroids, cyclophosphamide, and possibly plasma exchange.

For acute interstitial nephritis
Withdrawal of offending drugs, possibly steroids.

For infection
High-dose prolonged course of appropriate antibiotic (at least 4–6 weeks).

For haemolytic uraemic syndrome and thrombotic thrombocytopenic purpura
Plasma exchange with fresh frozen plasma and possible prostacyclin infusion (see Haemolytic uraemic syndrome for details).

For pigment nephropathy, myeloma kidney
Forced alkaline diuresis: N saline 500 ml alternating with 1.26% sodium bicarbonate solution 500 ml every 4 h; bumetanide 1–5 mg i.v. 8-hourly to maintain urine flow rate ≥100 ml/h; contraindicated in oliguria unresponsive to volume repletion and diuretics.

Treatment aims
To prevent development of acute tubular necrosis (vigorous resuscitation).
To relieve obstruction and prevent progressive renal damage.
To identify primary treatable renal disease.
To replace renal function.

Other treatments
- Acute tubular necrosis can be treated by renal replacement therapy, as follows:
Continuous arteriovenous or pumped continuous venovenous haemodiafiltration: preferred for immobile or intensive-care patients.
Intermittent haemodialysis (alternate-day): for mobile or general-ward patients.

Prognosis
- In acute tubular necrosis, the prognosis depends roughly on the number of additional organs that are failing, as follows: no other organs, survival is >80%; +1 organ (e.g. ventilation), 40–50%; +2 organs (e.g. ventilation, inotropes), <20%; +3 organs (e.g. ventilation, inotropes, total parenteral nutrition), <10%; +4 organs (e.g. ventilation, inotropes, total parenteral nutrition, liver), <5%.
- Many patients with acute tubular necrosis have near-complete recovery of renal function and do not develop chronic renal disease.
- Some patients make only a partial recovery, which may indicate that necrosis was cortical rather than acute tubular; these patients may recover renal function for some months or years before developing hypertension and progressive chronic renal failure.

Follow-up and management
- Long-term follow-up is recommended in patients with persistent hypertension, impaired renal function, haematuria, or proteinuria.

Key references
Bihari D, Neild G (eds): *Acute Renal Failure in the Intensive Therapy Unit.* Berlin: Springer-Verlag, 1990.

Rainford D, Sweny P (eds): *Acute Renal Failure.* London: Farrand Press, 1990.

Sweny P: Haemofiltration and haemodiafiltration: theoretical and practical aspects. *Curr Anaesth Crit Care* 1991, **2**:37–43.

Renal failure, chronic — A. Burns

Diagnosis

Definition
- Irreversible renal impairment is most often recognised by persistently high urea and creatinine concentrations; it often progresses to end-stage renal failure.

Mild: glomerular filtration rate (GFR) 20–50 ml/min; creatinine 150–300 µmol/L.
Moderate: GFR 10–20 ml/min; creatinine 300–700 µmol/L.
Severe: GFR <10 ml/min; creatinine >700 µmol/L.

Symptoms
Puritus, malaise, nausea, anorexia: early nonspecific symptoms.
Drowsiness, fits, coma, blunting of intellect, diarrhoea: late nonspecific symptoms.
Symptoms of underlying disease.

Signs
Anaemia.
Hypertension.
Leuconychia.
Brown line at distal end of nail.
Pigmentation.
Scratch marks.
Red eyes: high calcium X phosphate product.
Oedema.
Peripheral neuropathy: sensory.
Proximal myopathy: severe metabolic bone disease.
Kussmaul's respiration.
Pericarditis: causing tamponade.

Investigations
Serum electrolytes, urea, creatinine, creatinine clearance, 24-h urinary protein measurement.
Plain radiography of abdomen: to detect calculi and nephrocalcinosis.
Ultrasonography of kidneys: to measure size and exclude obstruction.
Intravenous urography: to delineate calyces and ureters and to show kidney size and any loss of renal cortex (only of value in mild chronic renal failure).
Kidney biopsy: for changes specific to underlying disease; contraindicated for small kidneys.
Immunoglobulin electrophoresis, Bence-Jones protein measurement: to diagnose multiple myeloma in elderly patients.
Radioisotope studies: captopril renography if renal artery stenosis suspected.

Complications
Anaemia.
Renal osteodystrophy.
Hypertension.
Puritus.
Peripheral neuropathy.
Pericarditis.
Acute on chronic renal failure: precipitated by hypovolaemia, hypertension, infection, toxic agents, overzealous control of blood pressure.
Accelerated atherosclerosis: increased risk of stroke, heart attack, and peripheral vascular disease.

Differential diagnosis
Acute renal failure: short history, examination shows features of underlying disease, normal haemoglobin, no evidence of renal osteodystrophy, normal or enlarged kidneys.

Aetiology
- The cause varies depending on the patient's age; the following may have a role:

Chronic glomerulonephritis in 28% of patients.
Chronic pyelonephritis (reflux nephropathy) in 17%.
Uncertain cause in 13%.
Amyloid, papillary necrosis in 11%.
Diabetes mellitus in 16%.
Polycystic kidney disease in 10%.
Renovascular disease in 8%.
Drugs in 2.5%.
Hypertension.
Chronic interstitial nephritis.
Hereditary nephritis.
In elderly patients: multiple myeloma, atherosclerotic renal artery stenosis, obstruction, and amyloid.
In children: congenital absence or dysplasia, obstruction: posterior urethral valves, juvenile nephronophthisis (cystic disease).
Family or previous history of renal disease (e.g. childhood urinary tract infection).

Epidemiology
- The incidence of chronic renal failure is difficult to estimate accurately.
- >60 in one million population each year are accepted for renal replacement in Europe.
- In the USA, >1 in 100 000 population each year develop end-stage chronic renal failure.

Progression
- Although chronic renal failure often progresses to end-stage renal failure, function may not deteriorate quickly and, in some patients, remains stable, although significantly impaired, for several years.
- Measurement of serum creatinine is the most useful clinical test in assessing progression (serum creatinine is related to muscle mass and renal function).
- Serum creatinine rises exponentially with deteriorating renal function.
- At least 50% of renal function is lost before serum creatinine begins to rise.
- Plotting reciprocal serum creatinine values against time is a useful indicator of progression of renal failure.

Renal failure, chronic
A. Burns

Treatment

Diet and lifestyle
- Patients should eat a high-energy diet, with potassium restriction and protein intake restricted to 0.5–0.75 g/kg body weight daily; in later stages of chronic renal failure, decreased protein intake can help to control symptoms of nausea, vomiting, and anorexia.
- Phosphate intake should be restricted, and absorption reduced by phosphate binders (calcium carbonate or aluminium hydroxide).
- Vitamin D supplementation is needed, using 1-hydroxylated preparations.

Pharmacological treatment
- Specific treatment is directed at the underlying cause.
- Nephrotoxic drugs and NSAIDs must be avoided, and doses of other drugs must be adjusted for the degree of renal failure.
- Angiotensin-converting enzyme inhibitors may help to control blood pressure, particularly in diabetic patients; diastolic pressure should be <90 mmHg. Care is needed with these agents when renal artery stenosis is suspected.
- Erythropoietin can be used to treat anaemia and improve well-being.
- Progression to end-stage chronic renal failure can be slowed by some or all of the following:

Obsessional control of systemic hypertension.

Reduction of glomerular blood pressure, using angiotensin-converting enzyme inhibitors.

Low-protein diets (in some patients).

Addressing the risk factors for accelerated atherosclerosis.

Non-pharmacological treatment
- Haemodialysis or peritoneal dialysis can be used (see Dialysis for details).

Treatment aims
To delay progression to end-stage renal failure.
To prevent renal bone disease.
To control hypertension.
To prevent acute on chronic renal failure (e.g. by avoiding urinary tract infection, correcting obstruction).

Prognosis
- Timely dialysis or transplantation greatly prolongs life.
- Extrarenal complications of multisystem diseases may limit survival.

Follow-up and management
- After chronic renal failure has been diagnosed, progress must be monitored at regular intervals; important parameters include the following:

Weight (for nutrition and fluid status).
Blood pressure (obsessional control may retard progression).
Urea (may alter with increased catabolism or protein intake).
Creatinine.
Haemoglobin.
Serum calcium (iatrogenic hypercalcaemia must be avoided: calcium is nephrotoxic).
Serum phosphate.
Serum alkaline phosphatase.
Albumin (particularly helpful in assessing nutrition).

Key references
El Nahas M, Mallick NP, Anderson S: *Prevention of Progressive Chronic Renal Failure*. Oxford: Oxford University Press, 1993.

Knan IH et al.: Chronic renal failure: factors influencing nephrology referral. *QJM* 1994, **87**:559–564.

Mogensen CE: Captopril delays progression to overt renal disease in insulin-dependent diabetes mellitus patients with microalbuminuria. *J Am Soc Nephrol* 1992, **3**:336.

Perneger TV, Whetton PK, Klag MJ: Risk of kidney failure associated with the use of acetaminophen, aspirin, and non-steroidal antiinflammatory drugs. *N Engl J Med* 1994, **331**:1675–1679.

Renal transplantation — R.H.H. Lord

Selection

Patient criteria
- Factors to check for include the following:

Age: biological age more important than chronological age, usual upper limit is 65–75 years.

Cancer: must be excluded.

Infection: i.e. Staghorn calculi, tuberculosis, bronchiectasis, HIV must be excluded.

Cardiovascular status: angina detected by stress test or coronary angiography; intermittent claudication detected by duplex doppler or digital vascular imaging; myocardial infarction remains the most common cause of death after transplantation; presence of peripheral vascular disease may compromise leg perfusion after transplantation.

Bladder function: positive urological history obtained by flow rate and residual bladder ultrasonography or video cystometrography, possibly with cystoscopy; bladder outflow tract obstruction may compromise graft function.

Donor criteria
- The criteria have been relaxed over the past 10 years because of a shortage of donors. Sepsis is no longer a contraindication if the organism is cultured. Diabetic donors may be considered, but frozen section of the kidney is needed before transplantation.

Age 2–75 years.

Absence of chronic renal disease.

Hepatitis B virus, HIV, and Hepatitis C virus negative.

No malignancies: except primary brain tumours.

- Live-related donors should always be sought: parents can only be a haplotype match (50%), but siblings can be HLA-identical (100%), a haplotype match (50%), or a complete mismatch (0%).

Matching

Tissue typing
HLA on chromosome 6. Class I = A and B, class II = DR.

- 1A, 1B, 1DR antigen is inherited from each patient.
- For matching, the importance is as follows: DR > B > A; i.e. 1A, 2B, 2DR match is better than 2A, 1B, 2DR match.

Direct cross match
- If donor lymphocytes combined with the patient's serum cause lymphocyte death, a positive cross match is implied, and the kidney is unsuitable.
- Highly sensitized patients have high levels of anti-HLA antibodies; this may be secondary to blood transfusion or pregnancies; the incidence of positive cross matches is increased.

Epidemiology
- 50% of patients on renal failure programmes are unsuitable for transplantation because of age or coexisting diseases (i.e. severe cardiovascular disease, cancer).
- 4800 people are on the UK kidney transplant waiting list (increasing every year).
- ~1200 kidney transplantations are done each year in the UK (static for past 6 years).
- Only 4–10% of transplants are taken from live-related donors in the UK.

Transplantation or dialysis?
Advantages of transplantation
Improved quality of life.
No dialysis.
Correction of anaemia.
Normal diet and fluid allowance.
Improved bone metabolism (however, increased osteoporosis from steroids).
Increased ease of travel.
Women of child-bearing age able to have children.
Cheaper.

Disadvantages of transplantation
Emotional stress.
Surgical and anaesthetic donor risks.

Approximate costs
Haemodialysis: £20 000/year.
Transplantation: £19 000 in the first year, £3500 in subsequent years.

Advantages of live-related donors
Improved graft survival.
Planned operation.
Shorter wait.
Lower incidence of postoperative acute tubular necrosis.
Usually, less rejection.

Treatment

Rejection

Clinical findings
Tenderness over graft.

Pyrexia.

Decreased urine output.

Fluid retention.

Hypertension.

Occasionally silent.

Investigation of graft dysfunction
Urine analysis: midstream urine, proteinuria, cytology.

Blood analysis: increased urea, creatinine, potassium, leucocyte count, interleukin 2R, cyclosporin A concentration, blood cultures.

Ultrasonography: to exclude obstruction, possibly to diagnose rejection.

Renal isotope scans: show decreased perfusion.

Renal biopsy: open, tru-cut, or needle aspiration.

Differential diagnosis
Acute tubular necrosis: 20–50% of grafts have primary nonfunction lasting 1–2 weeks.

Cyclosporin A toxicity.

Graft pyelonephritis.

Ureteric obstruction.

Renal artery stenosis.

Cytomegalovirus.

Histological features
Acute cellular rejection: lymphocyte infiltrate, macrophages, natural killer cells.

Acute vascular rejection: as above, with fibrinoid necrosis and infiltration of vessel walls.

Chronic rejection: fibrosis, chronic vascular changes (intimal proliferation) leading to vascular occlusion.

Treatment
Hyperacute rejection: extremely rare, usually due to error in tissue typing, no treatment.

Simple acute cellular rejection: pulse methylprednisolone.

Steroid-resistant cellular rejection and vascular rejection: antithymocyte globulin, antilymphocyte globulin, OKT3.

Chronic rejection: no effective treatment.

Immunosuppression

Agents
Combinations of prednisolone, azathioprine, cyclosporin A, and monoclonal and polyclonal antibodies.

New immunosuppressive drugs: rapamycin, tacrolimus, mycophenolate mofetil.

Side effects
All immunosuppressants: increased incidence of tumours (skin, reticuloendothelial system) and infection (e.g. opportunistic infections, cytomegalovirus).

Azathioprine: bone-marrow suppression (leucocytes, haemoglobin, platelets), hepatotoxicity.

Steroids: cushingoid facies, buffalo hump, central obesity, striae, thinning of skin, bruising, proximal myopathy, acne vulgaris, hirsuitism, osteoporosis, aseptic necrosis of the hips, diabetes, hyperlipidaemia.

Cyclosporin A: hirsuitism, tremor, gum hyperplasia, nephro-, neuro-, or hepatotoxicity.

OKT3 (anti-T-cell monoclonal antibody): first-dose effect (acute pulmonary oedema), increased incidence of lymphoproliferative disorders.

Cadaveric kidney storage
- The kidney should be perfused with buffered ice-cold fluid of high osmolarity.
- It should then be wrapped in two sterile bags and stored on crushed ice for up to 48 h.
- Prolonged storage times can be achieved using perfusion machines (expensive and rarely used in the UK).

Blood transfusion and transplantation
- Transfusion increases patient sensitization.
- The beneficial effect on transplantation outcome is less clear since the introduction of cyclosporin A.

Surgical complications
Early
Haemorrhage, renal vein and renal artery thrombosis, urinary leak.

Late
Renal artery stenosis, ureteric stenosis, ureteric reflux.

Prognosis
- 1-year kidney graft survival rates are 95% (live) and 70–90% (cadaveric); a few units achieve rates >90%.
- Most grafts are lost in the first 3 months.
- After the first year, ~4% of grafts are lost annually (mainly due to chronic rejection).

Follow-up and management
- Regular outpatient visits are needed (3 times weekly initially, decreasing to once a fortnight monthly and eventually once every 4 months).
- A 20% rise in creatinine is investigated initially with ultrasonography and biopsy.

Key references
Braun WE, Marwick TH: Coronary artery disease in renal transplant recipients. *Cleve Clin J Med* 1994, **61**:370–385.

Suthanthiran M, Strom TB: Renal transplantation. *N Engl J Med* 1994, **331**:365–376.

Renal tubular acidosis   J.E. Scoble

Diagnosis

Definition
- Renal tubular acidosis is a disorder of renal hydrogen secretion or bicarbonate reabsorption.
- The following subtypes have been defined:

Type 1 (distal): defect in distal hydrogen secretion, probably related to defect in hydrogen ATPase.

Type 2 (proximal): decreased proximal bicarbonate reabsorption, probably a defect in brush border sodium–hydrogen exchanger.

Type 3 (proximal and distal): described in older textbooks but does not exist.

Type 4 (hyporeninaemic hypoaldosteronism): decreased distal acidification due to aldosterone lack and decreased distal sodium reabsorption.

Symptoms
- Renal tubular acidosis has no specific symptoms.

Weakness, musculoskeletal pains, low back pain: in type 1 disease.

Failure to thrive: in children in type 2 disease; often associated with Fanconi syndrome and symptoms including bone pain from osteomalacia.

Symptoms of diabetes mellitus: in type 4 disease (frequent association).

Signs
- These are rare.

Weakness leading to paralysis: in type 1 disease.

Signs of diabetes mellitus: in type 4 disease.

Investigations
- The diagnosis of renal tubular acidosis is indicated by a hyperchloraemic metabolic acidosis defined from blood gas analysis with a normal plasma anion gap (*see box*), defined by $(Na^+ + K^+) - (Cl^- + HCO_3^-)$; this differentiates it from an increased anion gap acidosis such as in lactic acidosis.

Plasma potassium analysis: to detect hypokalaemia in patients with type 1 disease.

Short ammonium chloride loading test: if urine pH >6.0 to diagnose type 1 disease.

Sodium bicarbonate loading test: if urine pH <6.0 to diagnose type 2 disease.

Plain abdominal radiography: in type 1 disease, to look for nephrocalcinosis.

Parathyroid hormone measurement: to detect primary hyperparathyroidism.

Complications
- These can be renal as in type 1 disease or general complications of the underlying disease as in type 4 disease.

Nephrocalcinosis and nephrolithiasis: in type 1 disease.

Diabetes mellitus leading to renal failure from diabetic nephropathy: most common complication related to underlying disease in type 4 disease.

Differential diagnosis

Type 1 with nephrocalcinosis
Medullary sponge kidney, idiopathic hypercalciuria, hyperparathyroidism.

- Purgative abuse can lead to a hyperchloraemic acidosis with an abnormal short ammonium chloride loading test; this can be differentiated by the urinary ammonium excretion, which is normal in these patients but low in patients with type 1 disease.

Aetiology

Causes of Type 1 disease
Idiopathic, Sjögren's syndrome, SLE, primary biliary cirrhosis, amphotericin.

Causes of Type 2 disease
Idiopathic, cystinosis, Fanconi's syndrome, Wilson's disease, primary hyperparathyroidism, acetazolamide.

Causes of Type 4 disease
Diabetes mellitus (most important in clinical practice), urinary obstruction, sickle cell disease; mimicked by potassium-sparing diuretics.

Epidemiology
- Types 1 and 2 are rare; type 4 occurs relatively frequently.

Causes of normal anion gap acidosis
Failure of renal acidification due to renal tubular acidosis or acetazolamide.

Gastrointestinal loss of bicarbonate due to diarrhoea, purgative abuse, pancreatic fistula, ureteric diversion (e.g. ureterosigmoidostomy).

Ingestion of acid (e.g. hydrochloric).

Parenteral nutrition.

Treatment

Diet and lifestyle
- No special precautions are necessary.

Pharmacological treatment

For types 1 and 2 disease
- Patients should be given oral sodium bicarbonate up to 1–2 mmol/kg (type 1) or 3–5 mmol/kg (type 2) daily, titrated to improve acidosis.
- Potassium and, in type 2 disease, vitamin D supplements may also be needed.
- Acidosis can never be completely corrected by oral supplements.

For type 4 disease
- Fludrocortisone or loop diuretics with sodium bicarbonate are indicated.
- Potassium-sparing diuretics, NSAIDS, or angiotensin-converting enzyme inhibitors, which worsen hyperkalaemia, must be avoided.

Standard dosage	Fludrocortisone 100–400 µg daily. Bumetanide 1–5 mg and sodium bicarbonate up to 4 g daily.
Contraindications	*Fludrocortisone*: volume overload. *Bumetanide*: volume depletion. *Sodium bicarbonate:* volume overload.
Main drug interactions	None.
Main side effects	Fluid overload if inadequate diuretic given with sodium bicarbonate.

Treatment aims
To prevent nephrocalcinosis and nephrolithiasis in type 1 disease.

To treat bone disease with vitamin D if deficiency present in type 2 disease.

To avoid life-threatening hyperkalaemia caused by concomitant medication in type 4 disease.

Prognosis
- Type 1 disease can progress to renal failure (not usual).
- The prognosis for types 2 and 4 disease depends on the associated conditions.

Follow up and management
- Acidosis and, in type 1 disease, nephrocalcinosis and nephrolithiasis must be monitored.

Key references
Battle DC *et al.*: The use of the urinary anion gap in the diagnosis of hyperchloremic acidosis. *N Engl J Med* 1988, **318**:594–599.

Kurtzman NA: Disorders of distal acidification. *Kidney Int* 1990, **38**:720–727.

Maher ER, Scoble JE: Renal tubular acidosis. *Br J Hosp Med* 1989, **42**:116–119.

Urinary tract infection — K. Farrington

Diagnosis

Symptoms and signs

Lower urinary tract infection

Irritative voiding dysfunction, suprapubic tenderness: indicating cystitis.

Fever, perineal pain, irritative and obstructive voiding dysfunction, tenderness: indicating acute prostatitis.

Relapsing infection, voiding dysfunction, abdominal or back pain: indicating chronic prostatitis.

Upper urinary tract infection

Fever, chills, prostration, back or flank pain and tenderness, irritative voiding dysfunction: indicating acute pyelonephritis.

Fever and chills, flank pain and tenderness, flank or abdominal mass, irritative voiding dysfunction: indicating renal abscesses.

Symptomatic bacteraemia of urinary tract origin: clinical features of bacteraemia often overshadow those relating to urinary tract.

Investigations

To establish presence of infection

Urine culture: >10^2 colony-forming units (CFU) coliforms/ml or >10^5 CFU non-coliforms/ml in symptomatic women, 10^3 CFU bacteria/ml in symptomatic men, >10^5 CFU bacteria/ml in asymptomatic patients on two consecutive specimens, >10^2 CFU bacteria/ml in catheterized patients, any growth of bacteria from a suprapubic aspirate in symptomatic patients.

Urine microscopy: pyuria (>10 leucocytes/ml unspun urine) supportive evidence of urinary tract infection but not specific; pus cells in 'sterile' urine (sterile pyuria) may indicate fastidious organisms or previous antibiotic treatment; microscopic haematuria in 50% of patients.

Dipstick testing of urine: combined leucocyte esterase and nitrite test useful screening procedure, with negative predictive value of 96–97% at level of 10^5 CFU/ml.

To establish site of infection

- Whether infection is confined to the lower tract or has ascended to the upper tract has important treatment implications; the distinction is usually made clinically.

Fairley bladder washout technique and antibody-coated bacteria assays: show occult renal involvement in up to 30% of clinically judged lower urinary tract infection.

Radiography

- Radiography is used to identify structural abnormalities of urinary tract, including reflux nephropathy, obstruction, calculi, congenital abnormalities, and, in children, vesicoureteric reflux.

- It is indicated in children and men in first infection and in women with recurrent infections, upper urinary tract infection, unusual infecting organism, fever persisting >48 h after starting treatment, coexistent hypertension, or persistent microscopic haematuria.

Intravenous urography: investigation of choice in adults (usually delayed until after recovery); ultrasonography may be substituted or added in the case of renal impairment or when renal abscess or pelvic disease is suspected.

^{99m}Tc-DMSA (dimercaptosuccinic acid) scan: aids detection of scars if intravenous urography is doubtful.

^{99m}Tc-DMSA scan and ultrasonography: with either voiding cystourethrography or radionucleide cystography; investigation of choice in children.

Complications

Reflux nephropathy: cortical scarring and clubbing of underlying calyces in infants with bacteriuria associated with vesicoureteric reflux.

Renal damage, perinephric abscess formation, septicaemia: due to infection in presence of complicating factors (e.g. obstruction, stones, vesicoureteric reflux).

Differential diagnosis

Urethritis: chlamydia, gonorrhoea, herpes virus.

Vaginitis: bacteria, trichomonas, yeasts.

Perineal lesions: herpes virus, other sexually transmitted diseases, dermatological conditions, physical or chemical irritants.

Aetiology

- The common uropathogens are normal constituents of the colonic flora.
- *Escherichia coli* accounts for 85% of community-acquired urinary tract infection.
- Catheterization, instrumentation, cross infection, and selection of resistant bowel and environmental flora account for the different microbiological spectrum of hospital-acquired urinary tract infection.
- Almost always, infection is due to ascent of microorganisms through the urethra from the colonized perineum.

Epidemiology

- 3.7% of boys and 2% of girls in the first year of life have bacteriuria.
- 4–7% of pregnant women have bacteriuria, compared with 1–3% of young, non-pregnant women.
- Urinary tract infection is rare in young men except in practising homosexuals.
- 10–20% of elderly people living at home and up to 50% of institutionalized elderly people have bacteriuria.

Complicated or uncomplicated infection

- This distinction is useful for directing treatment.
- The following suggest occult renal involvement in apparent lower urinary tract infection or the presence of complicated urinary tract infection:

Male sex.
History of childhood urinary tract infection.
Symptoms for >7 days at presentation.
Recent antibiotic use.
Pregnancy.
Institutionalization: in elderly patients.
Recent instrumentation.
Indwelling catheter.
Underlying urinary tract abnormality.
Diabetes.
Immunosuppression.

Treatment

Diet and lifestyle
- A high fluid intake may help to alleviate dysuria during an acute episode; in the long term, it may be useful prophylactically.
- In women, post-coital voiding may be helpful; those using diaphragms and spermicides may benefit from changing to alternative contraceptive methods.

Pharmacological treatment

Indications
For lower urinary tract infections (uncomplicated): 3–5 day courses of trimethoprim, co-trimoxazole, nitrofurantoin, or co-amoxiclav; as effective as 7–14 day course; result in fewer relapses than single-dose treatment.

For lower urinary tract infections (complicated): chemotherapy as above continued for 7–14 days; short courses not suitable.

In pregnant women: 7–10 day course of amoxycillin, cephalexin, or nitrofurantoin; early screening and treatment of asymptomatic bacteriuria.

In men with prostatitis: trimethoprim, co-trimoxazole, or a quinolone for 4 weeks (longer for chronic prostatitis); non-bacterial prostatitis may respond to doxycycline or erythromycin.

For upper urinary tract infections (uncomplicated): severity of constitutional upset determines need for hospitalization.

In patients treated at home: oral trimethoprim, co-trimoxazole, co-amoxiclav, or quinolone for 14 days.

In hospitalized patients: initially, i.v. cefuroxime, cefotaxime, ciprofloxacin, co-amoxiclav, or co-trimoxazole; when fever subsides, oral treatment dictated by culture, continued for 14 days; relapses treated for 6 weeks.

For upper urinary tract infection (complicated):

In previously instrumented or catheterized patients: initially i.v. ceftazidime or amoxycillin with ciprofloxacin or gentamicin.

In patients with obstructed, infected upper tract: chemotherapy as above, with prompt drainage by percutaneous nephrostomy pending definitive surgery.

In patients with renal abscess: chemotherapy as above, with i.v. flucloxacillin, then 4–6 week courses of antibiotics based on cultures; percutaneous drainage usually needed.

Selected regimens
Amoxycillin 500 mg orally 3 times daily.
Cefotaxime 1 g i.v. 3 times daily.
Ceftazidime 1–2 g i.v. twice daily.
Cefuroxime 750 mg i.v. 3 times daily.
Cephalexin 500 mg orally 4 times daily.
Ciprofloxacin 500 mg orally or 200 mg i.v. twice daily.
Co-amoxiclav 750 mg orally or 1.2 g i.v. 3 times daily.
Co-trimoxazole 960 mg orally or i.v. twice daily.
Flucloxacillin 500 mg i.v. 4 times daily.
Gentamicin 80 mg i.v. 3 times daily.
Nitrofurantoin 100 mg orally 4 times daily.
Trimethoprim 200 mg orally twice daily.

Antibiotics: contraindications and side effects
Chronic renal failure: nitrofurantoin ineffective, causes neuropathy; tetracyclines worsen uraemia; aminoglycosides can be used but concentrations must be monitored; cause nephrotoxicity and auditory/vestibular toxicity.

Pregnancy: tetracyclines cause bone or teeth dystrophy; trimethoprim possibly teratogenic; quinolones possibly cause arthropathy; aminoglycosides cause auditory/vestibular toxicity.

Infancy: tetracyclines cause bone or teeth dystrophy; sulphonamides cause haemolysis.

Prophylaxis
- Post-coital or nightly: trimethoprim 100 mg, nitrofurantoin 100 mg, or cotrimoxazole 480 mg reduces recurrence in women with normal urinary tracts.
- Prophylaxis is also useful after acute pyelonephritis in pregnancy.

Treatment aims
To relieve symptoms.
To prevent increase in prematurity and perinatal mortality.
To prevent and eradicate life-threatening systemic sepsis.
To prevent progressive renal damage.

Prognosis
- Renal impairment in reflux nephropathy may progress without persisting infection and reflux.
- Adults with uncomplicated infection suffer minimal long-term sequelae if adequately treated.
- Complicated upper tract infections are potentially more damaging and may cause progressive renal scarring.

Follow-up and management
- Follow-up urine cultures are essential in pregnancy, after uncomplicated acute pyelonephritis, and after all complicated urinary tract infections.
- Any predisposing factors should be treated.
- Obstruction must be relieved by surgery or intermittent self-catheterization when indicated; calculi must be removed.

Recurrent infection

Relapse
- Relapse occurs soon after cessation of treatment.
- The same organism is involved.
- Relapse indicates inappropriate drug or duration of treatment, poor compliance, occult renal involvement, or underlying urinary tract abnormality.

Reinfection
- Reinfection occurs >6 weeks after cessation of treatment.
- A different organism is involved.
- Reinfection indicates failure of host defences.

Key references
Hooton TM, Stamm WE: Management of acute uncomplicated urinary tract infection in adults. *Med Clin North Am* 1991, **75**:339–357.

White RHR: Management of urinary tract infection and vesicoureteric reflux in children. *BMJ* 1990, **300**:1391–1392.

Wilkie ME *et al.*: Diagnosis and management of urinary tract infection in adults. *BMJ* 1992, **305**:1137–1141.

Index

A

abscess, perinephric 26
ACE inhibitors *see* angiotensin-converting enzyme inhibitors
acidosis, renal tubular 12, 14, 24
albumin, human, for hyponatraemia 11
albuterol *see* salbutamol
alphacalcidol for analgesic nephropathy 13
aluminium hydroxide for chronic renal failure 21
amoxycillin for urinary tract infection 27
amyloidosis 4, 20
anaemia 12
    haemolytic 6
analgesics for autosomal-dominant polycystic kidney disease 15
aneurysm 14
angiitis *see* vasculitis
angioplasty, percutaneous, for fibromuscular disease 17
angiotensin-converting enzyme inhibitors
    for chronic renal failure 21
    for renal artery stenosis 17
    for renal tubular acidosis 25
anodynes *see* analgesics
antibiotics
    for acute interstitial nephritis 13
    for autosomal-dominant polycystic kidney disease 15
    for infections in acute renal failure 19
antibodies for immunosuppression in renal transplantation 23
antihypertensive agents for analgesic nephropathy 13
anti-inflammatory drugs, nonsteroidal *see* NSAIDs
antimicrobial agents *see* antibiotics
antinociceptive agents *see* analgesics
antiplatelet drugs for haemolytic uraemic syndrome 7
antirheumatic agents *see* NSAIDs
ARDS *see* respiratory distress, adult
arrhythmia 8
arthralgia 12
ascites 4
aspirin for haemolytic uraemic syndrome 7
ataxia, cerebellar 6
atelectasis, congestive *see* respiratory distress, adult
ATG *see* globulin, antithymocyte
atherosclerosis, accelerated 20
atherosclerotic disease 16
azathioprine for immunosuppression in renal transplantation 23

B

Berger's disease *see* glomerulonephritis
Besnier–Boeck disease *see* sarcoidosis
beta blockers for renal artery stenosis 17
biopsy, renal 4, 12
bites, snake 6
bleeding *see* haemorrhage
blockage, urine 18
blood
    poisoning *see* septicaemia
    pressure, high *see* hypertension
Boeck's disease *see* sarcoidosis
Bourneville's disease *see* sclerosis, tuberous
breathing *see* respiration
Bright's disease *see* glomerulonephritis
bronchiectasis 22
bumetanide
    for acute tubular necrosis 19
    for hyperkalaemia 9
    for kidney myeloma 19
    for pigment myeloma 19
    for renal tubular acidosis 25

C

calcium
    carbonate for analgesic nephropathy 13
    gluconate for hyperkalaemia 9
    resonium for hyperkalaemia 9
calculi, Staghorn 22
CAPD *see* dialysis, continuous ambulatory peritoneal
cardiac arrest 8
cardiomyopathy 6
cardiovascular disease 3
cefotaxime for urinary tract infection 27
ceftazidime for urinary tract infection 27
cefuroxime for urinary tract infection 27
cephalexin for urinary tract infection 27
chlorambucil for glomerulonephritis 5
cholangiocarcinoma 14
ciprofloxacin for urinary tract infection 27
cirrhosis 4
    primary biliary 24
co-amoxyclav for urinary tract infection 27
coma 6
coning 10
convulsions *see* seizures
corticosteroids
    for acute interstitial nephritis 19
    for glomerulonephritis 5, 19
co-trimoxazole for urinary tract infection 27
crisis, scleroderma renal 4
cyclophosphamide for glomerulonephritis 5, 19
cyclosporin A
    for glomerulonephritis 5
    for immunosuppression in renal transplantation 23
cyst
    kidney
        benign noninherited 14
        rupture 14
    liver 14
cytomegalovirus 23

D

de Toni–Debre–Fanconi syndrome *see* Fanconi's syndrome
death, intrauterine 6
degeneration, hepatolenticular *see* Wilson's disease
diabetes
    insipidus, nephrogenic 8
    mellitus 4, 20, 24
dialysis 2, 13
    continuous ambulatory peritoneal 3
diarrhoea 6
    bloody 6
dipyridamole for haemolytic uraemic syndrome 7
disequilibrium 2
diuresis, forced alkaline
    for kidney myeloma 19
    for pigment nephropathy 19
diuretics
    for analgesic nephropathy 13
    loop
        for acute tubular necrosis 19
        for renal tubular acidosis 25
    potassium-sparing for renal tubular acidosis 25
dopamine for acute tubular necrosis 19
doxycycline for prostatitis 27
drowsiness 6, 20
dysrhythmia *see* arrhythmia

E

eicosapentanoic acid for glomerulonephritis 5
embolus, amniotic fluid 6
epilepsy *see* seizures
erythrocytosis *see* polycythaemia
erythropioetin for chronic renal failure 21
ESRD *see* renal failure, chronic

F

failure
    congestive heart 4
    renal
        acute 2, 4, 12, 18, 20
        chronic 2, 4, 12, 14, 20
        end-stage *see* chronic renal failure

Index

Fanconi's syndrome 12, 24
fever 26
  haemorrhagic
    dengue 6
    virus *see* hantavirus
fibrosis, myocardial 8
fits *see* seizures
flucloxacillin for renal abscesses 27
formication 8
frusemide for haemolytic uraemic syndrome 7

G

gentamicin for urinary tract infection 27
globulin, antithymocyte, for renal transplant rejection 23
glomerulonephritis 4
  chronic 20
  crescentic 19
  focal necrotizing 19
  non-proliferative 4
  proliferative 4
    endocapillary 4
    extracapillary 4
gonorrhoea 26
Goodpasture's syndrome 4
growth retardation 8

H

H_2 blockers for acute tubular necrosis 19
haematochezia *see* haemorrhage, gastrointestinal
haematuria 4, 14
haemodiafiltration for acute tubular necrosis
  continuous arteriovenous 19
  pumped continuous venavenous 19
haemodialysis 3
haemofiltration 3
haemolytic uraemic syndrome 6, 18
haemorrhage
  antepartum 6
  gastrointestinal 18
  subarachnoid 14
hantavirus 6
hepatorenal syndrome 18
herpes 26
hyperkalaemia 8, 18
hyperlipidaemia 10
hypernatraemia 10
hyperparathyroidism 24
hyperpotassaemia *see* hyperkalaemia
hypertension 16, 18, 20
  accelerated 6
  malignant 6
hyperthermia *see* fever
hypokalaemia 8

I

ileus 8
immunoglobulin A disease, mesangial 4
infarction, gut 6
infection
  Chlamydia 26
  Escherichia coli 6
  mycoplasma 6
  plasmodium *see* malaria
  renal 18
  urinary tract 26
    lower 26
    upper 26
intussusception 4
itching *see* pruritus

J

jaundice, haemolytic *see* anaemia, haemolytic

K

kidney *see also* renal
  cystic dysplasia of 14
  disease, polycystic 20
    autosomal-dominant 14
    autosomal-recessive 14
  medullary sponge 24

L

lactulose for hyperkalaemia 9
Legionnaires disease 18
leptospirosis 6, 18
Libman–Sacks disease *see* lupus erythematosus, systemic
Lignac–Fanconi's syndrome *see* Fanconi's syndrome
lupus erythematosus, systemic 6, 24

M

malaria 6
malnutrition 3
methylprednisolone
  for glomerulonephritis 5
  for renal transplant rejection 23
microangiopathy, thrombotic 4
misoprostol for analgesic nephropathy 13
mononeuropathy *see* neuropathy
muromonab-CD3 *see* OKT-3
mycophenolate mofetil for immunosuppression in renal transplantation 23
myelinosis, central pontine 10
myeloma
  kidney 19
  multiple 18, 20
  plasma cell *see* myeloma, multiple
myopathy, proximal 20

N

nephritic
  factor, C3 4
  illness, acute 4
nephritis 20
  haemolytic uraemic 4
  hereditary 20
  Heymann *see* glomerulonephritis
  interstitial 4, 8, 12
    acute 4, 12, 18
    chronic 12, 20
  salt-losing 378
  tubulointerstitial *see* nephritis, interstitial
nephrocalcinosis 14, 24
nephrolithiasis 14, 24
nephromegaly 14
nephronophthisis, juvenile 20
nephropathy
  analgesic 12
  Balkan 12
  diabetic 24
  pigment 18
  reflux 26
  tubulointerstitial 12
nephroso-nephritis virus, haemorrhagic *see* hantavirus
nephrotic syndrome 4
neuropathy, peripheral 20
nitrofurantoin for urinary tract infection 27
nocturia 14
nonsteroidal anti-inflammatory drugs *see* NSAIDs
NSAIDs
  as cause of acute interstitial nephritis 12
  for renal tubular acidosis 25

O

obstruction
  kidney 14
  renal artery *see* stenosis, renal artery
  ureteric 23
oedema 4
  noncardiogenic pulmonary 18
OKT3 for renal transplant rejection 23
ornithosis *see* psittacosis
osteodystrophy, renal 20

P

pericarditis 20
plasma exchange
  for glomerulonephritis 19
  for haemolytic uraemic syndrome 19
  for thrombotic thrombocytopenic purpura 19
pleuropneumonia-like organisms *see* infection, mycoplasma
polycythaemia 14
polydipsia 8

Index

polyuria 8
potassium for renal tubular acidosis 25
PPLO *see* infection, mycoplasma
prednisolone
    for acute interstitial nephritis 13
    for immunosuppression in renal transplantation 23
pre-eclampsia 4
prolapse, rectal 6
prostacyclin
    for haemolytic uraemic syndrome 7, 19
    for thrombotic thrombocytopenic purpura 19
prostatitis 26
protein, Bence–Jones 12
proteinuria 4
pruritus 18, 20
pseudohyponatraemia 10
pseudotuberculosis *see* sarcoidosis
psittacosis 6
purgative abuse 24
purpura 6
    thrombotic thrombocytopenic 6, 18
pyelonephritis
    bilateral 18
    chronic 20
    graft 23
pyonephrosis *see* pyelonephritis
pyrexia *see* fever

Q

quinolones for urinary tract infection 27

R

rapamycin for immunosuppression in renal transplantation 23
reflux, vesicoureteric 26
renal *see also* kidney
    insufficiency 6 *see also* failure, renal
    tubular dysfunction, proximal *see* Fanconi's syndrome
renovascular disease 20
respiration, Kussmaul's 20
respiratory distress, adult 18
rhabdomyolysis 8, 18
ricketts, renal *see* osteodystrophy, renal

S

salbutamol for hyperkalaemia 9
saline
    for haemolytic uraemic syndrome 7
    hypertonic for hyponatraemia 11
salivary gland disease *see* cytomegalovirus
salt wasting 12
Schaumann's disease *see* sarcoidosis
scleroderma 6
sclerosis, tuberous 14
seizures 6
Seoul virus *see* hantavirus
septicaemia 26
    Gram-negative 6
sicca syndrome *see* Sjögren's syndrome
Sjögren's syndrome 12, 24
SLE *see* lupus erythematosus, systemic
sodium
    bicarbonate
        for analgesic nephropathy 13
        for hyperkalaemia 9
        for renal tubular acidosis 25
    for analgesic nephropathy 13
spasm decerebrate 6
stenosis, renal artery 16, 20, 23
steroids *see* corticosteroids
stones *see* calculi

T

tacrolimus for immunosuppression in renal transplantation 23
thrombocytopenia 6
thrombopenia *see* thrombocytopenia
transplant rejection 12
transplantation 6
    renal 22
        for chronic renal failure 21
trimethoprim for urinary tract infection 27
TTP *see* purpura, thrombotic thrombocytopenic
tuberculosis 12, 22
twitches 6
    muscle 10

U

uraemia 18
urethritis 26
urography, intravenous 12
uveitis 12

V

vasculitis, large-vessel 16
ventricular dysfunction, left 16
vitamin D
    for chronic renal failure 21
    for renal tubular acidosis 25
volvulus *see* ileus

W

wasting, muscle 18
Wilson's disease 24
wound healing, poor 18

CURRENT DIAGNOSIS & TREATMENT

in

Neurology

Edited by
Anthony Schapira

Series editors
Roy Pounder
Mark Hamilton

A QUICK Reference for the Clinician

Contributors

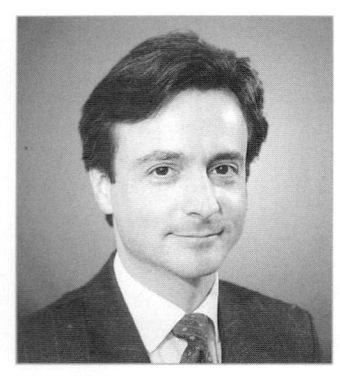

EDITOR

A H V Schapira

Professor Anthony Schapira is Chairman and Professor of Neurology at the Royal Free Hospital, London, and Professor of Neurology at the Institute of Neurology, London. His research interests are in Parkinson's disease and the biochemistry and molecular genetics of mitochondrial diseases.

REFEREES

Dr Russell Lane
Department of Neurology
Charing Cross Hospital
London, UK

Professor Adrian Williams
Department of Neurology
Selly Oak Hospital
Birmingham, UK

AUTHORS

CEREBRAL TUMOUR
Professor David GT Thomas
Department of Neurological Surgery
Institute of Neurology
London, UK

COMA
Dr David Bates
Department of Neurology
Royal Victoria Infirmary
Newcastle upon Tyne, UK

CRANIAL ARTERITIS
Dr Jeremy M Gibbs
Department of Neuroscience
Royal Free Hospital
London, UK

DEMENTIA
Dr Martin Rossor
Department of Neurology
St Mary's Hospital
London, UK

ENCEPHALITIS
Dr Tony Wilson
Department of Neurology
Royal Free Hospital
London, UK

EPILEPSY
Dr John S Duncan
Institute of Neurology
National Hospital for Neurology and Neurosurgery
London, UK

FACIAL PAIN, ATYPICAL
Dr JW Scadding
National Hospital for Neurology and Neurosurgery
London, UK

GUILLAN-BARRÉ SYNDROME
Dr Jeremy Rees
Department of Neurology
Guy's Hospital
London, UK

IDIOPATHIC POLYMYOSTITIS
Dr John A Morgan-Hughes
Department of Clinical Neurology
Institute of Neurology
London, UK

INTRACEBRAL HAEMORRHAGE
Dr K Ray Chaudhuri
Department of Neurology
Institute of Psychiatry
London, UK

Professor RIchard Frackowiak
MRC Cyclotron Unit
Hammersmith Hospital
London, UK

MENINGITIS, BACTERIAL
Dr Lionel Ginsberg
Department of Neurological Science
Royal Free Hospital
London, UK

Dr Dermot H Kennedy
Department of Infection and Tropical Medicine
Ruchill Hospital
Glasgow, UK

MIGRAINE
Professor Anthony HV Schapira
Department of Neurological Science
Royal Free Hospital
London, UK

MOTOR NEURONE DISEASE
Dr Catherine M Lloyd
Department of Neurology
Institute of Psychiatry
London, UK

Professor Nigel Leigh
Department of Neurology
Insitute of Psychiatry
London, UK

MULTIPLE SCLEROSIS
Professor W Ian McDonald
Department of Clinical Neurology
Institute of Neurology
London, UK

MYASTHENIA GRAVIS
Professor John Newsom-Davis
Institute of Molecular Medicine
John Radcliffe Hospital
Oxford, UK

NEURALGIA, POSTHERPETIC
Dr JW Scadding
National Hospital for Neurology and Neurosurgery
London, UK

NEURALGIA, TRIGEMINAL
Dr JW Scadding
National Hospital for Neurology and Neurosurgery
London, UK

NEUROPATHY, PERIPHERAL
Dr J Gareth Llewelyn
Department of Neurosciences
Royal Free Hospital
London, UK

PARKINSON'S DISEASE
Professor Anthony HV Schapira
Department of Neurological Science
Royal Free Hospital
London, UK

SLEEP DISORDERS
Dr David Parkes
Institute of Psychiatry
London, UK

SPINAL CORD AND CAUDA EQUINA COMPRESSION
Dr Andrew N Gale
Department of Neurology
Royal Free Hospital
London, UK

Mr RS Maurice-Williams
Department of Neurosurgery
Royal Free Hospital
London, UK

STROKE
Dr Richard Davenport
Department of Clinical Neurosciences
University of Edinburgh
Edinburgh, UK

TRANSIENT ISCHAEMIC ATTACKS
Dr Richard Davenport
Department of Clinical Neurosciences
University of Edinburgh
Edinburgh, UK

Professor Charles Warlow
Department of Clinical Neurosciences
Western General Hospital
Edinburgh, UK

TREMOR
Dr Philip D Thompson
University Department of Medicine
Royal Adelaide Hospital
Adelaide, Australia

Contents

2 Cerebral tumour

4 Coma

6 Cranial arteritis

8 Dementia
    degenerative dementias
    treatable dementias

10 Encephalitis

12 Epilepsy
    generalized epilepsy (absence, myoclonic, clonic, tonic, tonic–clonic, atonic)
    partial epilepsy (simple, complex, secondary generalized)

14 Facial pain, atypical

16 Guillain-Barré syndrome

18 Idiopathic polymyositis

20 Intracerebral haemorrhage
    cerebellar haemorrhage
    subarachnoid haemorrhage

22 Meningitis, bacterial

24 Migraine
    classic migraine (with aura)
    common migraine (without aura)
    hemiplegic migraine
    migrainous neuralgia (cluster headache)
    ophthalmoplegic migraine
    retinal migraine

26 Motor neurone disease

28 Multiple sclerosis
    progressive multiple sclerosis
    relapsing and remitting multiple sclerosis

30 Myasthenia gravis
    early-onset myasthenia gravis
    late-onset myasthenia gravis
    seronegative myasthenia gravis
    thymoma

32 Neuralgia, postherpetic

34 Neuralgia, trigeminal

36 Neuropathy, peripheral
    autonomic neuropathy
    chronic inflammatory demyelinating polyradiculoneuropathy
    focal/multifocal neuropathy
    motor neuropathies
    painful neuropathies
    sensorimotor polyneuropathy
    sensory polyneuropathy

38 Parkinson's disease

40 Sleep disorders
    circadian sleep disorders
    insomnia
    narcoleptic syndrome
    obstructive sleep apnoea
    parasomnia

42 Spinal cord and cauda equina compression

44 Stroke
    cerebral infarction (lacuna infarction, partial anterior circulation infarction, posterior infarction, total anterior circulation infarction)
    primary intracerebral haemorrhage
    subarachnoid haemorrhage

46 Transient ischaemic attacks

48 Tremor
    cerebellar tremor
    drug-induced tremor
    drug-withdrawal tremor
    dystonic tremor
    essential tremor
    exaggerated physiological tremor
    focal tremor
    hereditary tremor
    idiopathic tremor
    midbrain (rubral) tremor
    neuropathic tremor
    parkinsonian tremor
    physiological tremor
    primary orthostatic tremor
    symptomatic tremor
    task-specific action tremor
    toxin-induced tremor

50 Index

Cerebral tumour — D.G.T. Thomas

Diagnosis

Symptoms
- Symptoms generally include the following, alone or in combination:

Epilepsy: in >50% of patients by presentation; associated focal features may suggest localization of brain tumour; epilepsy of late onset (>25 years) indicates new brain lesion and should be investigated.

Dysphasia, hemiparesis, intellectual failure, personality change: due to brain dysfunction.

Headache, papilloedema, visual failure, vomiting: alone or in combination indicate raised intracranial pressure due to intracranial mass lesions.

Signs
Papilloedema, impaired visual acuity, visual field defects.

Diplopia: with or without clear III or VI nerve palsy.

Facial weakness.

Dysphasia.

Hemiparesis, hyper-reflexia, extensor plantar response, hemisensory loss.

Signs of primary malignancy in secondary brain tumours: e.g. site of previous melanoma excision visible in skin.

Investigations
Neuroradiography: primarily CT or MRI of brain; more invasive procedures (e.g. angiography or positron emission tomography) sometimes needed for further aspects of management.

Chest radiography: important as part of general screening for extracerebral primary or metastatic tumour in lungs.

EEG: possibly needed as secondary investigation to elucidate epileptic manifestations.

Blood tests: possibly needed to clarify differential diagnosis, e.g. blood cultures when metastatic brain abscess suspected.

Complications
Visual failure: papilloedema due to progressive raised intracranial pressure leads to blindness if unrelieved.

Coning: brain shift due to increasing mass of cerebral tumour can lead to brain herniation at tentorial hiatus, with irreversible ischaemic brain damage and fatal apnoea due to failure of mid-brain and brainstem function.

Differential diagnosis
Cerebrovascular disease.

Other organic brain disease (e.g. encephalitis or demyelination).

Other extracerebral intracranial tumours (e.g. meningioma).

Cerebral abscess: an important differential diagnosis; often no signs of acute infection in patients, despite relevant history of middle ear disease, bronchiectasis, or valvular heart disease.

Aetiology
- The cause of most cerebral tumours remains unknown, although the incidence is increased after exposure to radiation, in patients with neurofibromatosis, and in some rare inherited immunodeficiency diseases.
- Increasing evidence indicates that cerebral astrocytomas are associated with loss of tumour suppressor gene function from chromosomes 17 and 10 and with amplification of epidermal growth factor receptor.

Epidemiology
- Primary cerebral tumours account for ~55% of intracranial tumours in adults and are the tenth most common tumours in men.
- The annual incidence of cerebral tumour is ~10 in 100 000 population.
- The peak incidence is in the fifth decade, with a small male preponderance (55%).
- Secondary brain tumours are common and account for 15–20% of intracranial tumours in neurological series.

Treatment

Diet and lifestyle
- No special diet is necessary for patients with primary brain tumours.
- Impaired cognitive function and tiredness may limit work to part-time employment.

Pharmacological treatment

For epilepsy
- Anticonvulsant drug treatment is usually started in both epileptic and non-epileptic patients.

Standard dosage	Phenytoin 300–400 mg daily.
Contraindications	Hepatic impairment.
Main drug interactions	Analgesics, antibiotics, antidepressants.
Main side effects	Confusion, skin eruptions, gum swelling.

For raised intracranial pressure and stabilization of brain function

Standard dosage	Dexamethasone 4 mg every 6 h (adult) initially; up to 20 mg every 6 h may be useful for a few weeks as palliative terminal treatment.
Contraindications	Peptic ulcers.
Special points	When surgical decompression and adjuvant radiotherapy have been completed, steroids may be gradually withdrawn or reduced to a minimum level that keeps the patient asymptomatic. While the patient is taking dexamethasone, the risk of peptide ulceration is increased; H_2 antagonists such as ranitidine 150 mg twice daily are usually also prescribed.
Main drug interactions	Antidiabetics, diuretics.
Main side effects	Peptic ulceration, weight gain.

For acutely raised intracranial pressure
- In patients who are unconscious as a result of raised intracranial pressure from cerebral tumour or in those who have coned, with respiratory arrest, artificial ventilation, mannitol as an osmotic diuretic, and i.v. dexamethasone may be needed in an emergency department or intensive care unit setting.

Chemotherapy
- After surgery and adjuvant radiotherapy, anti-tumour chemotherapy may be indicated for malignant glioma, either as an adjuvant or at the time of relapse.
- Nitrosoureas and procarbazine are the agents chiefly used.
- Administration and monitoring must be done in a specialist oncology unit.

Treatment aims
To relieve symptoms; curing malignant primary or secondary brain tumours is generally not possible.

Other treatments
Surgery: almost always indicated to establish histological diagnosis and grading and, where possible, to reduce tumour bulk.
Radiotherapy: localized to tumour and surrounding area, usually given for malignant primary cerebral tumours; secondary metastatic cerebral tumours treated by whole-brain radiation.

Prognosis
- Prognosis is related to tumour type and histological grade, patient age, and functional performance at the time of treatment.
- The median survival with grade 4 astrocytomas is ~9 months and with grade 2 astrocytomas ~6 years.

Follow-up and management
- Clinical assessment of neurological and performance status, with follow-up brain scanning at intervals of 3–6 months, is used to monitor progress.
- At disease progression, further surgery is considered in 10–15% of patients, as are novel treatments, e.g. focused radiation or immunotherapy.
- The terminal phase is usually short, from a few days to 6 weeks, and patients may often be managed in the home, although hospice care may sometimes be preferable.

Driving regulations
- A patient who has epilepsy or who has had brain surgery for cerebral tumour is prohibited by the drivers licensing authority from driving for a variable period, sometimes indefinitely.

Key references
Apuzzo MLJ (ed): *Malignant Cerebral Glioma*. Illinois: American Association of Neurological Surgeons, 1990.
Mahaley MS: Neuro-oncology index and review (adult primary brain tumors). *J Neuro-Oncology* 1991, **11**:85–147.
Thomas DGT (ed): *Neuro-Oncology*. London: Arnold, 1990.

Coma D. Bates

Diagnosis

Definition
- Coma is a state of unrousable unresponsiveness in which the patient shows no psychologically understandable response to external stimulus or inner need.
- In practice, the condition may usefully be defined as a patient with a Glasgow coma scale of 2:4:2 or less (see box).

Symptoms
- Symptoms are usually unobtainable from the patient, but information is vital.

History from a witness: for evolution of coma, circumstances of patient's discovery, trauma, seizure, drugs.

Signs
Fever: indicating infection (meningitis, encephalitis, systemic).
Hypothermia: may be cause or effect.
Neck stiffness, Kernig's sign, papilloedema.
Cardiac abnormalities: indicating subacute bacterial endocarditis or emboli.
Hypertension or hypotension.
Slow, shallow respiration: suggesting drug intoxication.
Rapid respiration: suggesting infection or acidosis.
Anaemia, jaundice, rash.
Intoxication, diabetes, hepatic failure.
Organomegaly, polycystic kidneys, subarachnoid haemorrhage.
Meningitis, subarachnoid haemorrhage, raised intracranial pressure.

Investigations
Glasgow coma scale: for level of consciousness.
Brainstem function tests: pupillary response, spontaneous eye movements, oculovestibular responses.
Motor function tests: for lateralizing features.
Fundal examination: for papilloedema, haemorrhages, emboli.
Blood analysis: for biochemistry, e.g. glucose; renal, liver, and thyroid function, etc.
CT or MRI: for coma with focal signs or if the diagnosis is uncertain.
Lumbar puncture: for coma without focal signs but with meningism.
Haematological assays, chest radiography, EEG: for coma without focal signs or meningism (raised intracranial pressure must be excluded first).

The anatomy of consciousness.

Complications
Infections: particularly respiratory or renal, e.g. aspiration pneumonia.
Metabolic abnormalities.
Disseminated intravascular coagulation.
Decubitus ulcers.
Contractures.
Deep venous thromboses.
Death.

Differential diagnosis
Locked-in syndrome: voluntary response of eye opening and eye closure to command.
Vegetative state: spontaneous eye opening and sleep–wake cycles, but no evidence of cognition.
Pseudo-coma: intact oculovestibular responses and nystagmus to cold water caloric, blepharospasm.

Aetiology
- Causes include the following:
Drug or alcohol overdose.
Trauma.
Space-occupying intracranial lesions.
Infections: encephalitis, meningitis, septicaemia.
Intracranial haemorrhage and thrombosis.
Metabolic abnormalities.
Toxins.

Epidemiology
- 3% of emergency admissions to hospital are in coma.
- 40% of these patients have taken an overdose of sedative drugs.

Glasgow coma scale
Eye opening
1. Nil.
2. To pain.
3. *To speech.*
4. *Spontaneously.*

Motor response
1. Nil.
2. Extensor.
3. Flexor.
4. Withdrawal.
5. *Localizing.*
6. *Voluntary.*

Verbal response
1. Nil.
2. Groans.
3. *Inappropriate.*
4. *Confused.*
5. *Orientated.*

- Italics indicate no coma.

Treatment

Diet and lifestyle
Not relevant.

Pharmacological treatment
- Patients may need treatment for causative or concurrent disorders: antibiotics and antiviral agents, antifungal agents, correction of metabolic abnormalities, removal of toxic substances, treatment of mass lesions, s.c. heparin to prevent thrombotic complications.
- Steroids should not be given routinely in comatose patients but may help in specific instances when raised intracranial pressure, due to oedema, can be corrected.

Treatment aims
To correct cause.
To maintain hydration and nutrition.
To reverse coma and return normal physiological and psychological function.

Prognosis
- Sedative drugs or alcohol overdoses are not usually lethal, and the prognosis is good if the circulation and respiration are protected.
- The prognosis of other causes of non-traumatic coma depends on the cause (metabolic coma has better prognosis than hypoxic ischaemic coma), the depth (the deeper the coma, the worse the prognosis), the duration (the longer the coma, the worse the prognosis), and clinical signs, e.g. brainstem reflexes.
- Overall, only 15% of patients in non-traumatic coma for >6 h make a good or moderate recovery.

Follow-up and management
- The airway must be maintained.
- The patient must be given adequate nutrition.
- Skin, chest, bladder, and bowel must be protected.
- Progress must be monitored.

Key references
Bates D: The management of medical coma. *J Neurol Neurosurg Psychiatry* 1993, **56**:589–598.

Cranial arteritis — J.M. Gibbs

Diagnosis

Symptoms
Headache: present in 75% of patients; at any site, often throbbing, unilateral or asymmetrical, worse at night; scalp soreness and tenderness frequent.
Polymyalgia: proximal limb pain and stiffness in 58%.
Malaise, fatigue, weight loss: in 56%.
Jaw pain and fatigue: masticatory 'claudication' in 40%.
Fever: in 35%.
Cough: in 17%.
Amaurosis fugax: in 10%.
Permanent visual loss: in 8%.
Limb claudication: in 8%.
Transient ischaemic attack or stroke: in 7%.
Depression or confusional state: in 3%.
Diplopia: in 2%.

Signs
Abnormal temporal artery: tenderness, nodularity, thickening or reduced pulsation in 49% of patients.
Scalp tenderness elsewhere.
Tenderness of common carotid arteries.
Diminished carotid or limb pulses.
Ischaemic optic neuropathy: pale, swollen disc in a recently blinded eye.
Ophthalmoplegia: due to cranial-nerve or brainstem lesion.
Confusional state or encephalopathy.

Investigations
ESR measurement: substantially raised in most patients; mean, 85 ± 32 mm/h (<30 mm/h in 3% of patients); CRP or plasma viscosity no more sensitive or specific.
Full blood count: mild anaemia, thrombocytosis, and raised leucocyte count common.
Liver function tests: raised gamma glutamyl transferase, alkaline phosphatase, or aspartate transaminase in 15% of patients.
Lumbar puncture: necessary only if low-grade meningitis or cortical thrombophlebitis considered in differential diagnosis.
Temporal artery biopsy: essential when diagnosis not absolutely clear cut on clinical grounds; at least 2–3 cm length biopsy (longer segment more likely to yield positive result); occipital artery biopsy alternative in selected patients.
Angiography: necessary only to exclude arterial dissection or other arteritides in selected patients; may show abnormalities in all major branches of aortic arch in cranial arteritis; lacks sensitivity and specificity as diagnostic test.

Complications
Permanent blindness: in 8% of patients.
Brainstem or carotid territory infarction: in <5%.
Myocardial infarction.
Scalp necrosis.
Limb ischaemia.
Aortic rupture.

Differential diagnosis

Raised ESR
Other arteritides (rare in patients >70 years old).
Myeloma.
Other skull metastases.
Subacute meningitis.
Infection with venous sinus thrombosis.

Normal ESR
Migraine.
Tension headache.
'Occipital neuralgia'.
Cervical spine disease.
Paget's disease of the skull.
Vertebral or carotid dissection.
Temporomandibular joint disease.
Meningioma.

Aetiology
- Cranial arteritis is presumed to be an autoimmune disorder, but the antigen is not known (perhaps component of internal elastic lamina).
- Immunoglobulin and complement deposits have been shown at the internal elastic lamina; other histological features suggest that cell-mediated mechanisms are also involved.

Epidemiology
- The incidence is 9.3 in 100 000 population overall and 15–30 in 100 000 aged >50 years.
- The prevalence is 130 in 100 000 aged >50 years.
- Cranial arteritis rarely occurs in people aged <50 years.
- The median age of onset is 75 years (range, 56–92 years in published series).
- The female:male ratio is 3.7:1.

Pathology
- Cranial arteritis is an occlusive disease, involving large and medium-sized arteries arising from the aortic arch and sometimes the femoral arteries and aorta itself.
- Biopsy shows arterial luminal stenosis due to intimal proliferation, with disruption of the internal elastic lamina, mononuclear cell infiltration, necrosis of the media, giant cells, and granuloma formation; secondary thrombosis may be present. Involvement is patchy and may be missed by too small a biopsy.

Treatment

Diet and lifestyle
- No special precautions are necessary.

Pharmacological treatment

General principles
- Cranial arteritis requires prompt treatment by corticosteroids to prevent the rare but serious complications, particularly blindness.
- Presenting symptoms are often nonspecific and 'atypical' (e.g. pyrexia of unknown origin, weight loss, anaemia), so suspicion must be high and treatment initiated as soon as the diagnosis is seriously considered.
- Arterial biopsy is often taken after steroid treatment is started, but it should not be delayed by more than 2–3 days; the yield of positive histology in clinically probable cases falls from 60–80% with early biopsy to only 10% in patients biopsied 1 week after starting steroid treatment.
- Traditional high doses of prednisolone are justifiable in all patients with visual symptoms or signs and in those with features of cerebral or myocardial ischaemia.
- In critical cases (e.g. visual loss in one eye and early symptoms in the other), infusion of high-dose methylprednisolone probably reduces the risk of complete blindness.
- In patients without visual symptoms, prospective trials suggest that most respond to much lower doses (even less needed for polymyalgia without symptomatic arteritis).
- The rate of reduction depends on clinical severity at presentation, starting dose, symptom control, and ESR.
- A maintenance dose of 5–10 mg daily is usually needed for 2–3 years.
- An alternate-day regimen is sometimes possible, when the dose is very low.
- 30–50% of patients can discontinue treatment after 2 years.
- Some need treatment for several years, and a few apparently need long-term maintenance doses of 2–5 mg daily.

Steroid regimen
Initial dose: prednisolone 40–80 mg daily; methylprednisolone 1 g i.v. daily for 2–5 days in critical cases.
Months 1–2: reduced slowly to 20–40 mg daily.
Months 2–4: reduced slowly to 10–20 mg daily.
Months 4–24: reduced to maintenance dose 5–10 mg daily.
Months 24–36: withdrawal possible in ~50% of patients.

Complications of treatment
Vertebral compression fractures in 26%.
Other symptoms of osteoporosis.
Steroid myopathy in 11%.
Cataracts.
Gastrointestinal symptoms.
Other steroid side effects.

Other drugs
- Azathioprine has a modest steroid-sparing effect but is not of proven efficacy used alone.
- Cyclophosphamide is a possible third option but rarely used.

Treatment aims
To relieve symptoms.
To prevent complications.
To prevent and control steroid side effects.

Prognosis
- Prognosis is excellent with early and adequate steroid treatment, which is usually needed for at least 2–3 years.
- Subsequent morbidity is determined as much by steroid side effects as by the disease itself.

Follow-up and management
- Patients need regular monitoring of clinical symptoms, ESR, and potential steroid effects for at least 2 years, preferably in a specialist clinic (neurology or rheumatology).

Key references
Caselli RJ, Hunder GG, Whisnant JP: Neurologic disease in biopsy-proven giant cell (temporal) arteritis. *Neurology* 1988, **38**:352–359.

Hall S et al.: The therapeutic impact of temporal artery biopsy. *Lancet* 1983, **ii**:1217–1220.

Hayreh SS: Ophthalmic features of giant cell arteritis. *Baillières Clin Rheumatol* 1991, **5**:431–459.

Kyle V, Hazleman BL: Treatment of polymyalgia rheumatica and giant cell arteritis. Steroid regimens in the first two months. *Ann Rheum Dis* 1989, **48**:658–661.

Machado EB et al.: Trends in incidence and clinical presentation of temporal arteritis in Olmstead County, Minnesota, 1950–1985. *Arthritis Rheum* 1988, **31**:745–749.

Nordborg E, Bengtsson BA: Epidemiology of proven giant cell arteritis (GCA). *Intern Med* 1990, **227**:233–236.

Dementia — M.N. Rossor

Diagnosis

Definition
- Dementia is the syndrome of impairment in multiple domains of cognition, which must include memory, with intact arousal (compare with confusional state).
- Symptoms, signs, and investigations are used to differentiate potentially treatable causes of dementias from the degenerative dementias.

Symptoms
- Patients may be unaware of deficits and deny symptoms (anosagnosia); a history from a carer is therefore essential.

Memory loss: the most common presenting symptom.

Dysphasia, dyspraxia, visuospatial dysfunction, behavioural change: usually progressive and may occur in any order.

- Additional symptoms depend on the cause, e.g. the following:

Headache: due to space-occupying lesions.

Fatigue: due to systemic disease (e.g. HIV, hypothyroidism).

Weight loss: due to neoplasia.

Peripheral neuropathy: due to vitamin B_{12} deficiency, alcohol.

Seizures: may occur in patients with Alzheimer's disease or may have a focal cause.

Signs
- The primary degenerative dementias (e.g. Alzheimer's disease) have few signs other than those relating to higher cortical function.

Primitive reflexes (grasp, rooting, sucking), increased muscle tone: late in dementia.

More widespread dysfunction: in dementia plus syndromes, e.g. Huntington's disease (dementia plus chorea), multi-infarct dementia (dementia plus focal motor signs).

Papilloedema or focal neurology: suggesting a potentially treatable intracranial cause.

Investigations
- Few specific tests are available, and none for the most common cause, Alzheimer's disease.
- Investigations are aimed at excluding secondary causes, e.g. cerebral neoplasms, metabolic disturbances.

Psychometry: to assess pattern and severity of cognitive impairment.

Full blood count, ESR measurement, routine biochemistry.

Serum vitamin B_{12} and thyroid function tests.

Treponemal serology.

HIV antibody serology: in some patients.

Chest radiography.

ECG.

EEG.

CT or MRI: to exclude mass lesions, assess vascular changes, and determine regional atrophy.

Single-photon emission CT, positron emission tomography: if available, to assess regional metabolism.

Lumbar puncture: in selected patients to exclude inflammatory changes.

Cerebral biopsy: rarely used; can provide definitive histological diagnosis.

Complications
Progression of Alzheimer's disease and other degenerative dementias.

Death: usually due to bronchopneumonia.

Differential diagnosis
Acute confusional states or delirium with fluctuating impairment of arousal.

Korsakoff's and Wernicke's syndromes secondary to alcohol abuse.

Focal neuropsychological deficits, e.g. dysphasia.

'Pseudodementia' resulting from impairment of cognitive function by anxiety or depression.

Aetiology
- Any disease disrupting the function of cortico-cortical or subcortico-cortical connections can cause dementia, e.g. the following:

Causes of degenerative dementia
Alzheimer's disease, frontal-lobe degeneration, Pick's disease, cortical Lewy body disease, Huntington's disease, prion disease.

- Some hereditary dementias are associated with specific genetic markers, e.g. rare families with Alzheimer's disease and amyloid precursor protein (APP) gene mutations, later-onset disease with the apolipoprotein E4 genotype.

- Neuropathologically, dementia of Alzheimer's disease is associated with senile plaques and neurofibrillary tangles in the cerebral cortex.

- ~15% of Alzheimer's disease is familial.

Vascular causes
Multiple cortical or subcortical infarcts, small-vessel disease (Binswanger's disease).

Potentially treatable causes
Neoplasms, normal-pressure hydrocephalus, trauma, subdural and extradural haematomas, drugs or toxins.

Vitamin B_{12} deficiency, hypothyroidism, renal and hepatic dysfunction, inherited metabolic disease.

Multiple sclerosis, cerebral vasculitis, sarcoid.

HIV, neurosyphilis, chronic viral encephalitides, chronic meningitides, cerebral Whipples disease.

Epidemiology
- Dementia is common in elderly patients, occurring in 2–5% >65 years; 20–40% >80 years.
- Alzheimer's disease is the most common cause, accounting for 50% of dementia patients and a further 15–20% in association with vascular disease.

Treatment

Diet and lifestyle
- Patients must avoid fatigue, alcohol, and sedative drugs unless clearly indicated.
- Patients should ensure optimum general health (systemic illness, e.g. cardiac failure, can exacerbate dementia).
- Patients should use cognitive aids, e.g. clear labelling, diary.
- Medicalert bracelets should be worn.

Pharmacological treatment
- The treatment of dementia is firstly the treatment of the underlying cause when possible, e.g. removal of meningioma, vitamin B_{12} replacement.
- No drugs are known to alter disease progression of the degenerative dementias.
- The degeneration in Alzheimer's disease particularly affects the glutamatergic cortico-cortical association pyramidal neurones and the subcortico-cortical cholinergic projection neurones; cholinergic enhancement can improve memory in cholinergic deficit states. Various cholinergic muscarinic agonists, release enhancers and anticholinesterases are currently being developed.

Standard dosage	Tetrahydroaminoacridine (Tacrine) 40–160 mg daily in divided doses
Contraindications	Pregnancy.
Special points	Licensed in the USA and France. Improvements reported in 40% of patients.
Main drug interactions	None.
Main side effects	Cholinergic effects, hepatotoxicity.

Treatment aims
To treat the underlying cause, when possible.

Prognosis
- Prognosis depends on the causative disease.

Follow-up and management
- Management involves many disciplines: neurologists, psychiatrists, and geriatricians.
- Early involvement of social work and community psychiatric services is important.

Social support
The Alzheimer's Disease Society, Gordon House, 10 Greencoat Place, London SW1P 1PH, tel 0171 306 0606.

Legal issues
- The driving licensing authority must be notified.
- Patients should consider referring legal affairs to someone else (power of attorney).

Key references
Burns A, Levy R (eds): *Dementia*. London: Chapman Hall, 1994.

Corder EH *et al.*: Gene dose of apolipoprotein E type 4 allele and the risk of Alzheimer's disease in late onset families. *Science* 1993, **261**:921–923.

Knapp MJ *et al.*: A thirty week randomised controlled trial of high dose tacrine in patients with Alzheimer's disease. *JAMA* 1994, **271**:985–991.

Rossor MN: Management of neurological disorders: dementia. *J Neurol Neurosurg Psychiatry* 1994, **57**:1451–1456.

Encephalitis — L.A. Wilson

Diagnosis

Symptoms
Headache, behavioural abnormality, fever, photophobia, drowsiness.

Confusion, coma, convulsions: with progression.

Speech disturbance, limb weakness, incoordination, involuntary movements: indicating focal neurological disorder.

Signs
Drowsiness, confusion, irritability, coma.

Neck stiffness: due to associated meningeal inflammation (may be absent).

Associated focal cerebral hemisphere signs: e.g. hemiparesis and dysphasia; make herpes simplex encephalitis a probability.

Ataxia, nystagmus, myoclonus, involuntary movements, extensor plantar responses.

Investigations
CT and MRI of brain: help to exclude other causes and may show brain swelling; focal inferior temporal and orbital frontal damage with herpes simplex may take several days to become apparent on plain CT but may be seen earlier on contrast-enhanced CT.

CSF analysis: CSF may be under increased pressure and usually shows lymphocytic pleocytosis, modestly raised protein, and normal glucose concentration; showing a fourfold rise in specific viral antibody titres is only helpful in retrospect; enzyme-linked immunoassays for viral antigens and gene amplification with polymerase chain reaction are increasingly available to aid early specific diagnosis.

EEG: shows widespread slow activity with diffuse brain disorder and may show periodic complexes over temporal region in herpes simplex encephalitis.

Complications
Seizures: often occur and need vigorous treatment.

Cerebral oedema: may cause death and calls for measures to reduce intracranial pressure.

Differential diagnosis
Meningitis: bacterial, tuberculous, fungal, or viral.

Acute disseminated encephalomyelitis.

Toxic encephalopathy with systemic infection.

Metabolic encephalopathy: usually no fever, headache, or CSF abnormality.

Cerebral abscess, empyema, subdural haematoma, and other mass lesions.

Aetiology
- Viral invasion of the brain causes an inflammatory reaction of varying intensity, associated with perivascular cuffing with lymphocytes and other mononuclear cells and with destruction of nerve cells and glia; haemorrhagic necrosis may occur.

Epidemiology
- Herpes simplex virus is the most common cause of sporadic encephalitis.
- Other herpes viruses, especially herpes zoster, cytomegalovirus, and Epstein—Barr virus, are common causes, particularly when immunity is impaired, as in transplant or AIDS patients.
- Arboviral encephalitis occurs in epidemics where mosquitoes bite humans.
- Mumps encephalitis and subacute sclerosing encephalitis have declined in incidence with vaccination; the latter is a progressive late complication of measles infection.
- Progressive multifocal leukoencephalopathy, common in AIDS patients, is due to a human polyoma virus (JC) complicating immunodeficiency.
- HIV may cause meningoencephalitis at seroconversion and, later, a slowly progressive dementia.

Treatment

Diet and lifestyle
Not relevant.

Pharmacological treatment

- No effective treatment is available against many of the viruses causing encephalitis; often, the specific causative virus is not identified.
- Seizures need prompt anticonvulsant administration to reduce the deleterious effects of further seizures.
- Full supportive measures are necessary during what is often a self-limiting illness with good recovery.
- Intravenous acyclovir started early reduces the morbidity and mortality of herpes simplex encephalitis; treatment should not await the outcome of brain biopsy, which is seldom appropriate.

Standard dosage	Acyclovir 10 mg/kg i.v. infusion every 8 h for 10 days (adults), 500 mg/m^2 every 8 h (children aged 3 months to 12 years).
Contraindications	Hypersensitivity.
Special points	Renal impairment necessitates dose reduction.
Main drug interactions	Possible interaction with zidovudine.
Main side effects	Usually none.

- Ganciclovir may be of benefit when cytomegalovirus is the probable cause.
- Improvement of HIV encephalopathy has been reported with zidovudine.

Treatment aims
To treat herpes simplex encephalitis.
To prevent recurrent seizures.
To control raised intracranial pressure.
To provide optimal rehabilitation when necessary.

Other treatments
Ventilation, mannitol, and dexamethasone for cerebral oedema.
Fluid balance, nutrition, and airway maintenance.

Prognosis
- The outcome varies with different causative viruses, the age of the patient, and associated underlying disease.
- Death and serious residual disability are frequent with herpes simplex when the diagnosis and treatment are delayed.

Follow-up and management
- Specialized neurological rehabilitation may be important for patients with residual disability in the wake of the illness.

Key references
Aurelius E *et al.*: Rapid diagnosis of herpes simplex encephalitis by nested polymerase chain reaction assay of cerebrospinal fluid. *Lancet* 1991, **337**:189–192.
Whitley RJ: Viral encephalitis. *N Engl J Med* 1990, **323**:242–250.

Epilepsy — J.S. Duncan

Diagnosis

Symptoms
Seizures: usually abrupt onset, transient, stereotyped.
Loss of or altered awareness.
Abnormal posture, tone, movements: e.g. convulsion.
Somatic, visual, auditory, olfactory, gustatory symptoms.
Déjà vu, jamais vu.
Epigastric sensation.

Signs
- Usually no signs are manifest.
- Patients should be checked for the following:

Mental state and higher mental function.
Focal neurological deficit.
Evidence of raised intracranial pressure.
Evidence of adverse effects from antiepileptic drugs.
Cardiovascular abnormalities.

Investigations
EEG: routine, with hyperventilation and photic stimulation; if normal and diagnosis in doubt, sleep-deprived and sleep EEG, 24-h ambulatory tape, video-EEG telemetry can be considered (if episodes frequent).

Neuroimaging: if age at onset <1 year or >20 years, partial seizures on history, focal deficit on examination, focal EEG abnormality, difficulty obtaining control of seizures; MRI superior to CT, necessary for intractable partial seizures or focal deficit, if CT normal or unclear, or if surgical treatment of epilepsy contemplated.

Antiepileptic drug concentration measurement: if prescribed treatment, to check compliance and whether adverse effects are dose-related; may help assessment of scope for dose increases.

Blood chemistry: fasting glucose, liver, renal, and bone profiles.

Prolactin measurement: transient rise to 1000 mU/L in serum up to 20 min after tonic–clonic seizures; not raised if attack not epileptic; may rise after complex partial seizure.

Neuropsychology: if cognition or memory causes concern.

Chest radiography, ECG, HIV and syphilis serology: can also be considered.

Complications
Trauma.
Status epilepticus.
Sudden unexpected death.
Secondary cerebral damage.
Psychosocial handicap.

Differential diagnosis

Altered or lost awareness
Syncope, vagal overactivity, breath holding (children), arrhythmia, cardiac outflow obstruction, drug abuse, hypoglycaemia, toxic confusional state, narcolepsy or cataplexy, transient global amnesia, psychologically mediated disorders.

Abnormal movements
Paroxysmal movement disorder, oculogyric crisis, tetany from hyperventilation, psychologically mediated disorders.

Neurological deficit
Transient ischaemic attack, stroke, migraine, psychologically mediated disorders.

Sleep attacks
Parasomnias, paroxysmal nocturnal dystonia.

Aetiology
- Causes include the following:

Cryptogenic.
Idiopathic (often familial).
Hippocampal sclerosis (most frequent cause of refractory temporal-lobe epilepsy).
Cortical dysplasia.
Tumour.
Trauma.
Infection: encephalitis, bacterial meningitis.
Vascular: infarct, haemorrhage.
Hypoxia.
Granuloma: tuberculosis, cystercercosis (in developing countries).

Epidemiology
- 1 person in 40 has a non-febrile seizure at some time in their life.
- The annual incidence in the general population is 1 in 2000.
- The prevalence of active epilepsy (seizure within past 2 years) is 1 in 200 of the general population and 1 in 150 people <15 years.

Classification
- Classification is important for investigation, treatment, and prognosis.

Partial
Simple: aware, responsive, no amnesia.
Complex: impaired awareness, responsiveness, recollection; possible automatisms (orofacial, speech, motor).
Secondary generalized: evolves from partial seizures.

Generalized
Absence, myoclonic, clonic, tonic, tonic–clonic, atonic.

Treatment

Diet and lifestyle
- Patients must avoid excessive fatigue or alcohol excesses.
- Restrictions may be placed on driving and some occupations.

Pharmacological treatment
- Drug interactions are complex: data sheets must be consulted before treatment is started or stopped.
- The following doses are for adults.

First line
Carbamazepine: for simple, complex, or secondarily generalized partial seizures and for tonic or clonic generalized seizures; 100 mg initially, average maintenance dose 600–2400 mg daily in 2–4 doses (retard: 2 doses daily).

Clonazepam: for myoclonic seizures (second-line treatment for absences, atonic seizures); 0.5 mg initially, average maintenance dose 0.5–3.0 mg daily in 1–2 doses.

Ethosuximide: for absences; 250 mg initially, average maintenance dose 500–1500 mg daily in 1–2 doses.

Valproate: for any seizure; valproate 500 mg initially, average maintenance dose 1000–2500 mg daily in 1–2 doses.

Second line
Acetazolamide: for partial seizures, absence or atypical absence, and atonic or myoclonic seizures; 250 mg initially, average maintenance dose 500–1500 mg daily in 2 doses.

Clobazam: for atypical absences, atonic partial, tonic, clonic, or tonic–clonic seizures; 10 mg initially, average maintenance dose 10–30 mg daily in 1–2 doses.

Gabapentin:* for partial seizures; 300 mg initially, average maintenance dose 900–1800 mg daily in 3 doses.

Lamotrigine:* for partial seizures, tonic, clonic, tonic–clonic, or atonic seizures, and absence or atypical absence; 50 mg initially, average maintenance dose 100–500 mg daily in 2 doses; if combined with valproate, initial dosage should be 25 mg on alternate days.

Phenobarbitone: for partial seizures, tonic, clonic, tonic–clonic, atonic, or myoclonic seizures, and atypical absences; 60 mg initially, average maintenance dose 60–180 mg daily as single dose.

Phenytoin: for partial, tonic, clonic, or tonic–clonic generalized seizures; 200–300 mg initially, average maintenance dose 200–400 mg daily in 1–2 doses; zero-order kinetics: measurement of serum drug concentration needed for optimal dosing.

Piracetam: for myoclonic seizures; 12 g initially, average maintenance dose 12–24 g daily in 3 doses.

Vigabatrin: for partial and tonic, clonic, or tonic–clonic seizures; 500 mg initially, average maintenance dose 2000–4000 mg daily in 1–2 doses.

Not a licensed indication for generalized seizures in the UK (1994).

General adverse effects
Acute, dose-related: sedation, dizziness, nausea, headaches.

Idiosyncratic: skin rash, severe bone-marrow suppression, liver failure, behavioural disorder (especially barbiturates in children, vigabatrin), psychosis (vigabatrin).

Chronic: cosmetic, soft-tissue, osteomalacia (phenytoin, barbiturates), cognition.

Treatment aims
To control seizures without drug side effects.

Prognosis
- Remission occurs in 70–80% of patients in 2–5 years; patients have a 30% chance of remission if epilepsy is active for 5 years.
- After the patient is in remission, the overall risk of relapse is 20% in 2 years if the patient remains on medication, and 40% if medication is tapered.
- Risk factors for relapse include juvenile myoclonic epilepsy, generalized spike-wave on EEG, structural brain damage, and difficulty obtaining seizure control.

Follow-up and management
Staged treatment strategy
- This can be followed as far as necessary.
1. Minimizing of epileptogenic stimuli: fever (in children), alcohol, excessive fatigue, epileptogenic drugs, photosensitivity.
2. Initial small dose of first-line drug.
3. Dosage increase if needed, up to maximum tolerated dose.
4. Review of diagnosis, cause, and compliance if no response after treatment.
5. Trial of other first-line drugs alone or combined (80% of patients best treated by monotherapy, 10–15% by two drugs).
6. Second-line drugs considered.
7. Gradual withdrawal of unhelpful drugs or drugs causing adverse effects.
8. Referral for novel drugs.
9. Referral for possible neurosurgical treatment of partial or secondarily generalized seizures.
10. Gradual drug withdrawal considered in patients free of seizures for 2–3 years.

Essential counselling
- Patients should be advised of the need to take medication regularly, reasonable expectations, driving license regulations, contraception and pregnancy, safe bathing, and safe cooking with a microwave.

Key references
Duncan JS: Modern treatment strategies for patients with epilepsy. *J R Soc Med* 1991, **84**:159–162.

Laidlaw J, Richens A, Chadwick D (eds): *Textbook of epilepsy* edn 4. Edinburgh: Churchill Livingstone, 1993.

Shorvon SD: Medical assessment and treatment of chronic epilepsy. *BMJ* 1991, **302**:363–366.

Facial pain, atypical
J.W. Scadding

Diagnosis

Definition
- Atypical facial pain is defined as facial pain of psychogenic origin, i.e. pain that has no demonstrable organic basis and that is a symptom of underlying psychiatric disturbance, often depression.

Symptoms
Pain: usually starts unilaterally, becoming more extensive with time; bilateral pain frequent; unremitting (often present for years), continuous, not paroxysmal (although shooting pains are sometimes described); may have provoking factors (e.g. touching the face, eating, drinking).

Pain centred on the teeth: often related by the patient to previous or current dental problems (many patients have had extensive dental examinations and treatment before seeking other medical help).

Pain outside the trigeminal area: particularly behind ears or on neck anteriorly.

Associated symptoms of depression or anxiety: patients are frequently worried about underlying organic disease, despite reassurance.

Signs
- No physical signs are manifest, although many patients have had extensive dental procedures, sometimes including total dental clearance.

Investigations
- Usually no investigation is required.

Sinus and dental radiography, CT, referral to dentist or ear, nose, and throat surgeon: occasionally needed to exclude underlying organic disease when clinical doubt about diagnosis exists.

Complications
- Usually no complications develop.

Severe disruption of personal life: due to underlying disturbance in some patients.

Differential diagnosis
Temporomandibular joint pain or referred nasopharyngeal pain (occasionally) when pain is unilateral and focal.

Trigeminal neuralgia: should not cause confusion; can be distinguished by typical paroxysmal, short-lived episodes of pain and triggering factors and by the usual good response to carbamazepine.

Aetiology
- Causes include the following:
Underlying depression.
Somatization disorder (usually with other somatic complaints) or conversion disorder.

Epidemiology
- Women are affected much more often than men.
- Age at onset is usually >40 years.

Treatment

Diet and lifestyle
- No special precautions are necessary.

Pharmacological treatment
- A trial of antidepressant treatment at therapeutic dosage is justified in all patients suspected of having atypical facial pain

Standard dosage	Amitriptyline 10–25 mg at night initially, gradually increasing to 75–150 mg at night, as tolerated.
Contraindications	Recent myocardial infarction, heart block, mania, porphyria.
Special points	Up to maximum tolerated doses have been consistently shown in controlled trials to provide partial relief of pain. Other agents may be equally effective (e.g. paroxetine, fluvoxamine, lofepramine).
Main drug interactions	Sedation enhanced by other sedatives.
Main side effects	Drowsiness, constipation, urinary hesitancy, dry mouth, blurred vision, postural hypotension, tachycardia, sweating, tremor.

Treatment aims
To relieve pain.
To treat underlying psychiatric morbidity, as far as possible.

Other treatments
Psychiatric assessment in many patients, followed by appropriate psychotherapy or drug treatment.

Prognosis
- Most patients show some response to psychotherapeutic or antidepressant drug treatment, but a few are refractory to all interventions.

Follow-up and management
- All patients should be followed long enough for the diagnosis to be established, for underlying organic disease to be thoroughly excluded in cases of diagnostic doubt, and for a response to treatment to be monitored.

Key references
Feinmann C, Harris M, Cawley R: Psychogenic facial pain: presentation and treatment. *BMJ* 1984, **288**:436.

Sharau Y *et al.*: The analgesic effect of amitriptyline on chronic facial pain. *Pain* 1987, **31**:199–209.

Guillain–Barré syndrome J.H. Rees

Diagnosis

Symptoms
Ascending, symmetrical weakness in all limbs: legs usually affected first, with patient initially noticing difficulty climbing stairs, rising from sitting, and, eventually, walking and standing.
Paraesthesiae of extremities, with distal sensory loss: in 95% of patients.
Neck, shoulder, back, and sciatic pain: may be severe.
Diplopia, drooling, nasal regurgitation of food and drink, slurred speech, weak cough: indicating cranial nerve involvement.
Dyspnoea: late symptom, reflecting intercostal and diaphragmatic weakness.
Fatigue: possibly profound and often persisting after return of muscle strength.
Hesitancy and urinary retention: usually when weakness more advanced (as distinct from acute myelopathy, in which sphincter symptoms appear early).

Signs
Weakness in limbs: flaccid, usually symmetrical, arms usually less severely affected.
Cranial nerve palsies: facial nerve most often affected, followed by bulbar muscles.
Hyporeflexia, areflexia: early.
Sensory deficit: may be absent or minor despite prominent symptoms.
Profound sensory loss: in some patients.
Ataxia, ophthalmoplegia, areflexia, with little or no weakness: Miller–Fisher syndrome; rare.

Investigations
Initial
Lumbar puncture: classically, raised protein concentration associated with normal cell count (albuminocytological dissociation); protein possibly normal within first week.
Serum potassium measurement: to exclude hypo- or hyperkalaemic paralysis.
Antinuclear antibodies analysis: positive in cases associated with SLE.
Liver function tests: often abnormal.
Heavy metal screening: only if clinically indicated.
Porphyrin screening: positive in acute intermittent porphyria which may manifest like Guillain–Barré syndrome.

Specialist
Nerve conduction studies: to identify multifocal conduction block and slowed conduction, confirming demyelinating neuropathy; studies early in disease may be only mildly abnormal, e.g. delayed or absent F waves; axonal degeneration may also occur.
Electromyography: in patients without sensory involvement, to help to rule out neuromuscular conduction block or muscle disease and to document axonal degeneration.
Anti-ganglioside antibody analysis: anti-GM$_1$ antibodies present in 20–30% of patients and associated with poor prognosis; anti-GQ1b antibodies associated with Miller–Fisher syndrome.

Complications
Death: if airway not adequately protected.
Lung collapse, hypostatic pneumonia, deep-vein thrombosis, pulmonary embolism, joint stiffness and contractures, pressure sores, anxiety and depression, pain: due to prolonged immobility.
Cardiac arrhythmias, including bradycardic and asystolic episodes, labile blood pressure: due to autonomic instability.

Differential diagnosis
Brainstem encephalitis or infarct.
Acute myelopathy.
Poliomyelitis.
Other neuropathies: porphyria, vasculitis, critical-illness neuropathy, drug-induced neuropathy, toxins (e.g. heavy metals, organophosphates).
Neuromuscular conduction block: myasthenia gravis, botulism.
Muscle disease: hypokalaemia, polymyositis, acute rhabdomyolysis.
Functional disease: hysteria, malingering.

Aetiology
- The cause of Guillain–Barré syndrome is unknown, but, in 60–70% of patients, it is associated with antecedent infection.
- Inflammatory demyelination with variable axonal degeneration in the peripheral nervous system due to autoimmune mechanisms is triggered by many different agents, including the following:

Viruses: cytomegalovirus, Epstein–Barr virus, HIV (usually around seroconversion).
Bacteria: *Mycoplasma pneumoniae*, *Campylobacter jejuni*.
Vaccines against rabies or swine influenza.
Surgery.

Epidemiology
- Guillain–Barré syndrome has become the most frequent cause of acute generalized neuromuscular paralysis in developed countries since the virtual eradication of poliomyelitis.
- The incidence is 1–2 in 100 000 population.
- More men than women are affected.
- The disease occurs more often in young women and elderly patients.
- It is not contagious.
- No seasonal variation is evident.

Treatment

Diet and lifestyle
- No special precautions are necessary.

Pharmacological treatment

General measures
Frequent measurement of vital capacity and continuous ECG monitoring during progressive phase.

Admission to intensive care unit if vital capacity falling rapidly or patient unable to swallow saliva.

Regular turning, mouth and eye care, aspiration of secretions.

Heparin 5000 units s.c. twice daily (antiembolism stockings of dubious value in paralysed patients).

Nasogastric feeding if patient has bulbar palsy or is too weak to eat.

- High-dose steroids are ineffective.

Plasma exchange
- Plasma 50 ml/kg exchanged five times over 5–10 days is indicated for any patient unable to walk unaided.
- Treatment should be initiated as soon as the diagnosis is made because it is more effective in early disease.

Immunoglobulin

Standard dosage	Immunoglobulin 0.4 g/kg i.v. daily for 5 days or 1 g/kg daily for 2 days.
Contraindications	IgA deficiency due to circulating anti-IgA antibodies.
Special points	May cause aseptic meningitis and acute on chronic renal failure.
Main drug interactions	None.
Main side effects	Fever, hypersensitivity reactions, fluid overload.

Treatment aims
To prevent respiratory failure.
To relieve pain.
To prevent complications of immobility.
To optimize functional recovery.

Other treatments
Early tracheostomy: to assist tracheal toilet and increase patient comfort.

Ventilatory assistance: if vital capacity 20 ml/kg or falling rapidly (oxygen saturation best monitored by pulse oximetry, not arterial blood gas measurement) or patient unable to protect airway.

Endocardial pacemaker: for episodes of bradycardia or sinus arrest.

Prognosis
- ~5% of patients relapse; 80% make a good recovery (median time to full independence, 9 months); 20% have permanent disability; 5% die.
- Poor prognostic indicators include age >40 years, rapid onset of weakness, ventilation, high titres of IgG anti-ganglioside GM_1 antibodies, and previous diarrhoeal illness.

Follow-up and management
- A high level of vigilance must be maintained until recovery has started and the tracheostomy has been closed.
- The patient should be reassured that recovery is probable and is nearly complete in most cases.
- Rehabilitation, e.g. physiotherapy, must be continued after discharge.
- Immunization injections must be avoided, especially tetanus toxoid, which has been associated with relapse.

Key references
Hughes RAC, Bihari D: Acute neuromuscular respiratory paralysis. *J Neurol Neurosurg Psychiatry* 1993, **56**:334–343.

van der Meché FGA, Schmitz PIM, the Dutch Guillain–Barré Study Group: A randomised trial comparing intravenous immune globulin and plasma exchange in Guillain–Barré, syndrome. *N Engl J Med* 1992, **326**:1123–1129.

Idiopathic polymyositis
J.A. Morgan-Hughes

Diagnosis

Symptoms
Weakness of proximal limb muscles: evolving over weeks or months, with difficulty in lifting, running, climbing stairs, getting up from a squatting position or low chair.

Dysphagia: due to weakness of pharyngeal muscles.

Muscle pain and tenderness, flitting arthralgia, inability to raise head, Raynaud's phenomenon, dyspnoea and cough: rare.

Signs
Weakness of neck flexors and proximal limb muscles, with retained or hyperactive tendon reflexes: muscle wasting minimal or absent in early stages.

Investigations

General
Full blood count, autoantibody screen, thyroid function tests: to identify overlap myositis and autoimmune thyroid disease.

Chest radiography, pulmonary function tests, ventilation perfusion studies: in patients with respiratory-muscle involvement or interstitial lung disease.

Video barium swallow: in patients with dysphagia.

ECG: to identify cardiac conduction defects and arrhythmias.

Special
Analysis of autoantibodies to aminoacyl transfer RNA synthetases: e.g. Jo-1 antibody in patients with interstitial lung disease (positive in 70%).

Estimation of muscle creatine kinase activity in serum: activity usually increased 3–30-fold; serum creatine kinase concentration tends to reflect disease activity and is useful in monitoring treatment.

Needle electromyography: increased insertional activity with fibrillation potentials, positive sharp waves, and repetitive discharges; short and long duration, low amplitude, polyphasic motor unit action potentials.

Muscle biopsy: essential to establish diagnosis; samples from mildly to moderately affected proximal limb muscle (biceps or triceps brachii, vastus lateralis) that has not been needled for electromyography.

Light microscopy (cryostat sections): endomysial collections of inflammatory cells (lymphocytes, plasma cells, histiocytes) surrounding necrotic and non-necrotic muscle fibres; regenerating muscle fibres with basophilic cytoplasm and prominent nucleoli; variable increase in endomysial connective tissue; necrotic fibres may be invaded by macrophages and lymphocytes.

Complications
Aspiration.

Interstitial lung disease.

Weakness of respiratory muscles.

Raynaud's phenomena: more common in dermatomyositis.

Cardiac conduction defects and dysrhythmias: rare.

Differential diagnosis

General
Inclusion body myositis, sarcoid myopathy, mixed connective tissue disease, SLE, rheumatoid arthritis, Sjögren's syndrome, systemic sclerosis.

Dermatomyositis, paraneoplastic myositis.

Eosinophilic polymyositis.

Myositides from other causes
HIV, influenza A and B virus, coxsackie virus, echovirus, adenovirus.

Spirochaetes: *Borrelia burgdorferi* (Lyme disease).

Protozoa: toxoplasma.

Helminths: trichinella, cysticerca.

Genetic disorders
Limb girdle dystrophies, late-onset nemaline myopathy, late-onset acid maltase deficiency, spinal muscular atrophy, lipid storage myopathies.

Drug-induced myopathies
Corticosteroids, penicillamine, lovastatin, cholestyramine, zidovudine, procainamide, chloroquine, colchicine, pancuronium with corticosteroids.

Other
Lambert–Eaton myasthenic syndrome.
Polymyalgia rheumatica.

Aetiology
- The cause of idiopathic polymyositis is unknown; the increased incidence of HLA haplotype B8, DR3 suggests genetic susceptibility.

Epidemiology
- Idiopathic polymyositis affects all age groups but occurs most often in the 5th and 6th decades.
- The annual incidence is ~3 in one million population.
- It is slightly more common in women.

Pathogenesis
- Idiopathic polymyositis is a major histocompatibility complex class 1 restricted T-cell-mediated myotoxicity.
- $CD8^+$ cytotoxic T-lymphocytes expressing common alpha-beta receptor invade and destroy initially non-necrotic muscle fibres.
- In a rare polymyositis variant, non-necrotic fibres are invaded by $CD4^-$, $CD8^-$ T lymphocytes expressing the gamma-delta receptor, which interacts with heat-shock proteins.

Treatment

Diet and lifestyle
- Idiopathic polymyositis is unaffected by diet or smoking; alcohol consumption, however, should be restricted.

Pharmacological treatment

First line

Standard dosage	Prednisolone 30–60 mg orally single daily dose for 4–6 weeks initially, tapered by 2.5–5. mg every 2–4 weeks depending on response and serum creatine kinase concentration to maintenance dose 10–15 mg daily. Azathioprine 25–50 mg orally daily initially, increased to 2.5–3 mg/kg daily over 4 weeks; maintenance 1–2 mg/kg daily.
Contraindications	*Prednisolone:* caution in hypertension, peptic ulcer, diabetes mellitus, osteoporosis, glaucoma, psychosis, epilepsy, previous tuberculosis. *Azathioprine:* rare hypersensitivity, pregnancy and breast feeding.
Special points	*Prednisolone:* calcium and potassium supplements may be needed on long-term treatment. *Azathioprine:* full blood count, platelet count, liver and renal function monitoring weekly for first 2 months, monthly for next 6 months, at least 3-monthly thereafter.
Main drug interactions	*Prednisolone:* phenytoin, phenobarbitone, oral anticoagulants, NSAIDs. *Azathioprine:* allopurinol, neuromuscular blocking agents, cytostatics.
Main side effects	*Prednisolone:* dyspepsia, peptic ulcer, weight gain, hypertension, cushingoid changes, potassium loss, glucose intolerance, cataract, osteoporosis, vertebral fractures, avascular osteonecrosis, euphoria, psychosis, muscle weakness. *Azathioprine:* nausea, vomiting, diarrhoea, bone-marrow suppression, disturbed liver function.

Second line
Pulsed methylprednisolone 0.5–1 g i.v. daily for 5 days.
Human immunoglobulin 0.4 g/kg i.v. daily for 5 days.

Third line
- The following agents are indicated in refractory cases, usually with maintenance dose of oral steroids:

Methotrexate 7.5–30 mg orally or 0.4–0.8 mg/kg i.v weekly (adults).

Cyclophosphamide 1–4 mg/kg orally daily.

Cyclosporin 2–6 mg/kg orally daily (adults).

- All are contraindicated in hypersensitivity, pregnancy, and lactation.
- Monitoring of full blood count, platelet count, liver and kidney function is needed.
- Side effects include nausea, vomiting, diarrhoea, alopecia, bone-marrow suppression, and hepatic and renal toxicity.

Treatment aims
To halt progression of disease and improve muscle strength.

Other treatments
Low-dose whole-body irradiation.
Total nodal irradiation.
- Irradiation is indicated only in severe cases refractory to all of the drug treatments.

Prognosis
- Remission is usually achieved and maintained in 50–60% of patients with first-line treatment.
- Second-, third-, and fourth-line treatments have provided encouraging results in small uncontrolled trials, but their respective merits in cases refractory to first-line drugs have not yet been clearly established.
- Death is rarely due to muscle weakness and usually results from cardiopulmonary complications.

Follow-up and management
- Most patients need maintenance treatment for at least 1–2 years after remission has been achieved.

Key references
Cherin P *et al.*: Efficacy of intravenous gammaglobulin therapy in chronic refractory polymyositis and dermatomyositis: an open study with 20 adult patients. *Am J Med* 1991, **91**:162–168.

Dalakas MC: Clinical, immunopathologic, and therapeutic considerations of inflammatory myopathies. *Clin Neuropharmacol* 1992, **15**:327–351.

Hohlfeld R, Engel AG: The role of gamma-delta T-lymphocytes in inflammatory muscle disease. In *Heat Shock Proteins and Gamma-Delta T-cells* vol 3. Edited by Brosnan CF. Basel: Karger, 1992, pp 75–85.

Mastaglia FL, Walton JN (eds): Inflammatory myopathies. In *Skeletal Muscle Pathology.* Edinburgh: Churchill Livingstone, 1992, pp 453–491.

Soueidan SA, Dalakas MC: Treatment of inclusion-body myositis with high-dose intravenous immunoglobulin. *Neurology* 1993, **43**:876–879.

Intracerebral haemorrhage
K. Ray Chaudhuri and R.S.J. Frackowiak

Diagnosis

Symptoms
Headache, nausea, vomiting, drowsiness: due to raised intracranial pressure.
Seizure: due to lobar haematoma, in 28–30% of patients.
Diplopia: due to mesencephalic haematoma.
Hiccoughs, dysarthia, facial hyperaesthesia: due to medullary haematoma.

Signs
Confusion, coma, papilloedema: due to raised intracranial pressure.
Hemiplegia, aphasia, homonymous visual-field defects: due to cortical haematomas.
Vertical-gaze palsy, skew deviation of eyes, miotic unreactive pupils: due to thalamic haematoma.
III nerve palsy, skew deviation of eyes: due to midbrain haematoma.
Horizontal-gaze palsy, pin-point reactive pupil, hyperpyrexia: due to pontine haematoma.
Ipsilateral V–VII nerve palsy, ataxia or nystagmus: due to cerebellar haematoma.

Investigations
- Laboratory tests are not diagnostic but may identify underlying abnormalities.

Haematology profile: to identify bleeding disorders.
Clotting profile: to identify disorders of coagulation.
ESR and CRP measurement: to identify vasculitic disorders.
Skull radiography: to identify skull fractures in head injury.
CT of brain: to distinguish between haemorrhage (high density) and infarction; must be done within 2 weeks of event (otherwise, may be indistinguishable from infarct); helps diagnosis of hydrocephalus, cerebral oedema, and fractures.
MRI of brain: examination of choice for cavernous angiomas; may help in identifying multiple lesions in patients with intracerebral metastasis.
Four-vessel angiography: to identify aneurysms (causing subarachnoid haemorrhage) or arteriovenous malformations; four-vessel because, in 20–25% of patients, several aneurysms may be present.

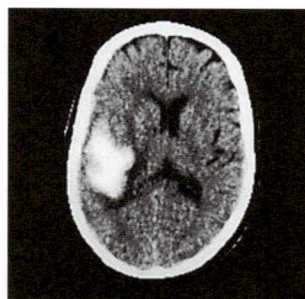

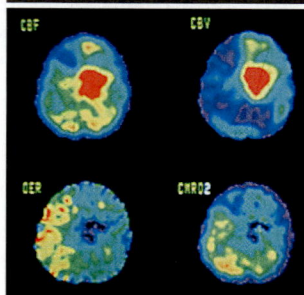

Intracerebral haemorrhage (top); fractional images of large arteriovenous malformation (bottom).

Complications
Tentorial herniation: with large supratentorial haematoma; herniation from below may occur rarely with large brainstem haematoma.
Foramen magnum herniation: preterminal event with large haematoma.
Hydrocephalus: with ventricular extension of haemorrhage from extrinsic pressure on CSF pathways, especially at aqueduct level and in cerebellar, caudate (75%), and thalamic haemorrhages.
Hyperpyrexia: usually in preterminal pontine haemorrhage.
Seizures: subcortical haematoma, which isolates strip of cortex.
Rebleed and vasospasm: in subarachnoid haemorrhage, risk of bleeding again is 35% within 1 month, with 42% mortality; vasospasm causing cerebral ischaemia occurs ~5 days after subarachnoid haemorrhage and may last ≥2 weeks.

Differential diagnosis
Haemorrhagic infarction: usually maximal neurodeficit from onset, raised intracranial pressure improbable, source of emboli present, CT showing mottled attenuation with minimal mass effect.
Subarachnoid haemorrhage: sudden (thunderclap) headache often preceded by warning (sentinel) headache (30–60%), meningism with possible neck stiffness, photophobia, III (posterior communicating artery aneurysm) or VI nerve palsies, confusion and emotional lability (anterior communicating artery aneurysm).
Haemorrhage into brain tumour: papilloedema, multiple-site haemorrhages, mass effect, non-contrasted CT showing high-density haemorrhage surrounding low-density centre.
Caudate haemorrhage: may cause headache, neck stiffness, and meningism.

Aetiology
- Causes include the following:

Hypertensive intracerebral haemorrhage.
Vascular malformations.
Bleeding into intracranial tumour.
Anticoagulant treatment (8–11% increased risk) and haemorrhagic disorders.
Sympathomimetic drugs (amphetamine, phenylpropanolamine).
Trauma.
Cerebral amyloid angiopathy (history of dementia in 10–30%, rare before 55 years).
Granulomatous vasculitis of CNS.
Necrotizing systemic vasculitis.

Epidemiology
- Intracerebral haemorrhage accounts for 10% of all strokes.
- Putaminal haemorrhage is the most usual variety of intracerebral haemorrhage (35%).

Treatment

Diet and lifestyle
- No special precautions are necessary.

Pharmacological treatment
- Lack of prospective data on randomized trials of intracerebral haemorrhage treatment has led to most patients being treated non-surgically.

For hypertension
- Severe hypertension should be treated to maintain mean arterial pressure between 60 and 70 mmHg.
- Intravenous beta blockers with additional alpha-blocking action (labetalol) and diuretics are useful.
- Nitroprusside, hydralazine, and calcium antagonists should be avoided; these are cerebral vasodilators and may worsen intracerebral pressure.

Standard dosage	Labetalol 2 mg/min i.v. infusion, 50–200 mg total.
Contraindications	Asthma, heart block.
Special points	Upright position must be avoided for 3 h after infusion.
Main drug interactions	Antiarrhythmics.
Main side effects	Postural hypotension.

For seizures
- Routine prophylaxis is not justified.
- Tonic–clonic convulsions need urgent control.

Standard dosage	Diazepam 10–20 mg i.v. and phenytoin 1 g i.v. over 30–45 min, with cardiac monitoring.
Contraindications	None of importance.
Special points	May precipitate in 5% glucose solution.
Main drug interactions	None of importance.
Main side effects	Nausea, vomiting, mental confusion.

For coagulopathies
- Patients should be given fresh frozen plasma, vitamin K, or platelet infusion.

For raised intracerebral pressure
- If facilities permit, intracerebral pressure can be monitored, and cerebral perfusion pressure (blood pressure minus intracerebral pressure) can be measured.
- Current techniques for measuring intracerebral pressure are invasive and have a 2–8% risk of intracranial infection.
- Intracerebral pressure should be maintained <20–25 mmHg.

Standard dosage	Mannitol 0.5 g/kg i.v. initially, with frusemide or subsequent albumin infusion.
Contraindications	Congestive cardiac failure, pulmonary oedema.
Special points	Mannitol should not be used when serum osmolality is >320 mOsm/L.
Main drug interactions	None of importance.
Main side effects	Chills, fever.

- Hyperventilation is indicated to maintain arterial carbon dioxide concentration at 3.5 kPa; excessive hyperventilation may produce cerebral ischaemia.
- Corticosteroids have no role in the management of raised intracerebral pressure caused by haemorrhage.

Treatment aims
To reverse neurodeficit.
To prevent complications.

Other treatments
- Direct evacuation of haematoma, ventricular drainage for hydrocephalus, or surgical obliteration for aneurysm is indicated for the following:
Cerebellar haemorrhage if signs of tegmental compression, haematoma 3 cm in diameter (on CT), hydrocephalus or obliteration of quadrigeminal cisterns.
Lobar haemorrhage (haematoma volume 20–40 ml), with progressive deterioration (100% mortality with medical treatment).
Acute hydrocephalus.
Subarachnoid haemorrhage: direct clipping aneurysms, thrombosis for giant aneurysms.
Haemorrhage from arteriovenous malformation: pre- and intraoperative embolization and staged resection.

Prognosis
- Large haematoma with progressive neurological deficits, coma at presentation, or ventricular extension have poor prognosis (overall mortality, 25–60%).
- Large pontine haemorrhage is usually fatal within 24–48 h.
- Caudate haemorrhage usually has a benign outcome despite ventricular extension and hydrocephalus.

Follow-up and management
- In patients needing anticoagulation, aspirin and dipyridamole treatment can be started a few days after surgery, warfarin probably after 1 month; earlier anticoagulation may be needed in certain types of aortic valve prosthesis.
- CT is mandatory if neurological deterioration occurs.

Key references
Kase CS: Intracerebral haemorrhage. In *Neurology in Clinical Practice*. Edited by W.G. Bradley *et al*. Oxford: Butterworth–Heinemann, 1991, pp 940–954.

Mohr JP *et al*.: The Harvard cooperative stroke registry: a prospective registry. *Neurology* 1978, **28**:754–762.

Meningitis, bacterial
L. Ginsberg and D.H. Kennedy

Diagnosis

Symptoms
Headache.
Neck and back pain and stiffness.
Vomiting.
Photophobia.
Fever.
Altered level of consciousness.
Seizures.

- Atypical clinical manifestations may occur in very young, elderly, or immunocompromised patients (highest-risk groups).

Signs
Nuchal rigidity: on flexion only, not on lateral rotation.
'Meningeal cry': high-pitched, in infants.
Kernig's sign: pain and hamstring spasm on passive knee extension with hip flexed.
Brudzinski's sign: spontaneous knee and hip flexion on attempted neck flexion.
Cranial nerve palsies and other focal signs.
Deteriorating level of consciousness: in up to 25% of patients.
Papilloedema, bulging fontanelle in infants: indicating raised intracranial pressure.
Pyrexia, tachycardia, shock, evidence of primary source of infection: e.g. pneumonia, endocarditis, sinusitis, otitis media.
Rash: in ~50% of patients with meningococcal infections, sometimes briefly erythematous before becoming petechial or purpuric.

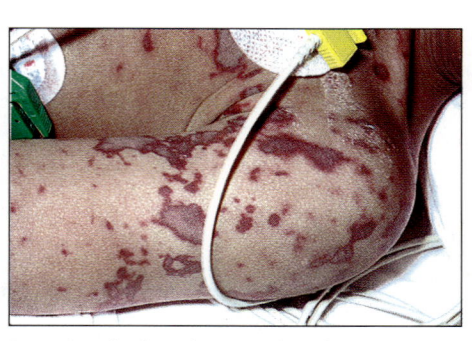

Purpuric rash of meningococcal meningitis.

Investigations
Lumbar puncture: in untreated acute bacterial meningitis, reveals turbid CSF under raised pressure, polymorph leucocytosis (hundreds or thousands of cells/µl), protein concentration usually >1 g/L, glucose concentration low. Specific tests for causative organisms include Gram stain, culture, sensitivity testing, fungal and tubercular microscopy and culture, and bacterial antigen immunoassay. Contraindications include papilloedema, deteriorating level of consciousness, and focal neurological signs; prepuncture cranial CT is needed in such patients to exclude mass lesion, e.g. in posterior fossa, that may mimic meningitis.
Full blood count: to detect neutrophil leucocytosis.
Coagulation screen and fibrin degradation product analysis: for disseminated intravascular coagulation.
Electrolyte analysis: to detect hyponatraemia.
Blood culture: may be positive when CSF sterile.
Chest and skull (sinus) radiography: to identify primary source of infection.

Complications
Seizures, focal CNS signs, raised intracranial pressure, subdural effusion, cerebral or subdural abscess formation, hydrocephalus (obstructive or communicating).
Septic shock, disseminated intravascular coagulation with adrenal haemorrhage: Waterhouse–Friderichsen syndrome, complication of meningococcal meningitis.
Inappropriate antidiuretic hormone secretion: in <10% of patients.
Arthritis: septic or immune complex, in <10% of meningococcal infections.
Behavioural disturbances, mental retardation, hearing loss, epilepsy, cranial nerve palsies, visual and motor deficits: long-term complications (more usual in *S. pneumoniae* infections; <30% of patients).

Differential diagnosis
- Few patients, even with severe headache and fever, have meningitis.

Viral meningitis, especially enteroviruses, mumps.
Intercurrent infections, especially influenza A and B with meningism.
Cranial infections: cerebral abscess, sinusitis, throat infections.
Noninfective meningitis: subarachnoid haemorrhage, leukaemic infiltration, Mollaret's meningitis (recurrent fever, meningeal signs, and CSF pleocytosis).
Autoimmune diseases, vasculitis.
Chemical meningitis, e.g. intrathecal drugs.

Aetiology
- 70–90% of cases of bacterial meningitis are due to one of three organisms:

Neisseria meningitidis (most common overall cause, mainly group B in UK).
Haemophilus influenzae (type b).
Streptococcus pneumoniae.

- Other organisms found in specific at-risk groups include the following:

Enterobacteriaceae, group B streptococci in neonates.
Listeria monocytogenes in neonates and immunocompromised patients.
Mycobacterium tuberculosis in patients from developing countries and immunocompromised patients.
Staphylococci in patients with head trauma or neurosurgical shunts.

Epidemiology
- The incidence of bacterial meningitis is ~5–10 in 100 000 annually in developed countries.
- The three common organisms have characteristic patterns of occurrence: *Neisseria meningitidis* in epidemics, *Haemophilus influenzae* in children <5 years, *Streptococcus pneumoniae* in patients aged >40 years (especially alcoholic, splenectomized, and sickle-cell anaemic patients).
- *H. influenzae* type b immunization is rapidly reducing the incidence of *H. influenzae* meningitis in the UK.

Treatment

Diet and lifestyle
- No special precautions are necessary.

Pharmacological treatment

General management
- Bacterial meningitis may prove fatal within hours; successful treatment depends on early diagnosis and i.v. administration of appropriate antibiotics in antimeningitic doses (intrathecal antibiotics not recommended); until the causative organism and its antibiotic sensitivities have been identified, broad-spectrum agents should be used (e.g. benzylpenicillin with chloramphenicol, cefotaxime, ceftriaxone).
- GPs should give patients with suspected meningococcal meningitis a single i.v. or i.m. injection of benzylpenicillin before urgent transfer to hospital.
- If lumbar puncture is delayed by the need for pre-puncture CT, antibiotic treatment should be started before the scan, after blood cultures.
- Other measures include bed-rest, analgesics, antipyretics, anticonvulsants for seizures (prophylactic use not recommended), and supportive measures for coma, shock, raised intracranial pressure, electrolyte disturbances, and bleeding disorders; routine corticosteroids are not recommended but may be beneficial in severely ill children, especially those with *Haemophilus influenzae* infection.
- Treatment should ideally be bactericidal with a high therapeutic ratio, the drug penetrating the CSF in adequate concentrations; very high i.v. doses may be needed despite damage to the blood–brain barrier in meningitis.

Against *Neisseria meningitidis* and *Streptococcus pneumoniae*

Standard dosage	*Adults:* benzylpenicillin 14.4 g (24 MU) i.v. daily in divided doses (usually 4 MU initially, then 2 MU 2-hourly; can be relaxed to 4- or 6-hourly regimen with evidence of clinical improvement, usually within 48–72 h); treatment should continue for 7 days after the patient has become afebrile (14 days for *S. pneumoniae* infection). *Children and infants:* benzylpenicillin 100–300 mg/kg daily depending on age, according to data sheet.
Contraindications	Penicillin hypersensitivity; caution in renal impairment, history of allergy.
Special points	Other options include cefotaxime, ceftriaxone, and chloramphenicol (*S. pneumoniae* with decreased penicillin sensitivity unusual in UK).
Main drug interactions	None.
Main side effects	Sensitivity reactions.

Against *Haemophilus influenzae*

Standard dosage	Chloramphenicol 50–100 mg/kg i.v. (orally when feasible) daily in 4 divided doses, reduced to 50 mg/kg daily as soon as clinically indicated. *Neonates:* 25 mg/kg daily (plasma concentrations must be monitored); treatment should continue for 7 days after the patient has become afebrile.
Contraindications	Porphyria; avoided in pregnancy and lactation; caution in hepatic or renal impairment (reduced dose).
Special points	Many now prefer cefotaxime or ceftriaxone.
Main drug interactions	Phenytoin.
Main side effects	Blood disorders including aplastic anaemia (rare: blood counts monitored), 'grey syndrome' in neonates (plasma concentrations monitored), peripheral and optic neuropathy (rare).

Prevention
- Chemoprophylaxis (using rifampicin or ciprofloxacin) is indicated for household contacts and index patients before hospital discharge.
- Immunization against *Haemophilus influenzae* infection (using *H. influenzae* type b vaccine) is recommended routinely for children at the ages of 2, 3, and 4 months.

Treatment aims
To secure survival and prevent persistent neurological complications.
To reduce the of recurrence by treating any predisposing cause.
To prevent spread to close contacts.

Prognosis
- Mortality is ~10% overall, 5–10% from *Haemophilus influenzae* infection, 5–10% from *Neisseria meningitidis* infection, and 10–30% from *Streptococcus pneumoniae* infection.
- Long-term sequelae are 9–22%, 4–6%, and 14–40%, respectively.

Follow-up and management
- Repeat lumbar puncture to monitor treatment is not necessary if the patient is improving.
- Bacteriological relapse needs immediate reinstitution of treatment.
- Acute meningitis is a notifiable disease in England and Wales; meningococcal infection is notifiable in Scotland.
- Adults should be reviewed at 3 months, children at 6–12 months, and neonates for longer to detect any long-term sequelae.

Causes of treatment failure
Wrong diagnosis: e.g. tuberculosis, abscess.
Wrong drug: poor CSF penetration, antimicrobial resistance.
Wrong route: intraventricular instillation needed for ventriculitis with 'resistant' infections.
Poor-risk patient: extremes of age, immunocompromise.
Unrecognized complication: treatable raised intracranial pressure, abscess or ventriculitis, subdural effusion or abscess (treatable); vasculitis, cerebritis (less treatable).
Shock.

Key references
Finch RG, Mandragos C: Corticosteroids in bacterial meningitis. *BMJ* 1991, **302**:607–608.
Quagliarello V, Scheld WM: Bacterial meningitis: Pathogenesis, pathophysiology and progress. *N Engl J Med* 1992, **327**:864–872.
Tunkel AR, Wispelweg B, Scheld M: Bacterial meningitis: recent advances in pathophysiology and treatment. *Ann Intern Med* 1990, **112**:610–623.

Migraine
A.H.V. Schapira

Diagnosis

Definition
Migraine with aura (classic migraine): characterized by aura followed by episodic unilateral throbbing headache, with gastrointestinal upset, photophobia, and phonophobia; auras usually last 10–20 min but can persist for up to 1 h; laterality of neurological disturbance not related to side of ensuing headache.

Migraine without aura (common migraine): characterized by episodic unilateral or bilateral headache, gastrointestinal upset, photo- or phonophobia, but no aura.

- Migraine headaches are paroxysmal, lasting from a few hours up to 3 days, but with periods of complete relief between attacks.

Migrainous neuralgia (cluster headache): 90% of sufferers men; paroxysmal very severe unilateral periorbital pain lasting 0.5–2 h, once or twice daily (often at night) for weeks, with months or years of relief between bouts; often associated with Horner's syndrome, lacrimation and nasal stuffiness ipsilateral to pain.

Ophthalmoplegic migraine: recurrent attacks of III or VI cranial-nerve palsies associated with headache; resolution of deficit may be delayed by several days.

Retinal migraine: uniocular visual loss involving scotoma or altitudinal defect followed by headache.

Hemiplegic migraine: recurrent attacks of hemiparesis of rapid onset followed by headache; weakness may last hours.

- Migraine variants are diagnoses of exclusion; other more serious causes of the clinical picture (e.g. stroke, aneurysmal leak, transient ischaemic attack) must be excluded before the diagnosis is accepted.

Symptoms
- The aura of classic migraine may be visual (in 50% of patients) or sensory (in 30%) or occasionally may involve dysphasia or motor deficit.

Visual auras: teichopsia, fortification spectra, fragmentation, scotoma, homonymous hemianopia.

Transient tingling or numbness: sensory symptoms; upper limbs more frequently involved than lower limbs.

Signs
- Common migraine may have no signs.
- The scotomas, hemianopia, and sensorimotor phenomena of classic migraine may be detected if the aura is still present at the time of examination.
- Prolonged deficit requires exclusion of other causes.

Investigations
- Investigation is not needed if the diagnosis of migraine is well founded; it is needed when the diagnosis is in doubt and in patients with residual neurological deficit after migraine.
- Investigation including the following is aimed at excluding alternative diagnoses:

ESR measurement: for temporal arteritis.
Radiography, MRI: for cervical spondylosis.
CT or MRI: for tumour, vascular malformation, hydrocephalus.
CSF analysis: for subarachnoid bleed, arteritis.
Angiography: for aneurysmal bleeding.

Complications
Migrainous infarction: rare, usually posterior parietal or occipital.

Differential diagnosis
Tension headache: continuous dull, pressure-like pain over vertex or around head; lasts weeks to years; nausea occasional, vomiting rare; may coexist with migraine to produce pattern of constant headache with episodic exacerbations.

Temporal arteritis: in patients usually aged >65 years with unilateral temporal pain and tenderness; visual disturbances may occur before blindness; high ESR.

Local disease: e.g. glaucoma, sinusitis, nasopharyngeal lesions, vascular abnormalities.

Tumour: cerebral tumours usually manifest with epilepsy, focal neurological deficits, clouded consciousness, and rarely headache, although this may develop later.

Haemorrhage: abrupt onset of severe headache, usually occipital and associated with neck stiffness and photophobia; aneurysms may produce pressure effects; no history of recurrent similar headaches.

Arteriopathies: SLE may manifest with migraine; polyarteritis nodosa may produce headache and transient neurological deficits.

Aetiology
- Migraine is probably due to a combination of genetic predisposition and environmental triggers (e.g. stress, certain foods) causing changes in neurotransmitter release (5-HT), with alteration in cerebral blood flow and pain in the distribution of the trigeminal nerve.

Epidemiology
- The prevalence is ~5% in men and 12–15% in women, although some investigators have quoted prevalence rates as high as 60–70%.
- The incidence increases from puberty to young adulthood; onset >50 years is unusual.

Treatment

Diet and lifestyle
- Dietary precipitants, e.g. chocolate, cheese, coffee, red wine, should be avoided in sensitive patients.
- Stress is a common precipitant of migraine: appropriate measures may reduce the frequency of attacks.
- The oral contraceptive pill should be avoided; it is contraindicated in migraine with focal neurological deficits.

Pharmacological treatment
- Many patients treat attacks satisfactorily with rest, darkness, and a simple analgesic.

For migraine with and without aura: acute
- Patients with gastrointestinal disturbance and more severe headache may benefit from a combination of analgesic and antiemetic; the antiemetic not only reduces vomiting but increases gastric emptying thereby improving absorption of the analgesic.
- More severe attacks unresponsive to this treatment may be treated by sumatriptan or ergotamine.

Standard dosage	Sumatriptan 50 mg or 100 mg orally at onset or 6 mg s.c. by autoinjector; maximum 200 mg tablet or 12 mg s.c. in 24 h. Ergotamine in varying doses according to route, e.g. 2 mg by suppository, tablet, or inhaler.
Contraindications	*Sumatriptan:* patients >65 years or with history of coronary disease; to be avoided in children or hemiplegic migraine. *Ergotamine:* vascular disease, active infection, hemiplegic migraine.
Special points	*Sumatriptan:* effective in 60% at 2 h and 80% at 4 h. *Ergotamine:* maximum dose of preparation must not be exceeded because of risk of vasospasm.
Main drug interactions	*Sumatriptan:* ergotamine, monoamine oxidase inhibitors, lithium. *Ergotamine:* beta blockers, methysergide, and sumatriptan all increase risk of vasospasm.
Main side effects	*Sumatriptan:* chest pain or tightness, light-headedness, transient pain at site of injection. *Ergotamine:* nausea, vomiting, headache (possible due to overuse), tingling, chest tightness.

For common and classic migraine: prophylactic
- Beta blockers or 5-HT antagonists should be considered for ≥2 attacks a month; 6–12 months' effective treatment may allow withdrawal at original frequency.

Standard dosage	Propranolol 20–80 mg daily may be sufficient; larger doses occasionally needed. Pizotifen 0.5 mg initially, with weekly increments of 0.5 mg to 1.5–3.0 mg maintenance dose. Other options: atenolol, nadolol, timolol, metoprolol, amitriptyline.
Contraindications	*Beta blockers:* asthma, cardiac failure, heart block.
Main drug interactions	See drug data sheets.
Main side effects	*Beta blockers:* bradycardia, heart failure, bronchospasm, vasoconstriction. *Pizotifen:* drowsiness, weight gain.

For migrainous neuralgia: acute
Sumatriptan or ergotamine.
Oxygen (>40%), if not contraindicated.
Prednisolone 60 mg (occasionally helpful).

For migrainous neuralgia: prophylactic
Short-term sumatriptan or ergotamine before predicted onset of attack.
Lithium and methysergide in refractory patients: regular monitoring of lithium concentrations and checking of thyroid function needed; methysergide used intermittently (4–5 months every 6 months) to reduce risk of retroperitoneal fibrosis.

Treatment aims
To provide adequate relief from symptoms.
To adjust treatment appropriately to severity and frequency of attacks.
To minimize effect of migraine on work and leisure activities.

Prognosis
- Most patients respond well to acute or prophylactic treatment, or both.
- The frequency of migraine often declines with age but only occasionally disappears.

Follow-up and management
- Regular follow-up in hospital is not required for uncomplicated migraine.
- GPs should assess the response to treatment until appropriate and successful treatment is established.
- Prophylactics should be continued for 6–12 months before withdrawal; subsequent re-use is possible for relapse.

Key references
Baumel B: Migraine. *Neurology* 1994, **44** (suppl 3):S13–S17.

Dalessio DJ: Diagnosing the severe headache. *Neurology* 1994, **44** (suppl 3):S6–S12.

Motor neurone disease
C.M. Lloyd and P.N. Leigh

Diagnosis

Definition
- Motor neurone disease is one of many motor neurone disorders. The term covers amyotrophic lateral sclerosis (the most usual form), progressive muscular atrophy, and progressive bulbar palsy (thought to be variants of the same disorder).
- The disorder is progressive and is characterized by degeneration of cortical, brainstem, and spinal-cord motor neurones.

Symptoms
Cramps or fasciculations: may precede other symptoms by months.
Asymmetrical weakness or wasting of proximal or distal upper limb muscles: presenting symptom in 40–60% of patients with upper limb involvement and 20% with lower limb involvement (unilateral foot drop common).
Dysarthria: presenting complaint in 25–30%, usually followed by limb involvement; 70–80% presenting with limb involvement develop dysarthria, culminating in anarthria.
Dysphagia: accompanying dysarthria.
Breathlessness: usually due to diaphragmatic weakness.
Minor sensory symptoms.
Changes in character and behaviour: in 5–10%.
Frontal-lobe dementia: in a few.

Signs
Typical disease
Fasciculations, wasting, depressed reflexes: lower motor neurone signs.
Spasticity, slowing of alternating movements, brisk tendon reflexes, Babinski responses: upper motor neurone signs.

- Typical motor neurone disease has lower and upper motor neurone signs in several regions (cranial nerves, arms, legs), with evidence of disease progression.
- Signs are usually asymmetrical in the early stages, with no evidence of sensory signs or bladder or bowel involvement.

Bulbar involvement
Emotional lability, with uncontrolled laughter and crying, brisk jaw jerk, spasticity of facial muscles, spastic dysarthria, dysphagia, spasticity of tongue: indicating upper motor neurone involvement (pseudobulbar palsy).
Wasting of facial and jaw muscles, fasciculation and wasting of tongue, nasal speech, dysphagia, bovine cough: indicating lower motor neurone involvement (bulbar palsy).

Investigations
- Laboratory results are usually normal (creatine kinase activity may be 2–3 times normal).
Electromyography: shows widespread anterior horn cell damage; nerve conduction studies usually normal; electrophysiology supports clinical diagnosis and excludes root and plexus lesions or motor neuropathy; characteristic abnormalities include fibrillation potentials and positive sharp waves, fasciculations, abnormal motor units of increased amplitude and duration.
MRI or myelography: may be needed to exclude spinal-cord or root compression; MRI may show altered signal in posterior limb of internal capsule in region of degenerating corticospinal-tract fibres.
Muscle biopsy: to exclude other diagnoses in atypical cases, not routinely indicated; confirms denervation, with small angular fibres and prominent fibre type grouping.

Complications
Depression: social and emotional isolation, especially in patients with severe dysarthria.
Dysphagia: leading to weight loss, malnutrition, dehydration, and aspiration.
Bronchopulmonary infections: related to aspiration and ventilatory muscle weakness.
Venous thrombosis and pulmonary embolism.
Constipation: due to pelvic and abdominal wall weakness and poor fluid intake.
Ventilatory failure: usual cause of death.

Differential diagnosis
Myasthenia gravis with bulbar onset.
Post-poliomyelitis muscular atrophy syndrome.
Cervical myelopathy.
Intramedullary spinal-cord lesions.
Motor neuronopathy.
Late-onset spinal muscular atrophy.
Kennedy's syndrome.
Late-onset hexosaminidase A deficiency.

Aetiology
- 5–10% of patients have a family history suggesting autosomal-dominant inheritance.
- Point mutations of the gene encoding Cu/Zn superoxide dismutase on chromosome 21q are present in 10–20% of families.
- X-linked bulbospinal neuronopathy (Kennedy's syndrome) is caused by a mutation of the gene encoding the androgen receptor.
- The cause of sporadic motor neurone disease is unknown; free radical damage and excitotoxicity have been implicated.

Epidemiology
- The incidence of motor neurone disease in Europe and North America is 2 in 100 000.
- The prevalence is 3–6 in 100 000.
- The male : female ratio is 1.5 : 1.
- The peak onset in sporadic disease is at 60 years, about a decade earlier in familial disease.
- The incidence may be increasing, especially in older age groups.

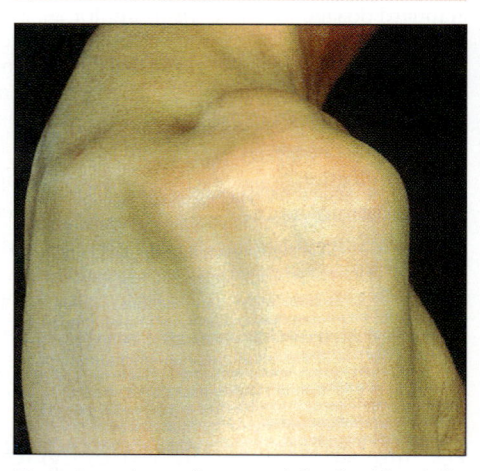

Marked muscle wasting around the shoulder girdle in a patient with motor neurone disease.

Treatment

Diet and lifestyle
- Dietary advice is needed for patients with dysphagia or who are being treated by percutaneous endoscopic gastrostomy.

Pharmacological treatment
- No drug treatment is known to alter the course of the disease; drugs are used to control the symptoms.

Benzhexol, hyoscine (orally or transdermal patches), atropine for drooling.

Quinine for cramps.

Baclofen, dantrolene sodium, diazepam for spasticity.

Amitryptyline, dothiepin, fluoxetine for depression.

Lactulose, danthron, isphagula husk for constipation (with increased fluid intake).

Opiates, diazepam for symptomatic relief of dyspnoea.

- The antiglutamate agent riluzole may slow disease progression; a definitive trial is in progress.

Non-pharmacological treatment
Physiotherapy.

Counselling for depression.

Percutaneous endoscopic gastrostomy for dysphagia (best considered early).

Radiotherapy to the parotid glands for excess saliva.

Assisted ventilation for respiratory failure: techniques available include nasal intermittent positive airway pressure ventilation, a rocking bed, a cuirasse, or, in exceptional circumstances, a tracheostomy and intermittent positive pressure ventilation.

Treatment aims
To maintain patient's independence and quality of life.
To alleviate symptoms.

Prognosis
- 80–90% of patients develop upper and lower motor neurone signs at some stage.
- 10% show only lower motor neurone signs (progressive muscular atrophy).
- The median survival is 4 years (2 years for bulbar onset).
- 5–10% of patients survive for 5 years or more; a few live for 15 years or more.
- Patients with only lower motor neurone signs tend to have a better prognosis than those with typical motor neurone disease.

Follow-up and management
- A multidisciplinary neuro-care team approach is recommended; the team comprises neurologist, physiotherapist, occupational therapist, speech therapist, dietitian, social worker, and other relevant health-care workers. Each patient may be allocated a 'key worker' to integrate the activities of the team.
- Communication and other aids should be provided, and the home adapted.
- Patients might require referral to a hospice.

Patient support
The Motor Neurone Disease Association, P.O. Box 246, Northampton NN1 2PR, tel 01604 250 505.

Key references
Bensimon G, Lacomblez V, Meininger V, the ALS/Riluzole Study group: A controlled trial of riluzole in amyotrophic lateral sclerosis. *N Eng J Med* 1994, **330**:585–591.

Leigh PN, Ray-Chaudhuri K: Motor neurone disease. *J Neurol Neurosurg Psychiatry* 1994, **57**:886–896.

Rosen DR *et al.*: Mutations in the Cu/Zn superoxide gene are associated with familial amyotrophic lateral sclerosis. *Nature* 1993, **362**:59–62.

Zeman S *et al.*: Excitatory amino acids, free radicals and the pathogenesis of motor neurone disease. *Neuropath Appl Neurobiol* 1994, **20**:219–231.

Multiple sclerosis — W.I. McDonald

Diagnosis

Symptoms

Relapsing and remitting
- 90% of patients initially have relapses and remissions of neurological disturbance attributable to CNS white matter lesions, including the following:

Visual loss.	Weakness.	Urinary urgency.
Diplopia.	Incoordination.	Pain.
Vertigo.	Paraesthesiae.	Impotence.

Progressive
- Progressive disease takes two forms.

Primary, in 10%: progressive from onset without remission.

Secondary, in 50%: progressive after an initially relapsing and remitting course.

Signs
- Signs are variable but include the following:

Optic atrophy.	Weakness.	Sensory loss.
Nystagmus.	Spasticity.	

Investigations
- The diagnosis is primarily clinical and depends on the demonstration of two or more necessarily separate CNS lesions in a patient with a history of two characteristic episodes.

- Investigations provide invaluable support, but none of the abnormalities is specific to multiple sclerosis.

Evoked potentials: especially visual and somatosensory, to detect subclinical involvement and provide evidence for demyelination.

MRI: to detect subclinical involvement and the characteristic pattern of lesions.

CSF analysis: for electrophoresis to show oligoclonal IgG, present in 90% of patients.

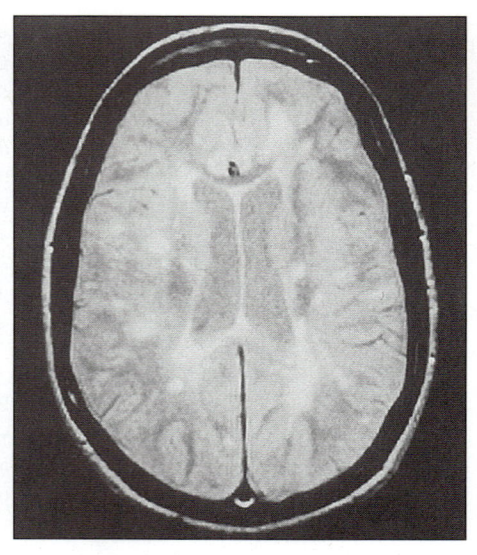

T_2 weighted MRI showing areas of abnormal signal in the cerebral hemispheres in a patient with multiple sclerosis.

Complications
Visual loss, paresis, tremor, incontinence: due to persistent neurological deficit.

Significant cognitive impairment: may occur late.

Differential diagnosis

Relapsing and remitting
Collagen vascular disease.
Neurosarcoidosis.

Progressive
Compression: e.g. tumour, craniocervical anomaly.
Spinocerebellar degeneration.
Motor neurone disease.

Aetiology
- Causes include the following:

Genetic predisposition: HLA association, but probably additional factors.

Extrinsic factor: probably infective, possibly viral.

Epidemiology
- 1 in 800 population in the UK is affected by multiple sclerosis.
- 20% of patients have an affected relative.
- The female:male ratio is 2:1.

Treatment

Diet and lifestyle

- Patients should be assessed for functional limitations to determine appropriate modifications in lifestyle (neurorehabilitation, physiotherapy, occupational therapy).
- A diet low in animal fat is often recommended, but convincing evidence of a specific effect is lacking.

Pharmacological treatment

For symptoms

Standard dosage	*For spasticity:* baclofen initially 5 mg 3 times daily; maximum 100 mg daily. *For urinary frequency, urgency, and incontinence:* oxybutynin 5 mg 2–3 times daily.
Contraindications	*Baclofen:* peptic ulceration. *Oxybutynin:* bladder outflow obstruction, glaucoma.
Main drug interactions	*Baclofen:* muscle relaxants. *Oxybutynin:* antimuscarinics.
Main side effects	*Baclofen:* weakness, sedation enhanced by alcohol. *Oxybutynin:* antimuscarinic effects.

- For impotence, patients should be referred to a specialist for intracorporal pharmacotherapy.

For relapse

- Steroids are indicated when functional impairment is significant.

Standard dosage	Methylprednisolone 1 g in 250 ml normal saline solution i.v. over 30 min daily for 3 days. Alternatively, oral steroids, although value uncertain: 3-week course, starting at 60 mg daily.
Contraindications	Hypertension, diabetes, peptic ulceration, systemic infection, history of tuberculosis, osteoporosis, history of psychiatric disorder.
Special points	Frequent use should be avoided.
Main drug interactions	Other drugs causing hypokalaemia, drugs inducing liver enzymes.
Main side effects	Fluid retention, hypokalaemia, depression, psychosis, hypertension, glucose intolerance, peptic ulceration, osteoporosis.

To modify the course

- Much interest is being taken at present in the use of beta interferon. The published evidence, however, shows only a modest reduction in relapse rate but a more marked effect on MRI activity. Beta interferon has not, however, been shown to affect the rate of progression of neurological impairment. Until more information is available, the widespread use of beta interferon cannot be recommended.

Treatment aims

To alleviate symptoms.
To control relapse.
To modify course.

Prognosis

- Prognosis is very variable, ranging from death in a few months to survival without disability for 50 years.
- At least one-third of patients have little disability after 15 years.

Follow-up and management

- Follow-up depends on the condition of the patient.
- In complete remission, regular follow-up is not needed.
- When significant disability is present, assessment in a comprehensive neurological rehabilitation clinic is useful as the condition changes.

Patient support

Multiple Sclerosis Society, 24 Effie Road, London SW6 1EE, tel 0171 736 6267.

Key references

Matthews WB *et al.* (eds): *McAlpine's Multiple Sclerosis.* Edinburgh: Churchill Livingstone, 1991.

McDonald WI: New treatments for multiple sclerosis. *BMJ* 1995, **310**:345–346.

Myasthenia gravis J. Newsom-Davis

Diagnosis

Symptoms
Painless muscle weakness increasing with exercise ('fatigue').

Drooping eyelids (one or both) and double vision.

- Weakness may characteristically also affect smiling, swallowing, chewing, speaking, neck muscles, arm elevation, elbow extension, hand movements, walking, and breathing.
- Symptoms are worst at the end of the day.

Signs
Fatiguable ptosis.

Variable limitation of eye movement.

Impaired eye closure.

Snarling smile.

Nasal speech.

Fatiguable weakness of affected muscles.

Wasting: rare.

Brisk tendon reflexes.

Investigations
Serum acetylcholine receptor antibody analysis: raised titre specific for myasthenia gravis.

Edrophonium ('Tensilon') test: if patient is seronegative.

Clinical electrophysiology: increased decrement; increased jitter on single fibre study.

CT of thymus: for thymoma.

Striated muscle antibody analysis: positive in 90% of patients with thymoma, 50% of patients with generalized myasthenia gravis.

Complications
Myasthenic crisis: acute respiratory or bulbar symptoms.

Cholinergic crisis: due to excess anticholinesterase treatment; causing hypersalivation, lacrimation, increased sweating, vomiting, and miosis.

Local or pleural spread of thymoma.

Differential diagnosis
Lambert–Eaton myasthenic syndrome.

Congenital myasthenia gravis.

Chronic fatigue syndrome.

Aetiology
- Antibodies to muscle acetylcholine receptors (AChRs) cause receptor loss.
- Immune response genes influence susceptibility.
- Penicillamine may induce AChR antibodies and typical myasthenia gravis.
- Placental transfer of AChR antibodies causes neonatal myasthenia gravis in the offspring of 12% of mothers with the disease.
- 'Seronegative' myasthenia gravis is antibody-mediated: the antigenic target is not known.

Epidemiology
- The prevalence is 8–9 in 100 000 people.
- The annual incidence is 0.4 in 100 000.
- All races are susceptible; restricted ocular myasthenia gravis is more frequent in Asian patients.
- The disease is manifest from infancy to extreme old age.

Clinical classification
- The clinical subgroup influences treatment selection; typical features are shown below.

Early onset (50%)
Symptom distribution: generalized.
Age at onset: <40 years.
Thymus pathology: hyperplasia.
Acetylcholine receptor (AChR) antibody titre: high.

Thymoma (10%)
Symptom distribution: generalized.
Age at onset: any.
Thymus pathology: thymoma.
AChR antibody titre: intermediate.

Late onset (25%)
Symptom distribution: generalized or ocular.
Age at onset: >40 years.
Thymus pathology: atrophy/normal.
AChR antibody titre: low.

Seronegative (15%)
Symptom distribution: ocular or generalized.
Age of onset: any.
Thymus pathology: atrophy/normal.
AChR antibody titre: absent.

Treatment

Diet and lifestyle
- No special precautions are necessary.

Pharmacological treatment

Management strategy
- Treatment should be given under specialist supervision and is usually attempted in the following order:

Anticholinesterase for immediate symptom control.
Plasma exchange in severe cases (see Other treatments).
Thymectomy in some patients (see Other treatments).
Prednisolone.
Prednisolone and azathioprine.
Other immunosuppressive treatment (cyclosporin, cyclophosphamide).

- Only if a particular treatment fails or is not indicated should the next one be tried.

Anticholinesterase
- This provides symptomatic relief in all patients.

Standard dosage	Pyridostigmine 30–120 mg 5 times daily. Propantheline 15 mg 3-4 times daily, if necessary, to control adverse gastrointestinal effects.
Contraindications	Intestinal or urinary obstruction.
Main drug interactions	Antiarrhythmics (quinidine), antibacterials (aminoglycosides, clindamycin, lincomycin and polymyxins), antimalarials (chloroquine), beta blockers (propanolol), lithium, muscle relaxants.
Main side effects	Diarrhoea, abdominal cramps, increased salivation, nausea and vomiting.

Prednisolone
- Prednisolone is indicated for restricted ocular myasthenia gravis (outpatients) and generalized disease of moderate severity unresponsive to other treatments (inpatients).

Standard dosage	*Outpatients:* prednisolone 5 mg single dose on alternate days, increased by 5 mg at weekly intervals to controlling dose or 0.75–1 mg/kg/day, whichever is lower. *Inpatients:* prednisolone 10 mg single dose on alternate days, increased by 10 mg increments to controlling dose or 1–1.5 mg/kg/day. In both groups, dose should be tapered by 5 mg/month when remission is established and adjusted to define effective minimal dose.
Contraindications	Osteoporosis, mental disturbance.
Main drug interactions	Antibacterials, e.g. rifampicin, antiepileptics.
Main side effects	Initial exacerbation of myasthenic symptoms, adrenal suppression, diabetes, osteoporosis, avascular necrosis of femoral head, mental disturbance, weight gain, cushingoid features, cataracts.

Azathioprine
- Azathioprine is indicated in combination with prednisolone for generalized moderate or severe disease (inpatients).

Standard dosage	Azathioprine 2.5 mg/kg/day orally.
Contraindications	Myelosuppression.
Special points	Full blood count and liver function tests weekly for 8 weeks, every 1–3 months thereafter.
Main drug interactions	Allopurinol enhances toxic effect.
Main side effects	Myelosuppression, hepatotoxicity, gastrointestinal symptoms, rashes, B-cell lymphoma (very rare).

Treatment aims
To allow patient to recover health.

Other treatments

Plasma exchange
- Plasma exchange is indicated for the following:

Symptomatic control in severe cases.
Myasthenic crisis.
Preparation for thymectomy.
After thymectomy while awaiting response.
Recurrently, in severe myasthenia gravis, while awaiting response to immunosuppressive drug therapy.

Thymectomy (by median sternotomy)
- Thymectomy is indicated for the following:

Thymoma (because of risk of local spread).
Early-onset generalized myasthenia gravis (outcome in subsequent 1–2 years 25% remission, 50% improvement, 25% neutral).

Prognosis
- Most patients achieve substantial improvement or full recovery.

Follow-up and management
- In patients treated by immunosuppressive drugs, continuing low-dose treatment and regular follow-up is usually needed to maintain disease control.

Key references
Newsom-Davis J: Myasthenia gravis. *Med Int* 1992, **100**:4168–4171.

Penn AS *et al.* (eds): Myasthenia gravis and related disorders. *Ann N Y Acad Sci* 1993, **681**:1–611.

Shillito P, Vincent A, Newsom-Davis J: Congenital myasthenic syndromes. *J Neuromusc Dis* 1993, **3**:183–190.

Verma P, Oger J: Treatment of acquired autoimmune myasthenia gravis. *Can J Neurol Sci* 1992, **19**:360–375.

Neuralgia, postherpetic — J.W. Scadding

Diagnosis

Symptoms
- Acute herpetic neuralgia merges into postherpetic neuralgia (persistent neuralgia at 3 months after acute eruption).
- The patient's emotional state, environmental temperature, and fatigue may all affect the severity of postherpetic neuralgia.

Continuous pain: often burning, raw, severe aching, or tearing.

Superimposed spontaneous paroxysmal pains: stabbing, shooting, or shock-like in many patients.

Pain in dermatome: often throughout affected dermatome but usually particularly severe within part of dermatome.

Pain accompanied by unpleasant skin sensitivity: hyperalgesia, and allodynia, sometimes with hyperpathia; these evoked pains are the most troublesome symptoms of postherpetic neuralgia for many patients.

Associated depression: common.

Weakness: caused by shingles affecting a limb dermatome at the same segmental level as the rash; on the trunk, anterior horn cell involvement may be present but difficult to detect and is clinically unimportant.

Signs
Scarring: usually; variable degree in affected dermatome; depigmented.

Hypoaesthesia in the scars, variable hyperalgesia, allodynia, and hyperpathia: in remainder of dermatome.

Investigations
- No investigation is needed in most patients.
- In younger patients, shingles, either isolated or with generalized zoster, may be a symptom of immunosuppression, particularly associated with lymphoma: appropriate investigation of such patients is needed.

Complications
Depression: common, sometimes severe.

Weakness in a limb: when an appropriate dermatome is affected.

Differential diagnosis
Other causes of sensory ganglion and root disease.

Aetiology
- Reactivation of herpes varicella zoster virus causes acute shingles.
- Corticosteroid treatment for an unrelated condition sometimes precipitates shingles.
- The mechanism of postherpetic neuralgia includes peripheral and CNS factors (abnormal impulse generation, partial deafferentation and loss of normal inhibition).
- Histopathology in postherpetic neuralgia shows damage to peripheral nerve, dorsal root ganglion, sensory root, and dorsal horn atrophy.

Epidemiology
- The female:male ratio is 3:2.
- The overall incidence of postherpetic neuralgia at 1 year is ~3% of all patients with acute shingles.
- The most common sites are the mid-thoracic dermatomes and the ophthalmic division of the trigeminal nerve: it may occur in any dermatome.
- Postherpetic neuralgia is rare after shingles in patients aged <50 years and becomes more common with increasing age >50 years.

Treatment

Diet and lifestyle
- No special precautions are necessary.

Pharmacological treatment
- No treatment for patients with acute shingles has yet been proved to prevent the development of postherpetic neuralgia. Treatment remains unsatisfactory.

Local
- Possibilities for local treatment must always be exhausted because simple measures may give partial relief and avoid the side effects so often seen with systemic drug treatment in this mainly elderly patient population.
- Treatments include the following:

Local anaesthetic ointment (5% lignocaine) 3 times daily: sometimes effective.

Capsaicin 0.075% ointment 3 times daily: may cause initial burning but helps some patients.

- Local anaesthetic, peripheral nerve or root blocks, and sympathetic blocks (occasionally) may temporarily relieve postherpetic neuralgia but have no long-term benefit.

Systemic

Standard dosage	Amitriptyline 10–25 mg at night, gradually increased to 75–150 mg at night, as tolerated. Dihydrocodeine 30–60 mg 3 times daily. Co-proxamol 2 tablets 3 times daily.
Contraindications	*Amitriptyline:* recent myocardial infarction, heart block, mania, porphyria.
Special points	*Amitriptyline:* up to maximum tolerated doses have been consistently shown in controlled trials to provide partial relief of postherpetic neuralgia.
Main drug interactions	Sedation enhanced by other sedatives.
Main side effects	*Amitriptyline:* drowsiness, constipation, urinary hesitancy, dry mouth, blurred vision, postural hypotension, tachycardia, sweating, tremor.

- Anticonvulsants, e.g. phenytoin, carbamazepine, sodium valproate, and clonazepam, have not been shown to relieve postherpetic neuralgia; any effect will probably be short-lived and consistent with a placebo response.
- Lignocaine 1–5 mg/kg i.v. relieves postherpetic neuralgia but is not a practical long-term treatment; oral mexiletine is ineffective.

Treatment aims
To relieve pain.

Other treatments

Local measures
- Cold packs applied for 15–20 min several times daily may produce partial analgesia, sometimes lasting a few hours after a single application.
- Transcutaneous electrical nerve stimulation, acupuncture, vibration, ultrasound may each be helpful in some patients.

Psychological measures
- Counselling by a clinical psychologist about coping strategies may help some patients.

Prognosis
- Most patients with troublesome postherpetic neuralgia at 1 year have the condition lifelong, although some patients slowly improve over long periods.
- After acute shingles, persistent, troublesome neuralgia gradually decreases over several months at least.

Follow-up and management
- ~50% of patients with postherpetic neuralgia benefit from regular long-term follow-up; the role of a sympathetic doctor who is prepared to listen should not be underestimated, even when all treatment options have apparently been exhausted.
- Many patients can be discharged from follow-up when treatment leads to partial relief of pain.
- The option of return visits should always be offered to patients if the pain becomes less tolerable in the future.

Key references
Watson CPN, Evans RJ: Post-herpetic neuralgia: a review. *Arch Neurol* 1986, **43**:836–840.

Watson CPN *et al.*: Post-herpetic neuralgia: 208 cases. *Pain* 1988, **35**:289–297.

Neuralgia, trigeminal — J.W. Scadding

Diagnosis

Symptoms
Pain: unilateral shooting, shock-like, usually from upper lip to eye or from corner of mouth to ear; rare in ophthalmic division; paroxysmal, lasting <1 min but may occur frequently; occurs spontaneously but often triggered by innocuous facial or oral stimulation, e.g. touching face, washing or shaving, brushing teeth, eating and drinking; bouts last weeks to months, with remissions of months to years; may become chronic in some patients; rarely develops on contralateral side; in chronic trigeminal neuralgia, some patients complain of background aching pain.

Signs
- Idiopathic trigeminal neuralgia has no signs.

Trigeminal sensory impairment: caused by a compressive lesion of the trigeminal root; such lesions may rarely lead to trigeminal neuralgia.

Investigations
- Investigation is not usually needed.

CT or MRI: in patients being considered for surgical treatment or in whom sensory impairment is present (symptomatic trigeminal neuralgia; rare).

Complications
Depression.

Differential diagnosis
- No other facial pain has the same stereotyped paroxysmal nature.
- Migrainous neuralgia, atypical facial pain, or ophthalmic postherpetic neuralgia should not cause confusion.

Aetiology
- The mechanisms of this unique paroxysmal neuropathic pain are poorly understood but involve peripheral and central factors.
- The following may play a role:

Mild compression of the trigeminal root by a blood vessel, usually an ectatic superior cerebellar artery, in chronic sufferers.

Minor degenerative changes in nerve ganglion or root.

Epidemiology
- The female:male ratio is 3:1.
- Onset usually occurs after the age of 50 years.
- The disease is associated with multiple sclerosis, but most young patients (<50 years) with trigeminal neuralgia do not develop multiple sclerosis.

Treatment

Diet and lifestyle
- No special precautions are necessary.

Pharmacological treatment

Carbamazepine
- Carbamazepine is the drug of choice.
- The slow-release preparation is better tolerated.

Standard dosage	Carbamazepine 100 mg twice daily initially, increased to a dose that controls pain or to maximum tolerated dose.
Contraindications	Hypersensitivity.
Special points	Blood level monitoring often helpful.
Main drug interactions	Sedation enhanced by other sedatives.
Main side effects	Drowsiness, nausea, ataxia, hypersensitivity rash (treatment must be stopped immediately).

Phenytoin
- Phenytoin should be used only when the patient does not respond to carbamazepine or with carbamazepine when pain is incompletely controlled.

Standard dosage	200–400 mg daily at night.
Contraindications	Hypersensitivity.
Special points	Blood levels must be monitored, particularly in elderly patients, because of non-linear metabolism kinetics.
Main drug interactions	Sedation enhanced by other sedatives.
Main side effects	Drowsiness, ataxia, hypersensitivity rash (rare), acneiform or seborrhoeic skin change, and gingival hypertrophy (all unusual in elderly patients).

Other drugs
- Baclofen and clonazepam are occasionally effective.

Treatment aims
To alleviate pain until onset of remission.

Other treatments

Surgery
- Surgery is indicated for patients with unremitting pain or who are unresponsive to or intolerant of medical treatment.

Controlled thermocoagulation gangliolysis
- This is a minimally invasive procedure, suitable for elderly, frail patients.
- It is effective, usually giving pain relief of at least 1–2 years, with low risk.
- It can be repeated if necessary.
- Morbidity includes facial sensory impairment; in rare instances, this is severe enough to lead to anaesthesia dolorosa and neuroparalytic keratitis.

Microvascular decompression
- This is effective, often permanently, and thus is more suitable for younger patients.
- Morbidity is the same as for thermocoagulation but also includes deafness and brainstem damage (rare).

Prognosis
- Some patients have bouts lasting weeks, with remissions of years.
- Some develop chronic trigeminal neuralgia.

Follow-up and management
- Frequent follow-up is needed until the pain is controlled.
- Withdrawal of treatment must be supervised to assess whether remission has occurred.

Key references
Loeser JD: Tic douloureux and atypical face pain. In *Textbook of Pain* edn 3. Edited by Wall PD, Melzack R. Edinburgh: Churchill Livingstone, 1994, pp 699–710.

Neuropathy, peripheral
J.G. Llewelyn

Diagnosis

Symptoms

General
Distal numbness.
Paraesthesiae, burning, lancinating pain.
Progressive distal weakness and wasting.
Foot and hand deformities, neuropathic ulcer, neuropathic arthropathy.

Of autonomic neuropathy
Impotence, orthostatic hypotension, dry eyes or mouth, urinary or faecal incontinence, nausea and vomiting, constipation or diarrhoea.

Signs

General
Muscle weakness and wasting.
Reduced or absent tendon reflexes.
Sensory ataxia, neuropathic tremor.
Nerve thickening.

Of autonomic neuropathy
Anhidrosis, unreactive or asymmetric pupils, postural hypotension (fall of 30 mmHg in systolic and 15 mmHg in diastolic pressure).

Investigations

Full blood count.
ESR measurement.
Glucose tolerance test: if random and fasting samples give equivocal results.
U&E analysis.
Liver function test.
Measurement of thyroid-stimulating hormone, vitamin B_{12}, serum protein electrophoresis, autoantibodies.
DNA analysis: for hereditary demyelinating neuropathies; chromosome 17 duplication in a subgroup of patients with HMSN type 1 (HMSN 1A); chromosome 17 deletion associated with hereditary liability to pressure palsies (tomaculous neuropathy).
Urinalysis: for glucose, Bence–Jones protein, porphyrins.
CSF analysis: raised protein concentration in inflammatory neuropathies.
Nerve conduction studies: diagnosis confirmed by slowing of motor or sensory conduction velocities (moderate in axonal type, marked in demyelinating type) and reduction in sensory action potential amplitude (small in axonal neuropathy).
Electromyography: characteristic pattern in denervated muscle.
Sensory threshold recording: thermal (useful in patients with small-fibre neuropathy) and vibration.
Imaging: screening for malignancy in patients with suspected paraneoplastic neuropathy; skeletal survey for suspected myeloma; chest radiography for suspected sarcoidosis.
Nerve biopsy: done in operating theatre under strict aseptic conditions using local anaesthetic; fascicular biopsy limits degree of sensory loss; full thickness biopsy indicated for suspected vasculitis; used to discover cause of progressive neuropathy not revealed by detailed investigation or to confirm presence of vasculitis, leprous neuropathy, or inflammatory infiltrates; sensory nerves (sural, superficial peroneal, superficial radial) usually biopsied.
Bone-marrow biopsy: for vitamin B_{12} deficiency or myeloma.
Formal autonomic function tests, endoscopy, colonoscopy, barium studies, urodynamic studies: for autonomic neuropathy.

Complications
Burns, cuts, bruising, neuropathic ulcers: unnoticed when sensory loss is severe.

Differential diagnosis
- The differential diagnosis depends on the cause.

Aetiology

Causes of sensory polyneuropathy
Diabetes, uraemia, hypothyroidism.
Amyloidosis.
Paraneoplastic, paraproteinaemic.
Thallium, isoniazid, vincristine, cisplatin, metronidazole.
Sjögren's syndrome.
Leprosy.
HIV, Lyme borreliosis infection.
Hereditary sensory and autonomic neuropathies.
Fabry's disease.
Vitamin B_{12} deficiency.

Causes of sensorimotor polyneuropathy
Hereditary motor and sensory neuropathies.
Alcohol.
Acute or chronic inflammatory demyelinating polyradiculoneuropathy.
Vasculitis.
Paraproteinaemic, paraneoplastic.
Diabetes, uraemia, hypothyroidism, acromegaly.
Sarcoidosis.

Causes of motor neuropathies
Acute or chronic inflammatory demyelinating polyradiculoneuropathy.
Porphyria, diphtheria, lead.
Hereditary motor neuropathies.

Causes of focal and multifocal neuropathies
Entrapment and compression syndromes.
Polyarteritis nodosa, connective tissue disorders,
Wegener's granulomatosis.
Lymphomatous and carcinomatous infiltration, neurofibromatosis.
Tuberculoid leprosy, herpes zoster, HIV, Lyme borreliosis.
Sarcoidosis: especially facial nerve.
Hereditary liability to pressure palsies.
Multifocal motor neuropathy with conduction block.

Epidemiology
- The epidemiology depends on the cause.

Treatment

Diet and lifestyle
- Patients with alcoholic neuropathy should abstain from drinking alcohol.
- Postural hypotension can be relieved by raising the foot of the bed.

Pharmacological treatment

For focal and multifocal neuropathies
For vasculitis: prednisolone 60 mg daily orally; azathioprine can be introduced to enable dose of steroids to be reduced; degree of immunosuppression and duration of treatment depend on clinical response.

For protection against peptic ulceration: H_2 antagonists

For alcoholic neuropathy: vitamin B supplements

For herpes zoster infection: acyclovir 800 mg orally 5 times daily for 1 week.

- Leprosy should be treated under specialist supervision.

For autonomic neuropathy
For postural hypotension: fludrocortisone 100–400 mg or ephedrine 15–60 mg daily.

For gastroparesis: erythromycin 125 mg daily, cisapride 10 mg 3 times daily, domperidone 10–20 mg 3 times daily, or metoclopramide up to 10 mg 3 times daily.

For diarrhoea: co-phenotrope (lomotil), loperamide (imodium), codeine phosphate.

For impotence: penile intracavernous papaverine injection

For painful neuropathy
- Treatment is extremely difficult and often unsatisfactory.

Regular simple analgesic, e.g paracetamol 1 g 4 times daily.

For burning diffuse pain and paraesthesiae: amitriptyline 25–75 mg at night or desimipramine 25–75 mg daily; a phenothiazine can be added if needed.

For shooting pain: carbamazepine 100 mg at night, increasing slowly to 600 mg daily in divided doses; mexiletine 100–400 mg daily may be worth trying.

For postherpetic neuralgia: topical capsaicin 0.075% after lesions have healed.

For chronic inflammatory demyelinating polyradiculoneuropathy
For acute disorder: see Guillain–Barré syndrome.

For mild to moderate disease: prednisolone 10 mg daily for 1 week, increasing by 10 mg/week to 30–40 mg daily; azathioprine may be added for steroid-sparing effect.

For progressive disease or relapses: i.v. immunoglobulin 0.4 g/kg/day for 5 days and possible replacement of azathioprine with either cyclosporin or cyclophosphamide.

Treatment aims
- Treatment aims depend on the type of neuropathy.

Other treatments

For focal and multifocal neuropathies
Conservative: wrist and foot support, elbow pad.
Surgical decompression:
Median and ulnar nerve entrapment with evidence of wasting or weakness of denervated muscles.
For persistent sensory symptoms when conservative measures have failed.

For chronic inflammatory demyelinating polyradiculoneuropathy
Plasma exchange for progressive neuropathy unresponsive to immunoglobulin.

Prognosis
- Prognosis depends on the underlying cause of the neuropathy.

Follow-up and management
- Regular follow-up is needed to assess progression.
- Patients requiring immunosuppression need frequent follow-up.

Key references
Chance PF et al.: DNA deletion associated with hereditary neuropathy with liability to pressure palsies. *Cell* 1993, **72**:143–151.

Dyck PJ, Thomas PK: *Peripheral Neuropathy* edn 3. Philadelphia: WB Saunders, 1993.

Lupski JR et al.: DNA duplication associated with Charcot–Marie–Tooth disease type 1A. *Cell* 1991, **66**:219–232.

van Doorn PA et al.: High dose intravenous immunoglobulin treatment in chronic inflammatory demyelinating neuropathy: a double blind, placebo controlled, crossover study. *Neurology* 1990, **40**:212–214.

Parkinson's disease A.H.V. Schapira

Diagnosis

Symptoms
Tremor: in ~70% of patients; unilateral and usually noted in hand first; may be seen in jaw or leg.

Poverty of movement, difficulty initiating movements and with repetitive movements: e.g. shuffling gait, drooling, difficulty turning in bed, micrographia, softness of voice, constipation.

Rigidity: e.g. poor balance, falls, muscle stiffness, pain.

Signs
Tremor: asymmetric, resting, 'pill-rolling' at 3–5 Hz; usually disappears on intention; increased by anxiety; possibly postural tremor at 6–8 Hz.

Rigidity and bradykinesia: stooped, flexed posture; shuffling gait with poor swing of affected arm; cogwheel rigidity, may be enhanced by synkinesis; immobile facies, reduced blink and swallowing rates; rigidity usually noted first in axial muscles, e.g. neck and shoulder.

Investigations
- No tests are available for Parkinson's disease; the diagnosis is based on clinical features alone.
- Investigation is indicated only if the diagnosis is in doubt or presentation is atypical.

Testing of autonomic function, including sphincter electromyography: patients with multiple system atrophy may show abnormalities.

MRI: can show abnormal hypointensity in the putamen of patients with multiple system atrophy.

Copper and caeruloplasmin measurement: in all patients with young-onset or atypical Parkinson's disease.

Complications
Depression, anxiety.

Postural imbalance.

Cognitive and psychiatric problems: frontal lobe dysfunction, bradyphrenia, fluctuating confusional state (dementia in 25% of patients); possible overlap with other syndromes, e.g. diffuse Lewy body disease, senile dementia of Lewy body type.

Complications of L-dopa.

Differential diagnosis
Drug-induced parkinsonism: e.g. phenothiazines, butyrophenones; usually symmetrical and reversible.

Essential tremor: bilateral; absent at rest, exacerbated by intention, or maintaining posture; improved by alcohol; possible family history; should be treated with beta blockers or primidone when necessary.

Multiple system atrophy or progressive supranuclear palsy: symptoms and signs usually symmetrical; tremor less usual; falls frequent; additional features, e.g. pyramidal or cerebellar deficits, gaze palsies, or autonomic involvement including postural hypotension, and bladder dysfunction.

Wilson's disease: 40% present with neurological features, mainly parkinsonism; liver cirrhosis or psychiatric disease also occur; Kayser–Fleischer rings visible by slit lamp in most; low serum caeruloplasmin, high urinary copper; liver biopsy shows high copper and evidence of liver cell damage; should be treated with penicillamine.

Toxin-induced parkinsonism.

Mitochondrial disorders; abnormal movements, usually dystonia or chorea.

Aetiology
- >80% dopamine depletion occurs in the striatum at presentation; neurones are lost in the substantia nigra (dopaminergic), locus coeruleus (noradrenergic), and substantia innominata (cholinergic). Intracytoplasmic inclusions, Lewy bodies, are found in surviving neurones.
- The cause of Parkinson's disease is not known, but environmental toxins and genetic susceptibility may play a role alone or in combination.

Epidemiology
- The incidence is ~20 in 100 000, with an overall prevalence of 150 in 100 000 (500 in 100 000 for those aged >50 years).
- The male : female ratio is equal.
- Parkinson's disease occurs world wide but is possibly less frequent in China and Africa than in the United States and Europe.

Parkinson's disease
A.H.V. Schapira

Treatment

Diet and lifestyle
- Maintaining activity is important: a multidisciplinary approach, with physiotherapy, occupational therapy, speech therapy, and social work contact is helpful; patients and carers may need support.
- Dietary protein should be reduced during the day; a main meal at night allows more predictable absorption of L-dopa.

Pharmacological treatment

At diagnosis
- Most neurologists advocate selegiline, although early use is debated.

Standard dosage	Selegiline (Deprenyl) 10 mg/day.
Contraindications	Possible interaction with tricyclic antidepressants or 5-HT reuptake inhibitors.
Special points	Delays requirement for L-dopa by about 1 year, although mechanism of action uncertain.
Main drug interactions	Concurrent L-dopa dose may need to be decreased 20–50%.
Main side effects	Gastrointestinal upset, hypotension.

At review
- Treatment is essentially symptomatic.
- L-Dopa has medium to long-term side effects, so treatment is prescribed when clinical features interfere with life.
- Tremor and bradykinesia respond well, postural instability less well.
- The use of controlled-release L-dopa offers some improvement in patients with medium to advanced disease, especially in decreasing 'off time'; transition to these drugs should be gradual because the bioavailability is different from the standard preparations; some neurologists use controlled-release preparations early to provide a more 'physiological' prolonged drug exposure to dopaminergic neurones.
- Dopaminergic agonists may be used alone (early) or in combination with L-dopa.

Standard dosage	L-Dopa with a dopa decarboxylase inhibitor, initially at low dose and frequency, e.g. 50–100 mg twice daily; increased as necessary. Dopaminergic agonists, e.g. bromocriptine, lyseride, pergolide in low doses initially and built up gradually.
Contraindications	L-Dopa: closed angle glaucoma. Dopaminergic agents: hypotension, cardiac arrhythmias.
Special points	L-Dopa: generally, frequent small doses (up to every 2–3 h) are better than infrequent large doses. Dopaminergic agents: may be used alone, but tolerance to these drugs develops quickly.
Main drug interactions	Dopaminergic agents: combination with L-dopa may improve control and potentially delay onset of side effects associated with L-dopa.
Main side effects	L-Dopa: gastrointestinal upset, postural hypotension, confusion, hallucination, dyskinesias and dystonia (excess L-dopa), fluctuations, including dyskinesias, freezing, and unpredictable 'on–offing' in 50–60% of patients 3–5 years after starting treatment; neuropsychiatric side effects best treated by dose modification, but clozapine may be used (possible development of agranulocytosis). Dopaminergic agents: hypotension, hallucinations, confusion, gastrointestinal symptoms (may be helped by pretreatment by domperidone).

- Apomorphine, as pen-jet or infusion introduced under medical supervision, can significantly improve control in suitable patients; rapidity of onset is helpful to improve ability to perform certain tasks.
- Amantidine may be useful in patients with medium to advanced disease; anticholinergics are now rarely used, although they may help to decrease salivation.

Treatment aims
To improve functional disability.
To avoid or minimize drug-related side effects.
To treat fluctuations when present.

Other treatments
- Fetal implant therapy continues to be developed, but substantial and sustained benefit has not yet been shown.
- Adrenal implants are rarely performed and are of questionable efficacy.
- The benefit of antioxidant treatment has not yet been shown.
- Posteroventral pallidotomy may be useful in selected patients to improve tremor and rigidity.

Prognosis
- Parkinson's disease progresses at variable rates and reduces life-expectancy, with relative survival being 66% of the matched general population.

Follow-up and management
- The need for symptomatic treatment should be assessed.
- Correct use and titration of drugs should be monitored.
- Medical and support needs should be assessed.

Key references
Calne DB: Treatment of Parkinson's disease. *N Engl J Med* 1993, **329**:1021–1027.
Marsden CD: Parkinson's disease. *J Neurol Neurosurg Psychiatry* 1994, **57**:672–681.

Sleep disorders   J.D. Parkes

Diagnosis

Symptoms

Insomnia
Daytime fatigue.
Depression.
Subalertness.

Obstructive sleep apnoea
Obstructive snoring.
Breath holding.
Partial arousal.
Excessive daytime sleepiness.

Narcoleptic syndrome
Excessive daytime sleepiness.
Abnormal floppiness or paralysis: with laughter or expectation of sudden event (cataplexy).
Short night sleep latency.
Insomnia.
Excessive motor activity during sleep: leg kicking and sleep-walking.
Sleep paralysis, loss of muscle tone, and pre-sleep dream-timing.

Parasomnias
Hypnic jerks: at sleep onset.
Sleep-walking and night terrors: 60–90 min after sleep onset, during non-rapid eye movement sleep.
Cluster headache, painful erections, nightmares: during rapid eye movement sleep; accompanied by dreaming.
Enuresis, sleep-talking, leg-kicking: common.
Bruxism, head-banging: less common.

Circadian sleep disorders
Persistent late timing of sleep: e.g. 04.00–14.00 h.
- Sleep quality is normal in circadian sleep disorders.

Signs
- No abnormal physical signs are manifest in most sleep disorders.

Investigations
Polysomnography: unnecessary in most sleep–wake disorders, including the narcoleptic syndrome.
Advantages: allows detailed scientific sleep study and may occasionally clarify diagnosis of sleep disorder, particularly when combined with video monitoring.
Disadvantages: expensive, time-consuming, scarce facility.
Sleep oxymetry: useful in evaluation of sleep apnoea and review of treatment.
Advantages: cost-effective, freely available, skilled technician unnecessary.
Disadvantages: determines oxygen saturation not sleep structure or arousal, misses some cases of obstructive sleep apnoea.
Multiple sleep latency test: in narcoleptic syndrome and other forms of daytime sleepiness, mean sleep latency is short.
Plasma and urinary screen: for hypnotic or CNS stimulant drugs, occasionally useful in suspected drug abuse or poor drug compliance.

Complications
- Sleep disorders may be as disabling as epilepsy.

Daytime fatigue, subalertness, depression.
Work and social problems: major cause of road traffic accidents.

Differential diagnosis
Not applicable.

Aetiology
- Insomnia is often multifactorial, with abnormal lifestyle, physical and psychological factors and sometimes hypnotic-stimulant drug or alcohol misuse.
- Familial insomnia is not uncommon.
- The narcoleptic syndrome has 99% association with HLA DR2 and DQw1; only 1 in 500 HLA DR2 positive patients, however, has the narcoleptic syndrome.
- Circadian sleep disorders are due to shift work or psychological factors (e.g. avoiding school).

Epidemiology
- Chronic insomnia occurs in up to 20% of adults; it is more common in women than in men.
- Persistent excessive daytime sleepiness is usually caused by obstructive sleep apnoea or the narcoleptic syndrome.
- Parasomnias including bed wetting and sleep walking are common, most frequent in childhood.
- Circadian sleep disorders caused by shift work occur in one-third of the European workforce; shift work is tolerated better by younger people.
- The delayed sleep phase syndrome has an incidence of 1 in 10 000 people.

Treatment

Diet and lifestyle

- Regular bedtime, a comfortable quiet bed, pre-sleep relaxation, a warm drink, and avoidance of rumination may improve insomnia.
- In the narcoleptic syndrome, 2–3 planned short naps during the day, coffee drinking, and herbal stimulants, e.g. guarana, may improve alertness.
- Sleep regularity with fixed stable bedtime and wake-time is useful in the management of many parasomnias.

Pharmacological treatment

For insomnia

Standard dosage	Short-term (3–6 months) benzodiazepine or non-benzodiazepine hypnotic, e.g. temazepam, 2–3 times weekly can be considered.
Contraindications	Pregnancy, psychiatric illness, sleep apnoea.
Special points	Long-term nightly use to be avoided; can be combined with psychological support, although hypnotics not main-line treatment for most forms of chronic insomnia.
Main drug interactions	Enhanced sedative effect with many other drugs; metabolic interactions.
Main side effects	Waking sedation, tolerance.

For narcoleptic syndrome: daytime sleepiness

Standard dosage	Dexamphetamine maximum 60 mg daily, pemoline, mazindol, methylphenidate; exact dose titration and timing essential.
Contraindications	Vascular disease, hypertension, pregnancy, prostatism, breast-feeding.
Special points	Stimulants ineffective for cataplexy. Regular monitoring of patients on long-term treatment needed.
Main drug interactions	Sympathomimetics, monoamine oxidase inhibitors.
Main side effects	Talkativeness, euphoria, gastrointestinal irritation, sweating, constipation.

For narcoleptic syndrome: cataplexy

Standard dosage	Clomipramine 10–50 mg once daily.
Contraindications	Recent myocardial infarction, heart block.
Special points	Cataplexy does not respond to stimulants, but these can be used in combination with clomipramine.
Main drug interactions	As for tricyclic antidepressants.
Main side effects	Delayed ejaculation, sexual malfunction in men, appetite increase and gradual weight gain.

Treatment aims

To restore normal waking alertness and mood.

To prevent sleep hypoxia, arousal, and cor pulmonale.

To alleviate symptoms of narcolepsy.

Other treatments

Continuous positive airways pressure: effective in patients with obstructive sleep apnoea.

Consideration of surgery.

Prognosis

- The prognosis varies widely between the different sleep disorders.
- The narcoleptic syndrome does not remit.
- In many forms of insomnia, the prognosis is poor.

Follow-up and management

- Assessment of insomnia requires medical, psychiatric, and psychological review; a written treatment plan should be drawn up with the patient, aiming for sustained benefit in 3–6 months of treatment
- In patients with the narcoleptic syndrome, progress should be monitored using a sleep–wake diary; drug compliance should be ensured by monitoring plasma and urine concentrations.

Patient support

Narcolepsy Association (UK), 1 Brook Street, Stoke on Trent ST4 1JN, tel/fax 01782 416 417.

Driving regulations

- The licensing authority must be notified.
- In the UK currently, the general guideline is that driving ability with excessive daytime sleepiness depends on the success of and degree of compliance with treatment.

Key references

Douglas NJ, Thomas S, Jan MA: Clinical value of polysomnography. *Lancet* 1992, **339**:347–350.

Hill NS: Noninvasive ventilation. *Am Rev Respir Dis* 1993, **147**:1050–1055.

Thorpy MJ: *Handbook of Sleep Disorders*, New York: Marcel Dekker, 1990.

Spinal cord and cauda equina compression
A.N. Gale and R.S. Maurice-Williams

Diagnosis

Symptoms
- The neurological symptoms are progressive.

Localized back pain: if worse at night, tumour should be suspected.
Root pain.
Numbness or paraesthesiae, weakness: below level of lesion; may be asymmetrical.
Loss of control of sphincters.

Signs

At level of lesion
Spinal tenderness or deformity: depending on the disease.
Weakness, wasting, reflex loss: root lesion.

Below level of lesion
- Signs may be asymmetrical, e.g. Brown–Sequard syndrome.
- With spinal cord lesions, sacral sensation may be relatively 'spared'.

Weakness.
Sensory loss.
Spasticity, clonus, hyper-reflexia, extensor plantars: if above L1, i.e. spinal cord.
Flaccidity, areflexia: if below L1, i.e. cauda equina.

Investigations
- Laboratory investigations may indicate cause, suggest alternative diagnosis, or help in preparation for surgery.
- Neuroimaging is best done in a neurosciences unit.

Full blood count and ESR measurement: may identify anaemia or suggest infection.
Serum vitamin B_{12}, syphilis serology, serum acid phosphatase measurement, plasma protein electrophoresis: may be helpful in some patients.
Chest radiography: may show mass or infection.
Plain radiography of spine: may show loss of pedicle or vertebral collapse.
Myelography, CT myelography, MRI: may be needed urgently; CSF should always be saved, particularly if a compressive lesion is not identified.
Plain CT: in some patients.

Complications
Irreversible neurological damage: due to infarction of cord or roots.
Urinary infection: due to neurogenic bladder.
Deep venous thrombosis and pressure sores: from immobility.

Differential diagnosis

Spastic paraparesis
Inflammatory myelopathies: acute transverse myelitis, multiple sclerosis, HIV infection, tropical spastic paraparesis (human T-cell leukaemic virus I).
Vascular myelopathies: spinal stroke (anterior spinal artery distribution), vascular malformation.
Malformations: Arnold Chiari (possible lower brainstem or cerebellar signs), syringomyelia (absent arm reflexes and suspended sensory loss).
Cerebral lesions: bilateral strokes, para-sagittal tumour.

Flaccid paraparesis
Flaccidity and absent reflexes (spinal shock) caused by acute spinal cord lesions; rare in compression.
Acute Guillain–Barré syndrome: symmetrical, distal sensory loss, areflexia.

Aetiology
- Causes include the following:

Extradural tumours: secondary carcinoma, lymphoma, myeloma.
Intradural–extramedullary tumours: meningioma, neurofibroma.
Intramedullary tumours: glioma, ependymoma, lipoma.
Disc protrusions: usually cervical or lumbar, usually spontaneous, often sudden onset.
Osteophytic ridges: may combine with narrow spinal canal, i.e. cervical or lumbar canal stenosis.
Infection: pyogenic epidural abscess, tuberculosis.
Trauma: fractures or dislocations of vertebrae.
Haematomas: epidural and subdural (rare).

Epidemiology
- No data are available.

Treatment

Diet and lifestyle
Not relevant.

Pharmacological treatment
Chemotherapy or radiotherapy: after decompression or biopsy of malignant lesion.

Steroids: before and after surgery to minimize spinal-cord oedema (e.g. dexamethasone 16 mg daily in divided doses).

Non-pharmacological treatment
- If acute spinal-cord compression is suspected, the patient must be referred to a neurosurgical unit immediately.
- Any delay may lessen the chance of recovery.

Decompression
- Lesions lying posterior to the spinal cord or within the dura mater should be removed from behind through a laminectomy.
- Lesions lying anterior to the dura mater, with the exception of lumbar disc protrusions, should be removed from the front.

Spinal stabilization
- Lesions that cause collapse of the vertebral bodies cause forward angulation; stabilization should be by insertion of a graft from the front or instrumental stabilization attached to laminae in extension e.g. Hartshill rectangle.

Treatment aims
To establish the diagnosis.
To reverse neurological deficit while preserving spinal stability, if lesion removable.
To prevent progression or recurrence, if lesion not removable.

Prognosis
- The prognosis depends on the underlying cause, the rate rather than degree of compression, and the delay in decompression.
- Patients with long-established myelopathy due to hard disc material or osteophytic bars have poor prognosis; those with soft disc protrusions do well.
- Myelopathies due to prostatic secondaries have a relatively good prognosis.
- Metastases from breast or bronchus have a poor prognosis; direct invasion from bronchus has a very poor prognosis.
- Good recovery even from severe neurological deficit may follow successful surgical removal of benign tumours.
- Prognosis is good if decompression occurs before the onset of severe paraparesis.

Follow-up and management
- Patients need subsequent physiotherapy, rehabilitation, surgical appliances (e.g. walking aids, orthoses, wheelchair), occupational therapy, and home assessment.
- Patients should be referred to a spinal unit if the residual deficit is severe.
- Complications can be prevented by anti-embolism stockings, low-dose s.c. heparin, prevention of pressure sores, bladder care, and early treatment of intercurrent infection.

Key references
Maurice-Williams RS, Richardson PL: Spinal cord compression: delay in the diagnosis and referral of a common neurological emergency. *Br J Neurosurg* 1988, **2**:55–60.

Stroke — R.J. Davenport and C.P. Warlow

Diagnosis

Definition
- Stroke is defined as rapidly developing (usually over minutes) clinical symptoms or signs of focal and, at times, global loss of cerebral function, with symptoms lasting >24 h or leading to death, with no apparent cause other than that of vascular origin.

Symptoms
- Symptoms depend on the vascular territory involved.

Anterior (carotid) circulation
Speech, visuospatial, motor, or sensory loss: indicating cortical lesions.

Isolated contralateral sensory or motor loss: indicating deeper hemispheric lesions.

- Extensive hemispheric involvement may lead to altered consciousness due to cerebral oedema.

Posterior circulation
Homonymous hemianopia or brainstem disturbance: e.g. diplopia, vertigo, imbalance, altered consciousness.

- Headache, loss of consciousness, and seizures are more common presenting features in subarachnoid or primary intracerebral haemorrhage than in cerebral infarction.

Signs
- Signs range from none or very subtle (e.g. subjective sensory disturbance) to brain-death.

Investigations
- Diagnosis of stroke remains clinical, based predominantly on the history.
- Primary investigations are aimed at identifying abnormalities that may further compromise cerebral function (in patients admitted to hospital) or provide aetiological clues.
- Secondary investigations are aimed at detecting the cause of stroke, which influences early management.
- Tertiary investigations are aimed at preventing recurrence and excluding unusual causes (see Transient ischaemic attacks).

Primary investigations
Full blood count, ESR, U&E and glucose measurement, ECG, chest radiography.

Secondary investigations
CT: sensitive at differentiating haemorrhage from infarction immediately; may appear normal early in infarction; final topographical distribution of any infarction best seen at days 7–10.

Lumbar puncture: for suspected subarachnoid haemorrhage if CT normal.

- Other specific tests indicated by clinical setting (e.g. blood cultures).

Complications
Infections (e.g. pneumonia, urinary tract infection).

Venous thromboembolism.

Cardiac arrhythmias, cardiac failure, myocardial infarction.

Fluid imbalance.

Pressure sores.

Spasticity, contractures, frozen shoulder.

Mood disorders.

Seizures.

Falls, fractures.

Differential diagnosis
Intracranial tumour.
Subdural haematoma.

Aetiology

Causes of cerebral infarction
As for transient ischaemic attacks (see separate entry).

Causes of intracranial haemorrhage
Hypertension.
Aneurysm or arteriovenous malformation.
Bleeding diathesis.

Epidemiology
- The annual incidence in the UK is 2 in 1000 population.
- 100 000 patients annually in the UK suffer their first stroke.
- Stroke is the third most common cause of death in industrialized countries.
- It is the largest single cause of severe disability in people living at home.

Classification
- Stroke can be classified as follows:

Cerebral infarction: in 80% of patients.
Primary intracerebral haemorrhage: in 10%.
Subarachnoid haemorrhage: in 5%.
Uncertain: in 5%.

- Cerebral infarction may be further classified on clinical criteria, as follows:

Total anterior circulation infarction: hemiplegia, hemianopia, new cortical deficit.
Partial anterior circulation infarction: two of the above three, new cortical deficit alone, or motor or sensory deficit more restricted than lacunar infarction.
Lacunar infarction: pure motor or sensory stroke, sensorimotor stroke, or ataxic hemiparesis; thought to be caused by intrinsic disease of single perforating artery.
Posterior circulation infarction: evidence of brainstem lesion or homonymous hemianopia.

Treatment

Diet and lifestyle
- Although convincing evidence to support lipid lowering therapy is absent, patients should be advised to adopt a low-animal-fat diet; reduction in dietary salt may lower blood pressure.
- Excess alcohol can cause hypertension and should be reduced.
- Smokers should stop, and moderate exercise be encouraged where possible.

See also Transient ischaemic attacks.

Pharmacological treatment
- No effective medical intervention currently exists for most strokes.
- Trials investigating the roles of antithrombotic and thrombolytic treatment are in progress.
- No evidence supports blood pressure lowering in the acute phase unless hypertensive encephalopathy or aortic dissection is present.

Non-pharmacological treatment

Surgery
- Some patients with intracerebral haematomas may benefit from surgical drainage, although no universally acceptable selection criteria exist.
- Patients with subarachnoid haemorrhages should be referred to a clinical neuroscience unit.

Rehabilitation
- Stroke units combining physiotherapy and occupational and speech therapy save lives.
- Immobilized patients should wear anti-embolism stockings.
- Support from the social services is an important but often neglected element in a patient's recovery.

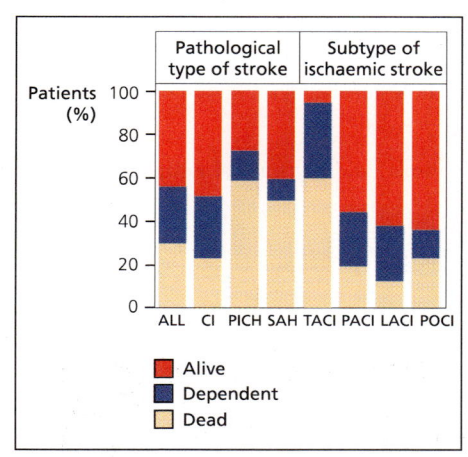

Outcome at 1 year for first stroke according to type or subtype of stroke. CI, cerebral infarction; LACI, Lacunar infarction; PACI, partial anterior circulation infarction; PICH, primary intracerebral haemorrhage, POCI, posterior circulation infarction; SAH, subarachnoid haemorrhage; TACI, total arterior circulation infarction.

Treatment aims
To prevent further cerebral damage or secondary complications.

To treat the cause of the stroke, where possible.

To enable survivors to achieve independence.

Prognosis
- For cerebral infarction, the overall 30-day case fatality is 10%.
- ~50% of survivors remain dependent.
- Important prognostic indicators include type and extent of stroke (*see figure*), age, and presenting level of consciousness.
- Intracranial haemorrhage carries a notably worse prognosis.

Follow-up and management
- The key aim is to identify and modify treatable risk factors (e.g. hypertension, smoking).
- Starting 1–2 weeks after cerebral infarction, lifelong antiplatelet treatment is indicated (aspirin 75–150 mg daily).
- Anticoagulation is effective as primary and secondary prophylaxis for cerebral infarction when atrial fibrillation is present.
- For patients who recover well from a carotid distribution stroke, endarterectomy may be indicated.

Key references
Bamford J: Clinical examination in diagnosis and subclassification of stroke. *Lancet* 1992, **339**:400–402.

Dennis M, Langhorne P: So stroke units save lives: where do we go from here? *BMJ* 1994, **309**:1273–1276.

Humphrey P: Stroke and transient ischaemic attacks. *J Neurol Neurosurg Psychiatry* 1994, **57**:534–543.

Langhorne P *et al.*: Do stroke units save lives? *Lancet* 1993, **342**:395–398.

Warlow CP: Disorders of the cerebral circulation. In *Brain's Disease of the Nervous System* edn 10. Edited by Walton J. Oxford: Oxford University Press, 1993, pp 197–268.

Transient ischaemic attacks
R.J. Davenport and C.P. Warlow

Diagnosis

Definition
- A transient ischaemic attack is abrupt loss of focal cerebral or monocular function with symptoms lasting <24 h, which, after adequate investigations, is presumed to be due to embolic or thrombotic vascular disease.

Symptoms
- Symptoms such as syncope, confusion, convulsions, incontinence, and isolated dizziness are not acceptable for transient ischaemic attacks.

Carotid territory
- This is the site of 80% of transient ischaemic attacks.

Unilateral paresis: weakness, heaviness, or clumsiness.
Unilateral sensory loss.
Aphasia.
Transient monocular visual loss: amaurosis fugax.

Vertebrobasilar territory
- This is the site of 20% of transient ischaemic attacks.

Bilateral or alternating weakness or sensory symptoms.
Vertigo, diplopia, dysphagia, ataxia: patients must have two or more simultaneously.
Sudden bilateral blindness: in patients aged >40 years.

Uncertain arterial distribution
Hemianopia alone.
Dysarthria alone.

Investigations
- Investigations are of little help in the recognition of transient ischaemic attacks; they are directed at determining the cause of the attack.
- Baseline tests should be done in most cases; further investigations depend on the clinical situation, age of the patient, and results of the baseline tests.

Baseline tests
Full blood count: to detect anaemia, polycythaemia, leukaemia, and thrombocythaemia.
ESR measurement: to detect vasculitis, infective endocarditis, and hyperviscosity.
Plasma glucose measurement: to detect diabetes and hypoglycaemia.
Plasma cholesterol measurement: to detect hypercholesterolaemia.
Syphilis serology: to detect syphilis.
Urinalysis: to detect diabetes and renal disease.
ECG: to detect left ventricular hypertrophy, arrhythmia, and myocardial ischaemia or infarction.

Non-routine investigations
Electrolytes analysis: in patients on diuretics, to detect hyponatraemia and hypokalaemia.
Urea analysis: in hypertensive patients, to detect renal impairment.
Thyroid function test: in patients in atrial fibrillation, to detect thyrotoxicosis.
Chest radiography: to detect enlarged heart, calcified valve, and pulmonary arteriovenous malformation.
Cranial CT or MRI: to detect infarct and structural lesion.
Carotid ultrasonography or angiography: to detect carotid stenosis, in patients with carotid transient ischaemic attacks.
Temporal artery biopsy: to detect giant-cell arteritis.
Blood culture: to detect infective endocarditis.
Cardiac enzyme analysis: to detect acute myocardial infarction.

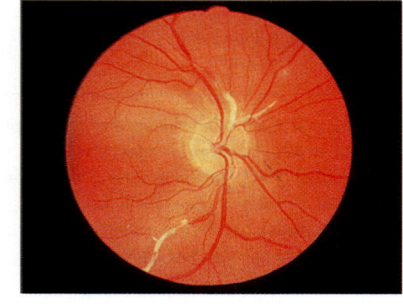

Cholesterol emboli seen on fundoscopy in a patient with amaurosis fugax.

Complications
Stroke.

Differential diagnosis
Migraine with aura.
Partial epileptic seizures.
Structural intracranial lesions: tumour, vascular malformation, chronic subdural haematoma, giant aneurysm.
Multiple sclerosis: in patients aged <40 years.
Labyrinthine disorders: e.g. Meniere's disease, benign positional vertigo.
Peripheral nerve or root lesion.
Metabolic disorders: e.g. hypoglycaemia.
Psychological disorders: e.g. hyperventilation.

Aetiology

Causes
Embolism complicating atherosclerosis of arteries to brain (50% of attacks).
Intracranial small-vessel disease (lipohyalinosis) (20%).
Embolism from the heart (20%).
Inflammatory arterial disease (e.g. giant-cell arteritis).
Arterial dissections.
Haematological disorders (e.g. polycythaemia).

Risk factors
- Factors that increase the risk of degenerative arterial disease in general include the following:

Age, hypertension, diabetes mellitus, cigarette smoking, plasma cholesterol, plasma fibrinogen, excess alcohol consumption (via hypertension).

- Markers for arterial disease include the following:

Ischaemic heart disease, peripheral vascular disease, cervical arterial bruit, left ventricular hypertrophy.

- Evidence of cardiac embolic source includes the following:

Atrial fibrillation, recent myocardial infarction, valvular disease, prosthetic heart valves.

Epidemiology
- 15% of patients suffering their first stroke have had preceding transient ischaemic attacks; only half of these attacks will have been seen or recognised by a doctor.
- The annual incidence of patients with attacks who present for further investigation and treatment is about 0.5 in 1000.
- The incidence increases with age.
- More men are affected than women.

Treatment

Diet and lifestyle

- Treating raised blood pressure reduces the risk of stroke by 50%, even after only a few years; the effect on coronary events is less impressive. Targets should be a systolic and diastolic pressure of below about 180 mmHg and 100 mmHg respectively. Treatment should involve non-pharmacological methods initially, followed by drugs if necessary.
- The effect of stopping smoking is most marked on reducing cardiac events, and all patients should be encouraged vigorously to stop.
- Reducing serum cholesterol leads to a reduced risk of cardiac events, but no reliable data for stroke are available; treatment may have risks. A diet low in saturated fats should be advised, and drugs should only be considered for serum cholesterol concentrations persistently >7.5 mmol/L.
- Physical exercise should be encouraged and probably helps by facilitating weight, cholesterol, and blood pressure control.

Pharmacological treatment

Antiplatelet drugs

- Antiplatelet drugs have shown clear evidence of benefit in a meta-analysis of all trials: the risk of non-fatal myocardial infarction and stroke is reduced by one-third; the risk of all fatal vascular events is reduced by one-sixth.
- Aspirin is the best agent currently available.

Standard dosage	Aspirin 75–150 mg.
Contraindications	Active peptic ulceration.
Special points	As effective as higher doses, with a lower risk of gastrointestinal toxicity.
Main drug interactions	Increased risk of bleeding with warfarin.
Main side effects	Gastrointestinal haemorrhage.

Anticoagulants

- Anticoagulants are indicated when a definite cardiac source of emboli has been identified (e.g. mitral valve disease with atrial fibrillation, prosthetic heart valve, recent myocardial infarction, dilated cardiomyopathy).
- In non-rheumatic atrial fibrillation, warfarin is superior to aspirin.
- Where the source or the emboli is of uncertain relevance (e.g. mitral valve prolapse, aortic sclerosis), aspirin is probably best.
- Short-term warfarin may be used empirically for symptomatic treatment of frequent attacks resistant to aspirin.
- Possible benefits of warfarin must always be weighed against definite side effects in individual patients, particularly if the risk of stroke is not high.

Standard dosage	Warfarin sufficient to maintain INR at 2–4.
Contraindications	Bleeding diathesis, active peptic ulceration.
Special points	Not tolerated well by patients aged >75 years; regular blood monitoring needed.
Main drug interactions	Alcohol, NSAIDs, antiepileptics, antidepressants.
Main side effects	Haemorrhage.

Treatment aims

To prevent stroke or other serious vascular events (secondary prevention).

Other treatments

Carotid endarterectomy: for symptomatic carotid stenoses >70% only.

Prognosis

- The risk of stroke in the first year after a transient ischaemic attack is 12%.
- Thereafter, the risk is 7% each year (seven times the risk in the normal population).
- The greatest risk occurs in the first month after the attack.
- Cardiac death occurs more often than stroke death after an attack.
- The combined risk of all serious vascular events (stroke, myocardial infarction, other vascular death) is ~9% annually.

Follow-up and management

- Risk factors (e.g. hypertension) must be adequately controlled, and antiplatelet therapy maintained.

Key references

Dennis M *et al.*: The prognosis of transient ischaemic attacks in the Oxfordshire community stroke project. *Stroke* 1990, 21:848–853.

European Carotid Surgery Trialist's Collaborative Group: MRC European Carotid Surgery Trial: interim results for symptomatic patients with severe (70–99%) or with mild (0–29%) carotid stenosis. *Lancet* 1991, 337:1235–1243.

Hankey GJ, Warlow CP: *Major Problems in Neurology 27: Transient Ischaemic Attacks of the Brain and Eye*. London: WB Saunders, 1994.

Tremor P.D. Thompson

Diagnosis

Definition
- Tremor is an involuntary, rhythmic, smooth, sinusoidal oscillation of a body part. Faster tremors (6–12 Hz) are usually of fine amplitude; slower tremors (2–5 Hz) are coarse and of large amplitude. Tremors may be described according to the following:
Cause or underlying diagnosis.
Clinical circumstances of occurrence: rest (limb supported), postural (limb outstretched), kinetic (during voluntary movement), task-specific action (e.g. during writing), intention (in terminal stages of movement).
Affected body part: e.g. head, voice, hand, leg.
Frequency (cycles/s or Hz, considerable overlap).

Symptoms
Shaking and trembling of hands: resulting in clumsiness and loss of manual dexterity.
Slow voluntary movement (with rest tremor): suggesting Parkinson's disease.
Weakness or sensory symptoms: suggesting neuropathic tremor.
Twisting movements (with tremor): suggesting dystonic tremor.
Unsteadiness when standing (shaking legs), relieved by walking or sitting: suggesting primary orthostatic tremor.

Signs

Parkinsonian
Rest ('pill-rolling'), possibly with postural tremor: 4–5 and 5–6 Hz, respectively; arms affected more than legs, which are affected more than jaws or lips.

Midbrain (rubral)
Rest, postural, intention tremor: 2–5 Hz; particularly affecting arms.

Cerebellar
Postural, intention, kinetic tremor: 3–6 Hz; arms and trunk more than legs; titubation.

Essential
Postural, kinetic tremor: 5–8 Hz; arms more than head more than legs; isolated.

Neuropathic
Postural, kinetic tremor: 4–6 Hz; arms more than legs.

Dystonic
Postural, kinetic tremor: 2–6 Hz; arms more than legs; exacerbated in certain postures.

Primary orthostatic
Tremor of legs and trunk when standing: 14–16 Hz.

Physiological
Postural tremor: 8–12 Hz; affecting arms; normal finding.

Exaggerated physiological
Postural tremor: 8–12 Hz; affecting arms; larger amplitude than physiological tremor.

Focal
Postural tremor: 4–8 Hz; affecting head, face, jaw, chin, tongue, voice, trunk (alone).

Task-specific action
Kinetic tremor during specific tasks: ~6 Hz; affecting arms, lips, and head.

Investigations
- Investigations are needed to exclude symptomatic tremor or identify the cause.
Serum caeruloplasmin, thyroid function, blood glucose measurement: for Wilson's disease, thyrotoxicosis, and hypoglycaemia, respectively.
Nerve conduction studies, electromyography, serum immunoglobulin measurement: in patients with suspected neuropathy.
Brain imaging: if clinical suspicion of structural lesion, e.g. hemitremor, focal neurological signs, midbrain or cerebellar tremor.

Complications
Clumsiness, loss of manual dexterity, difficulty writing, embarrassment.

Differential diagnosis
Repetitive myoclonus: brisk, abrupt jerks.
Chorea: flowing random variable movements.

Aetiology

Hereditary
Essential tremor (50% of cases inherited autosomal-dominant).

Idiopathic
Physiological tremor.
Primary orthostatic tremor.
Task-specific action tremors.

Symptomatic
Parkinson's disease.
Akinetic rigid syndromes.
Dystonic tremor.
Thyrotoxicosis.
Cerebellar disease: multiple sclerosis, degenerative ataxias.
Midbrain lesions: multiple sclerosis, vascular.
Wilson's disease.
Peripheral neuropathy (especially demyelinating).
Exaggerated physiological tremor.
Drug-induced tremor.
Toxins.

Epidemiology
- Essential tremor occurs in 300 in 100 000 population.
- Parkinson's disease occurs in 200 in 100 000 population (increasing with age).

Diagnostic difficulties

Drug-induced tremor
Beta-2 agonists, caffeine, theophylline, tricyclic antidepressants, 5-HT reuptake inhibitors, lithium, neuroleptics, amphetamines, valproate, steroids, thyroxine.

Toxin-induced tremor
MPTP (1-methyl-4-phenyl-1,2,3,6-tetrahydropyridine), mercury.

Drug-withdrawal tremor
Alcohol, barbiturates, benzodiazepines, opiates.

Exaggerated physiological tremor
Drugs (as above), drug withdrawal (as above), metabolic disease: thyrotoxicosis, hypoglycaemia, phaeochromocytoma, anxiety, fatigue.

Treatment

Diet and lifestyle
- Caffeine and fatigue may exacerbate tremor.
- Alcohol may help essential tremor, but addiction is a possibility.
- Aids for stability when standing (e.g. shooting stick) help orthostatic tremor.

Pharmacological treatment

For essential tremor
Standard dosage	Propranolol 40–120 mg twice daily. Primidone up to 250 mg 2–3 times daily.
Contraindications	*Propranolol:* obstructive airways disease, heart failure.
Special points	*Primidone:* at least 20% of patients develop nausea, vomiting and unsteadiness at beginning of treatment; initial dose should be small (62.5 mg syrup or one-quarter of a standard tablet), taken at bedtime.
Main drug interactions	None.
Main side effects	*Propranolol:* hypotension, bradycardia, bronchospasm. *Primidone:* nausea, vomiting, unsteadiness.

For parkinsonian tremor
L-Dopa, anticholinergic, amantadine, dopamine agonists in doses as for Parkinson's disease *(see* Parkinson's disease *for details).*

For dystonic tremor
Standard dosage	Benzhexol 2 mg daily, increased by 2 mg daily each week, as side effects permit; doses up to 15 mg daily may be needed to realize maximum benefit.
Contraindications	Glaucoma, prostatic hyperplasia.
Special points	Side effects common in elderly patients.
Main drug interactions	None.
Main side effects	Dry mouth, blurred vision, confusion, constipation, urinary outflow obstruction.

For primary orthostatic tremor
Clonazepam, primidone, phenobarbitone: response generally poor.

Treatment aims
To identify and remove causes of exaggerated physiological tremor.
To identify and treat causes of symptomatic tremor.

Other treatments
Thalamotomy or thalamic stimulation: in severe tremors refractory to drugs.

Prognosis
- The prognosis depends on the cause of the tremor.

Follow-up and management
- Follow-up depends on the cause of the tremor.

Key references
Cleeves L, Findley LJ, Marsden CD: Odd tremors. In *Movement Disorders* 3. Edited by Marsden CD, Fahn S. Oxford: Butterworth Heinemann, 1994, pp 434–498.

Findley LJ: Tremors: differential diagnosis and pharmacology. In *Parkinson's Disease and Movement Disorders.* Edited by Jankovic J, Tolosa E. Baltimore: Williams and Wilkins, 1993, pp 293–313.

Index

A

abscess
   brain 2, 10, 22
   epidural 42
   subdural 22
absence 12
acetazolamide for epilepsy 13
acromegaly 36
acupuncture for postherpetic neuralgia 33
acyclovir for encephalitis 11
adrenal implants for Parkinson's disease 39
albumin for intracerebral haemorrhage 21
altitudinal defect 24
Alzheimer's disease 8
amantadine
   for parkinsonian tremor 49
   for Parkinson's disease 39
amaurosis fugax 6 see also blindness
amitriptyline
   for atypical facial pain 15
   for migraine 25
   for motor neurone disease 27
   for painful peripheral neuropathy 37
   for postherpetic neuralgia 33
amnesia 12 see also memory loss
amyloidosis 36
anaesthetics for postherpetic neuralgia 33
analgesics
   for bacterial meningitis 23
   for migraine 25
   for painful peripheral neuropathy 37
anarthria 26
aneurysm, giant 46
angiography, carotid 46
anhidrosis 36
antibiotics for bacterial meningitis 23
anticholinergic drugs
   for parkinsonian tremor 49
   for Parkinson's disease 39
anticholinesterase for myasthenia gravis 31
anticoagulants for transient ischaemic attacks 47
anticonvulsants
   for bacterial meningitis 23
   for encephalitis 11
   for postherpetic neuralgia 33
antidepressants for atypical facial pain 15
antidiuretic hormone secretion, inappropriate 22
antiemetics for migraine 25
antithrombotic treatment for stroke 45
anxiety 14, 38
aphasia 20, 46 see also dysphasia
apomorphine for Parkinson's disease 39
areflexia 42
arrhythmia, cardiac 16, 44
arteriopathy 24
arteritis
   cranial 6
   giant-cell see arteritis, temporal
   temporal 24
arthritis
   immune complex 22
   infectious see arthritis, septic
   rheumatoid 18
   septic 22
arthropathy, neuropathic 36
aspirin for transient ischaemic attacks 47
astrocytomas, cerebral 2
asystole 16
ataxia 10, 16, 20, 46
   sensory 36
ataxis, spinocerebellar see degeneration, spinocerebellar
atrophy
   multiple system 38
   muscular
      spinal 18, 26
      syndrome, post-poliomyelitis 26
   optic 28
atropine for motor neurone disease 27
aura 24
awareness, altered 12
azathioprine
   for idiopathic polymyositis 19
   for peripheral neuropathies 37

B

baclofen
   for motor neurone disease 27
   for multiple sclerosis 29
   for trigeminal neuralgia 35
behaviour disorder 22
benzhexol
   for dystonic tremor 49
   for motor neurone disease 27
benzodiazepines for insomnia 41
benzylpenicillin for meningitis 23
beta blockers for migraine 25
Binswanger's disease 8
biopsy
   bone-marrow 36
   temporal artery 46
bleeding see haemorrhage
blindness 46 see also amaurosis fugax
block, neuromuscular conduction 16
blood pressure
   labile 16
   low see hypotension
bradycardia 16
bradykinesia 38
bradyphrenia 38
brain see also cerebral
   disease, organic 2
breath, holding of 12
bromocryptine for Parkinson's disease 39
Brown–Sequard syndrome 42
Brudzinski's sign 22
bruising 36 see also haematoma
burns 36

C

caeruloplasmin 48
calcium antagonists for intracerebral haemorrhage 21
capsaicin
   for painful peripheral neuropathy 37
   for postherpetic neuralgia 33
carbamazepine
   for epilepsy 13
   for neuralgia
      postherpetic 33
      trigeminal 35
   for painful peripheral neuropathy 37
cataplexy 40
cataracts 7
cerebral see also brain
   arterial attack see transient ischaemic attack
   damage 12
cerebrovascular accident see stroke
chemotherapy
   for cauda equina compression 43
   for cerebral tumour 3
   for spinal cord compression 43
chorea 8, 38, 48
clobazam for epilepsy 13
clomipramine for cataplexy 41
clonazepam
   for epilepsy 13
   for neuralgia
      postherpetic 33
      trigeminal 35
   for primary orthostatic tremor 49
coagulation, disseminated intravascular 22
cognitive impairment 28
coma 4, 10, 20
compression
   nerve 28
   of cauda equina 42
   of spinal cord 42
confusion 8
confusional state, toxic 12
coning 2
connective tissue disease 18
convulsions 10 see also epilepsy, seizures
co-proxamol for postherpetic neuralgia 33
corticosteroids
   for bacterial meningitis 23
   for cauda equina compression 43
   for cranial arteritis 7
   for Guillain–Barré syndrome 17
   for multiple sclerosis 29
   for spinal cord compression 43

Index

crisis
  cholinergic 30
  myasthenic 30
  ocyloguric 12
cry, meningeal 22
cyclophosphamide for idiopathic polymyositis 19
cyclosporin A
  for chronic inflammatory demyelinating polyradiculoneuropathy 37
  for idiopathic polymyositis 19
cytomegalovirus 10

D

danthron for motor neurone disease 27
dantrolene for motor neurone disease 27
deafness *see* hearing loss
deformity
  foot 36
  hand 36
degeneration
  hepatolenticular *see* Wilson's disease
  spinocerebellar 28
déjà vu 12
delirium 8
dementia 8
  degenerative 8
  frontal-lobe 26
  multi-infarct 8
  senile, of Lewy body type 38
demyelination 36
depression 14, 32, 34, 38
dermatomyositis 18
dexamethasone
  for cauda equina compression 43
  for cerebral tumour 3
  for encephalitis 11
  for raised intracranial pressure 3
  for spinal cord compression 43
dexamphetamine for daytime sleepiness 41
diabetes 36
diazepam
  for intracerebral haemorrhage 21
  for motor neurone disease 27
dihydrocodeine for postherpetic neuralgia 33
diphenylhydantoin *see* phenytoin
diphtheria 36
diplopia 2, 16, 20, 28, 46
disorientation *see* confusion
domperidone for peripheral neuropathy 37
L-dopa
  for Parkinson's disease 39
  for Parkinsonian tremor 49
dopamine agonists
  for parkinsonian tremor 49
  for Parkinson's disease 39
dosulepin *see* dothiepin
dothiepin for motor neurone disease 27
drug abuse 12
dyskinesia *see* movement disorder
dysphagia 46
dysphasia 2, 8, 18, 24, 26 *see also* aphasia
dyspraxia 8
dysrhythmia *see* arrhythmia
dystonia 38
  paroxysmal nocturnal 12
dystrophy, limb girdle 18

E

Eaton–Lambert syndrome 18 *see also* myasthenic syndrome, Lambert–Eaton
EBV *see* Epstein–Barr virus
effusion, subdural 22
embolism, pulmonary 16, 26
encephalitis 10, 12
  herpes 10
  subacute sclerosing 10
encephalomyelitis 10
  myalgic *see* fatigue syndrome, chronic
encephalopathy, toxic 10
enuresis 40
ependymoma 42
epilepsy 2, 12, 22 *see also* convulsions, seizures
  atonic 12
  clonic 12
  focal *see* epilepsy, partial
  generalized 12
  localization-related *see* epilepsy, partial
  myoclonic 12
  partial 12
    complex 12
    secondary generalized 12
    simple 12
  tonic 12
  tonic–clonic 12
Epstein–Barr virus 10
ergotamine for migraine 25
erythromycin for peripheral neuropathy 37
ethosuximide for epilepsy 13

F

Fabry's disease 36
failure
  heart 44
  ventilatory 26
fainting *see* syncope
fasciculations 26
fatigue
  daytime 40
  syndrome
    chronic 30
    postviral *see* fatigue syndrome, chronic
fetal implant therapy for Parkinson's disease 39
fibrillation, atrial 46
fibrosis, pulmonary *see* lung disease, interstitial
fits *see* epilepsy, seizures
fludrocortisone for peripheral neuropathy 37
fluid imbalance 44
fluoxetine for motor neurone disease 27
fluvoxamine for atypical facial pain 15
fontanelle, bulging 22
Foresteir–Certonciny syndrome *see* polymyalgia rheumatica
frusemide for intracerebral haemorrhage 21

G

gabapentin for epilepsy 13
ganciclovir for encephalitis 11
gangliolysis, controlled thermocoagulation, for trigeminal neuralgia 35
gastroparesis for peripheral neuropathy 37
glaucoma 24
glioma 42
grand mal *see* epilepsy
granulomatosis, Wegener's 36
Guillain–Barré syndrome 16, 42

H

haematoma 10 *see also* bruising
  cerebellar 20
  midbrain 20
  pontine 20
  subdural 44, 46
  thalamic 20
haemorrhage 24
  brain tumour 20
  caudate 20
  intracerebral 20, 44
  pontine 20
  subarachnoid 4, 20, 22, 24, 44
headache 10, 20, 22
  cluster 40
  tension 6, 24
  throbbing 24
hearing loss 22
hemianopia 24, 46
hemicrania *see* migraine
hemiparesis 24
hemiplegia 20
herniation
  foramen magnum 20
  tentorial 20
HIV 36, 42
5-HT
  antagonists for migraine 25
  reuptake inhibitors *see* antidepressants
Huntington's disease 8
hydralazine for intracerebral haemorrhage 21
hydrocephalus 20, 22
hyoscine for motor neurone disease 27
hyperpathia 32

Index

hyperventilation 46
hypnotics for insomnia 41
hypoaesthesia 32
hypoglycaemia 12, 46
hypokalaemia 16
hypotension
    orthostatic 36
        postural 36
hypothermia 4
hypothyroidism 36
hysteria 16

I

immunization against *Haemophilus influenzae* for prevention of bacterial meningitis 23
immunoglobulin
    for chronic inflammatory demyelinating polyradiculoneuropathy 37
    for Guillain–Barré syndrome 17
    for idiopathic polymyositis 19
impotence 28, 36
incontinence 28, 36
incoordination 28
infarction
    brainstem 6
    cerebral 44
    haemorrhagic 20
    lacunar 44
    myocardial 41, 44
infection
    bronchopulmonary 26
    respiratory 4
    urinary tract 44
insomnia 40
ischaemia, transient cerebral *see* transient ischaemic attacks
ispaghula husk for motor neurone disease 27

J

jerks, hypnic 40
joint
    disease, temperomandibular 6
    disorders *see* arthritis

K

Kennedy's syndrome 26
Kernig's sign 22
Korsakoff syndrome *see* psychosis, Korsakoff's

L

labetalol for intracerebral haemorrhage 21
labyrinthine disorder 46
lactulose for motor neurone disease 27
lamotrigine for epilepsy 13
leprosy 36

lesion
    cerebral 42
    intracranial 46
    intramedullary spinal cord 26
    nasopharyngeal 24
    peripheral
        nerve 46
        root 46
leukaemic infiltrates 22
levodopa *see* L-dopa
Lewy body disease *see* Parkinson's disease
Libman–Sacks disease *see* lupus erythematosus, systemic
lidocaine *see* lignocaine
lignocaine for postherpetic neuralgia 33
lithium for migrainous neuralgia 25
locked-in syndrome 4
lofepramine for atypical facial pain 15
loperamide for peripheral neuropathy 37
lung disease, interstitial 18
lupus erythematosus, systemic 18, 24
Lyme disease 36
lyseride for Parkinson's disease 39

M

Machado–Joseph disease *see* degeneration, spinocerebellar
malformation
    Arnold–Chiari 42
    arteriovenous 44
    vascular 42
malingering 16
mannitol
    for encephalitis 11
    for intracerebral haemorrhage 21
Marinesco–Sjögren syndrome *see* degeneration, spinocerebellar
mazindol for daytime sleepiness 41
memory loss 8 *see also* amnesia
Menière's disease 46
meningioma 2, 6, 9, 42
meningitis 4
    bacterial 10, 12, 22
    fungal 10
    Mollaret's 22
    noninfective 22
    tuberculous 10
    viral 10
meningoencephalitis 10
mental retardation 22
metabolic disorder 46
methotrexate for idiopathic polymyositis 19
methylprednisolone
    for cranial arteritis 7
    for multiple sclerosis 29
methysergide for migrainous neuralgia 25
metoprolol for migraine 25

mexiletine for peripheral neuropathy 37
migraine 6, 12, 24, 46
    classic 24
    common 24
    hemiplegic 24
    ophthalmoplegic 24
    retinal 24
    with aura 24
    without aura 24
Miller–Fisher syndrome 16
mitochondrial disorder 38
motor neurone disease 26, 28
movement
    disorder, paroxysmal 12
    twisting 48
myasthenia gravis 26, 30
myasthenic syndrome, Lambert–Eaton 30 *see also* Eaton–Lambert syndrome
myelitis, transverse 42
myelopathy 16
    acute inflammatory 42
    cervical 26
    vascular 42
myoclonus 10
    repetitive 48
myopathy
    lipid storage 18
    nemaline 18
    sarcoid 18
myositides 18
myositis
    inclusion body 18
    multiple *see* polymyositis
    paraneoplastic 18

N

nadolol for migraine 25
narcolepsy 12, 40
nerve
    conduction studies 16, 36, 48
    stimulation, transcutaneous electrical for postherpetic neuralgia 33
neuralgia
    migrainous 24, 34
    occipital 6
    postherpetic 32, 34
    trigeminal 14, 34
neurofibroma 42
neurofibromatosis 2
neuronopathy, motor 26
neuropathy
    axonal 36
    drug-induced 16
    hereditary motor 36
    ischaemic optic 6
    peripheral 36
        autonomic 36
        focal/multifocal 36
        painful 36

Index

neurosarcoidosis 28
nimodipine for intracerebral haemorrhage 21
nitroprusside for intracerebral haemorrhage 21
nitrosoureas for cerebral tumour 3
nystagmus 10, 20, 28

O

oedema, cerebral 10
Ondine's curse *see* sleep apnoea, obstructive
ophthalmoplegia 16
opiates for motor neurone disease 27
opioids *see* opiates
oxybutynin for multiple sclerosis 29
oxygen for acute migrainous neuralgia 25

P

pacemaker, endocardial, for Guillain–Barré syndrome 17
pain
 atypical facial 14, 34
 periorbital unilateral 24
 temporomandibular joint 14
pallidotomy, posteroventral for Parkinson's disease 39
palsy
 bulbar 26
 nerve
  cranial 16, 22
  ipsilateral 20
  oculomotor *see* palsy, third nerve
  third 20
 progressive supranuclear 38
 pseudobulbar 26
papaverine for peripheral neuropathy 37
papilloedema 2, 8, 20, 22
paraesthesiae 28, 36
paralysis
 agitans *see* Parkinson's disease
 in narcoleptic syndrome 40
 oculomotor *see* ophthalmoplegia
  nerve *see* palsy, third nerve
 third nerve *see* palsy, third nerve
paraparesis, spastic 42
paraproteinaemia 36
parasomnia 12, 40
paresis 28
 unilateral 46
Parkinson's disease 38
paroxetine for atypical facial pain 15
pemoline for daytime sleepiness 41
pergolide for Parkinson's disease 39
petit mal *see* epilepsy
phenobarbitone
 for epilepsy 13
 for primary orthostatic tremor 49
phenothiazines for peripheral neuropathy 37

phenytoin
 for epilepsy 3, 13
 for intracerebral haemorrhage 21
 for neuralgia
  postherpetic 33
  trigeminal 35
phonophobia 24
photophobia 22, 24
pizotifen for migraine 25
plasma exchange
 for Guillain–Barré syndrome 17
 for myasthenia gravis 31
 for progressive neuropathy 37
pneumonia 44
 hypostatic 16
poliomyelitis 16
polyarteritis nodosa 24
polymyalgia 6
 rheumatica 18
polymyositis 16, 18
 eosinophilic 18
polyradiculoneuritis *see* Guillain–Barré syndrome
polyradiculoneuropathy, chronic inflammatory demyelinating 36
porphyria 16, 36
postural imbalance 38
prednisolone
 for acute migrainous neuralgia 25
 for chronic inflammatory demyelinating polyradiculoneuropathy 37
 for cranial arteritis 7
 for giant-cell arteritis 329
 for idiopathic polymyositis 19
 for myasthenia gravis 31
 for peripheral neuropathy 37
pressure
 intracranial, raised 3, 4, 20
 subarachnoid *see* pressure, intracranial
primidone for tremor 49
procarbazine for cerebral tumour 3
propantheline for myasthenia gravis 31
propranolol
 for essential tremor 49
 for migraine 25
pseudocoma 4
pseudodementia, depressive 8
pseudopolyarthritis, rhizomelic *see* polymyalgia rheumatica
psychological disorder 46
psychosis, Korsakoff's 8
psychosocial handicap 12
ptosis, fatiguable 30
pyridostigmine for myasthenia gravis 31

Q

quinine for motor neurone disease 27

R

radiotherapy
 for cauda equina compression 43
 for spinal cord compression 43
Ramsey–Hunt syndrome *see* Parkinson' disease
Raynaud's phenomenon 18
reflexes, primitive 8
rheumatism, peri-extra-articular *see* polymyalgia rheumatica
rifampicin for prevention of bacterial meningitis 23

S

sarcoidosis 36
sclerosis
 disseminated *see* sclerosis, multiple
 hippocampal 12
 multiple 28, 42, 46
 systemic 18
scotoma 24
seizures 10, 12, 20, 22, 44, 46 *see also* epilepsy
selegiline for Parkinson's disease 39
sensory
 impairment, trigeminal 34
 loss, unilateral 46
serotonin *see* 5-HT
shock 22
shoulder, frozen 44
sicca syndrome *see* Sjögren's syndrome
sinusitis 22, 24
Sjögren's syndrome 18, 36
SLE *see* lupus erythematosus, systemic
sleep
 apnoea, obstructive 40
 disorders 40
  circadian 40
sodium valproate for postherpetic neuralgia 33
spasticity 44
spectra, fortification 24
status epilepticus 12
steroids *see* corticosteroids
stroke 6, 12, 42, 44
sumatriptan for migraine 25
syncope 12
syringomyelia 42

T

teichopsia 24
tetany 12
tetrahydroaminoacridine for dementia 9
thrombolytic treatment for stroke 45
thrombosis 16
 venous 4, 26
thymectomy for myasthenia gravis 31

Index

thymoma 30
timolol for migraine 25
transient ischaemic attack 6, 12, 44, 46
tremor 28, 38, 48
   cerebellar 48
   dystonic 48
   essential 38, 48
   focal 48
   midbrain 48
   neuropathic 36, 48
   parkinsonian 48
   physiological, 48
   primary orthostatic 48
   rubral 48
   task-specific action 48
tuberculosis 12
tumour
   cerebral 2, 24
   extracerebral intracranial 2
twitches, muscle *see* fasciculation

U

uraemia 36
urgency, urinary 28

V

vagal overactivity 12
valproate for epilepsy 13
vasculitis 16, 36
vasospasm, cerebral *see* transient ischaemic attack
vertigo 28, 46
   aural *see* Menière's disease
   benign positional 46
vigabatrin for epilepsy 13
vision, double *see* diplopia
visual
   field defect, homonymous 20
   loss 24, 28
      transient monocular 46
vitamin B_{12} 42
   deficiency 36
   for dementia 9

W

warfarin for transient ischaemic attacks 47
Waterhouse–Friderichson syndrome 22
weakness 48
   alternating 46
   limb 32
Wernicke's syndrome 8
Wilson's disease 38

Z

zidovudine for encephalitis 11

CURRENT DIAGNOSIS & TREATMENT

in

Psychiatry

Edited by
Neil Holden

Series editors
Roy Pounder
Mark Hamilton

A QUICK Reference for the Clinician

Contributors

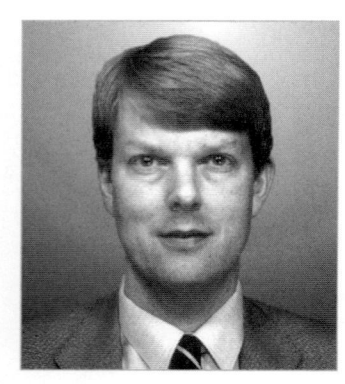

EDITOR

N L Holden

Dr Neil Holden is Consultant Psychiatrist and Director of Postgraduate Education at the Nottingham Healthcare NHS Trust. He is on the Editorial Board of the British Journal of Hospital Medicine and examiner for the Royal College of Psychiatrists and Leicester University. His research and clinical interests are in eating disorders and general psychiatry.

REFEREES

Dr Klaus Bergmann
Consultant Psychiatrist
The Maudesley Hospital
London, UK

Dr Sidney Crown
Consulting Psychiatrist
Royal London Hospital
London, UK

AUTHORS

ALCOHOL WITHDRAWAL SYNDROME

Dr Prakash Naik
Consultant Psychiatrist
Solihull Healthcare
Solihull, UK

Mr John Lawton
Clinical Service Pharmacist
Mapperley Hospital
Nottingham, UK

ATTEMPTED SUICIDE

Dr Eleanor Feldman
Department of Psychiatry
University Hospital
Queen's Medical Centre
Nottingham, UK

BULIMIA NERVOSA

Dr Janet Treasure
Eating Disorders Unit
Institute of Psychiatry
London, UK

DEPRESSION AND MANIA

Dr Conor Duggan
Department of Psychiatry
Mapperley Hospital
Nottingham, UK

OBSESSIVE COMPULSIVE DISORDER

Dr Shashi Rani
Department of Behavioural Cognitive Psychotherapy
Springfield Hospital
London, UK

Dr Lynne M Drummond
Department of Behavioural Cognitive Psychotherapy
St George's Hospital
London, UK

PANIC AND GENERALIZED ANXIETY DISORDER

Professor Peter Tyrer
Department of Community Psychiatry
St Charles Hospital
London, UK

PERSONALITY DISORDERS

Dr Brian Ferguson
Consultant Psychiatrist
Stonebridge Centre
Nottingham, UK

POSTNATAL MENTAL ILLNESS

Dr Margaret Oates
Department of Psychiatry
Queen's Medical Centre
Nottingham, UK

SCHIZOPHRENIA

Dr Richard Mullen
Department of Psychiatry
Maudesley Hospital
London, UK

Dr Anthony S David
Department of Psychological Medicine
Maudesley Hospital
London, UK

Contents

2 **Alcohol withdrawal syndrome**
  delirium tremens
  uncomplicated alcohol withdrawal

4 **Attempted suicide**
  high risk of completed suicide
  low risk of completed suicide

6 **Bulimia nervosa**

8 **Depression and mania**
  dysthymia
  hypomania
  major depression
  mania

10 **Obsessive compulsive disorder**

12 **Panic and generalized anxiety disorder**

14 **Personality disorders**
  eccentric personality (paranoid/schizoid)
  fearful personality (anankastic, anxious/avoidant, dependent)
  flamboyant personality (dissocial, histrionic, impulsive/borderline)

16 **Postnatal mental illness**
  mild depressive illness (neurotic or reactive)
  puerperal psychosis (bipolar or manic–depressive)
  severe depressive illness (unipolar)

18 **Schizophrenia**

20 **Index**

Alcohol withdrawal syndrome   P. Naik and J. Lawton

Diagnosis

Symptoms and signs

Uncomplicated alcohol withdrawal
- Patients may continue to have physical signs and symptoms of long-term alcohol abuse (e.g. peripheral neuropathy, calf tenderness, liver failure).
- Symptoms appear within several hours of reduction or cessation of alcohol intake and last 5–7 days.

Nausea or vomiting.

Anxiety, irritability, insomnia.

Illusions and poorly formed transient hallucinations.

Autonomic hyperactivity: e.g. tachycardia, raised blood pressure.

Coarse tremor of hands, tongue, or eyelids.

Alcohol withdrawal delirium (delirium tremens)
- Symptoms develop 1–7 days after reduction or cessation of intake and last 2–3 days.
- The following features differentiate delirium tremens from uncomplicated alcohol withdrawal:

Disorientation and confusion.

Vivid hallucinations: visual, auditory, tactile.

Delusions.

Investigations

Routine
Full blood count: to identify anaemia and macrocytosis.

Vitamin B_{12} and serum folate measurement: to detect deficiencies.

U&E and creatinine measurement: to assess level of hydration.

Liver function tests: to diagnose evidence of liver damage.

Chest radiography: to detect chest infections and cardiomyopathy.

Indicators of long-term excessive alcohol use
Alcohol history: most sensitive and important indicator; elicits amount and duration of intake and evidence of complications.

Mean cell volume measurement: raised volume 20% sensitive and nonspecific.

Gamma glutamyltransferase measurement: increased concentration 60% sensitive and nonspecific.

Complications
Tonic–clonic seizures.

Physical injury.

Wernicke's encephalopathy: acute onset, characterized by ataxia, ophthalmoplegia, and confusion; syndrome underdiagnosed but should be considered in all comatose patients.

Korsakoff's psychosis: irreversible brain damage; main defect is loss of recent memory, leading to confabulation.

Differential diagnosis
Withdrawal from sedatives (benzodiazepines, barbiturates).
Diabetic ketoacidosis.
Hypoglycaemia.

Aetiology
- Alcohol withdrawal syndrome is caused by stopping or reducing alcohol intake in patients dependent on alcohol.

Epidemiology
- 1.5 million people in the UK consume alcohol at dangerous levels.
- 300 000 people in the UK suffer from alcohol dependence.
- 25% of acute medical admissions in the UK are alcohol-related.

Definitions

Units
Safe levels: for women, <14 units/week; for men, <21 units/week.
Hazardous levels: for women, 14–35 units/week; for men, 21–50 units/week.
Dangerous levels: for women, >35 units/week; for men >50 units/week.

Alcohol abuse
Regular daily intake of a large amount of alcohol.
Regular heavy drinking limited to weekends or in binges lasting weeks or months.
No evidence of withdrawal symptoms.

Alcohol dependence
Subjective awareness of a compulsion to drink.
Prominence of drink-seeking behaviour.
Evidence of tolerance.
Presence of withdrawal symptoms after reduction or cessation of alcohol ingestion.
Use of alcohol to relieve or avoid development of withdrawal symptoms.
Social, psychological, and physical consequences of alcohol use.

Treatment

Diet and lifestyle
- No special precautions are necessary, beyond modifying alcoholic lifestyle.

Pharmacological treatment
- Pharmacological treatment is needed for patients showing evidence of alcohol withdrawal; treatment of alcohol abuse is not necessary.

Setting for treatment
- No evidence suggests that inpatient treatment is superior to outpatient treatment; inpatient treatment is, however, recommended for the following patients:

Those who may develop delirium tremens and severe withdrawal complications (fits, Wernicke's–Korsakoff's psychosis).

Those who are considered a high suicide risk.

Those who require respite from disorganized social settings.

Benzodiazepines
- These are the first-line treatment to relieve withdrawal symptoms and protect against complications.

Standard dosage	Chlordiazepoxide 20 mg or diazepam 10 mg 4 times daily, gradually reduced over 7–10 days, then stopped.
Contraindications	Respiratory depression, acute pulmonary insufficiency.
Special points	Dose should be reduced if signs of oversedation or respiratory depression; long-term use to be avoided. Oxazepam (short-acting, no active metabolites) is agent of choice in liver failure. Patients in whom oral route is inadequate should be given slow i.v. diazepam emulsion according to drug data sheet.
Main drug interactions	Sedatives, cimetidine.
Main side effects	Drowsiness, ataxia, amnesia.

Chlormethiazole
- Chlormethiazole is the second-line choice to relieve withdrawal symptoms and protect against complications.

Standard dosage	Chlormethiazole 3 capsules 4 times daily, gradually reduced over 7–10 days, then stopped.
Contraindications	Acute pulmonary insufficiency, continued alcohol consumption.
Special points	Oral administration not recommended for outpatient use because combination with alcohol can be fatal; i.v. administration indicated when benzodiazepines fail to control withdrawal symptoms and seizures. Long-term use to be avoided.
Main drug interactions	Sedatives, cimetidine.
Main side effects	Nasal congestion, conjunctival irritation.

Thiamine

Standard dosage	*For uncomplicated alcohol withdrawal:* thiamine 10–30 mg orally daily. *For imminent or diagnosed Wernicke's encephalopathy:* thiamine 200–300 mg orally daily in divided doses or, if oral route inadequate, 250 mg i.m. or i.v. slowly (as 1 pair Pabrinex ampoules); increased or repeated as necessary.
Contraindications	Known hypersensitivity to thiamine.
Main drug interactions	None.
Main side effects	Hypersensitivity reactions have been reported after repeated injections.

Treatment aims
To relieve withdrawal symptoms.
To prevent withdrawal complications.
To help patient to plan long-term goals.

Prognosis
- If the patient is adequately treated, in the absence of medical complications, the prognosis is good.
- 5–20% of patients with delirium tremens die from complications, e.g. infection, hypothermia, aspiration, and vascular collapse.
- Wernicke's encephalopathy, if untreated, can lead to irreversible brain damage.

Follow-up and management
- Individual patients' needs vary, and the regimen must be tailor-made.
- Anxiety and depressive illness must be excluded.
- Recently detoxified patients can be given long-term prophylactic treatment with thiamine 10 mg daily.
- Disulfiram may be helpful in maintaining abstinence.

Patient support
- Support should come from three sources: individual therapy (providing support, encouraging abstinence), group therapy (e.g. Alcoholics Anonymous), and outpatient and day-hospital support.

Key references
Naik P, Lawton J: Pharmacological management of alcohol withdrawal: a review. *Br J Hosp Med* 1993, **50**:265–269.

O'Brien MD: Management of major status epilepticus in adults. *BMJ* 1990, **301**:918.

Attempted suicide — E. Feldman

Diagnosis

Symptoms and signs

History: high risk of completed suicide

Presence or previous history of major mental illness: especially endogenous depression, mania, and schizophrenia.

Evidence of planning: time spent in preparation of the means of death, e.g. buying and hoarding tablets, precautions taken against discovery or intervention by others, acts in anticipation of death, e.g. making or updating will, writing suicide note.

Continuing wish to die: no help sought after attempt, continued wish to die after resuscitation, hopelessness.

Violent method chosen: e.g. hanging, jumping from height.

History: low risk of completed suicide

No history or presence of major mental illnesses.

Little or no preparation or precautions: decision to attempt suicide taken within 1 h of the act or after ingestion of alcohol, act performed in front of another.

No continuing wish to die: help sought after act, no wish to die after resuscitation, optimism about future.

Non-violent means: method perceived by patient as having a low risk of real harm; patients may not understand the toxic effects of drugs taken and may mistakenly consider paracetamol and aspirin harmless because they are available over the counter and benzodiazepines dangerous because they are prescription-only drugs.

Mental state

- Orientation and memory must be checked first because the toxic effects of drugs or alcohol must be allowed to wear off before further assessment is attempted.
- An acute organic brain syndrome, including visual hallucinations can be caused by overdose of tricyclic antidepressants.

Features of major mental illness, especially endogenous depression or psychosis: patient should be asked about persistent low mood, worse in mornings, sleep disturbance with early morning wakening, appetite and weight loss, lack of energy, pessimism, low self-esteem, guilt, excessive worrying, delusions, and hallucinations.

Investigations

- Available databases should be checked for evidence of previous or present psychiatric care.
- Further history should be obtained from available informants.
- Physical investigations appropriate for the type of self-harm should be made.

Complications

- No overall physical complications are seen; complications depend on the nature of the self-harm.

Differential diagnosis

Self-cutting or self-damage to relieve tension: often multiple superficial cuts on forearms.

Self-mutilation in context of psychotic illness: especially schizophrenia.

Accidental ingestion of toxic substances: e.g. tablets that look like sweets to children, weedkiller stored in a lemonade bottle.

Aetiology

- Causes include the following:

High risk of completed suicide
Major depression, schizophrenia, mania.
Alcoholism and drug abuse.
Chronic physical ill health.
Recent bereavement.

Low risk of completed suicide
Poorly developed coping skills.
Relationship problems.
Social stressors.

Epidemiology

- Trends vary widely over time and across different cultures.
- Risk factors for completed suicide are male sex, poor physical health, unemployment or retirement, being separated, widowed, or divorced, living alone.
- A recent trend in men <35 years has been noted in the UK.
- Patients at low risk of completed suicide are usually female, <45 years, from a low socioeconomic class, and living in urban areas with social deprivation and crowding.
- The rate in people aged 12–15 years is increasing in the UK.
- In the UK, the rates for attempted suicide were 363 in 100 000 women >15 years and 272 in 100 000 men >15 years in 1990 (Oxford city).
- The UK rate for completed suicide was 11.1 in 100 000 in 1990.
- Suicide is the second most common cause of death in men <35 years in the UK and one of the 10 most common causes of death overall in the UK.

Treatment

Diet and lifestyle
- High alcohol intake, social isolation, and lack of employment are all high risk factors for repetition of suicide attempts, so efforts should be made to change the lifestyle of the patients through therapeutic intervention.

Pharmacological treatment
- The physical consequences of self-harm must be treated first.
- Except in emergencies, psychotropic drugs should be given only for treatment of specific mental illness under close psychiatric supervision, usually as an inpatient.
- Tranquillizing drugs must be avoided unless absolutely necessary for the safety of patients or others.
- For the emergency management of violently mentally disturbed patients, a short-acting antipsychotic, e.g. droperidol or haloperidol in 5 mg increments i.m. every 15 min, should be used until symptoms are controlled, unless seizures are a risk. An antiparkinsonian drug, e.g. procyclidine 5–10 mg i.m., can be added to avoid dystonic reactions. Drugs should not be given i.v. when the cause of the mental disturbance is not known.
- When seizures are a risk, a benzodiazepine, e.g. diazepam as diazemuls in 5 mg increments i.v. or lorazepam 2–5 mg i.m., can be used. Benzodiazepines must be avoided in patients with severe respiratory impairment. Antipsychotic agents and benzodiazepines combined have an additive tranquillizing effect.

Non-pharmacological treatment

Counselling
- Most patients are cooperative, and many are not suffering from mental illness. Low-risk patients should be offered brief problem-orientated counselling, where available.
- Patients with alcohol or substance abuse problems should be referred to the relevant specialist services.
- Relationship therapy should be offered to patients with relationship problems if both partners are agreeable.
- Open access or a telephone help-line may be offered, if available.

Psychiatric referral
- High-risk patients need psychiatric referral.
- Patients with major mental illness need urgent psychiatric treatment, usually on an inpatient basis. The provisions of the Mental Health Act (1983) (England and Wales) should be used if voluntary treatment is declined.

Detention and emergency treatment
- Patients threatening discharge who have not been assessed or who have been assessed and are considered to be at immediate risk may have to be detained for further assessment or treatment.
- If a patient refuses to talk, information to make an assessment must be obtained from other informants before the patient can be discharged.
- Compulsory detention in hospital must be considered in cases of psychiatric illness or serious suicide risk.
- Common law allows emergency action in the patient's best interests and presumes a duty of care; failure to act may be construed as negligent.
- The Mental Health Act (1983) (England and Wales) does not apply to alcoholism, substance abuse, and the treatment of physical illness.

Treatment aims
To treat any underlying mental disorder.
To help patient to solve problems and to provide support through current crisis.
To strengthen patient's future coping skills.

Prognosis
- Repetition occurs most often within the first 3 months of an episode.
- Repetition with increased suicidal intent may herald completed suicide.
- Long-term risk of completed suicide overall is ~1% at 1 year and ~2.8% at 8 years.
- ~7% of patients make 2 or more attempts, 2.5% 3 or more, and 1% 5 or more.

Follow-up and management
- Low-risk patients do not need special care.
- High-risk patients and those with mental illness need close monitoring.

Factors associated with repetition
- Factors that indicate a greater risk of repetition include previous psychiatric treatment, alcohol problems, previous deliberate self-harm, sociopathic traits, living alone, and unchanged problems and circumstances.
- Chronic repeaters invariably have severe personality difficulties, chaotic lifestyles, deprived backgrounds, and great difficulty in engaging in any form of therapy.

Dealing with violent mentally disturbed patients
- Aggressive patients are often frightened.
- Keep calm and gentle in voice and actions.
- Do not corner, crowd, or threaten the patient.
- Give clear explanations of what is happening.
- Do not see or leave the patient alone.
- Call for adequate extra staff, porters, security staff, or police as necessary backup.

Key references
Anonymous: Management of behavioural emergencies. *Drug Ther Bull* 1991, **29**:62–64.
Hawton K, Fagg J: Trends in deliberate self poisoning and self injury in Oxford, 1976–90. *BMJ* 1992, **304**:1409–1411.
Vassilas CA, Morgan HG: General Practitioners' contact with victims of suicide. *BMJ* 1993, **307**:300–301.

Bulimia nervosa — J. Treasure

Diagnosis

Symptoms
Behaviour disguised because of shame and guilt.
Preoccupation with diets: in a woman of normal weight.
Vomiting: with atypical symptoms.
Oedema: in young women.
Fullness and bloating after meals.
Preoccupation with constipation.
Amenorrhoea or irregular menstruation.
Low mood, anxiety, drug or alcohol abuse.
Sports injury.

Signs
Tooth enamel loss, caries, prostheses.
Enlarged salivary glands.
Mouth abrasions.
Callus on dorsum of hand: Russell's sign, due to gag reflex causing a bite.

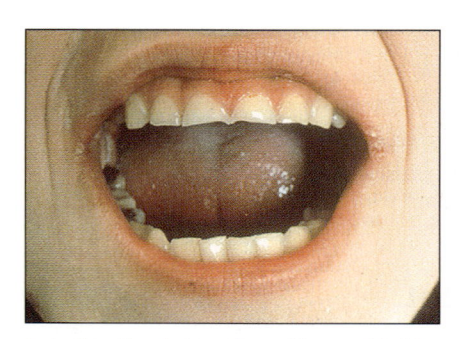

Loss of tooth substance in an 18-year-old girl who had vomited since the age of 15 years.

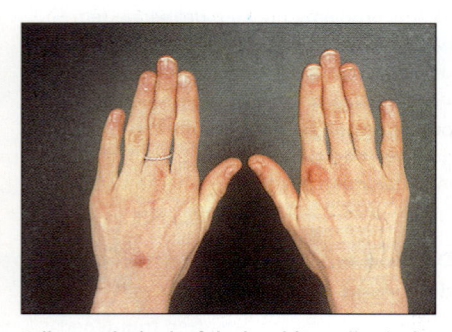

Callus on the back of the hand (Russell's sign).

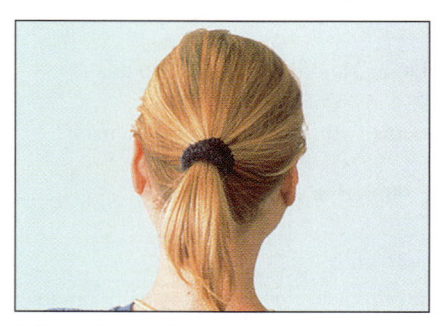

Salivary gland enlargement in a young woman vomiting twice each day.

Investigations
History: for psychological, nutritional, and weight-control measures.
U&E analysis: vomiting causes low potassium and high bicarbonate; laxatives cause low sodium, low potassium, and low bicarbonate; urea increased with dehydration.

Complications
• Complications occur in <1% of sufferers.
Gastrointestinal bleeding.
Cardiac dysrhythmia.
Renal failure.

Differential diagnosis
• After the history has been obtained, it is characteristic.
Anorexia nervosa.
Depression.

Aetiology
• Causes include the following:
Dieting: risk increased 8-fold.
Psychosocial: poor parenting experiences, life events.
Genetic: family history of depression, obesity, and alcoholism.

Epidemiology
• 2% of women between the ages of 15 and 25 years suffer from bulimia nervosa.
• The prevalence is increasing in generations born after 1950.
• 5% of sufferers are men.
• All social classes are affected.

Treatment

Diet and lifestyle
- Patients must be helped to eat a regular, well balanced diet; this is achieved by pharmacological and non-pharmacological treatment.

Pharmacological treatment
- Drugs are less effective than psychological therapy but can produce a window of remission during which psychological therapy can begin.

Standard dosage	Fluoxetine 60 mg.
Contraindications	Hypersensitivity, renal failure, lactation, unstable epilepsy; caution in liver failure, renal impairment, cardiac disease, diabetes, pregnancy.
Special points	Produces 20% abstinence rates.
Main drug interactions	Monoamine oxidase inhibitors, tryptophan, tricyclic antidepressants, lithium, flecainide, encainide, vinblastine, carbamazepine.
Main side effects	Asthenia, fever, neurological effects (including headache), pharyngitis, dyspnoea, rash, nausea (paradoxically).

Non-pharmacological treatment
- Psychological approaches are the treatment of choice because they are more effective in the short term, probably also in the long term, but 9–19 hourly sessions of specialist therapy may be needed. Self-treatment manuals are available.
- The effective components include the following:

Educational: nutritional, weight control.

Behavioural: food and purging diary, prescription of regular meals, stimulus control to limit meal size, distraction or relaxation to interrupt symptomatic behaviour.

Cognitive: modification of distorted beliefs about shape and weight, strengthening of coping resources, stress management, problem solving, communication and assertiveness skills.

- Abstinence rates of 50–60% are achieved.

Treatment aims
To restore normal eating patterns.
To provide psychological support and treatment.

Prognosis
- 50–60% of patients are asymptomatic after treatment.
- Relapse is common in the first year after treatment.
- 70% are asymptomatic after 2 years.
- Self-harm is common in the 30% of patients with borderline personality disorders (i.e. ~30% of these or ~10–20% of all patients).

Follow-up and management
- 6-monthly follow-up is needed.

Key references
American Psychiatric Association: Practice guidelines for eating disorders. *Am J Psychiatry* 1993, **150**:212–228.

Cooper PJ: *Bulimia Nervosa: A Guide to Recovery.* London: Robinson Publishing, 1993.

Kendler KS *et al.*: The genetic epidemiology of bulimia nervosa. *Am J Psychiatry* 1991, **148**:1627–1637.

Schmidt U, Treasure J: *Getting Better Bit(e) by Bit(e).* Hove: Laurence Erlbaum, 1993.

Szmucker G, Dare C, Treasure J: *Handbook of Eating Disorders. Theory, Treatment and Research.* Chichester: John Wiley and Sons, 1995.

Depression and mania   C. Duggan

Diagnosis

Symptoms and signs
- In both mania and major depression, mood-congruent delusions may arise; these may be accompanied by auditory hallucinations.

Mania
Distinct periods of elevated expansion or irritable mood, with the following:

Hyperactivity.

Pressure of speech.

Flight of ideas.

Subjective self-esteem, euphoria, grandiosity.

Reduced sleep.

Distractability.

Recklessness.

Major depression
Distinct periods of dysphoric mood, loss of interest or pleasures in usual activities, with the following:

Change in appetite or weight.

Sleep disturbance.

Psychomotor agitation or retardation.

Anergia.

Difficulty in concentrating or making decisions.

Hopelessness.

Suicidal thoughts or attempts.

Dysthymia
Chronic disturbance with depressed mood, lasting 2 years: similar symptoms to a major depressive episode but less severe.

- A major depressive episode may be imposed on dysthymia ('double depression').

Investigations
- Laboratory investigations are of limited use because of the frequency of false-positive and false-negative results.

- In middle-aged and elderly patients, however, investigations to rule out secondary depression (e.g. associated with occult neoplasm or endocrine disturbance) may be warranted if the patient's symptomatology suggests physical illness.

Assessment of severity of episode: presence of delusions or hallucinations, prominent vegetative symptoms, and large number of symptoms indicate increasing severity; rating scales, e.g. Beck or Hamilton, useful because they give quantitative measurement of severity and can be repeated to produce a serial profile of the episode.

Assessment of probability of suicide: indicated by level of hopelessness, social isolation, presence of delusions, suicide planning or previous attempts, concurrent personality disorder, alcoholism, or drug abuse.

Assessment of impact of episode: on social relationships, work.

Complications
High suicide rate: 15%.

Distress to others in the patient's social network: e.g. spouse, children.

Impairment in occupational function: e.g. reduced productivity, absenteeism, unemployment.

Death due to dehydration and malnutrition: in elderly patients.

Differential diagnosis

Mania or hypomania
Organic affective syndrome: e.g. amphetamines or steroids.
Schizoaffective disorder.
Cyclothymia.

Major depression
Organic affective syndrome: e.g. steroids.
Dementia: in elderly patients.
Schizophrenia, schizoaffective disorder.
Dysthymia, cyclothymia.
Chronic anxiety state.
Uncomplicated bereavement.

Dysthymia
Major depression.
Personality disorder: e.g. dependent, borderline, histrionic.
Normal fluctuation of mood.

Aetiology
- Causes include the following:

Biological factors
Genetic: bipolar and major depressive disorders are familial; increased evidence of inheritability for bipolar disorder.
Neurochemical: activity of biogenic amines (i.e. 5-HT, noradrenaline) decreased in depression, increased in mania.

Psychosocial factors
Psychoanalytic: introjection of an ambivalently viewed lost object leads to a rigid superego punishing person for sexual or aggressive impulses.
Cognitive: depression results from habitual maladaptive ways of thinking or from a perceived inability to control events (learned helplessness).
Adverse life event: current adversity (especially loss events) leads to depression by interacting with other vulnerability factors and temperament.

Epidemiology
- The lifetime expectancy of suffering from major depression is 10% in men and 20% in women; for mania, the expectancy is 1% for men and women.

- The female:male ratio is 2:1 for major depression and 1:1 for mania.

Treatment

Diet and lifestyle
- No special precautions are necessary.

Pharmacological treatment

For depression
- Depression is a recurrent disorder; hence the impact of treatment must be evaluated in terms of the following:

Response: reduction of symptoms with treatment.
Remission: resolution of symptoms for a continuous period in an episode.
Recovery: a stable remission lasting at least 4–6 months.
Relapse: symptoms recur during remission.
Recurrence: a new episode after recovery.

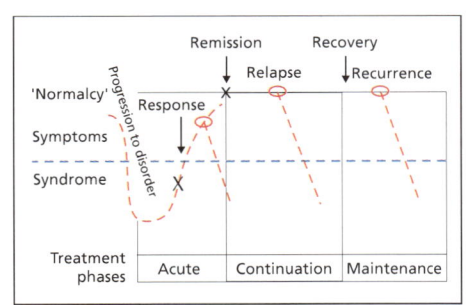

Stages of evaluation for major depression.

Standard dosage	Tricyclic antidepressants, e.g. imipramine 75 mg, increasing to 150 mg, or specific 5-HT re-uptake inhibitor, e.g. fluoxetine 20 mg, to obtain remission.
Contraindications	Recent myocardial infarction, heart block.
Special points	Response in ~70% of patients (30% respond to placebo), may take 4–6 weeks; failure may be due to inadequate level of treatment or poor compliance. Medication at full dose or psychotherapy continued for at least 6 months after resolution of symptoms to prevent relapse. The World Health Organization recommends prophylaxis for anyone with more than one severe episode in the preceding 5 years.
Main drug interactions	Hypertensive crises with monoamine oxidase inhibitors.
Main side effects	Anticholinergic effects, sedation, weight gain, sexual dysfunction.

- In patients who do not respond to two successive trials of different medications given for an adequate duration, diagnosis, previous treatment, and compliance must be reviewed.
- Failure to obtain remission is associated with increased duration of symptoms, severity of episode, 'double depression', and secondary depression.
- Further interventions include augmentation of the antidepressant regimen with lithium or carbamazepine, thyroid supplementation, simultaneous use of several antidepressants, or electroconvulsive therapy.

For mania or hypomania

Standard dosage	*For acute episode:* combination of major tranquillizer, e.g. haloperidol 2–10 mg i.m., benzodiazepine, e.g. lorazepam 2 mg i.m., and lithium to achieve blood concentration 0.8–1.2 mmol/L. *For maintenance treatment:* lithium to achieve blood concentration 0.4–1 mmol/L.
Contraindications	Pregnancy, Addison's disease, renal impairment.
Special points	~50% of patients relapse with monotherapy, so drug may be combined with carbamazepine, clomazepam, or valproic acid; antidepressants (which may cause a relapsing cycle) and antipsychotics generally unhelpful.
Main drug interactions	Thiazide diuretics increase lithium concentration; specific 5-HT re-uptake inhibitors increase CNS toxicity.
Main side effects	Gastrointestinal disturbances, fine tremor, polyurea, polydipsia.

- Complications include hypothyroidism, glomerulonephropathy, and nephrogenic diabetes insipidus.

Treatment aims
To obtain remission and prevent relapse of major depression.
To prevent exacerbation of mania.

Other treatments

Electroconvulsive therapy
- This is indicated for depressed patients with delusions, catatonic stupor, and severe suicidal tendencies or severely depressed patients in whom pharmacotherapy is not indicated.
- Side effects are cognitive: a transient postictal confusional state, longer-term memory impairment.

Psychotherapy
- Cognitive behavioural therapy or interpersonal psychotherapy are no more effective than pharmacotherapy in obtaining remission but may be more effective in preventing relapse.
- Psychotherapy is less effective when depression is severe.

Prognosis
- 50% of patients suffering from major depression may be in remission by 6 months; 12% fail to remit by 5 years.
- The rate of recurrence of major depression varies widely, with a possible subgroup of patients who have an especially poor outcome and who need long-term maintenance treatment.
- Patients with bipolar disorders have a poorer prognosis than those with major depression, with recurrence and rehospitalization the norm.
- Only 15% of patients with bipolar disorders remain well.

Follow-up and management
- The recognition that bipolar patients and some depressed patients have a chronic disorder needing life-long treatment has encouraged the setting up of specialized mood disorder clinics where patients are seen throughout their lives; this improves compliance, encourages early intervention, and encourages group or peer support.

Key references
Anonymous: AMA practice guideline to major depressive disorder in adults. *Am J Psychiatry* 1993, **150** (suppl 4):1–26.

Obsessive compulsive disorder
R.S. Rani and L.M. Drummond

Diagnosis

Symptoms
Obsessions: involuntary unwanted intrusive thoughts, images, or impulses; accompanying feelings of anxiety.

Compulsions: overt actions, e.g. checking or cleaning; voluntary covert (mental) actions, e.g. neutralizing thoughts; reduced anxiety.

Ruminations: obsessional thoughts without overt compulsions; compulsions are covert.

Signs
Patient recognition of obsessional thoughts as senseless, their own thoughts, alien to their personality.

Resistance to compulsive behaviour: may be seen, at least initially.

Investigations
- The aim is to allow formulation of problems and to assess suitability for treatment by ruling out depression, drug and alcohol abuse, psychosis, and organic causes.

Behavioural analysis: problems reviewed in detail, e.g. using Lazarus mnemonic (*see box*); in addition, maintaining factors, avoidance behaviours, full psychiatric and medical history, and mental state must be elicited; self-monitoring by patient over time, e.g. with diary, used at initial assessment stage and then to monitor subsequent changes, useful for measuring duration and frequency of problem behaviours.

Questionnaires: specific questionnaires used to measure problem and monitor progress during treatment.

Behavioural tests: help therapist to observe problem behaviour directly, e.g. test for patient with 'fear of contamination by germs' would be to ask him or her to touch a contaminated area, e.g. carpet, and to note the rituals performed, e.g. checking, washing.

Complications
Episodes of depression: frequent, although fewer suicides than in other depressive patients.

Differential diagnosis
Phobia.
Anankastic personality disorder.
Schizophrenia.
Anorexia nervosa.
Gilles de la Tourette syndrome.
Brain damage or learning disability.

Aetiology
- Causes may include the following:

Biological theories
Reduction in neurotransmitters, particularly 5-HT in the limbic system.
Gross brain disease: abnormal activity in the limbic system, abnormality in frontal lobe and basal ganglia system, or feedback system between limbic area and central connections.
Increased genetic concordance more probable in monozygotic than dizygotic twins.

Psychoanalytic theories
Regression to anal eroticism.
Defense mechanisms: isolation, undoing, and reaction formation.
Protection against underlying psychosis.

Sociological theories
Environment: modelling.
Life events: bereavement, head injury.
Strict religious training.

Behavioural and cognitive theories
Learned response to specific situations.
Theory of prepotency.

Epidemiology
- The male:female ratio is equal.
- Obsessive compulsive disorders usually affect people in early adult life.
- They are seen in different cultures.
- Large-scale epidemiological surveys in the USA have shown a 6-month incidence of 1.3–2.0% and a lifetime incidence of 1.9–3.3%.

Lazarus mnemonic
For rapid behavioural assessment
B = behaviour.
A = affect.
S = sensations.
I = imagery.
C = cognitions.
I = interpersonal relationships.
D = drugs.

Treatment

Diet and lifestyle
- No special precautions are necessary.

Pharmacological treatment
- Drugs can be useful when the patient is depressed, although 40–60% of patients derive no significant benefit from drugs.

Standard dosage	Clomipramine 150 mg daily. Fluvoxamine 100 mg daily, increased to 300 mg daily, possibly with a neuroleptic, e.g. sulpiride 100 mg twice daily, increased to 200 mg twice daily. Fluoxetine 20 mg daily, increased to 60 mg daily.
Contraindications	*Clomipramine:* myocardial infarction, heart block, severe liver disease, pregnancy. *Fluvoxamine, fluoxetine:* pregnancy, lactation, epilepsy, severe renal failure. *Sulpiride:* phaeochromocytoma; avoided in breast feeding and renal impairment.
Special points	Many patients relapse on stopping the drug; treatment may need to be continued for years.
Main drug interactions	*Clomipramine:* monoamine oxidase inhibitors, barbiturates, alcohol, anticholinergics, local anaesthetics, cimetidine, antihypertensives, oestrogen. *Fluvoxamine:* propranolol, theophylline, phenytoin, warfarin, monoamine oxidase inhibitors, alcohol, lithium, tryptophan. *Fluoxetine:* monoamine oxidase inhibitors, tryptophan, lithium. *Sulpiride:* alcohol, antihypertensives, anticonvulsants, antidiabetics, antidepressants.
Main side effects	*Clomipramine:* significant anticholinergic effects, e.g. dry mouth, blurred vision, constipation, urine retention. Sexual disturbances, e.g. impotence, common. *Specific 5-HT reuptake inhibitors:* lower overall incidence of adverse effects than clomipramine. Nausea and headaches.

Non-pharmacological treatment

Behavioural and cognitive therapy
- This is the treatment of choice.

Exposure and response prevention: should be prolonged, *in vivo*, graduated (as far as the patient can tolerate), and self-imposed.
Other techniques: modelling, shaping, prompting and pacing, and thought-stopping.
Habituation training: deliberate thought evocation, writing the thought down repeatedly, and listening to a loop tape.
Cognitive therapy: overvalued ideation may be amenable.

Psychosurgery
Stereotactic limbic leucotomy: for patients with severe obsessive compulsive disorder who have not responded to other forms of treatment (rarely used).

Psychodynamic psychotherapy
- This is only useful for patients with obsessional traits, not for obsessive compulsive disorders.

Treatment aims
To reduce or abolish obsessional thoughts and actions.
To decrease restrictions in lifestyle.
To reduce depression and anxiety.

Prognosis
- Success rates have ranged from 75% to 85% of patients.
- The outcome for obsessional ruminations is less favourable.
- Gains are maintained for at least 4 years.

Follow-up and management
- Follow-up appointments are generally 1, 3, and 6 months after discharge.
- Patients are educated to become their own therapists, to draw up their own programme, and to use the principles when they encounter difficulties.

Causes of treatment failure
Depression.
Overvalued ideation.
Exposure sessions too short.
Neutralizing by seeking reassurance, etc.
Non-compliance.

Key references
Abel JL: Exposure with response prevention and serotonergic antidepressants in the treatment of obsessive compulsive disorders: a review and implications for interdisciplinary treatment. *Behav Res Ther* 1993, 31:463–478.

De Silva P, Rachman S: *Obsessive Compulsive Disorders – The Faults*. Oxford: Oxford University Press, 1992.

Rasmussen SA, Eisen JL, Pato MT: Current issues in the pharmacologic management of obsessive compulsive disorders. *J Clin Psychiatry* 1993, **54 (suppl)**:4–9.

Stern RS, Drummond LM: *The Practice of Behavioural and Cognitive Psychotherapy*. Cambridge: Cambridge University Press, 1991.

Panic and generalized anxiety disorder
P. Tyrer

Diagnosis

Symptoms

Panic
Recurrent attacks of severe unprovoked anxiety: starting suddenly, reaching a peak within a few minutes, and lasting at least 20 min, with at least two of the following:

Palpitations.
Stomach churning.
Hot or cold flushes.
Shaking or trembling.
Choking or difficulty breathing.
Dry mouth.
Fear of dying.
Feelings of unreality.
Fear of losing control.

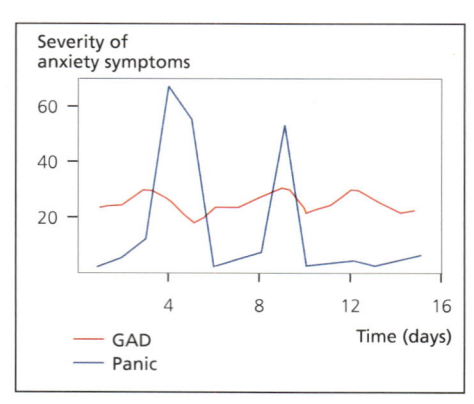

Course of pure panic disorder and pure generalized anxiety disorder (GAD).

Generalized anxiety disorder
Relatively persistent anxiety: at least 6 months, associated with worrying and apprehension about events and other matters that do not justify excessive worry; the anxiety and worry are associated with at least four of the following symptoms:

Palpitations.
Hot or cold flushes.
Choking or difficulty breathing.
Fear of dying.
Fear of losing control.
Stomach churning.
Shaking or trembling.
Dry mouth.
Feeling of unreality.
Irritability.
Being easily startled.
Mental tension.
Muscle tension.
Difficulty in getting to sleep.
Difficulty in swallowing.
Difficulty in concentrating.

Signs

Panic
• Doctors seldom see a panic attack *in vivo* because patients usually feel more secure in a medical setting. Features present on examination include the following:

Fear of having a panic attack.
Reassurance that a heart attack or other physical catastrophe is not imminent.
Wish to be physically examined.
Physiological evidence of anxiety: usually no different from generalized anxiety disorder.

Generalized anxiety disorder
Furrowed brow, hunted look, lack of confidence: evidence of long-standing anxiety.
Tachycardia: pulse 80–100 beats/min.
Sweating.
Dilated pupils.
Observed tremor.

Investigations

• Investigations should not be entered into lightly in patients with anxiety disorders because they may cause hypochondriacal concern and increased anxiety. If, however, anxiety appears for the first time in middle age or later, it may have an organic cause.

Thyroid function tests, full blood screening, neurological assessment: may sometimes be indicated if anxiety is episodic, diurnally varied, or linked to specific somatic symptoms persistently; epilepsy and phaeochromocytoma are rare but remediable causes of anxiety.

Complications

Alcohol dependence: with persistent anxiety (alcohol provides temporary relief).
Hypochondriasis: due to anxiety about bodily complaints.
Agoraphobia: due to persistent severe anxiety, particularly after panics in public places.
Social phobia: due to self-consciousness of anxiety attacks.

Differential diagnosis

Adjustment disorder, phaeochromocytoma, thyrotoxicosis: anxiety related to physical disease.

Post-traumatic stress: anxiety due to major unusual event (e.g rape, major disaster).

Hypochondriasis, somatoform disease: anxiety due entirely to fear of disease or preoccupation with bodily symptoms.

Organic psychoses, schizophrenia, affective psychoses: anxiety due to psychotic symptoms, e.g. delusions or hallucinations.

Agoraphobia, social or simple phobias: anxiety due to specific stimuli, accompanied by avoidance of the stimuli.

Mixed anxiety and depressive disorder, depressive episode: anxiety due to depressive symptoms.

Substance abuse disorders: anxiety due to alcohol or drug abuse.

Aetiology

• The immediate cause of anxiety in panic and generalized anxiety disorder is unknown.

• The episodes of anxiety are unfocused or 'free-floating' (generalized anxiety disorder) or spontaneous (panic).

• Both disorders are associated with life changes and events and may sometimes be a delayed reaction to the events.

• A genetic component is possible.

Epidemiology

• Panic attacks are most frequent in the 15–24-year age range and have an annual prevalence of ~2% in this group, with ~1% in the total population.

• Generalized anxiety disorder is much more common, with an annual prevalence of ~6%.

Treatment

Diet and lifestyle
- A good square meal is sometimes said to be the best tranquillizer in the world; unsurprisingly therefore, some anxious people resolve their anxiety by overeating and getting fat. This may relieve their anxiety (good studies show that fat people are less anxious generally than thin people) but does not improve their health overall.
- Because anxious people fear trouble around every corner, they often restrict their lifestyles; this is seen to its extreme in the housebound agoraphobic.

Pharmacological treatment
- The patient's view must be taken into account: some refuse drug treatment, others are equally negative about psychological treatment.
- Less effective treatments, e.g. beta blockade and relaxation training, should be avoided in patients with panic disorder.
- Combined drug and psychological treatments are acceptable and may even be more effective than individual treatments alone.
- Patients must be warned against self-medication with alcohol for anxiety and pain: it provokes worse symptoms in the longer term.
- The duration of treatment should be set in advance, whenever possible.

Standard dosage	Benzodiazepines, e.g. diazepam 2–10 mg daily. Chloral hydrate, e.g. Noctec 500–1000 mg at night. Beta blockers, e.g. propranolol 40–120 mg daily. Tricyclic antidepressants, e.g. amitriptyline 100–150 mg daily. Specific 5-HT reuptake inhibitors, e.g. fluoxetine 20 mg daily.
Contraindications	*Benzodiazepines:* caution with previous or present evidence of dependent personality or behaviour.
Special points	*Benzodiazepines:* rapid and more effective in short term than other treatments, but tolerance and dependence makes them generally unsuitable for regular treatment; may interfere with success of behaviour therapy. *Chloral hydrate:* useful if insomnia is a major symptom. *Beta blockers:* useful if somatic symptoms of anxiety are prominent but not severe (more useful in generalized anxiety disorder). *Tricyclic antidepressants:* more effective than benzodiazepines when given for more than 4 weeks, but slow onset of anti-anxiety effects.
Main drug interactions	Additive effects with alcohol.
Main side effects	Sedation (not beta blockers).

Non-pharmacological treatment
- Psychological treatments include the following:

Relaxation training: of some value (but less than other more intensive therapies) and can be very cheap.

Cognitive therapy: effective in both disorders, may be superior to other psychological treatments; aimed at altering unproductive dysfunctional thinking that helps to generate and maintain anxiety; patients with panic disorders learn to decatastrophize thinking, so that attacks are avoided.

Behaviour therapy: effective in treating maladaptive behaviours associated with anxiety, mainly by gradual exposure to more adaptive situations.

Combination therapies: cognitive behaviour therapy, anxiety management training.

Hypnosis and alternative therapies (yoga, meditation): sometimes useful but not as effective as cognitive and behaviour therapies.

Treatment aims
To alleviate symptoms.
To teach patient to recognise anxiety early.
To teach patient stress management and relaxation techniques.

Prognosis
- Prognosis is generally good except when symptoms begin early in adult life and are associated with personality disturbance.

Follow-up and management
- Drug treatment is best regarded as a temporary measure, except in patients who are persistently anxious; long-term treatment should be psychological because relapse is less likely and self-esteem is improved.

Key references
Durham RC, Allan T: Psychological treatment of generalized anxiety disorder: a review of the clinical significance in outcome studies since 1980. *Br J Psychiatry* 1993, **163**:19–26.

Tyrer P, Hallstrom C: Antidepressants in the treatment of anxiety disorder. *Psychiatr Bull* 1993, **17**:75–76.

Personality disorders — B. Ferguson

Diagnosis

Definition
- Personality disorders are dysfunctional patterns of thinking and behaviour that reflect persistent ways of relating to self and others, which deviate markedly from the norm and are invariably accompanied by impairment of social role or major subjective distress.
- The specific personality disorders that appear in adolescents can be broadly categorized into three main areas:

Flamboyant: histrionic, emotionally unstable (borderline or impulsive), dissocial.

Eccentric: paranoid/schizoid.

Fearful: anankastic, anxious/avoidant, dependent.

- Others are acquired later in life and arise as a result of organic insult, psychiatric illness, or catastrophic stress.

Symptoms and signs
Suspicion, oversensitivity, querulousness, unforgiving: paranoid.

Emotional coldness, solitude, social insensitivity: schizoid.

Impulsiveness, emotional instability, poor self-control: emotionally unstable (impulsive or borderline).

Obsessions, perfectionism, rigidity, self-doubt: anankastic.

Social sensitivity, apprehension, feelings of social inferiority: anxious, avoidant.

Reliance on others, subordination of own needs, fear of abandonment: dependent.

Callousness, irresponsibility, blaming others, aggressiveness: dissocial.

Dramatics, suggestibility, seeking centre stage, shallowness: histrionic.

Investigations
History: should be corroborated with other sources if possible (with patient's permission): personality characteristics of parents, early development, adverse life events and upbringing; school/social services (history of neglect, impoverishment, or abuse); legal sources (e.g. probation office); spouse, cohabitee (partners may also have personality disorders); employer.

Standardized questionnaires: usually time-consuming but highly reliable; patients are asked tightly worded questions covering specific areas of personal and social function in order to avoid biassed judgement on the part of the therapist; this is particularly important in the case of disorders with antisocial characteristics.

Munich Checklist for ICD-10: a good alternative.

EEG: finding may be abnormal in patients with dissocial disorder.

Complications
High suicide rate.

Self-harming behaviour: may lead to frequent presentations in a wide variety of health-care settings, e.g. casualty, medical wards.

Alcohol addiction and drug abuse.

Harm to others: e.g. violent assault or sexual abuse of children.

Differential diagnosis
Comorbidity with mental illness (AXIS I): cross-sectional studies show that ~40% of patients also manifest AXIS I disorders when they present in clinical settings.

Schizotypal disorder: frequently overlaps with borderline and schizoid disorders.

Prodromal or residual phase of schizophrenia.

Affective disorders: hypomania may mimic dissocial disorder; depression is frequent in patients suffering from borderline disorder.

Aetiology
- Causes include the following:

Genetic inheritance.

Abnormal developmental biology.

Failure to negotiate critical stages of emotional development.

Childhood trauma: sexual abuse is a more frequent feature in borderline disorders.

Social theories: abnormal parenting or lack of an appropriate role model.

Epidemiology
- Schizoid personality disorder appears to be rare because sufferers avoid society.
- The prevalence in the general population is 2–6%; in primary care settings, 15–34%; in psychiatric outpatients, 20–40%; in psychiatric inpatients, 40–60%; in forensic settings, 50–90%.

Treatment

Diet and lifestyle
- No special precautions are necessary.

Pharmacological treatment
- All drugs must be used with caution because of the dangers of overdose and abuse.
- Neuroleptics, e.g. thioridazine, haloperidol, fluoperazine in low doses, can alleviate symptoms, e.g. hostility, anger, suspiciousness, and depressed mood in borderline or dissocial conditions.
- Monoamine oxidase inhibitors may be useful in borderline conditions.
- Long-term use of benzodiazepines must be avoided because of the probability of addiction; they may cause paradoxical disinhibition.
- Mood stabilizers (lithium and carbamazepine) are most useful when mood swings or family history of affective disorder are evident.

Non-pharmacological treatment

Psychotherapy
- Interpretative psychotherapies for flamboyant disorders are effective in mild to moderate conditions.

Behaviour or cognitive therapy
- This is being developed but is not widely available; it is similar to therapies used in the treatment of depression and anxiety.

Supportive therapy
- This includes social support and is most useful for patients with severe disruptive personality disorders.
- Patients are encouraged to find practical solutions to present problems, e.g. relationship difficulties, accommodation, other personal needs.

Group therapy
- Group therapy may help patients with some forms of personality disorders.
- It includes the use of therapeutic communities.

Treatment aims

To alleviate subjective distress and reduce impact of dysfunctional behaviour.

Prognosis

- Prognosis is usually poor in severely affected patients, but most improve with age (4th or 5th decade); improvement is more noticeable for the flamboyant group.
- The outcome is invariably worse when comorbid mental illness is present.
- Good prognostic features include intelligence and the presence of positive adaptive traits, e.g. candour and introspectiveness.

Follow-up and management

- No treatment has universally proven effectiveness; the most useful approach is based on long-term supportive contact and crisis intervention when needed.
- Patients tend to arouse strong feelings in therapists; staff working in crisis situations particularly need regular support.

Danger

- Most patients with personality disorders are no more dangerous than unaffected people.
- A few people with severe disorders, especially those with paranoid or dissocial traits, can exhibit considerable aggression towards others; safety and surveillance is paramount in such circumstances.
- In community settings, the police should be involved to make the situation safe.
- Admission to secure units or forensic facilities may be needed.

Key references

Anonymous: *ICD-10 Classification of Mental and Behavioural Disorders. Clinical Descriptions and Diagnostic Guidelines.* Geneva: World Health Organization, 1992.

McGuffin P, Thapar A: The genetics of personality disorder. *Br J Psychiatry* 1992, **160**:12–23.

Stone M: Long term outcome in personality disorders. *Br J Psychiatry* 1993, **162**:299–313.

Tyrer P, Casey P, Ferguson B: Personality disorder in perspective. *Br J Psychiatry* 1991, **159**:463–471.

Tyrer P, Stein G (eds): *Personality Disorder Reviewed.* London: Royal College of Psychiatrists, 1993.

Postnatal mental illness — M.R. Oates

Diagnosis

Definition
- Postnatal mental illness is defined as a new episode of mental illness in a woman who has been well for at least the previous 6 months, with onset in the first 90 days *post partum*.
- The illness may be manifest later in the puerperium.

Symptoms and signs

Puerperal psychosis (bipolar or manic depressive psychosis)
- Onset is abrupt and occurs between days 3 and 16 in most women.
- Within a week, the picture settles to become clearly that of an acute severe affective psychosis.

Variable acute undifferentiated psychosis, with lucid intervals, perplexity, agitation, confusion: for first few days.

Hallucinations and delusions, emotional and behavioural disturbance, disrupted sleep and appetite.

Overactivity, elation, pressure of talk, flight of ideas: in one-third of patients.

Agitation, psychological retardation, self-neglect, depressive delusions about baby: in two-thirds; such patients may become stuperosed and stop eating and drinking.

Severe depressive illness (unipolar depressive illness)
- Onset is early, with more gradual deterioration.
- One-third of patients, the most severely ill, verging on psychotic, present early (within first 6 weeks); two-thirds, those most likely to be missed, present later (between 10 and 20 weeks).

Disrupted sleep and early morning wakening, diurnal variation of mood.

Marked slowing of psychological functioning, impaired concentration, indecisiveness.

Prominent loss of pleasure and spontaneity: everything is an effort, particularly the baby.

Overvalued ideas or delusions of unworthiness, incompetence, and guilt.

Frequent intrusive, obsessional thoughts of failure as mother or harm coming to child.

See Depression and mania *for details*.

Mild depressive illness (neurotic or reactive depressive illness)
- Onset is within the first 90 days, but presentation is later (between 3 and 8 months).
- No classic biological features of severe depressive illness are seen.
- The patient improves in company and can be distracted.

Variable levels of distress, anxiety, irritability, tiredness, and difficulty coping with baby.

Investigations
- No special clinical investigation is needed beyond the normal physical postnatal investigations.

Complications
Delayed detection and treatment of severe mental illness, physical morbidity.

Suicide and infanticide: rare but tragic and often avoidable.

Prolonged morbidity.

Failure to establish relationship with child.

Removal of child by family or social services.

Lasting problems in child's social, emotional, and cognitive development and physical health.

Marriage breakdown.

Differential diagnosis
The blues: tearfulness between days 3 and 5; spontaneous resolution within a few days.

Acute confusional state (delirium, organic brain syndrome): rare, caused by infection, eclampsia, or other neurological disorder.

Distress: caused by social, marital, or relationship problems.

- Severe depressive illness may follow major life stresses.

Aetiology
- Biological factors are of greater importance than psychological factors in the cause of severe conditions; the reverse is true for the mild conditions.
- No current evidence suggests that the hormonal profile of mentally ill mothers differs from that of normal women; the post-partum drop to low progesterone concentrations is probably responsible for 'the blues'; puerperal psychosis may be related to a predetermined hypersensitivity of dopamine receptors to the post-partum fall in oestrogen.
- Manic depressive illness in a first-degree relative indicates a 1 in 3 risk for puerperal psychosis.
- Previous manic depressive illness (whether *post partum* or not) indicates a 1 in 2 risk after every delivery; previous severe postnatal depression indicates a 1 in 3 risk after subsequent deliveries; previous non-post-partum depression or other neurotic condition indicates a 1 in 5 risk or higher.
- Emergency caesarian section increases the risk of puerperal psychosis in primiparus women; infertility, assisted reproduction, previous obstetric loss, or traumatic delivery may contribute to severe depressive illness.
- Marital conflict, social adversity, lack of confidante, single status, and ambivalence about the baby all increase the risk of a mild depressive illness.

Epidemiology
- 10% of all women delivered suffer from a depressive illness.
- 3% of all women delivered suffer from a severe depressive illness.
- 2 in 1000 women delivered are admitted to a mental hospital suffering from a puerperal psychosis.
- Similar rates have been found in many cultures throughout the world.

Treatment

Diet and lifestyle
- No special precautions are necessary apart from providing social support while the patient is recovering.

Pharmacological treatment
- Women with puerperal psychosis or suffering from severe depression, with suicidal despair, must be admitted to a Mother and Baby Unit.
- Most postnatal depressive illnesses can be managed at home, with the involvement of a specialized community psychiatric nurse.

For puerperal psychosis
- The immediate priority is to sedate the patient with neuroleptics to a level that makes her safe, allows adequate nutrition, and reduces her perplexity and fear.

Standard dosage	Chlorpromazine 50 mg 3 times daily with 75 or 100 mg at night, titrated to suit individual; alternatively, trifluoperazine or haloperidol. *For early-onset depressive psychoses:* tricyclic antidepressants.
Contraindications	*Neuroleptics:* hypersensitivity; caution in cardiovascular disease, hepatic impairment, epilepsy.
Special points	If no response occurs within 7 days, electroconvulsive therapy or lithium carbonate can be tried (lithium serum concentration ~0.8–1 mg/L within 1 week; normal thyroid and renal function must be established first). *Neuroleptics:* post-partum women are very sensitive to extrapyramidal side effects, so monitoring needed. *Tricyclic antidepressants:* effect takes 10–14 days; should be started at same time as electroconvulsive therapy (may be sufficient alone for less severe illness).
Main drug interactions	*Neuroleptics:* antagonize anticonvulsants.
Main side effects	*Neuroleptics:* sedation, extrapyramidal effects, acute dystonias, akasthesia, parkinsonism.

For severe depressive illness
- Most women respond satisfactorily to antidepressants; 60% respond to first-choice tricyclic antidepressant.
- Excessive sedation should be avoided because of childcare responsibilities.
- Women should always be referred to a psychiatrist if they are severely distressed, in a state of hopeless despair, or suicidal.

See Depression and mania *for details*.

Drugs and breast feeding
- No psychotropic drug is of proven safety.

Tricyclic antidepressants, fluvoxamine: yes.
Other specific 5-HT reuptake inhibitors, monoamine oxidase inhibitors, lithium: no.
Neuroleptics in small oral doses: probably yes.

Treatment aims
To provide early detection and prompt treatment in the setting most appropriate for safe recovery.
To give priority to the needs of the baby.
To avoid unnecessary separation of mother and baby.
To provide social and psychological support.

Other treatments
- Psychosocial treatment includes the following:

Adjunctive psychotherapy and specific counselling for all patients.

Non-directive or cognitive therapy (6 sessions at weekly intervals) effective for mild depressive illness.

Practical social support and addressing of concurrent problems: essential for resolution of all illnesses.

- Psychosocial treatment is as effective as antidepressants for mild depressive illness.

Prognosis
- With early intervention and effective treatment, the prognosis is excellent; improvement beginning within 2 weeks and recovery within 6–8 weeks.
- Without treatment, the illness may be prolonged, although 60% of patients recover spontaneously within 6 months.

Follow-up and management
- Treatment should continue for at least 6 months after the patient has recovered, longer in the case of a relapse.
- Patients with previous manic depressive episodes should take lithium for 2 years.

The next baby
- For serious mental illness, the risk follows every childbirth.

Puerperal psychosis, 1 in 2 risk.
Postnatal depression, 1 in 3–5 risk.

Key references
Oates MR: Management of major mental illness in pregnancy and puerperium. *Baillières Clin Obstet Gynaecol* 1989, 3:906–920.

Schizophrenia
R. Mullen and A. David

Diagnosis

Symptoms and signs

Prodromal
- Prodromal symptoms and signs are not always manifest.

Deteriorating social and occupational performance.

Odd behaviour.

Depression.

Schizotypal personality.

First-rank
- First-rank symptoms and signs are of particular diagnostic value.

Hearing own thoughts spoken aloud.

Third-person auditory hallucinations.

Voices commenting on patient's actions.

Thought broadcast, insertion and withdrawal.

Passivity: feelings or actions experienced, made, or influenced by external agents.

Hallucinations of somatic passivity.

Delusional perception.

Other symptoms

Other delusions.

Hallucinations: any modality, especially auditory.

Abnormal speech: vague, loose associations, neologisms.

Irritable and over-aroused or incongruous mood.

Suspicious and preoccupied appearance.

Violent or odd behaviour.

Poor insight.

Mannerisms and stereotypes.

Autochthonous delusions or delusional mood.

The chronic syndrome

Lack of drive and initiative.

Self neglect, blunted affect, poor concentration.

Persisting delusions and hallucinations: possibly.

Investigations
- None is diagnostic, but organic causes must be excluded and a baseline set before treatment.

Drug screen: for cannabis and stimulants especially.

Full blood count, electrolyte measurement, liver function tests, EEG, CT of head (if available), syphilis serology, thyroid function tests: routine tests to rule out organic causes.

Complications

Increased criminality: e.g. the risk of murder is doubled.

Suicide: 10% of deaths.

Depression: common after an acute episode.

Water intoxication: rare but lethal.

Catatonic stupor: rare but lethal.

Deterioration: often renders patient vulnerable to unscrupulous manipulation.

Differential diagnosis

Drug-induced psychoses.

Affective disorders.

Other paranoid disorders.

Psychomotor seizures.

Other diffuse or focal brain disorders.

Abnormal personality.

Culturally sanctioned behaviour and beliefs: may be mistaken for mental illness by someone not familiar with that culture.

Aetiology
- The cause of schizophrenia remains unknown, but the following may have a role:

Genetics: influences well established; 50% concordance in monozygotic twins.

In-utero and perinatal complications.

Physical brain disorder.

Increased risk in temporal lobe epilepsy.

Epidemiology
- The lifetime risk of suffering from schizophrenia is 1%.
- The median age of onset is 30 years; onset is earlier in men.
- The incidence is 15–20 in 100 000 population annually.

Treatment

Diet and lifestyle
- Careful social management is crucial.
- Overstimulation leads to relapse and understimulation worsens negative symptoms.
- High expressed emotion in the family (hostility, critical comments, emotional over-involvement) worsens the prognosis; patients may fare better in a hostel or have an improved prognosis after specific family interventions designed to reduce expressed emotion.
- Various day-care facilities are available.
- Patients must be encouraged to avoid illicit drugs.

Pharmacological treatment
- Antipsychotic drugs are usually needed for acute illness and help to prevent relapse.

Chlorpromazine
- This controls psychotic symptoms and can rapidly calm an agitated patient.

Standard dosage	Chlorpromazine 75–300 mg daily, up to 1 g for severe illness.
Contraindications	Coma, bone-marrow depression, closed-angle glaucoma.
Special points	Neuroleptic malignant syndrome is rare but lethal.
Main drug interactions	Enhanced sedative effect with other CNS depressants.
Main side effects	Antimuscarinic effects, dystonia, parkinsonism, sedation, menstrual disturbance, tardive dyskinesia, hypotension.

- Trifluoperazine 10–20 mg and haloperidol 1.5–20 mg are less sedating but cause worse extrapyramidal effects.

Other drugs
Depot antipsychotics: parenterally every 1–4 weeks; preferable for poorly compliant patients.

For violent patients: droperidol or haloperidol 10–20 mg parenterally, with diazepam 10–20 mg slow i.v. infusion; zuclopenthixol acetate 50–150 mg i.m. a longer-acting alternative.

Clozapine: for selected patients resistant to other drug treatment; more effective but risk of agranulocytosis necessitates specialized monitoring.

Anticholinergic drugs: procyclidine 5 mg daily or twice daily relieves acute extrapyramidal effects of neuroleptics; not for routine prescription (may worsen tardive dyskinesia and are abused); propranolol an alternative for akathisia.

Lithium: particularly when affective symptoms are prominent.

Treatment aims
Acute: to ensure safety and resolve psychotic symptoms.

Long-term: to provide social rehabilitation and prevent relapse and deterioration.

Other treatments
Electroconvulsive therapy: particularly for stupor.

Intensive psychotherapy: unhelpful but a supportive relationship is necessary.

Cognitive and behavioural approaches: can be of use for persistent symptoms and unwanted behaviour.

- Mental Health Act sections may be needed.

Prognosis
- 16% of patients have a single episode.
- 32% have a relapsing and remitting illness.
- 52% pursue a chronic course.

Follow-up and management
- Schizophrenia usually requires lifelong management.
- The help of a social worker and a Community Psychiatric Nurse should be sought.
- The Care Programme approach provides a framework for follow-up of the vulnerable and designates a key worker.
- The risk of suicide and aggression must be monitored.
- Careful advice on appropriate accommodation and employment is invaluable.
- Maintenance neuroleptics help in the long term.
- Patients and carers benefit from support and education.

Key references
Johnstone EC: Schizophrenia: problems in clinical practice. *Lancet* 1993, **341**:536–538.

Waddington JL: Schizophrenia: developmental neuroscience and pathobiology. *Lancet* 1993, **341**:531–536.

Index

A

affective
  disorder 15, 18
    psychotic see psychosis, affective
  syndrome, organic 8
aggression 15
agoraphobia 12
alcohol
  abuse 2, 12
  addiction see alcohol dependence
  amnestic disorder see psychosis, Korsakoff's
  dependence 2, 12, 14
  in generalized anxiety disorder 13
  in panic 13
  withdrawal syndrome 2
alcoholism see alcohol dependence
amitriptyline
  for generalized anxiety disorder 13
  for panic 13
anorexia nervosa 6, 10
anticholinergic drugs for schizophrenia 19
antidepressants see also 5-HT reuptake
  inhibitors, monoamine oxidase inhibitors
  for hypomania 9
  for mania 9
  tricyclic
    for depression 9
    for generalized anxiety disorder 13
    for panic 13
    for puerperal psychosis 17
    for severe postnatal depressive illness 17
    in breast feeding 17
antipsychotics see also tranquillizers,
  neuroleptics
  for schizophrenia 19
anxiety 8, 12
  disorder, generalized 12
AXIS 1 disorder 14

B

behaviour disturbance 16
behavioural
  analysis 10
  therapy for obsessive compulsive disorder 11
benzodiazepines
  for alcohol withdrawal syndrome 3
  for generalized anxiety disorder 13
  for hypomania 9
  for mania 9
  for panic 13
  for personality disorders 15
bereavement 8
beta blockers
  for generalized anxiety disorder 13
  for panic 13
brain syndrome, organic 4, 16
  psychotic see psychosis, organic
bulimia nervosa 6

C

carbamazepine
  for depression 9
  for hypomania 9
  for mania 9
  for personality disorders 15
chloral hydrate
  for generalized anxiety disorder 13
  for panic 13
chlordiazepoxide for alcohol withdrawal
  syndrome 3
chlormethiazole for alcohol withdrawal
  syndrome 3
chlorpromazine
  for puerperal psychosis 17
  for schizophrenia 19
claustrophobia see phobia
Clerambault syndrome see psychosis, organic
clonazepam
  for hypomania 9
  for mania 9
clozapine for schizophrenia 19
compulsions 10
confusional state, acute 16
convulsions see seizures

D

delusions 16, 18
dementia 8
  praecox see schizophrenia
depression 6, 8, 10, 15, 18
  endogenous 4
  psychotic reactive see psychosis, affective
depressive
  disorder and anxiety, mixed 12
  illness, postnatal
    mild 16
    neurotic 16
    reactive 16
    severe 16
    unipolar 16
development of child 16
diazepam
  for attempted suicide 5
  for generalized anxiety disorder 13
  for panic 13
  for schizophrenia 19
droperidol
  for attempted suicide 5
  for schizophrenia 19
drug abuse 15 see also substance abuse
dysthymia 8

E

eclampsia 16

F

fits see seizures
fluoperazine for personality disorders 15
fluoxetine
  for bulimia nervosa 7
  for depression 9
  for generalized anxiety disorder 13
  for obsessive compulsive disorder 11
  for panic 13
fluvoxamine
  for obsessive compulsive disorder 11
  in breast feeding 17

H

hallucination 16
  auditory 18
  somatic passivity 18
hallucinosis see psychosis, organic
haloperidol
  for attempted suicide 5
  for hypomania 9
  for mania 9
  for personality disorders 15
  for puerperal psychosis 17
  for schizophrenia 19
harm
  to others 14
  to self 14
5-HT reuptake inhibitors see also antidepressants, monoamine oxidase inhibitors
  for depression 9
  in breast feeding 17
hyperthyroidism see thyrotoxicosis

I

imipramine for depression 9
impulsiveness 14
infanticide 16
initiative, lack of 18

K

Kandinsky syndrome see psychosis, organic
Korsakoff syndrome see psychosis, Korsakoff's

L

lithium
  for depression 9
  for personality disorders 15
  for puerperal psychosis 17
  for schizophrenia 19
  in breast feeding 17
lorazepam
  for attempted suicide 5
  for hypomania 9
  for mania 9

Index

M

mania 8
MAOIs *see* monoamine oxidase inhibitors
mental illness, postnatal 16
monoamine oxidase inhibitors *see also* antidepressants, 5-HT reuptake inhibitors
   for personality disorders 15
   in breast feeding 17
mood
   disorder
      nonpsychotic *see* affective disorder
      psychotic *see* psychosis, affective
   dysphoric 8
   stabilizers for personality disorders 15
   variation, diurnal 16

N

neuroleptics *see also* antipsychotics, tranquillizers
   for obsessive compulsive disorder 11
   for personality disorders 15
   for puerperal psychosis 17
neurosis
   hypochondriacal *see* hypochondriasis
   obsessive–compulsive *see* obsessive compulsive disorder
   post-traumatic *see* stress, post-traumatic
   phobic *see* phobia, social

O

obsessions 10, 14
obsessive compulsive disorder 10

P

panic 12
paranoia *see* paranoid disorder
paranoid
   disorder 18
   psychoses *see* paranoid disorder
personality
   disorder 8, 14
      anankastic 10, 14
      anxious/avoidant 14
      dependent 14
      dissocial 14
      eccentric 14
      fearful 14
      flamboyant 14
      histrionic 14
      hysterical *see* personality disorder, histrionic
      impulsive/borderline 14
      paranoid 14
      passive-dependent *see* personality disorder, dependent
      schizoid 14
      schizotypal 18
phaeochromocytoma 12
phobia 10
   social 12
procyclidine
   for schizophrenia 19
   with antipsychotic drugs for attempted suicide 5
propranolol
   for generalized anxiety disorder 13
   for panic 13
   for schizophrenia 19
psychosis 4
   affective 12
   drug-induced 18
   Korsakoff's 2
   organic 12
   paranoid *see* paranoid disorder
   postnatal manic depressive 16
   puerperal 16
   traumatic *see* psychosis, organic
psychosurgery 11
psychotherapy for depression and mania 9

R

ruminations 10

S

schizoaffective disorder 8
schizophrenia 8, 10, 12, 14, 18
   incipient *see* personality, schizotypal
   latent *see* personality, schizotypal
   pseudoneurotic *see* personality, schizotypal
   pseudopsychopathic *see* personality, schizotypal
schizophrenic disorders *see* schizophrenia
seizures
   psychomotor 18
   tonic–clonic 2
self
   harm 14
   mutilation 4
   neglect 18
serotonin *see* 5-HT
sleep disturbance 8
somatoform disease 12
stress, post-traumatic 12
substance abuse 12 *see also* alcohol abuse, drug abuse
suicide 8, 16, 18
   attempted 4
   high risk of completed 4
   low risk of completed 4
   rate, high 8, 14

T

thiamine for alcohol withdrawal syndrome 3
thioridazine for personality disorders 15
thymoanaleptics *see* antidepressants
thymoleptics *see* antidepressants
thyroid supplementation for depression 9
thyrotoxicosis 12
tranquillizers *see also* antipsychotics, neuroleptics
   for hypomania 9
   for mania 9
trifluoperazine
   for puerperal psychosis 17
   for schizophrenia 19

V

valproic acid
   for hypomania 9
   for mania 9

W

water intoxication 18

Z

zuclopenthixol for schizophrenia 19

CURRENT DIAGNOSIS & TREATMENT

in

Respiratory disorders

Edited by
Anthony Frew

Series editors
Roy Pounder
Mark Hamilton

A QUICK Reference for the Clinician

Contributors

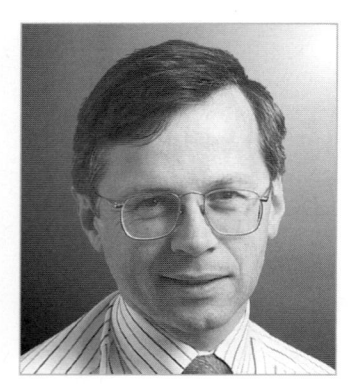

EDITOR

A J Frew

Dr Anthony Frew is Senior Lecturer in Medicine at the University of Southampton and Consultant Chest Physician to the Southampton University Hospital. His research interests are the mechanisms of asthma and allergic disease, especially the role of T lymphocytes. He is secretary of the British Society for Allergy and Clinical Immunology.

REFEREES

Dr CFA Pantin
Department of Respiratory Medicine
City General Hospital
Stoke-on-Trent, UK

Dr Neil Thompson
Department of Respiratory Medicine
Western Infirmary
Glasgow, UK

AUTHORS

ADULT RESPIRATORY DISTRESS SYNDROME

Dr David G Sinclair
Army Chest Unit
Cambridge Military Hospital
Aldershot, UK

Dr Timothy W Evans
Unit of Critical Care
National Heart and Lung Institute
London, UK

ASTHMA

Dr Anthony J Frew
University Medicine
Southampton General Hospital
Southampton, UK

ASTHMA, OCCUPATIONAL

Dr Anthony J Frew
University Medicine
Southampton General Hospital
Southampton, UK

BRONCHIECTASIS AND CYSTIC FIBROSIS

Dr David R Baldwin
Department of Respiratory Medicine
North Staffordshire Hospital
Stoke-on-Trent, UK

Dr CFA Pantin
Department of Respiratory Medicine
City General Hospital
Stoke-on-Trent, UK

CHRONIC OBSTRUCTIVE AIRWAY DISEASE

Dr Jonathan Michael Corne
University Medicine
Southampton General Hospital
Southampton, UK

FIBROSING ALVEOLITIS

Dr KT Khoo
Department of Respiratory Medicine
City General Hospital
Stoke-on-Trent, UK

Dr Monica Spiteri
Department of Respiratory Medicine
City General Hospital
Stoke-on-Trent, UK

GRANULOMATOSES

Dr Christopher Higgs
Palliative Medicine
Dorothy House Foundation
Bath, UK

LUNG CANCER

Dr Anthony J Frew
University Medicine
Southampton General Hospital
Southampton, UK

PLEURAL EFFUSION

Dr Anthony J Frew
University Medicine
Southampton General Hospital
Southampton, UK

PNEUMONIA

Dr Mark A Woodhead
Department of Respiratory Medicine
Manchester Royal Infirmary
Manchester, UK

SARCOIDOSIS

Dr Monica Spiteri
Department of Respiratory Medicine
City General Hospital
Stoke-on-Trent, UK

Dr KT Khoo
Department of Respiratory Medicine
City General Hospital
Stoke-on-Trent, UK

SLEEP APNOEA, OBSTRUCTIVE

Dr Robert Davies
Osler Chest Unit
John Radcliffe Hospital
Oxford, UK

TUBERCULOSIS, PULMONARY

Dr Ian Pavord
Respiratory Medicine Unit
City Hospital
Nottingham, UK

Dr John T McFarlane
Respiratory Medicine Unit
City Hospital
Nottingham, UK

Contents

2   Adult respiratory distress syndrome

4   Asthma

6   Asthma, occupational

8   Bronchiectasis and cystic fibrosis

10   Chronic obstructive airway disease

12   Fibrosing alveolitis

14   Granulomatoses
      Wegener's granulomatosis
      Churg–Strauss syndrome
      Lymphomatoid granulomatosis
      Necrotizing sarcoid or bronchocentric granulomatosis

16   Lung cancer

18   Pleural effusion

20   Pneumonia

22   Sarcoidosis

24   Sleep apnoea, central, hypoventilation, periodic breathing

26   Sleep apnoea, obstructive

28   Tuberculosis, pulmonary

30   Index

Adult respiratory distress syndrome
D.G. Sinclair and T.W. Evans

Diagnosis

Symptoms
Dyspnoea: variable severity, developing abruptly or gradual onset some days after initial insult.

Signs
Tachypnoea.

Warmth and peripheral vasodilatation.

Signs of pulmonary oedema: on auscultation.

Other signs of underlying disease.

- Cyanosis may not be apparent.

Investigations
Chest radiography: for bilateral pulmonary infiltrates; to confirm pulmonary oedema in presence of predisposing condition.

Pulmonary artery catheterization: to measure pulmonary artery occlusion pressure (normally <15 mmHg) and plasma oncotic pressure to exclude cardiogenic oedema.

Arterial blood gas analysis: refractory hypoxaemia unresponsive to increased inspired oxygen concentration (partial arterial oxygen pressure <8.0 kPa, fractional inspired oxygen concentration 0.4, arterial–alveolar oxygen tension ratio <0.25); low total respiratory compliance (<30 ml/cm H_2O).

Fibreoptic bronchoscopy and lavage or biopsy, upper respiratory tract cultures, skeletal survey, CT and nuclear imaging, specialized blood tests (e.g. plasma amylase): to establish underlying condition.

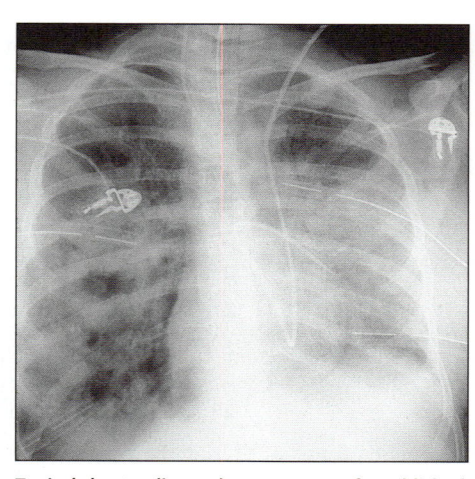

Typical chest radiograph appearance of established adult respiratory distress syndrome, showing pneumothoraces, position of endotracheal tube, intercostal chest drains, and pulmonary artery flotation catheter.

Complications
Death.

Pneumothorax.

Renal failure.

Debilitation in period after intensive care: survivors usually recover fully within 12 months.

Differential diagnosis
- The diagnostic criteria exclude other diagnoses.

Aetiology
- Causes include the following:

Aspiration of gastric contents.

Inhalation of toxic fumes.

Trauma resulting in direct pulmonary contusion.

Oxygen toxicity.

Bacterial, viral, or drug-induced pneumonia.

Massive burns or major trauma.

Disseminated intravascular coagulation.

Massive haemorrhage or multiple transfusion.

Pre-eclampsia.

Amniotic fluid embolism.

Sepsis from any cause.

Acute pancreatitis.

Head injury or raised intracranial pressure.

Epidemiology
- Adult respiratory distress syndrome may be less common than was previously thought (1000–1500 cases identified each year in the UK), although cases of acute lung injury not meeting the diagnostic criteria occur much more often.
- The prevalence varies according to the predisposing illness (2–25%).

Pathophysiology
- Adult respiratory distress syndrome may be the pulmonary manifestation of a pan-endothelial insult resulting from the activation of many humoral and cellular events.
- It is uniformly characterized by increased permeability of the alveolar–capillary membrane, leading to pulmonary oedema.
- Deranged cellular use of oxygen occurs as part of the syndrome and may result in widespread multiorgan failure of variable severity.

Treatment

Diet and lifestyle
- Patients need nutritional support by parenteral or enteral route while on the ventilator.

Pharmacological treatment
- Underlying conditions should be fully investigated and steps taken to correct any reversible disorders.
- Nosocomial infection and supra-added sepsis should be managed aggressively.
- Vasodilator, inodilator, and chronotropic agents should be used to support circulation and urine output.
- Enteral nutrition and gastrointestinal cytoprotective agents (e.g. sucralfate) should be given when possible.

Non-pharmacological treatment
- The involvement of multiple organ systems in the disease process means that supportive measures are not confined to the respiratory system.
- All patients with severe lung injury and established adult respiratory distress syndrome should be managed in the intensive care unit.
- Full respiratory and invasive haemodynamic monitoring and urinary catheterization are needed.

Respiratory support
- The aim is to maintain partial arterial oxygen pressure >8 kPa using continuous positive airways pressure applied via a face mask or mechanical ventilation.
- New techniques (e.g. pressure-controlled, inverse-ratio ventilation) are aimed at recruiting collapsed alveoli while reducing peak airway pressures (and therefore the risk of barotrauma) and raising mean airway pressures (thereby improving oxygenation).

Cardiac and circulatory support
- The aim is to maximize oxygen delivery to tissues.
- Haemoglobin should be maintained at 10–12 g/dl, with a haematocrit of 30–35%.
- Cardiac output and oxygen delivery should be measured and optimized by the judicious manipulation of filling pressures and the use of inotropic drugs.

Fluid balance
- The aim of manipulating fluid balance is to reduce circulating volume as much as possible in an effort to reduce further extravasation of oedema into the alveoli.
- Pulmonary artery occlusion pressure should be maintained at 8–10 mmHg.
- Diuretics may be needed to maintain urine output >0.5 ml/kg/h.

Treatment aims
To provide definitive treatment (if available) for the underlying condition.
To support affected systems, e.g. respiratory and cardiovascular, until spontaneous resolution occurs, by optimizing oxygen delivery.

Prognosis
- Mortality depends on the underlying condition, being ~50% in patients with adult respiratory distress syndrome after trauma and ~90% after sepsis.
- 90% of survivors recover 90% of their pre-morbid lung function after 12 months and suffer little or no respiratory impairment.
- Supportive treatments carry appreciable morbidity (e.g. pneumothorax, renal failure).
- Survivors are invariably debilitated after the prolonged stay in intensive care.

Follow-up and management
- The aim of follow-up is to maximize recovery from the effects of both the initial illness and the adult respiratory distress syndrome.
- Attention to physical rehabilitation, with nutritional advice, physiotherapy, and controlled exercise when appropriate, is needed for patients and their families.

Key references
Bone RC et al.: Adult respiratory distress syndrome: sequence and importance of multiple organ failure. *Chest* 1992, **101**:320–326.

Fowler AA et al.: Adult respiratory distress syndrome: risk with common predispositions. *Ann Intern Med* 1983, **98**:593–597.

MacNaughton PD, Evans TW: Management of the adult respiratory distress syndrome. *Lancet* 1992, **339**:469–472.

Murray JF et al.: An expanded definition of the adult respiratory distress syndrome. *Ann Rev Respir Dis* 1988, **138**:720–723.

Asthma   A.J. Frew

Diagnosis

Symptoms
- Symptom severity shows considerable temporal variation; they are often worse at night or in early morning.

Wheeze.

Breathlessness on exertion.

Chest tightness: not pain.

Cough: with or without sputum; may be the only symptom, especially in children.

Signs
Diffuse polyphonic wheeze.

Costal recession: due to high negative intrapleural pressure or rapid respiratory rate.

Tachycardia: in severe attack.

Pulsus paradoxus: in severe attack.

Cyanosis or confusion: signs of impending respiratory arrest; wheeze may be absent.

Investigations

On presentation
Dynamic spirometry: forced expiratory volume in 1 s (FEV_1) and forced vital capacity; response to beta-2 agonist (>15% improvement in FEV_1 confirms reversible airflow obstruction; failure to improve does not exclude asthma).

Serial peak flow monitoring: early peak flow often low in asthma; >15% diurnal variation strongly suggests asthma, peak flow reduced after work or exposure to sensitizing agent.

Skin tests: to assess role of airborne allergens (~50% of patients have positive immediate skin tests).

Steroid response test: >15% increase in FEV_1 after 2-week course of oral prednisolone 30 mg daily.

Airways hyper-responsiveness test: increased sensitivity to histamine, shown by 20% fall in FEV_1 to abnormally small doses of nebulized histamine.

For acute episodes
Peak flow rate measurement: to assess severity.

Arterial blood gas analysis: partial oxygen pressure reduced; partial carbon dioxide pressure usually low in acute episode; rising or raised partial carbon dioxide pressure suggests exhaustion and impending respiratory arrest; different patterns in acute exacerbations of chronic obstructive airway disease (see Chronic obstructive airway disease for details).

Chest radiography: to check for pneumothorax or pneumonia and to exclude heart failure.

ECG: if cause of breathlessness unclear.

Sputum culture: good samples often difficult to obtain; most exacerbations due to viral not bacterial infection.

Complications
Retarded growth rate: in children.

Thoracic cage deformity.

Pneumothorax.

Recurrent bronchial infection.

Respiratory arrest and death.

Fixed airway obstruction.

Differential diagnosis
- The diagnosis is usually obvious and easily confirmed.

Acute or chronic bronchitis.

Irreversible airway obstruction.

Rhinitis with post-nasal drip.

Left ventricular failure.

Aetiology
- Asthma has an important genetic component, which is inherited separately from the genetic tendency to atopy.
- ~50% of patients have associated atopic allergy, especially children.
- Breastfed babies appear to be protected against the development of atopy and asthma.
- All grades of asthma show airway inflammation, with eosinophils, mononuclear cells, and epithelial desquamation.
- Viral infections are clearly linked to exacerbations of asthma and may be responsible for initiating asthma in patients with adult-onset disease.
- Exposure to environmental chemicals and pollution is blamed for the current increase in prevalence: clear evidence of a causal relationship is awaited.

Epidemiology
- The prevalence of asthma appears to be increasing; in the UK, an estimated 10% of children and 5% of adults are affected.
- The male:female ratio in children is 1.5:1.
- The peak onset occurs between the ages of 5 and 10 years.
- Up to 70% of children with asthma remit by the age of 20 years.

Treatment

Diet and lifestyle

- Special diets are not usually needed; patients with salicylate sensitivity should avoid foods containing natural salicylates (advice from dietitian).
- Exercise is encouraged; swimming is often better tolerated than outdoor sports (exercise-induced asthma is triggered by cold dry air).

Pharmacological treatment

Corticosteroids

Standard dosage	*Inhaled corticosteroids:* starting dose varies according to severity, e.g. beclomethasone 200–400 µg twice daily (maximum, 1000 µg twice daily); dosage should be maintained or increased in patients needing oral steroids. *Oral corticosteroids:* prednisolone 30 mg daily for 5 days; longer courses may be needed if improvement is slow; dose need not be tapered if course lasts <14 days.
Contraindications	None.
Special points	Rinsing mouth after inhaling steroids reduces risk of oropharyngeal side effects. Spacer device must be used if dose >1000 µg daily.
Main drug interactions	None.
Main side effects	*Inhaled steroids:* hoarse voice, oropharyngeal candidiasis. *Oral steroids:* cushingoid features, especially osteoporosis, bruising, weight gain.

Xanthines

Standard dosage	Theophylline, dose adjusted to give blood concentrations of 55–110 µmol/L.
Contraindications	Liver disease, heart disease, epilepsy, porphyria.
Special points	Narrow therapeutic margin, so dose should be low initially and adjusted with aid of plasma drug concentrations.
Main drug interactions	Plasma concentration increased with many other drugs, e.g. antibiotics (ciprofloxacin, erythromycin), cimetidine, antidepressants, diltiazem, verapamil, fluconazole.
Main side effects	Nausea, reflux oesophagitis, tremor.

Short-acting beta-2 agonists

Standard dosage	Depends on agent and device, e.g. salbutamol, terbutaline 1–2 puffs as needed.
Contraindications	None.
Special points	Frequent use of short-acting beta-2 agonists suggests suboptimal control.
Main drug interactions	Beta blockers must be avoided.
Main side effects	Tremor.

For severe attacks

Hospital admission.
Severity assessment (especially blood gases).
Oxygen administration.
Bronchodilatation (nebulizer).
Oral prednisolone administration.
Intravenous hydrocortisone administration.
Intravenous aminophylline administration.
Ventilation if patient is tired or weakening or if blood gases show rising arterial blood pressure.

Treatment aims

To find minimum level of treatment to suppress symptoms.

To enable patients to take responsibility for day-to-day management of the condition.

To enable patients to avoid days off work or school.

To reduce the frequency of exacerbations and to avoid hospital admissions.

Prognosis

- Many children with asthma experience spontaneous remission in their second decade of life.
- Adult-onset asthma rarely remits.
- Most asthmatic patients cope well with their disease and have a normal life expectancy.
- A few severely ill or unstable asthmatic patients are at risk of respiratory arrest or sudden death; often, these patients need large doses of oral corticosteroids to control the disease.

Follow-up and management

- Exacerbations should be treated by the following:

Increased dose of inhaled corticosteroid.
Oral prednisolone 30 mg daily for 5–7 days.
Antibiotics if patient is febrile or sputum discoloured.
Nebulized bronchodilatation.

Key references

Anonymous: Guidelines on the management of asthma. *Thorax* 1993, **48**:S1–S24.

Djukanovic R *et al.*: Mucosal inflammation in asthma. State of the art. *Am Rev Respir Dis* 1990, **142**:434–457.

Goldstein RA *et al.*: NIH conference: asthma. *Ann Intern Med* 1994, **121**:698–708.

Kay AB: Asthma and inflammation. *J Allergy Clin Immunol* 1991, **87**:893–910.

Packe GE *et al.*: Bone density in asthmatic patients taking high dose beclomethasone diprorionate and intermittent systemic corticosteroids. *Thorax* 1992, **47**:414–417.

Tattersfield AE: Long-acting β_2-agonists. *Clin Exp Allergy* 1992, **22**:600–605.

Asthma, occupational — A.J. Frew

Diagnosis

Symptoms
Breathlessness at rest or on exertion, wheeze, worsening after work, improvement at weekends or during holidays.

Signs
Diffuse polyphonic wheeze.

Costal recession: due to high negative intrapleural pressure or rapid respiratory rate.

Tachycardia: in severe attack.

Pulsus paradoxus: in severe attack.

Cyanosis or confusion: signs of impending respiratory arrest; wheeze may be absent.

Investigations
Baseline spirometry: response to beta-2 agonist.

Bronchial hyper-responsiveness test: using histamine PC_{20}.

Detailed peak flow monitoring: at work and on days off or holidays.

Cross-shift spirometry: >10% change suggests occupational cause.

Specific challenge tests: to confirm role of new agent in causing asthma or to determine responsible agent when several agents are present in the workplace.

Challenge test: <20% fall in forced expiratory volume in 1 s, with no such change on control day.

Bronchial response test: twofold increase, with no such change on control day.

Complications
Respiratory failure.

Chronic breathlessness.

Differential diagnosis
Asthma due to non-occupational causes.
Other causes of breathlessness.
Irritant effect of chemical at work.

Aetiology
- Causes include the following:

Animal hair.
Laboratory animals.
Chemicals.
Food processing.
Enzymes (detergents).
Hairdressing.

Epidemiology
- The incidence of occupational asthma is increasing and now accounts for >50% of industrial lung disease.

Treatment

Diet and lifestyle
- Exposure should be reduced (to zero if possible) by moving to low-exposure zone, provision of personal respirator, or leaving employment.

Pharmacological treatment
- Treatment is the same as for other forms of asthma (see Asthma *for details*).
- All cases of occupational lung disease need specialist assessment to ensure that the correct diagnosis is reached and appropriate treatment instituted.
- Most patients need inhaled corticosteroids and bronchodilators.

Standard dosage	Beclomethasone 400–800 µg daily (maximum, 1000 µg twice daily).
Contraindications	None.
Special points	Rinsing of mouth after inhaling steroids reduces risk of oropharyngeal side effects. Spacer device must be used if dose exceeds 1000 µg daily.
Main drug interactions	None.
Main side effects	Hoarse voice, oropharyngeal candidiasis.

Treatment aims

To control symptoms of asthma and restore normal levels of activity.

To reduce risk of developing chronic asthma.

Prognosis

- Most patients improve when withdrawn from exposure.
- >40% should have no residual signs or symptoms of asthma, but up to 30% have chronic persistent symptoms, despite full withdrawal from exposure.
- Persistent asthma is especially frequent with low molecular weight sensitizers but can also occur with high molecular weight (protein) antigens.

Follow-up and management

- Patients should be followed carefully to check whether asthma resolves with time.
- Regular radiographic monitoring is necessary for patients with interstitial fibrosis.

Key references

Bernstein IL *et al.* (eds): *Asthma in the Workplace.* New York: Marcel Dekker, 1993.

Salvaggio JE: The impact of allergy and immunology on our expanding industrial environment. *J Allergy Clin Immunol* 1990, **85**:689–699.

Bronchiectasis and cystic fibrosis
D.R. Baldwin and C.F.A. Pantin

Diagnosis

Symptoms

Bronchiectasis and cystic fibrosis

Cough, purulent, large-volume sputum, episodic fever or malaise, night sweats, nasal discharge, possibly with purulent sinusitis, dyspnoea, recurrent haemoptysis, pleuritic chest pain.

Cystic fibrosis: additional symptoms

Diarrhoea or steatorrhoea, abdominal pain, constipation: in adults.

Meconium ileus: 10% of childhood presentations.

Failure to thrive: in children.

Prolonged neonatal jaundice, rectal prolapse.

Signs

Bronchiectasis and cystic fibrosis
- Frequently few signs are manifest except a few crackles.

Clubbing, coarse crackles, tachypnoea, hyperinflation, signs of weight loss, halitosis: in more florid cases.

Cystic fibrosis: additional signs

Greasy smelly faeces, steatorrhoea, abdominal distension, poor growth.

Investigations

Sputum culture: for *Staphylococcus aureus*, *Haemophilus influenzae*, and *Pseudomonas* spp. (especially *P. aeruginosa* and *P. cepacia*) and to exclude active tuberculosis.

Sputum cytology: to exclude malignancy.

Serum immunoglobulin measurement.

Chest radiography: shows hyperinflation, tramlines, crowded lung markings, and ring shadows.

High-resolution CT: shows ring and cystic lesions and bronchial wall thickening.

Sinus radiography: shows mucosal thickening and fluid levels.

Respiratory function tests: for normal, obstructive, or mixed ventilatory defect.

Aspergillus skin and precipitin tests.

Nasal mucociliary clearance test.

Sweat test, fludrocortisone suppression test, gene analysis: to diagnose cystic fibrosis; sweat chloride >60 mmol/L in 98% of patients; failure of fludrocortisone suppression in adults.

Complications

Bronchiectasis and cystic fibrosis

Infective exacerbations: viral or bacterial.

Pneumothorax.

Respiratory failure.

Cor pulmonale.

Empyema.

Amyloidosis.

Chest pain: usually pleuritic, associated with an area of bronchiectasis.

Haemoptysis.

Metastatic spread of infection: now rare; brain abscess was classic complication.

Arthropathy: rheumatoid arthritis and nonspecific seronegative arthritis related to activity of disease.

Cystic fibrosis: additional complications

Diabetes mellitus, biliary cirrhosis, heat exhaustion, intussusception in children, cholelithiasis, azoospermia, volvulus in children, oesophageal reflux, distal intestinal obstruction syndrome.

Differential diagnosis

Bronchiectasis

Asthma.
Fibrosing alveolitis.
Chronic bronchitis.
Lung carcinoma.
Cyanotic heart disease.
Sinusitis with chronic cough.

Cystic fibrosis

Coeliac disease.
Giardiasis.

Aetiology

- Bronchiectasis results from failure of the airway protective mechanisms, including mucociliary clearance mechanisms, and the inflammatory response.
- Further damage may be due to the host response and the infecting microbes.
- Causes include the following:

Bronchiectasis

Impaired clearance: defective mucociliary clearance, congenital, bronchial obstruction, immunodeficiency.

Inflammation: inflammatory pneumonitis, fibrotic or granulomatous lung disease, previous severe infection, allergic aspergillosis.

Cystic fibrosis

Gene (chromosome 7) mutations that produce abnormal cystic fibrosis transmembrane conductance regulator, causing viscid secretions.

Epidemiology

- The estimated prevalence of bronchiectasis in the UK is 1–2 in 1000 (probably an underestimate); it is more common in developing countries.
- Cystic fibrosis is the most common serious inherited disease.
- In the UK it is present in 1 in 2500.
- 1 in 25 people carries the abnormal gene.
- 290 babies are born with cystic fibrosis, and 146 people die of it annually.

Associated diseases

Rheumatoid arthritis.
Ulcerative colitis.
Purulent sinusitis.
Alpha-1 antiprotease deficiency.
Yellow nail syndrome.
Primary lymphoedema.
Malignancy.
Connective tissue disorders.
Vasculitis.
Infertility.

Treatment

Diet and lifestyle
- Patients should keep as fit as possible.
- Patients with cystic fibrosis need pancreatic supplements with snacks and meals, high energy intake to maintain weight, overnight nasogastric feeding or feeding gastrostomy, and fat-soluble vitamin supplements.

Pharmacological treatment

General guidelines
- Treatment specific to the underlying cause includes the following:

Removal of foreign body or inspissated mucus.

Treatment of active tuberculosis.

Replacement of immunoglobulins: for panhypogammaglobulinaemia, selective IgM and IgG, and possibly IgG_2 deficiency, but not for selective IgA deficiency (risk of anaphylaxis).

Treatment of associated conditions, e.g. rheumatoid arthritis.

For bronchiectasis
Antibiotics: drug choice based on sputum culture; given either for exacerbations or at regular intervals; courses should last 2–3 weeks, and antimicrobial agents should be given in high doses; for patients colonized with *Pseudomonas* spp., specific antipseudomonal antibiotics should be given, including nebulized antibiotics, e.g. colistin, for maintenance treatment between courses.

Bronchodilators: for patients with demonstrable airflow obstruction.

Steroids: improved morbidity in short term, but effects on prognosis not known; inhaled steroids recommended for patients with prominent or reversible airflow obstruction.

Mucolytics: nebulized rh DNAase is effective in many patients with viscid sputum.

For cystic fibrosis
Lactulose, oral acetylcysteine, and oral gastrografin with nasogastric aspiration and i.v. fluids: for distal intestinal obstruction syndrome.

H_2 antagonist or proton-pump inhibitor: for oesophageal reflux.

Non-pharmacological treatment

Physiotherapy
- Physiotherapy is the main form of non-pharmacological treatment.
- Methods include postural drainage, deep cough, and forced expiratory manoeuvres twice daily.

Other options
For haemoptysis: bed-rest and antibiotics, selective embolization, intubation and balloon tamponade, or local resection.

For pneumothorax: aspiration, intercostal drainage, pleurodesis or partial pleurectomy (if recurrent or unresponsive).

For respiratory failure: supplemental oxygen therapy, nasal ventilation.

For nasal polyps: polypectomy.

For severe localized disease: surgery.

Lung or heart–lung transplantation, especially in cystic fibrosis.

Treatment aims
To minimize lung damage by limiting pulmonary infection and increasing clearance of pulmonary secretion.

Prognosis
- The prognosis of bronchiectasis depends on the severity of the disease.
- The median survival with cystic fibrosis is 25 years in the UK.

Follow-up and management
- All patients with moderate to severe bronchiectasis need regular care from a respiratory physician.
- All patients with cystic fibrosis should attend a recognised cystic fibrosis centre.

Patient support
Assistance with claims for attendance and mobility allowances.

Counselling regarding lung transplantation, fears of dying, reproduction, etc.

Information about Cystic Fibrosis Trust.

Key references
Cole PJ: Bronchiectasis. In *Respiratory Medicine*. Edited by Brewis RAL, Gibson GJ, Geddes DM. London: Baillière Tindall, 1990, pp 726–759.

Davis PB: Evolution of therapy for cystic fibrosis. *N Engl J Med* 1994, **331**:672–673.

Fiel SB: Clinical management of pulmonary disease in cystic fibrosis. *Lancet* 1993, **341**:1070–1074.

Koch C, Hoiby N: Pathogenesis of cystic fibrosis. *Lancet* 1993, **341**:1065–1069.

Orenstein DM: Cystic fibrosis. *Curr Probl Pediatr* 1993, **23**:4–15.

Chronic obstructive airway disease
J.M. Corne

Diagnosis

Symptoms
Cough: chronic bronchitis is defined as a cough productive of sputum on most days for at least 3 consecutive months in 2 successive years.

Increasing shortness of breath.

Weight loss.

Signs
Barrel-shaped chest, tracheal tug, decreased cardiac dullness and reduced breath sounds, palpable liver due to hepatic displacement: signs of hyperexpansion.

Increased respiratory rate, use of accessory muscles of respiration, paradoxical movement of costal margins, 'pursed lip' breathing, reduced breath sounds: signs of airflow obstruction.

Cyanosis, hypercapnic flap, peripheral vasodilatation: signs of respiratory failure.

Right ventricular heave, raised jugular venous pressure, peripheral oedema: signs of pulmonary hypertension.

Fine inspiratory crackles: frequently found in chronic obstructive airway disease and do not necessarily imply coexistent heart failure.

Investigations
Full blood count: polycythaemia found in a few patients.

ECG: to detect right axis deviation or signs of right-sided strain.

Chest radiography: to detect signs of chronic obstructive airway disease (low flat diaphragms, long thin heart), emphysema (hypodense bullae, large retrosternal airspace on lateral radiography), or pulmonary hypertension (prominent hilum, with reduced peripheral vascular shadows).

Spirometry: to confirm obstructive picture and to show degree of reversibility to therapeutic agents.

Arterial blood gas measurement: to check for hypoxia and carbon dioxide retention; high bicarbonate concentration suggests more chronic carbon dioxide retention.

Walking test: a sensitive test of therapeutic response; the patient is asked to walk a 10 m distance at increasing speeds, and the test is terminated when he or she cannot walk the distance any faster.

Complications
Infective exacerbations.

Pulmonary hypertension.

Respiratory failure.

Pneumothorax.

Differential diagnosis

Shortness of breath
Asthma.
Left ventricular failure.
Large airway obstruction, e.g. proximal tumour.

Recurrent chest infections
Aspiration secondary to oesophageal disease.
Immunosuppression.

Aetiology
- Causes include the following:
Cigarette smoking.
Atmospheric pollution: much less important than smoking, but mortality from chronic obstructive airway disease increases in areas of atmospheric pollution.
Alpha-1 antitrypsin deficiency: rare; homozygous form present in 1 in 5000 people, and not all of these develop chest disease; causes basal emphysema.
Intravenous drug abuse.

Epidemiology
- Epidemiological studies are hampered by lack of an accepted definition; in a study of GPs conducted in 1961, however, a prevalence of 8% in men and 3% in women was found.
- Chronic obstructive airway disease is estimated to cause the loss of 31 000 000 working days each year.

Asthma or chronic obstructive airway disease?
- Many smokers who develop airway disease in later life have late-onset asthma rather than smoking-induced chronic obstructive airway disease.
- Features suggesting asthma include a family history of atopic disease, good response to beta-2 agonists, and raised IgE concentrations.
- Many patients with chronic obstructive airway disease have a reversible element and are often regarded as being at the asthmatic end of the spectrum.

Treatment

Diet and lifestyle
- Stopping smoking reduces the rate of deterioration of lung function to that of non-smokers and, at an early stage, may improve symptoms.
- Loss of weight improves functional capacity.
- Patients' homes can be assessed for the need for aids to daily living.

Pharmacological treatment
- Inadequate inhaler technique is one of the main reasons for treatment failure; inhaler technique must always be checked before treatment is initiated or changed.

Inhaled beta-2 agonists
Standard dosage	Salbutamol inhaler 200 µg or nebulizer 2.5–5 mg up to 4 times daily.
Contraindications	Hypersensitivity.
Special points	Patient responses vary; clinical improvement may occur but may not be detected on spirometric assessment.
Main drug interactions	None.
Main side effects	Tremor, hypokalaemia after high doses.

Inhaled anticholinergics
Standard dosage	Ipratropium bromide inhaler 20–40 µg or nebulizer 100–500 µg 4 times daily.
Contraindications	Hypersensitivity; caution in glaucoma (nebulized solutions).
Main drug interactions	None.
Main side effects	Dry mouth (rare).

Inhaled steroids
- Inhaled steroids are indicated for patients who have shown an objective response.

Standard dosage	Beclomethasone dipropionate 200–2000 µg twice daily.
Contraindications	Hypersensitivity.
Special points	Systemic absorption can be reduced with a spacer device.
Main drug interactions	None.
Main side effects	Oral candidiasis.

Oral steroids
- Oral steroids are indicated for exacerbations of chronic obstructive pulmonary disease and for maintenance treatment in severely ill steroid-responsive patients.

Standard dosage	Prednisolone 30 mg in the morning for exacerbations; lowest possible dose for maintenance treatment.
Contraindications	None.
Special points	Steroid responsiveness should be shown by >10% improvement in forced expiratory volume in 1 s after 3 weeks of prednisolone 30 mg.
Main drug interactions	None.
Main side effects	Osteoporosis, diabetes, steroid psychosis.

Theophyllines
- These have been shown to improve exercise tolerance.

Standard dosage	Theophylline 375–500 mg daily.
Contraindications	None.
Special points	Plasma concentrations must be monitored; they should be maintained at 10–20 µg/L.
Main drug interactions	Cimetidine, erythromycin, ciprofloxacin, and oral contraceptives reduce metabolism; cigarettes, alcohol, phenytoin, and rifampicin increase metabolism.
Main side effects	Tachycardia, arrythmias.

Treatment aims
To maximize functional capacity.
To reduce decline in lung function.

Other treatments

Long-term oxygen therapy (>15 h daily)
- Indications include the following:

Partial pressure of oxygen <7.3 kPa on two successive occasions when patient is stable.
Forced expiratory volume in 1 s <1.5 L.
Non-smoking patient.
Failure to show carbon dioxide retention after a trial of oxygen.
At least one episode of peripheral oedema.

Nasal intermittent positive pressure ventilation
- This may be suitable in patients who retain carbon dioxide with oxygen therapy.

Venesection
- Venesection is indicated if packed cell volume is >0.55.

Prognosis
- If forced expiratory volume in 1 s is <1L, 5-year survival is 69%.

Follow-up and management
- Forced expiratory volume in 1 s must be monitored.
- Response to treatment must be assessed.

Key references
Ferguson GT, Cherniak RM: Management of chronic obstructive pulmonary disease. *N Engl J Med* 1993, **328**:1017–1022.

Pride N: The natural history of chronic bronchitis and emphysema. *Med Int* 1991, **89**:3718–3721.

Fibrosing alveolitis — K.T. Khoo and M.A. Spiteri

Diagnosis

Symptoms
Dyspnoea: on exertion, progressive.
Cough: usually unproductive and irritating.

Signs
Clubbing: in 65–85% of patients.
Fine late inspiratory crackles: at lung base, later throughout lungs.
Cyanosis: especially on effort.
Late right ventricular heave, right ventricular gallop, loud pulmonary second sound, raised jugular venous pulse, peripheral oedema: signs of cor pulmonale.

Investigations
Chest radiography: shows small lung fields, irregular nodular or reticulonodular opacities; often maximal in lower zones, honeycombing in severely ill patients, pulmonary artery enlargement, and cardiomegaly with cor pulmonale.
High-resolution CT: sensitive; may detect disease when chest radiograph normal; characteristically shows subpleural 'rind' of increased density, with central sparing; distortion of bronchi and cystic air spaces in advanced disease.
Radionuclide scanning: ^{67}Ga taken up by macrophages appears as hot spots but not specific to cryptogenic fibrosing alveolitis; ^{99m}Tc DTPA (diethylenetriaminepenta-acetic acid) enhanced clearing in assessing lung permeability, occurs early before lung function deterioration detected.
Pulmonary function tests: restrictive ventilatory defect, with low lung volumes, decreased lung compliance, and reduced carbon monoxide transfer.
Arterial blood gas analysis: may be normal in patients with mild disease; partial oxygen pressure typically falls on exercise.
Bronchoalveolar lavage: increased cell counts in bronchoalveolar fluid; raised lymphocyte count may indicate better response to treatment.
Lung biopsy: open lung biopsy gold standard but inappropriate in very ill or elderly patients; transbronchial, percutaneous, or drill biopsy may produce smaller specimens, inadequate for useful histological analysis.
Haematology and biochemistry: usually unhelpful; ESR may be raised; globulin or immunoglobulin (one or more classes) concentrations often raised; 30% of patients positive for rheumatoid or antinuclear antibody.

Complications
Death: ~60% of patients die as direct consequence of fibrosing lung disease (some with terminal infection, others from respiratory failure).
Pulmonary hypertension, right heart failure: clinically evident in some patients.
Lung cancer: apparent excess in patients with fibrosing alveolitis (smokers and non-smokers).

Differential diagnosis
- Many conditions of known cause have a tendency to alveolar-wall fibrosis.
Fibrogenic dust inhalation: e.g. silica, asbestos.
Granulomas: due to extrinsic allergic alveolitis, berylliosis, sarcoidosis.
Chronic exudates: e.g. chronic left ventricular failure, drugs, chronic renal failure.

Aetiology
- The cause of fibrosing alveolitis is unknown.
- The disease is characterized by an inflammatory exudate of the alveolar wall, with a tendency to fibrosis.
- Cryptogenic fibrosing alveolitis can occur alone or be associated with connective tissue disorders of unknown cause, e.g. systemic sclerosis, SLE, rheumatoid arthritis, polymyositis.
- Certain drugs, e.g. bleomycin, methotrexate, and amiodarone, can produce a picture similar to cryptogenic fibrosing alveolitis.
- Certain viral agents, e.g. influenza A2 virus, have been reported as inducing fibrosing alveolitis.

Epidemiology
- Fibrosing alveolitis is manifest mostly in the fifth or sixth decade.
- The prevalence is estimated to be 2–5 in 100 000 population.

Treatment

Diet and lifestyle
- Morbidity is increased, with progressive restriction of daily activities.
- Diet has no effect.

Pharmacological treatment
- The minimum duration of treatment is unknown

Corticosteroids
- ~50% of patients have some symptomatic benefit, at least short-term, from steroids; no more than 20% show objective radiographic or physiological improvement.

Standard dosage	Prednisolone 60 mg daily for 1–2 months; reduced slowly to maintenance dose if condition responsive.
Contraindications	Uncontrolled hypertension, diabetes mellitus, infection, severe osteoporosis.
Main drug interactions	Antihypertensive drugs.
Main side effects	Weight gain, oedema, bruising, purple striae in skin (especially of abdomen), moon face, osteoporosis, collapse of vertebrae, diabetes mellitus, hypertension, myopathy (especially proximal girdle muscles), hirsutism, menstrual disturbances, psychotic reactions, cataracts, withdrawal phenomena.

Cyclophosphamide
- Many patients fail to respond to high-dose steroids alone; in patients who continue to deteriorate, low-dose prednisolone can be combined with cyclophosphamide, an immunosuppressant drug.

Standard dosage	Cyclophosphamide 125 mg daily with prednisolone 20 mg on alternate days.
Contraindications	Severe renal impairment, porphyria.
Special points	Clinical improvement not expected within 2 months of starting treatment.
Main drug interactions	Allopurinol, muscle relaxants.
Main side effects	Haemorrhagic cystitis, bone-marrow suppression, alopecia.

Other drugs
- D-Penicillamine and methotrexate have proved disappointing.

Supportive treatment
Supplemental oxygen.
Diuretics for heart failure.
Opiates for suppression of cough and alleviation of breathlessness.

Treatment aims
To improve quality of life by preventing deterioration of lung function.
To relieve symptoms.
To give maximum supportive care, including counselling, when symptomatic relief not possible.

Other treatments
- Single-lung transplantation is indicated for patients with rapidly progressive disease and young patients who do not respond to conventional treatment.

Prognosis
- Mortality within 5 years of diagnosis is 50%.
- Probable responders usually have a more cellular histological response.
- Improved survival may be achieved if the disease is detected early and more precise predictors of progression are developed to prevent high-risk patients, in whom more aggressive treatment would be justified.
- The 1-year survival rate after single-lung transplantation is 50%.

Follow-up and management
- The response should be assessed by clinical, subjective and objective changes in chest radiography and pulmonary function tests.

Key references

Johnston ID et al.: The management of cryptogenic fibrosing alveolitis in three regions of the United Kingdom. *Eur Hosp J* 1993, **6**:891–893.

Schwartz DA et al.: Determinants of progression in idiopathic pulmonary fibrosis. *Am J Respir Crit Care Med* 1994, **149**:444–449.

Schwartz DA et al.: Determinants of survival in idiopathic pulmonary fibrosis. *Am J Respir Crit Care Med* 1994, **149**:450–454.

Terriff BA et al.: Fibrosing alveolitis: chest radiography and CT as predictors of clinical and functional impairment at follow-up in 26 patients. *Radiology* 1992, **184**:445–449.

Granulomatoses — C.M.B. Higgs

Diagnosis

Symptoms
- Symptoms are often nonspecific, with a wide variety of manifestations.

Initial or indolent phase
Cough, dyspnoea.

Nasal and ocular symptoms: in Wegener's granulomatosis.

Wheeze or asthma, abdominal pain: in Churg–Strauss syndrome.

Active or aggressive phase
Fever, malaise, anorexia, weight loss.

Cough, dyspnoea, haemoptysis, chest pain.

Skin rash, arthralgia.

Signs
- Manifestations are widely varied.

Chest signs: often little, compared with extent of radiographic changes.

Wheeze: feature of Churg–Strauss syndrome and bronchocentric granulomatosis.

Nasal inflammation and granulation: in Wegener's and lymphomatoid granulomatoses.

Ocular inflammation or proptosis: in Wegener's granulomatosis.

Vasculitic or nonspecific skin rash.

Peripheral or cranial neuropathy.

Investigations
Full blood count: anaemia common; eosinophilia $>1.5 \times 10^9/L$ in Churg–Strauss syndrome.

ESR and plasma viscosity measurement: usually raised values.

Renal function test: abnormalities frequent in Wegener's granulomatosis.

Chest radiography: varied appearances; can show mass lesion, consolidation, or diffuse shadowing; cavitating nodules typical of Wegener's granulomatosis.

Anti-neutrophil cytoplasmic antibodies (ANCA): cANCA present in 90% of patients with active Wegener's granulomatosis, pANCA present in some Churg–Strauss, lymphomatoid, or Wegener's sufferers; other autoserology usually negative.

Biopsy: ideally open lung biopsy; bronchoscopic or renal biopsy may give specific histology; nasal and skin biopsy usually nonspecific.

Complications

General
Pulmonary haemorrhage: uncommon.

Infection: common.

Peripheral or cranial neuropathy, mononeuritis multiplex.

Wegener's granulomatosis
Renal impairment: in 40% of patients.

Deafness: in 30%.

Churg–Strauss syndrome
Cardiac involvement: in 50% (most common cause of death).

Differential diagnosis

General
Collagen-vascular diseases.
Other systemic vasculitides, subacute bacterial endocarditis, atrial myxoma.

Pulmonary disease alone
Sarcoid, tuberculosis, neoplasm, infection.

Pulmonary and renal disease
Goodpasture's syndrome, SLE.

Eosinophilic disease
Eosinophilic pneumonia, bronchopulmonary aspergillosis, hypereosinophilic syndrome, drug reaction.

Aetiology
- The cause is unknown but may be a granulomatous or vasculitic response to infection or neoplasm.
- Bronchocentric granulomatosis is associated with aspergillus infection.
- Lymphomatoid granulomatosis may be a form of lymphoma.

Epidemiology
- Granulomatoses are rare conditions, of which Wegener's is by far the most common.
- They occur at all ages but mainly in people aged 35–55 years.

Diagnostic pointers
- Histology is often unavailable or inconclusive; diagnosis therefore rests on a combination of clinical features, investigations, and histology.

Wegener's granulomatosis
Necrotizing, granulomatous vasculitis, involving upper and lower respiratory tract and kidneys; c-anti-neutrophil cytoplasmic antibody positive.

Churg–Strauss syndrome
Asthma, eosinophilia, and vasculitis; p-anti-neutrophil cytoplasmic antibody often positive.

Lymphomatoid granulomatosis
Non-necrotizing, involving upper and lower respiratory tract; rare.

Necrotizing sarcoid or bronchocentric granulomatosis
Lung shadows without extrapulmonary features.

Treatment

Diet and lifestyle
- Stopping smoking should be encouraged in view of the risk of chest infection from disease and treatment.

Pharmacological treatment

Prednisolone
- Prednisolone is important in all initial treatment and in maintenance for Churg–Strauss syndrome, necrotizing sarcoid granulomatosis, and bronchocentric granulomatosis.

Standard dosage	Prednisolone 60–80 mg orally daily initially. Optional initial pulse methyl prednisolone 1 g i.v. on 3 alternate days. Steady dose reduction and alternate-day use after 1 month. Wegener's patients should be weaned off drug entirely after remission.
Contraindications	Caution in diabetes mellitus, hypertension, or peptic ulceration.
Special points	Patients must be given a steroid-warning card; blood glucose and blood pressure must be checked.
Main drug interactions	Rifampicin, carbamazepine, phenytoin, phenobarbitone.
Main side effects	Fluid retention, hypertension, proximal myopathy, mental disturbance, osteoporosis, skin fragility, increased risk of infection.

Cyclophosphamide
- Cyclophosphamide is essential in Wegener's granulomatosis, advised in lymphomatoid granulomatosis, and sometimes needed in Churg–Strauss syndrome.

Standard dosage	Cyclophosphamide 2 mg/kg orally daily. Optional initial pulse cyclophosphamide 0.5 g i.v., followed by 0.5–1 g i.v. monthly, according to leucocyte count.
Contraindications	Porphyria, pregnancy.
Special points	Dose reduced in patients with renal impairment; should be adjusted according to regular leucocyte counts and side effects; usually continued for 1 year after remission has been induced.
Main drug interactions	Allopurinol, suxamethonium.
Main side effects	Bone-marrow suppression, nausea and vomiting, hair loss, cystitis, sterility, bladder cancer, lymphoma.

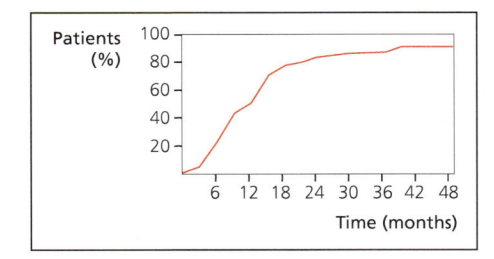

Cumulative remission rate on standard treatment for Wegener's granulomatosis (in the 75% of patients who achieve complete remission).

Treatment aims
To achieve remission and prevent relapse.

Prognosis

Wegener's granulomatosis
- Long-term survival is >80%, but relapse is common, and >80% of patients suffer permanent morbidity.

Churg–Strauss syndrome
- Long-term survival is high, but cardiac complications are the main cause of death.

Lymphomatoid granulomatosis
- The 5-year survival rate is 50%, less if lymphoma is present.

Necrotizing sarcoid or bronchocentric granulomatosis
- The prognosis and response to steroids are good.

Follow-up and management
- Long-term monitoring is required; ESR or plasma viscosity and chest radiography are guides of disease activity.
- Anti-neutrophil cytoplasmic antibody titres are helpful guides in Wegener's granulomatosis; they do not rise in infective episodes but may rise some time before relapse occurs.
- Renal function in Wegener's granulomatosis should be monitored.

Key references
Hoffman GS et al.: Wegener's granulomatosis: an analysis of 158 patients. *Ann Intern Med* 1992, **116**:488–498.

Lanham JG: Churg–Strauss syndrome. *Br J Hosp Med* 1992, **47**:667–673.

Pisani RJ, DeRemee RA: Clinical implications of the histopathologic diagnosis of pulmonary lymphomatoid granulomatosis. *Mayo Clin Proc* 1990, **65**:151–163.

Lung cancer   A.J. Frew

Diagnosis

Symptoms
Cough, haemoptysis, breathlessness, hoarseness.
Chest pain, lymphadenopathy.
Weight loss, general malaise.
Intellectual impairment, headache, focal neuropathy, tremor.

Signs
- Signs are not always manifest.

Lobar or lung collapse, consolidation, pleural effusion, monophonic wheeze.
Cervical lymphadenopathy, hepatomegaly, local chest-wall tenderness, Horner's syndrome, neurological deficit.
Finger clubbing, cerebellar degeneration, peripheral neuropathy.

Investigations

For diagnosis
Chest radiography: shows mass, collapse, distal infection, abscess, adenopathy, metastases.
Sputum cytology: shows malignant cells.
Bronchoscopy: tumour often directly visible; operability can be assessed, and samples obtained for cytology and histology.
Pleural aspiration and biopsy: primary test if effusion present; malignant cells indicate inoperable tumour.

For staging
Bronchoscopy: to assess presence of central disease.
CT of thorax: to assess presence of hilar or mediastinal adenopathy.
Mediastinoscopy: to evaluate lymphadenopathy.
Biochemistry: may indicate bone or liver involvement; sodium and calcium disturbance may occur without metastasis.
Liver ultrasonography: disease often spreads to liver.
CT of brain: disease often spreads to brain.

Complications
Lobar collapse, obstruction of superior vena cava.
Pneumonia, abscess.
Pain, pleural effusion.
Pericardial effusion, direct invasion.
Metastases: especially bone, brain, liver, adrenal glands.
Local neurological invasion, neuropathies.
Cushing's syndrome, inappropriate antidiuretic hormone secretion, hypercalcaemia.
Recurrent venous thrombosis.
Clubbing, hypertrophic osteoarthropathy.

LOOK FOR:- Cachexia,
Clubbing.
Nicotine stained fingers.
Lymph nodes.
Signs of intrathoracic involvement
1. Pleural Effusion
2. Collapse
3. Recurrent Chest Infection.

Differential diagnosis
Simple pneumonia.
Benign tumour or cysts.
Tuberculosis.
Pulmonary metastases.
Other causes of lung abscess.
Other causes of pleural effusion.

Aetiology
- Causes include the following:

Cigarette smoking: lung cancer was rare in the 19th century, and its increase is closely linked to the increasing popularity of cigarettes in the 20th century.
Atmospheric pollution: increased rates in urban areas.
Radioactivity: mining pitchblend, uranium.
Manufacturing: chromate, asbestos, nickel, arsenic, haematite.

Epidemiology
- Lung cancer is the most common cancer in men.
- It is the second most common cancer in women.

SPIROMETRY → TO ASSESS OPERABILITY. IF $FEV_1 < 1L$ CAN NOT OPERATE. IN ORDER TO ASSESS RELATIVE LUNG FEV_1 ISOTOPE VENTILATION STUDIES MAY BE PERFORMED.

Lung cancer
A.J. Frew

Treatment

Diet and lifestyle
- Anorexia is a common feature; no specific diet is needed, but oral corticosteroids often lead to improved mood and appetite.
- Patients should be encouraged to be active.
- Most patients stop smoking after diagnosis, but this does not alter prognosis significantly.

Pharmacological treatment
- Chemotherapy is the treatment of choice for small-cell cancer; various regimens are available.
- No satisfactory regimen has yet been found for large-cell tumours (i.e. adenocarcinoma, squamous-cell or anaplastic tumours).
- The local oncology service should be consulted.

Non-pharmacological treatment

Surgical resection
- Surgical resection is possible in only a few patients.
- It is limited by the frequent involvement of mediastinal nodes and central structures.
- Adequate lung function is needed (forced expiratory volume in 1 s >1.2 L for lobectomy, >1.5 L for pneumonectomy).
- Surgical resection is rarely appropriate for small-cell lung cancer (usually has extensive central disease, even if endoscopically resectable).

Radiotherapy
- Palliative radiotherapy is useful in the management of haemoptysis and bony deposits.
- 'Radical' radiotherapy is no longer favoured for limited disease because few cures result.
- 'Local' (endobronchial) radiotherapy, a novel experimental treatment, has yet to show any superiority to palliative external beam radiotherapy.

Endobronchial laser resection
- This is a palliative procedure for tracheal or main bronchus disease.
- It is available in only a few specialist centres.

Treatment aims
1. To identify patients who can be treated surgically.
2. To identify patients with small-cell cancer and treat them by chemotherapy.
3. To provide palliative treatment, guided by symptoms, to the remaining patients.

Prognosis
- Prognosis is generally poor unless the tumour is resectable.
- When patients are technically resectable, the 5-year survival rate is ~28%.

Follow-up and management
- Surgical cure is possible in 5–10% of patients.
- In patients who are inoperable, the main goal is palliation.
- Local symptoms are usually best treated by radiotherapy.

Key references
Capewell S *et al.*: Lung cancer in young men. *Resp Med* 1992, **86**:499–502.

Hazuka MB, Bunn PA: Controversies in the nonsurgical treatment of stage III non-small cell lung cancer. *Am Rev Resp Dis* 1992, **145**:967–977.

Pierce RJ: Lasers, brachytherapy and stents – keeping airways open. *Resp Med* 1991, **85**:263–265.

Pleural effusion — A.J. Frew

Diagnosis

Symptoms
- Patients are often asymptomatic if the effusion is small.

Breathlessness.

Chest pain: increased on deep inspiration or movement.

Positional discomfort or pain: with large effusions, causing mediastinal shift.

Symptoms of underlying disease.

Fever.

Signs
- Signs are clinically detectable only if the volume is ≥ 300 ml; loculated effusion may be very difficult to detect.

Decreased movement of chest wall on affected side.

Dull percussion note: 'stony dull'.

Absent breath sounds in area of dullness.

Occasional bronchial breathing at upper margin of area of dullness.

Displaced trachea: large effusions only.

Investigations
Chest radiography: to assess extent of effusion and possible underlying disease.

Ultrasonography: if doubt about nature of shadowing and to define loculated area for aspiration.

Aspiration: for cytology, Gram stain and Ziehl–Neelsen stain for acid-fast bacilli, culture, protein content.

Pleural biopsy: in experienced hands, much more reliable for diagnosis of tuberculosis and malignancy than simple aspiration.

Repeat radiography: after drainage of effusion, to visualize underlying lung.

Thoracoscopy: if doubt remains, to obtain better samples for histology.

CT: for visualizing loculated effusions and pleural and parenchymal disease.

Complications
Constrictive fibrosis of pleura and restricted lung function: caused by empyema and postpneumonic effusions.

Iatrogenic secondary infection.

Iatrogenic pneumothorax.

Unilateral pulmonary oedema: after injudiciously rapid drainage.

Haemorrhage: damage to intercostal vessels, especially after pleural biopsy.

Differential diagnosis

Infections: postpneumonic, tuberculosis, extension from subphrenic sepsis.

Inflammation: pancreatitis, rheumatoid arthritis, SLE, polyarteritis nodosa.

Primary malignancy: mesothelioma.

Secondary malignancy: bronchogenic carcinoma, metastatic spread (especially breast, stomach, pancreas), lymphoma.

Infarction secondary to pulmonary embolism.

Aetiology
- Causes include the following:

Exudates

Unknown in ~20%, despite extensive investigation.

Infections: viral pleurisy, bacterial pneumonia, tuberculosis, empyema.

Secondary malignancy or secondary cancer (e.g. lung, breast, stomach), leukaemia or lymphoma.

Vascular: pulmonary infarction.

Collagen disorders: rheumatoid arthritis.

Primary pleural malignancy (mesothelioma).

Transudates

Congestive heart failure, hypoalbuminaemia (nephrotic syndrome and hepatic cirrhosis), constrictive pericarditis.

Abdominal disease: subphrenic abscess, pancreatitis.

Epidemiology
- In the UK, pleural effusion is frequently found with lung cancer and after pneumonia.
- Tuberculosis is declining in importance in the UK but remains one of the most common causes of pleural effusion world wide.
- Mesothelioma is rare but is associated with asbestos exposure.

Treatment

Diet and lifestyle
- No special precautions are necessary.

Pharmacological treatment

Principles
- The principal aim is to treat any underlying cause and to treat the local problem by drainage, possibly with chemical pleuradhesis.
- For transudates, the underlying disease must be treated.
- For infective causes (empyema, pneumonia), systemic antibiotics are indicated and intercostal drainage is essential; surgical drainage and decortication of pleura can be done if thick pleural rind develops.
- For tuberculosis, standard oral antituberculosis chemotherapy is indicated. The effusion should be aspirated to dryness. Tube drainage and surgery should be avoided if possible. See Tuberculosis, pulmonary *for details*.
- For malignant effusions, pleural effusion indicates inoperability; treatment is guided by symptoms. Intermittent aspiration is usually helpful. Tube drainage is the best method of preventing recurrence and achieving pleuradhesis. In mesothelioma, tube drainage is best avoided if possible because of the risk of seeding tube tract.
- Pulmonary infarcts usually resolve without needing drainage.
- For non-infective non-malignant causes, the effusion should be drained to dryness and followed with repeated chest radiographs.
- Pulmonary infarcts usually resolve without needing drainage, but formal anticoagulation with warfarin is usually appropriate (*see* Pulmonary embolism *for details*).

Chemical pleuradhesis
- Chemical pleuradhesis is best done by specialists, who can consider the advantages and disadvantages in each individual case.

Standard dosage	Tetracycline in saline solution for injection after pleural cavity has been drained by an intercostal drain. Bleomycin is an acceptable alternative for malignant effusions.
Contraindications	Transudate, bronchopleural fistulae, infection.
Main drug interactions	None.
Main side effects	Local pain, transient fever.

Treatment aims
To achieve resolution of pleural effusion without residual fibrosis or functional deficit.

Prognosis
- Prognosis varies widely according to the underlying cause.
- If cleared by drainage, most bacterial effusions resolve, leaving some pleural scarring, which may need surgery if severe.
- Malignant effusions have poor prognosis, and treatment is mainly palliative, guided by symptoms.

Follow-up and management
- Serial chest radiographs should be taken, usually at 4–6 week intervals to assess recurrence.
- Lung function tests are needed to assess residual restrictive deficit if radiographic changes persist.

Key references
Arvastson B *et al.*: Mepacrine in malignant pleural effusion. *Scand J Resp Dis* 1973, **54**:132.

Collins TR, Sahin SA: Thoracentesis: complications, patient experience and diagnostic value. *Chest* 1987, **91**:817–819.

Harley HRS: Malignant pleural effusions and their treatment by intercostal talc pleuradhesis. *Br J Dis Chest* 1979, **73**:173.

Keller SM: Current and future therapy for malignant pleural effusion. *Chest* 1993, **103 (suppl)**:63S–67S.

Seaton A, Seaton D, Leitch AG: *Crofton & Douglas's Respiratory Diseases* edn 4. Oxford: Blackwell Scientific Publications, 1981, pp 1094–1096.

Pneumonia   M.A. Woodhead

Diagnosis

Symptoms

Common
- Onset may be abrupt or over days.

Cough: with sputum, which may be purulent, in two-thirds of patients.

Fever: possibly with rigors.

Pleuritic chest pain.

Dyspnoea.

Less common
Haemoptysis, vomiting, diarrhoea, myalgia.

Mental confusion: especially in patients with severe pneumonia and in elderly patients.

Falls and new urinary incontinence: in elderly patients.

Signs
Pyrexia, herpes labialis.

Mental confusion, cyanosis, hypotension: suggesting severe illness.

Raised respiratory rate: suggesting severe illness.

Dullness on percussion.

Increased vocal fremitus.

Crackles.

Bronchial breathing: aegophony and whispering pectoriloquy; in one-third of patients.

Investigations

To confirm diagnosis
Chest radiography: shows consolidation.

To assess severity
Arterial blood gas analysis: low partial oxygen pressure, raised partial carbon dioxide pressure, low pH.

Blood U&E analysis: high risk associated with raised blood urea and low sodium.

Full blood count: leucocyte count <4 or >20 × 10^9/L indicates high risk.

Liver function tests: low albumin indicates high risk.

To assess cause
Blood culture: for bacteraemia.

Sputum Gram stain and culture.

Pleural-fluid Gram stain and culture.

Serology: acute and convalescent sera for antibodies to viruses, chlamydia, mycoplasma, coxiella, and legionella.

Bronchoscopy: for lower respiratory secretions; often needed in immunocompromised patients but rarely in others.

Complications
Empyema, lung abscess, pulmonary embolus, adult respiratory distress syndrome.

Acute renal failure, haemolysis.

Differential diagnosis
Pulmonary oedema.
Exacerbation of chronic bronchitis.
Pulmonary embolus.
Lung cancer.

Aetiology
- Pneumococcal infection is the cause of 75% of community-acquired pneumonias.
- Gram-negative enterobacteria (e.g. *Escherichia coli*) are the cause of 50% or more of nosocomial pneumonias.
- Anaerobic bacteria (e.g. bacteroides) are important in aspiration pneumonia.
- Immunocompromised patients may be infected by a huge range of microorganisms, e.g. unusual bacteria and fungi, many of which would not cause infection in immunocompetent patients.

Epidemiology
- Pneumonia occurs at all ages but is most frequent in very young and very old patients.
- GPs see on average 10 cases annually.
- One patient in every five seen needs hospital admission.
- Most cases occur in the winter months.
- Mycoplasma infection occurs in 4-yearly epidemics and affects mainly teenagers and young adults.
- 50% of legionella infections are acquired abroad, especially in Mediterranean countries.
- Legionella infection may occur in epidemics related to water systems in buildings.
- Psittacosis is often acquired from birds, especially parrots.
- Q fever is usually acquired from sheep.

Classification
Community-acquired pneumonia.

Nosocomial pneumonia: e.g. after cerebrovascular accident or major surgery.

Aspiration pneumonia: caused by inhalation of oropharyngeal secretions, during vomiting, or when consciousness is depressed, e.g. during epileptic fit.

Immunocompromised pneumonia: e.g. with HIV infection, organ transplantation, cytotoxic chemotherapy.

Treatment

Diet and lifestyle
- Smoking and smoking-related diseases are the main risk factor for pneumonia; smoking education is therefore important.

Pharmacological treatment

General guidelines
Oxygen: to maintain partial oxygen pressure in arterial blood >8 kPa (60 mmHg); may cause hypercapnia in patients with chronic obstructive pulmonary disease, so arterial blood gases should be monitored.

Oral or parenteral fluids: to correct dehydration.

Non-sedative analgesia: for pleuritic chest pain.

Physiotherapy: only if large sputum volumes are difficult to expectorate.

Intensive care, including assisted ventilation: valuable for patients in whom respiratory failure worsens despite treatment.

Antibiotics
- Initial treatment must be empirical; this can be modified later if indicated by microbiological results.
- Oral antibiotics are appropriate in mild infection, parenteral if infection is severe or accompanied by vomiting.
- Treatment should be for at least 5 days; severely ill patients need treatment for up to 3 weeks.

For mild community-acquired disease: aminopenicillin (e.g. amoxycillin) or erythromycin.

For severe community-acquired disease: 2nd- or 3rd-generation cephalosporin (e.g. cefuroxime), possibly with erythromycin.

For nosocomial infection: 2nd- or 3rd generation cephalosporin, possibly with aminoglycoside.

For aspiration: aminopenicillin with metronidazole.

For immunocompromised disease: individually determined by causative pathogen.

Standard dosage	Amoxycillin 500 mg 3 times daily.
	Erythromycin 500 mg 4 times daily.
	Cefuroxime 750 mg 3 times daily.
	Aminoglycoside guided by blood level.
	Metronidazole 400 mg 3 times daily.
Contraindications	Hypersensitivity.
Main drug interactions	Warfarin.
Main side effects	Phlebitis diarrhoea.

Prophylaxis
Annual influenza vaccination: for patients with chronic heart or lung disease, renal failure, or diabetes mellitus and for immunosuppressed patients.

Pneumococcal vaccination: for patients who are asplenic or have sickle cell disease, chronic renal failure, or chronic lung, heart, or liver disease, and those with diabetes mellitus or who are immunocompromised.

Treatment aims
To improve oxygenation.
To achieve rapid resolution of pneumonia and return to normal activities.
To prevent death.
To relieve symptoms.

Prognosis
- Pyrexia usually settles within 48 h of starting treatment.
- Lethargy after pneumonia often lasts weeks or months.
- Radiographic shadowing is slow to clear and lags behind clinical recovery.
- Death is unusual in patients managed at home.
- 5–10% of patients admitted to hospital die.
- Up to 50% reaching intensive care die.
- The mortality in nosocomial pneumonia is up to 30% and may be higher in immunocompromised patients.

Follow-up and management
- Patients should be seen 6 weeks after presentation, and chest radiography repeated to confirm recovery and exclude underlying lung disease, especially lung cancer.

Key references
British Thoracic Society: Guidelines for the management of community acquired pneumonia in adults admitted to hospital. *Br J Hosp Med* 1993, **49**:346–350.

Hopkin JM: Respiratory disease in the immunocompromised host: non-AIDS. In *Respiratory Medicine*. Edited by Brewis RAL, Gibson GJ, Geddes DM. London: Baillière Tindall, 1990.

Macfarlane JT et al.: Prospective study of aetiology and outcome of adult lower-respiratory-tract infections in the community. *Lancet* 1993, **341**:511–514.

Woodhead MA: Management of pneumonia. *Respir Med* 1992, **86**:459–469.

Sarcoidosis
M.A. Spiteri and K.T. Khoo

Diagnosis

Symptoms
- Patients may have no respiratory symptoms.

Dyspnoea: on exertion.
Cough: usually unproductive.
Chest discomfort: vague intermittent ache.
Fatigue, malaise, weight loss, fever.
Symptoms of the complications of sarcoidosis.

Signs
Fine inspiratory crackles and wheezes: rarely.
Lymphadenopathy.
Uveitis, keratoconjunctivitis sicca, retinopathy.
Erythema nodosum, skin nodules, maculopapular rash, lupus pernio.
Nasopharyngitis.
Hepatomegaly, splenomegaly, portal hypertension.
Bone cysts, polyarthralgia, myopathy.

Investigations
Chest radiography: 90% of patients have abnormal radiographs, which show a wide variety of appearances (*see* Clinical staging).
Pulmonary function tests: may be entirely within normal limits, despite extensive radiographic shadows, or may show significant physiological dysfunction with clear radiographical lung fields.
Tuberculin skin text: negative in two-thirds of patients, despite previous bacille Calmette–Guérin immunization.
Blood tests: leucocyte count may show lymphopenia; ESR may be raised; serum immunoglobulins and electrophoresis may show panhyperglobulinaemia; serum angiotensin-converting enzyme increased in two-thirds of acute patients; hypercalcaemia in ~18% of patients; liver function indices in a few may show intrahepatic cholestasis.
24-h urine collection: hypercalciuria may be present despite normal serum calcium concentration.
ECG: arrhythmias, bundle branch block pattern in some patients.
Biopsy of lymph node, lung tissue, skin, liver, or other tissue: shows non-caseating epithelioid granulomata.
Kveim–Siltzbach test: may be helpful when other histological material unavailable.
Bronchoalveolar lavage: may be helpful adjunct to diagnosis; many patients with 'active' sarcoidosis show increased percentage of lymphocytes, predominantly of the 'helper' T-cell type; as fibrosis develops, an increase in neutrophils occurs.
- Special situations may call for the following: ^{67}Ga scans (often positive in sarcoidosis); radioactive ^{201}Tl (taken by sarcoid tissue and by ischaemic myocardium); high resolution CT scan (with MRI, may be particularly useful in unusual or difficult diagnostic circumstances such as neurosarcoidosis); ophthalmological assessment, including slit lamp examination and fluorescein angiography (needed in patients with associated occular symptoms).

Complications
Peripheral neuropathy, facial-nerve palsy, other cranial-nerve palsies, papilloedema, meningitis, space-occupying lesions, epilepsy, cerebellar ataxia, hypopituitarism, diabetes insipidus.
Bundle branch block, arrhythmias, congestive cardiac failure, pericarditis, cardiomyopathy, cor pulmonale.
Disordered calcium metabolism, hypercalcaemia, hypercalciuria, nephrocalcinosis.
Enlarged parotid and lacrimal glands.
Glaucoma, cataract: complication of chronic uveitis.

Differential diagnosis

Hilar lymphadenopathy
Tuberculosis, Hodgkin's lymphoma, infectious mononucleosis, leukaemia, metastases, enlarged pulmonary arteries.

Hilar lymphadenopathy with pulmonary infiltration
Tuberculosis, pneumoconiosis, lymphangitic carcinoma, idiopathic haemosiderosis, pulmonary eosinophilia, alveolar-cell carcinoma, histiocytosis X.

Diffuse pulmonary infiltration
The above and also chronic beryllium disease, honeycomb lung, rheumatoid lung, fibrosing alveolitis, Sjögren's syndrome, extrinsic allergic alveolitis.

Non-caseating granulomata
Tuberculosis and other mycobacterial infections, fungal infections, leprosy, syphillis, cat-scratch disease, berylliosis, hypersensitivity pneumonitis or extrinsic allergic alveolitis, foreign-body reactions, lymphoma, carcinoma, biliary cirrhosis, Crohn's disease, hypogammaglobulinaemia, granulomatous vasculitides, parasitic infection.

Aetiology
- The cause is unknown, but the following may have a role:
Transmittable agents.
An atypical reaction to tuberculosis or other mycobacteria.
Genetic predisposition.

Epidemiology
- Sarcoidosis is usually manifest in the 20–40-year age group.
- It is more usual in temperate than in tropical climates.
- The prevalence rates are difficult to establish because the disease is often asymptomatic; in the UK, the incidence is 10–20 in 100 000 population; the frequency in Ireland is higher.
- Sarcoidosis is more prevalent and tends to be more chronic in blacks, who have higher risk of nonrespiratory manifestations.

Clinical staging
Stage 0: normal chest (5–10% of patients).
Stage I: bilateral hilar adenopathy (50%).
Stage II: bilateral hilar adenopathy and peripheral pulmonary infiltration; paratracheal nodes may also be enlarged (25%).
Stage III: parenchymal infiltration only (15%).

Treatment

Diet and lifestyle
- No special precautions are necessary.

Pharmacological treatment
- Treatment is not needed in many patients because the disability is mild and remission is usual.

Corticosteroids
- These can suppress the manifestations of acute sarcoidosis, with rapid clearing of radiographic lesions; whether they alter the long-term outcome or prevent development of late fibrosis if started early remains unproven.

Standard dosage	Prednisolone 30 mg daily for 4 weeks; reduced by 5 mg every month to 15 mg daily if patient improves; reduced by 2.5 mg every 1–2 months to 10 mg daily if patient stable; reduced gradually, aiming to stop after completing 12 months of continuous treatment, if sarcoid activity in remission.
Contraindications	Uncontrolled hypertension, diabetes mellitus, infection, severe osteoporosis.
Special points	Relapses treated by increased dose; some patients with objective evidence of relapse on >3 occasions may need long-term low-dose maintenance prednisolone.
Main drug interactions	Antihypertensive drugs.
Main side effects	Weight gain, oedema, bruising, purple striae in skin (particularly abdomen), moon face, osteoporosis, collapse of vertebrae, diabetes mellitus, hypertension, myopathy (especially proximal girdle muscles), hirsutism, menstrual disturbances, psychotic reactions, cataracts, withdrawal phenomena.

Immunosuppressants
- Treatment should be given under specialist supervision.
- Chloroquine can control some cases of chronic fibrotic sarcoidosis involving lungs and skin; it is especially helpful in the management of lupus pernio and pulmonary fibrosis.
- Methotrexate can be helpful in the treatment of chronic skin lesions, e.g. lupus pernio.

Standard dosage	Chloroquine 200 mg on alternate days for up to 9 months. Methotrexate 10 mg once weekly for 3 months; repeated courses every 6 months, possibly with oral steroids or chloroquine, may be necessary in some patients.
Contraindications	Hepatic and renal impairment.
Special points	Chloroquine usually given with low-dose steroids.
Main drug interactions	Alcohol, NSAIDs, antacids.
Main side effects	*Chloroquine:* visual disturbances, irreversible retinal damage, corneal opacities. *Methotrexate:* hepatic fibrosis, acute bone-marrow suppression.

NSAIDs
- Anti-inflammatory agents are usually used in acute 'exudative' sarcoidosis, e.g. in patients with acute uveitis, phlyctenular conjunctivitis, polyarthritis, and erythema nodosum.

Standard dosage	Indomethacin 50–200 mg daily in divided doses, with food.
Contraindications	Active peptic ulceration, severe renal, cardiac, and hepatic failure.
Main drug interactions	Angiotensin-converting enzyme inhibitors, anticoagulants, antidiabetics, antidepressants, 4-quinolones.
Main side effects	Gastrointestinal disturbances, ulceration, and bleeding, blood disorders (thrombocytopenia), headache, dizziness.

Treatment aims
To prevent development of irreversible pulmonary fibrosis.

Prognosis
- 70% of patients remit spontaneously.
- Accompanying hilar adenopathy usually regresses within ~1 year.
- ~10% of patients develop parenchymal lesions, of which many resolve within 1 year.
- ~40% of patients resolve spontaneously within 1 year; the rest may progress with varying speed to irreversible fibrosis, which, in severely ill patients, may be complicated by upper-zone bullous disease and aspergillomas, with recurrent infection and haemoptysis.

Follow-up and management
- Regular clinical review is needed for patients being treated by steroids or immunosuppressants.

Key references
Mitchell IC, Turk JL, Mitchell DN: Detection of mycobacterial rRNA in sarcoidosis with liquid-phase hybridisation. *Lancet* 1992, **339**:1015–1017.

Nakata K *et al.*: Gamma-delta T-cells in sarcoidosis. Correlation with clinical features. *Am J Respir Crit Care Med* 1994, **149**:981–988.

Panel of the World Association of Sarcoidosis and other Granulomatous Diseases: Consensus Conference: activity of sarcoidosis. *Eur Respir J* 1994, **7**:624–627.

Spiteri MA, Clarke SW, Poulter LW: Alveolar macrophages that suppress T-cell responsiveness may be crucial to pathogenic

Sleep apnoea, central, hypoventilation, periodic breathing — R.J.O. Davies

Diagnosis

Definition
- Central sleep apnoea is a clinical syndrome with a range of causes, which can be loosely divided into two groups:

Neuromuscular weakness or chest-wall disease: the primary problem is inefficiency of the respiratory pump; patients may develop daytime ventilatory failure.

Periodic respiration (Cheyne–Stokes breathing): the primary problem is disordered respiratory feedback control; patients do not develop daytime ventilatory failure.

Symptoms
Daytime sleepiness, restless sleep, transient breathlessness: during the arousal and tachypnoea that follow an apnoea; symptoms of sleep disturbance.

Morning headache and nausea, poor exercise tolerance, ankle swelling, daytime breathlessness: only with neuromuscular or chest-wall disease; symptoms of respiratory failure.

Symptoms of primary causative disease.

Signs
Cyanosis, peripheral oedema, raised venous pressure, signs of pulmonary hypertension or right ventricular hypertrophy: signs of ventilatory failure and cor pulmonale.

Raised venous pressure and oedema: signs of heart failure.

Muscle fasciculation, weakness, loss of tendon reflex: signs of myopathy, dystrophy, motor neurone disease, post-poliomyelitis syndrome.

Supine breathlessness and paradoxical abdominal movement on sniffing: signs of diaphragm weakness due to bilateral phrenic palsy, acid maltase deficiency, or other muscular disease.

Upper motor neurone and brainstem signs: signs of stroke.

Chest-wall deformity: signs of scoliosis, thoracoplasty.

Investigations

Initial
Awake arterial oxygen saturation and blood gas analysis: for possible hypercapnia; alveolar–arterial oxygen gradient often normal.

Spirometry: to exclude chronic obstructive airway disease and assess lung volume; daytime ventilatory failure with central sleep apnoea rare if vital capacity >1.5 L standing; supine fall in forced vital capacity of >20% suggests marked diaphragm weakness.

Haemoglobin analysis: for polycythaemia.

Nerve physiology, muscle biopsy, ECG, echocardiography: can also be considered.

Sleep studies
- These are used to exclude obstructive sleep apnoea, show characteristic apnoeas without continuing respiratory effort, show worsening hypoventilation during rapid eye movement sleep, and quantify the severity of the abnormality present.
- Interpretation can be difficult because some patients with apnoea due to pharyngeal collapse make little respiratory effort and some patients with a primary failure of respiratory drive have secondary airway collapse.

Complications
Ventilatory failure, cor pulmonale, pneumonia: in patients with neuromuscular or chest-wall disease.

Accidents: particularly motor accidents, due to poor daytime vigilance.

Differential diagnosis

Daytime sleepiness
Obstructive sleep apnoea.
Narcolepsy.
Idiopathic hypersomnolence.
Periodic movements of legs during sleep.
Inadequate sleep.

Respiratory failure
Chronic obstructive lung disease.
Obstructive sleep apnoea.

Aetiology

Neuromuscular or chest-wall disease
- Patients just able to sustain normal ventilation while awake hypoventilate as respiratory drive falls at onset of sleep.
- This worsens further with the muscle atonia of rapid eye movement sleep.
- How this contributes to the daytime ventilatory failure is not clear.
- The sleeping hypoxaemia probably accelerates blunting of ventilatory drive, which allows further daytime ventilatory deterioration.
- Thoracic wall stiffness and respiratory muscle fatigue are probably also important.

Periodic respiration
- This develops when the feedback loop controlling respiration has an excessive feedback gain or delay.
- Contributing factors include excessive central drive levels (CNS disease), circulatory delay (heart failure), hypoxaemia, hypocapnia, and arousal from sleep (high altitude).

Epidemiology
- Neuromuscular causes of central sleep apnoea are unusual.
- Sleeping periodic respiration affects >50% of patients with severe chronic heart failure and >20% of inpatients with neurological disease.

Treatment

Diet and lifestyle
- Changing diet and lifestyle do not alter central sleep apnoea.
- Patients should not smoke: concurrent lung disease worsens respiratory failure.

Pharmacological treatment

For neuromuscular or chest-wall disease
- The mainstay of treatment for these conditions is nocturnal ventilatory support.
- Tricyclic antidepressants have a small role in controlling nocturnal hypoxaemia (thus ameliorating respiratory failure) by decreasing the amount of rapid eye movement sleep.

Standard dosage	Protryptiline 10–20 mg orally at night.
Contraindications	Cardiac disease, epilepsy, mania, liver disease, glaucoma.
Main drug interactions	Alcohol, monoamine oxidase inhibitors, antihistamines, anticonvulsants.
Main side effects	Anticholinergic effects, arrhythmias, impotence, urinary retention.

For periodic respiration
- Many patients with periodic respiration are asymptomatic and need no treatment; treatment of symptomatic periodic respiration remains experimental.
- Underlying heart failure should be controlled.
- Oxygen, low-dose carbon dioxide, positive airway pressure, or acetazolamide may have a role.

Non-pharmacological treatment

Nocturnal ventilatory support
- This is indicated for patients with central sleep apnoea, daytime ventilatory failure and an otherwise good quality of life.
- It improves daytime symptoms, respiratory failure, and cor pulmonale, thereby improving prognosis.
- Techniques include nasal positive pressure ventilation, the rocking bed, tank and cuirass ventilators.

Advantages: corrects sleep disruption, daytime sleepiness, and respiratory failure.

Disadvantages: need for specialist care to acclimatize patient to ventilator and for follow-up.

Causes of treatment failure: ventilator or mask failure due to mechanical failure or air leaks, poor compliance due to mouth air leak, nasal obstruction, claustrophobia, inadequate patient education, or poor mask fit, upper airway collapse secondary to extrathoracic negative-pressure (tank or cuirass) ventilation, incorrect diagnosis (respiratory failure due to obstructive lung disease).

Improvements in awake arterial blood gases in seven patients with neuromuscular or chest-wall disease and ventilatory failure after nocturnal ventilatory support.

Oxygen
- Overnight oxygen (24–28%) may improve symptoms of patients in whom ventilatory support is not appropriate; it has not been shown to improve prognosis in this group and may worsen daytime ventilatory failure.

Treatment aims

Neuromuscular or chest-wall disease
To improve symptoms and quality of life.
To correct respiratory failure and cor pulmonale.
To improve mortality and morbidity.

Periodic respiration
To improve sleep disturbance symptoms.

Prognosis

Neuromuscular or chest-wall disease
- Untreated patients with significant daytime respiratory failure and central sleep apnoea have a limited life expectancy (usually only a few months).
- With successful nocturnal ventilatory support, the prognosis approaches that of the underlying condition.

Periodic respiration
- Cheyne–Stokes breathing is not now thought to predict mortality independently of the severity of the underlying disease.

Follow-up and management
- Patients with neuromuscular or chest-wall disease and an otherwise good prognosis, but not in daytime ventilatory failure, need review so that overnight ventilation can be started with onset of daytime hypercapnia.
- Patients on domiciliary nocturnal ventilation need long-term support.

Patient support
The Sleep Apnoea Trust, Warwick Lodge, Piddington Lane, Piddington, High Wycombe, HP14 3BD, tel 01494 881369.

Driving regulations
- The licensing authority must be notified.
- In the UK currently, the general guideline is that driving ability with excessive daytime sleepiness depends on the success of and degree of compliance with treatment.

Key references
Hill NS: Noninvasive ventilation. *Am Rev Respir Dis* 1993, **147**:1050–1055.

Khoo MCK, Gottschalk A, Pack AI: Sleep-induced periodic breathing and apnea: a theoretical study. *J Appl Physiol* 1991, **70**:2014–2024.

Kryger MH: Sleep and heart failure. *Eur Respir J* 1990, **3**:1103–1104.

Sleep apnoea, obstructive — R.J.O. Davies

Diagnosis

Definition
- Obstructive sleep apnoea is a recurrent obstruction to breathing due to upper-airway narrowing or collapse during sleep.

Symptoms
- Symptoms are often manifest for several years before diagnosis.

Daytime sleepiness, snoring, restless sleep: usual adult presentation, often with history of witnessed apnoeas from partner.

Nocturnal choking or panic attacks, irritability, nocturia, enuresis, impotence, cognitive dysfunction, memory loss, social disharmony, emotional disturbances: less common.

Behavioural disturbance, failure to thrive: nonspecific features in children, in addition to adult symptoms.

Signs
Obesity: particularly neck; characteristic but not invariable.
Small crowded pharynx with mucosal oedema.
Retrognathia.
Tonsil hypertrophy: usual cause of obstructive sleep apnoea in children.
Nasal obstruction.
Respiratory failure or cor pulmonale: in 10% of patients.
Features of hypothyroidism or acromegaly: rare.

Investigations

Initial
Awake arterial oxygen saturation or blood gas analysis, spirometry, haemoglobin analysis: for ventilatory failure (arterial oxygen and blood gases), obstructive airways disease (spirometry), and polycythaemia (haemoglobin).

Thyroid or growth hormone estimations: can be considered.

Sleep studies
- Sleep studies are needed to establish the diagnosis by showing upper-airway obstruction with continuing respiratory efforts; no ideal combination of physiological signals exists, but markers of respiratory effort, apnoea, and sleep disturbances are all needed.

Polysomnography: gold standard; includes EEG sleep staging, oronasal airflow assessment, and measurement of thoracoabdominal movement or oesophageal pressure; accurately identifies obstructive apnoeas but time-consuming and expensive and disturbs patient's sleep.

Limited sleep studies: common in UK; usually include pulse oximetry and video recording to assess respiratory disturbance and an alternative to EEG as marker of arousal (e.g. movement, heart rate, blood pressure); limited studies often adequate but need subjective interpretation and depend on experience of interpreter.

Complications
Respiratory failure, cor pulmonale: usually in patients with peripheral airways obstruction (often mild).
Accidents: particularly motor accidents, due to poor daytime vigilance.
Cardiovascular disease: increased vascular mortality (improves with effective treatment).

Differential diagnosis

Daytime sleepiness
Narcolepsy.
Idiopathic hypersomnolence.
Central sleep apnoea.
Periodic breathing.
Periodic movements of legs during sleep.
Inadequate sleep.

Respiratory failure
Chronic obstructive pulmonary disease.
Neuromuscular weakness.
Scoliosis.

Aetiology
- Causes include the following:

Pharyngeal narrowing due to obesity, endopharyngeal masses (including tonsils), retrognathia, micrognathia, hypothyroidism, acromegaly.

Reduced pharyngeal muscle activity due to alcohol, sedative drugs, neuromuscular disorders.

Nasal obstruction.

Epidemiology
- The peak age of presentation is 40–60 years.
- The male:female ratio is 10:1.
- 3 in 1000 randomly selected UK men have severe obstructive sleep apnoea.
- The sleep apnoea/hypopnoea syndrome may affect 4% of men and 2% of women.

Variants of obstructive sleep apnoea
Simple snoring: in 20% of men.
Snoring with arousals from sleep: severe sleep fragmentation and daytime sleepiness after heavy snoring without apnoeas or hypoxaemia.
Obstructive sleep hypopnoea: airflow does not entirely cease.
Central variant: patients do not make efforts to breathe during the apnoeas, particularly while lying supine; snoring or typical obstructive sleep apnoea usually occurs in other postures.
Laryngeal sleep apnoea: sleeping stridor due to laryngeal disease or denervation or Shy–Drager syndrome.

Treatment

Diet and lifestyle
- Weight loss can correct obstructive sleep apnoea, but most patients also need other treatment.
- Reduced alcohol intake helps simple snoring and mild obstructive sleep apnoea.
- Obstructive sleep apnoea only present supine is improved by avoiding this posture.

Pharmacological treatment
- Drug treatment is secondary to continuous airways pressure.

Nasal steroids and decongestants
- These reduce simple snoring but have little effect on obstructive sleep apnoea; they may be needed during continuous positive airways pressure therapy.

Standard dosage	Beclomethasone 100–200 mg, budesonide 100–200 mg, or ipratropium bromide 40–80 mg, all twice daily in both nostrils.
Contraindications	*Ipratropium:* caution in glaucoma.
Special points	Vasoconstrictor decongestants worsen nasal obstruction with sustained use and should be avoided.
Main drug interactions	None.
Main side effects	Nasal dryness.

Tricyclic antidepressants
- Antidepressants have a minor role in mild obstructive sleep apnoea by suppressing rapid eye-movement sleep, when sleep apnoea often worsens

Standard dosage	Protriptyline 10–20 mg orally at night.
Contraindications	Cardiac disease, epilepsy, mania, liver disease, glaucoma.
Main drug interactions	Alcohol, monoamine oxidase inhibitors, antihistamines, anticonvulsants.
Main side effects	Anticholinergic effects, arrhythmias, impotence, urinary retention.

Non-pharmacological treatment

Continuous positive airways pressure
- This is the main treatment in most patients with substantial daytime sleepiness.

Advantages: dramatic correction of sleep disruption, daytime sleepiness, snoring, and apnoeas.

Disadvantages: unsightly, mask may be claustrophobic or cause nasal ulceration if badly fitted.

Causes of treatment failure: machine or mask failure; poor compliance due to nasal obstruction, claustrophobia, inadequate patient education, poor mask fit (air leaks or nasal ulceration), mouth air leak; incorrect diagnosis (central sleep apnoea, narcolepsy, respiratory failure from another cause).

Surgery
- Surgery is indicated for patients with the following:

Structural nasal obstruction (e.g. polyps, deviated septum).
Tonsil hypertrophy.
Facial maldevelopment.
Severe obstructive sleep apnoea with continuous positive airways pressure failure.
- Tracheostomy is rarely indicated.
- Soft-palette resection is not consistently curative and is not currently recommended.

Treatment aims
To relieve symptoms.
To correct respiratory failure.
To reduce excess vascular mortality.

Prognosis
- After effective treatment, patients are symptom-free and have a similar prognosis to weight-matched controls.
- Few patients reduce their weight sufficiently to stop continuous positive airways pressure treatment.

Follow-up and management
- Patients on continuous positive airways pressure treatment need review including maintenance of their equipment, replacement of masks and consideration of reducing their airway pressure or stopping treatment after weight loss.

Patient support
The Sleep Apnoea Trust, Warwick Lodge, Piddington Lane, Piddington, High Wycombe, Bucks HP14 3BD, tel 01494 881 369.

Driving regulations
- The licensing authority must be notified.
- In the UK currently, the general guideline is that driving ability with excessive daytime sleepiness depends on the success of and degree of compliance with treatment.

Key references
Davies RJO, Stradling JR: The acute effects of obstructive sleep apnoea. *Br J Anaesth* 1993, **71**:725–729.

Douglas NJ, Thomas S, Jan MA: Clinical value of polysomnography. *Lancet* 1992, **339**:347–350.

Findley LJ, Weiss J, Jabour EP: Drivers with untreated sleep apnoea. *Arch Intern Med* 1991, **151**:1451–1452.

McNamara SG, Grunstein RR, Sullivan CE: Obstructive sleep apnoea. *Thorax* 1993, **48**:754–764.

Polo O et al.: Management of obstructive sleep apnoea/hypopnoea syndrome. *Lancet* 1994, **344**:.656–660.

Tuberculosis, pulmonary — I. Pavord and J.T. Macfarlane

Diagnosis

Symptoms

Primary infection

- 90% of patients have no symptoms; the following are seen rarely:

Malaise, fever, erythema nodosum, phlyctenular conjunctivitis.

Post-primary infection

- Often no symptoms are seen.

Malaise, weight loss, fever, night sweats.

Cough, mucoid or mucopurulent sputum, haemoptysis, dyspnoea, dull chest ache, pleuritic chest pain.

Enlarged neck glands.

Haematuria, infertility.

Abdominal pain, chronic diarrhoea, weight loss.

Meningism.

Progressive back pain, paraspinal swelling, swollen joints.

Malaise, weight loss, fever, meningism: symptoms of miliary tuberculosis; may be nonspecific, particularly in elderly patients.

Signs

- Physical examination is often unhelpful.

Evidence of weight loss, pyrexia, erythema nodosum: in primary infection.

Signs of pulmonary collapse, consolidation, or effusion, crackles (upper zones, increased after coughing), amphoric breath sounds over a large cavity.

Lymphadenopathy, palpable kidney, right iliac fossa mass, swollen joint, meningism.

Hepatosplenomegaly, choroid tubercles, meningism: signs of miliary tuberculosis.

Investigations

Chest radiography:

Primary: normal in 70% of patients; more often abnormal in children <5 years; typically shows unilateral hilar lymphadenopathy; bronchial compression can produce segmental or lobar collapse or hyperinflation, particularly in lower, lingula, and middle lobes; ulceration into bronchial tree, producing distal patchy consolidation, or into pleura, producing effusion.

Post-primary: classically shows bilateral upper-zone consolidation progressing to cavitation, fibrosis, and upper-lobe contraction; chronic tuberculosis lesions often calcified.

Tuberculin testing: positive test implies current or past infection or previous bacille Calmette–Guérin vaccination; positivity increases with age in UK; useful in identifying primary disease in younger patients; strongly positive response (e.g. heaf grade 3 or 4) with previous vaccination suggests previous primary infection.

Bacteriology: samples stained (fluorescent auramine or Ziehl–Neelsen) and cultured (e.g. in Lowenstein–Jensen medium); useful in establishing diagnosis in post-primary disease and in guiding management; sputum smear often positive in cavitating disease; examination of two good early-morning sputa allows identification of 90% of smear-positive cases; smear-positive sputum implies significant risk of infection; culture and sensitivity testing takes 4–8 weeks.

Complications

Lobar or segmental collapse or consolidation, pleural effusion, pericardial involvement, tuberculoma formation: in primary tuberculosis.

Post-primary or miliary tuberculosis, later infection at distant sites: caused by blood dissemination at time of primary infection.

Differential diagnosis

- Radiographic and some clinical features can be mimicked by the following:

Lung cancer.

Sarcoidosis.

Some bacterial pneumonias.

Allergic bronchopulmonary aspergillosis.

Pneumoconiosis.

Actinomycosis.

Aetiology

- Causes include the following:

General disease

Inhalation of *Mycobacterium tuberculosis* either from the cough of a patient with sputum-positive disease or from infected droplets in a microbiology laboratory.

Post-primary disease

Reactivation of dormant *M. tuberculosis* disseminated at the time of primary infection; risk increased in patients with diseases causing depressed immunity (e.g. malnutrition, alcoholism, diabetes, AIDS).

Epidemiology

- The estimated annual incidence in the UK in 1983 was 12.2 in 100 000 people.
- The annual incidence in Indian, Pakistani, and Bangladeshi ethnic groups is ~170 in 100 000.
- Recently, the overall incidence has increased slightly.

Atypical tuberculosis

- The frequency of atypical tuberculosis is increasing in elderly men with pre-existing lung disease.
- It is mostly caused by *Mycobacterium kansasaii, malmoense, xenopi, avium,* or *avium intracellulare* (*M. avium intracellulare* particularly in later stages of AIDS).
- Presentation is similar to that of *M. tuberculosis* infection: 10–40% of patients may be asymptomatic.
- Management is complicated, involving prolonged multidrug treatment, including rifampicin and ethambutol; expert advice is needed.

Tuberculosis, pulmonary

Treatment

Diet and lifestyle
- Smoking must be stopped, and nutrition improved.

Pharmacological treatment
- Treatment must be supervised by a physician experienced in all aspects of tuberculosis management.
- Patients must be educated about the disease and the importance of prolonged treatment.
- Sputum-positive patients must be advised that they remain infectious for the first 2 weeks of treatment.

Standard 6-month unsupervised regimen

Standard dosage	Isoniazid 300 mg daily (child, 10 mg/kg daily; maximum, 300 mg) for 6 months, rifampicin 450–600 mg daily (child, 10 mg/kg daily) for 6 months, and pyrazinamide 1.5–2 g daily (child, 35 mg/kg daily) for 2 months.
Contraindications	*All:* previous severe adverse event. *Isoniazid:* drug-induced liver disease, porphyria; caution in liver or renal disease. *Rifampicin:* jaundice, porphyria; caution in liver disease. *Pyrazinamide:* liver disease, porphyria; caution in renal impairment, gout, or diabetes.
Special points	*Isoniazid:* isoniazid-resistant *Mycobacterium tuberculosis* present in 4–6% of patients. *Rifampicin:* colours urine and tears orange; may stain soft contact lenses.
Main drug interactions	*Isoniazid:* binds to pyridoxine and may produce deficiency; inhibits phenytoin metabolism. *Rifampicin:* hepatic enzyme induction increases metabolism and reduces effect of anticonvulsants, oral contraceptive pill, steroids, and digoxin. *Pyrazinamide:* interferes with renal testing for ketones; reduces renal excretion of uric acid.
Main side effects	*Isoniazid:* gastrointestinal intolerance, exacerbation of acne, hepatotoxicity (in 1–2% of patients; can be severe), peripheral neuropathy (in 2%; prevented by pyridoxine supplements 10 mg daily). *Rifampicin:* nausea, abnormal liver function tests (usually mild and reversible), influenza-like reaction. *Pyrazinamide:* hepatotoxicity, arthralgia, precipitation of gout, urticaria.

- Ethambutol should be considered if resistance is suspected.
- Longer periods are needed for meningitis and with extensive disease.
- Pyridoxine 10 mg daily may be added when deficiency is a possibility.

Supervised regimen
Isoniazid 15 mg/kg 3 times weekly (adult and child) for 6 months.
Rifampicin 600–900 mg (child, 15 mg/kg) 3 times weekly for 6 months.
Pyrazinamide 2–2.5 g (child, 50 mg/kg) 3 times weekly for 2 months.

Other drugs
Corticosteroids: improve outcome in pericarditis and meningitis; of value in patients with severe infection, persistent pyrexia, or weight loss; higher doses needed if rifampicin used.

Streptomycin, capreomycin, cycloserine, ethionamide for multiresistant or atypical infection: specialist advice must be sought.

Treatment aims
To achieve bacteriological and clinical cure.
To prevent resistance (with combination treatment).
To prevent or treat disease in contacts.

Prognosis
- ~6% of adults with pulmonary tuberculosis die of it before finishing chemotherapy.
- Only ~3% relapse if the full course of chemotherapy is taken; the rate is higher if compliance is poor.

Follow-up and management
- Close supervision is necessary throughout chemotherapy.
- Compliance must be checked; urine must be checked for rifampicin.
- The patient must be checked for adverse effects.
- Response must be assessed: symptoms, weight gain, radiographic changes.

Prevention
- Notification of new cases to the district consultant for communicable disease control is a legal requirement.
- Care is needed in people with close contact with sputum-positive disease: 10% develop tuberculosis, mostly identified by initial tuberculin testing or chest radiography.
- Bacille Calmette–Guérin vaccination has a protective efficacy of ~70%.

Key references
Joint Tuberculosis Committee of the British Thoracic Society: Chemotherapy and management of tuberculosis in the United Kingdom. *Thorax* 1990, 45:403–408.

Subcommittee of the Joint Tuberculosis Committee of the British Thoracic Society: Control and prevention of tuberculosis in Britain: an updated code of practice. *BMJ* 1990, 300:995–999.

Index

A

abscess
   lung 16, 20
   subphrenic 18
acetazolamide for periodic respiration 25
acetylcysteine for cystic fibrosis 9
acromegaly 26
actinomycosis 28
adult respiratory distress syndrome 2-3, 20
airway disease, chronic obstructive 10
airway obstruction
   fixed 4
   irreversible 4
airways hyper-responsive test 4
airways pressure, continuous positive, for obstructive sleep apnoea 27
allergic alveolitis, extrinsic 12, 22
alpha-1 antitrypsin deficiency 10
alveolar cell carcinoma 22
alveolitis
   extrinsic allergic 12, 22
   fibrosing 8, 12-13, 22
aminoglycosides for pneumonia 21
aminophylline, intravenous, for asthma 5
amiodarone 12
amoxycillin for pneumonia 21
amyloidosis 8
analgesics for pneumonia 21
ANCA 14
antibiotics for bronchiectasis 9
   antibodies, antineutrophil cytoplasmic 14
anticholinergic drugs for chronic obstructive airway disease 11
antidepressants for sleep apnoea
   central 25
   obstructive 27
antidiuretic hormone secretion, inappropriate 16
antineutrophil cytoplasmic antibodies 14
antitrypsin deficiency, alpha-1 10
apnoea, sleep
   central 24, 26
   obstructive 24, 26
arrhythmia 22
arterial blood gas analysis 4
arthritis, rheumatoid 12, 18
arthropathy 8
Aspergillus infections, bronchopulmonary 14

asthma 4-5, 8, 10
   occupational 6-7
atrophy syndrome, post-poliomyelitis muscular 24
azoospermia 8

B

bacterial endocarditis, subacute 14
Bacteroides 20
beclomethasone
   for asthma 5
   for chronic obstructive airway disease 11
   for obstructive sleep apnoea 27
   for occupational asthma 7
berylliosis 12, 22
beryllium disease
   chronic 22
beta-2 agonists
   for asthma 5
   for chronic obstructive airway disease 11
biopsy, lung 12
bleomycin for chemical pleuradhesis 19
brain metastases 16
breathing
   Cheyne-Stokes 24
   periodic 24, 26
breathlessness 4, 6, 18
bronchiectasis 8-9
bronchitis 4
   acute, chronic 4
   exacerbation 20
bronchoalveolar lavage 12
bronchocentric granulomatosis 14
bronchodilators
   for asthma 5
   for bronchiectasis 9
   for occupational asthma 7
bronchopulmonary aspergillosis 14
   allergic 28
budesonide for obstructive sleep apnoea 27
bundle branch block 22

C

cancer, lung 12, 16, 21, 28
carbon dioxide for periodic respiration 25
carcinoma 18, 22
   alveolar cell 22
cardiac failure
   congestive 22
   right 12
cardiomyopathy 22

cardiovascular disease 26
cat-scratch disease 22
cataract 22
cefuroxime for pneumonia 21
central sleep apnoea 24, 24-25, 26
cephalosporins for pneumonia 21
cerebellar
   ataxia 22
   degeneration 16
chest
   pain 18
      pleuritic 8, 20
   tightness 4
Cheyne-Stokes, breathing 24
chloroquine for sarcoidosis 23
choking, nocturnal 26
cholelithiasis 8
chronic obstructive airway disease 10-11
chronic obstructive lung disease 24, 26
Churg-Strauss syndrome 14
cirrhosis 18, 22
   biliary 8
clubbing 12, 16
COAD see chronic obstructive airway disease
collagen, vascular 14
collapse
   lobar 16, 28
   lung 16
   segmental 28
computed tomography *see* CT
congestive
   atelectasis *see* adult respiratory distress syndrome
   cardiac failure 22
constrictive pleural fibrosis 18
continuous positive airways pressure for obstructive sleep apnoea 27
COPD see chronic obstructive airway disease
cor pulmonale 8, 22, 24, 26
corticosteroids
   for asthma 5
   for bronchiectasis 9
   for chronic obstructive airway disease 11
   for fibrosing alveolitis 13
   for obstructive sleep apnoea 27
   for occupational asthma 7
Crohn's disease 22
cryptogenic fibrosing alveolitis 12
CT, high-resolution 12
Cushing's syndrome 16

Index

cyanosis 4, 6, 8, 12
cyclophosphamide
  for fibrosing alveolitis 13
  for granulomatoses 15
cycloserine for pulmonary tuberculosis 29
cystic fibrosis 8-9
cytoplasmic antibodies, antineutrophil 14

D

deafness 14
decongestants for obstructive sleep apnoea 27
degeneration, cerebellar 16
diabetes insipidus 22
diarrhoea, chronic 28
distal intestinal obstruction syndrome 8
diuretics for fibrosing alveolitis 13
dust inhalation, fibrogenic 12
dyspnoea 2, 28

E

ECG, in asthma 4
effusion, pleural 16, 18
embolism 18
embolus 20
emphysema 10
empyema 8, 20
endocarditis, bacterial, subacute 14
eosinophilia
  pulmonary 22
  tropical see eosinophilia pulmonary
epilepsy 22
erythema nodosum 22
erythromycin for pneumonia 21
extrinsic allergic alveolitis 12, 22

F

failure
  heart, congestive 22
  renal 2
  respiratory 10
fever 28
fibrogenic dust inhalation 12
fibrosing alveolitis 8, 12-13, 22
fibrosis, cystic 8
focal neuropathy 16
foreign-body reaction 22
fungal infection 22

G

glaucoma 22
Goodpasture's syndrome 14
granuloma 12
  Hodgkin's see Hodgkin's disease
granulomatoses 14-15
granulomatosis 14
  bronchocentric 14
  lymphomatoid 14
  necrotizing sarcoid 14
granulomatous vasculitis 22

H

H_2 blockers for cystic fibrosis 9
haematuria 28
haemoptysis 8, 16, 20, 28
haemorrhage, pulmonary 14
haemosiderosis, idiopathic 22
Hamman–Rich syndrome see alveolitis, fibrosing
Hansen's disease see leprosy
headache, morning 24
hearing loss see deafness
heart see also cardiac
  failure, right 12
herpes labialis 20
histiocytosis X 22
hoarseness 16
hypercalcaemia 16
hypercalciuria 22
hypereosinophilic syndrome 14
hypersomnia with periodic respiration see sleep apnoea, obstructive
hypersomnolence, idiopathic 24, 26
hypertension
  portal 22
  pulmonary 10, 12, 24
hypertrophy, right ventricular 24
hypogammaglobulinaemia 22
hypopituitarism 22
hypoventilation 24

I

immunoglobulin
  for bronchiectasis 9
  for cystic fibrosis 9
infarction, pulmonary 18
infection

actinomyces see actinomycosis
  parasitic 22
  pneumococcal 20
  postpneumonic 18
infertility 28
ipratropium
  for chronic obstructive airway disease 11
  for obstructive sleep apnoea 27
isoniazid for pulmonary tuberculosis 29

L

lactulose for cystic fibrosis 9
legionella 20
leprosy 22
lesion, space-occupying 22
leukaemia 22
Libman–Sacks disease see lupus erythematosus, systemic
Loeffler syndrome see eosinophilia, pulmonary
lobar
  collapse 16, 28
  consolidation 28
lung
  abscess 16, 20
  biopsy 12
  cancer 12, 16, 20, 28
  collapse 16
  honeycomb 22
  rheumatoid 22
  shock see respiratory distress, adult
  transplantation, single, for fibrosing alveolitis 13
lupus
  erythematosus, systemic 12, 18
  pernio 22
lymphadenopathy 16
lymphoma 22
  Hodgkin's 22
lymphoreticulosis, inoculation see cat-scratch disease

M

meningism 28
meningitis 22
mesothelioma 18
methotrexate
  for fibrosing alveolitis 13
  for sarcoidosis 23
metronidazole for pneumonia 21
mononeuritis multiplex 14
mononucleosis, infectious 22

Index

motor neurone disease 24
mucolytics for bronchiectasis 9
mucoviscidosis *see* fibrosis, cystic
myositis, multiple *see* polymyositis
myxoma, atrial 14

N

narcolepsy 24, 26
narcotics *see* opiates
neoplasm, pulmonary 14
neuropathy 14
   focal 16
   peripheral 16, 22

O

obesity 26
obstruction, superior vena cava 16
oedema 24
   peripheral 24
   pulmonary 18, 20
Ondine's curse *see* sleep apnoea, obstructive
opiates for fibrosing alveolitis 13
opioids *see* opiates
osteoarthropathy, hypertrophic 16
oxygen
   for central sleep apnoea 25
   for fibrosing alveolitis 13
   for periodic respiration 25
   for pneumonia 21

P

pain, chest 18
   pleuritic 8, 20
pancreas, fibrosing disease of *see* fibrosis, cystic
pancreatitis 2, 18
papilloedema 22
penicillamine for fibrosing alveolitis 13
pneumoconiosis 22, 28
pneumonia 16, 20
   bacterial 28
   eosinophilic 14 *see also* eosinophilia, pulmonary
   interstitial *see* alveolitis, fibrosing
pneumonitis, hypersensitivity 22 *see also* alveolitis, extrinsic allergic
pneumothorax 2, 4, 8, 10
polyarteritis nodosa 18

polymyositis 12
prednisolone
   for asthma 5
   for chronic obstructive airway disease 11
   for fibrosing alveolitis 13
   for granulomatoses 15
   for sarcoidosis 23
pre-eclampsia 2
proton-pump inhibitors for cystic fibrosis 9
protryptiline for sleep apnoea
   central 25
   obstructive 27
pseudotuberculosis *see* sarcoidosis
psittacosis 20
pulmonary *see* lung
pyrazinamide for pulmonary tuberculosis 29

Q

Q fever 20

R

renal
   failure 2
     acute 20
   impairment 14
respiration *see also* breathing
   periodic 24
respiratory
   distress, adult 2, 20
   failure 10
retrognathia 26
rifampicin for pulmonary tuberculosis 29

S

salbutamol
   for asthma 5
   for chronic obstructive airway disease 11
sarcoidosis 12, 22, 28
Schaumann's disease *see* sarcoidosis
sclerosis, systemic 12
scoliosis 26
sepsis, subphrenic 18
SIADH *see* antidiuretic hormone secretion, inappropirate
sicca syndrome *see* Sjögren's syndrome
Sjögren's syndrome 22
SLE *see* lupus erythematosus, systemic
sleep
   apnoea

sleep *cont.*
     central 24, 26
     obstructive 24, 26
     inadequate 26
snoring 26
spirometry 24
steatorrhoea 8
steroids *see* corticosteroids
streptomycin for pulmonary tuberculosis 29
sweat, night 28
syphilis 22

T

tachypnoea 2
terbutaline for asthma 5
tetracycline for chemical pleuradhesis 19
theophylline
   for asthma 5
   for chronic obstructive airway disease 11
thrombophlebitis *see* thrombosis, venous
thrombosis, venous 16
tracheostomy for obstructive sleep apnoea 27
transplantation, single lung, for fibrosing alveolitis 13
tuberculin testing 28
tuberculoma formation 28
tuberculosis 14, 22
   miliary 28
   pulmonary 28

V

vaccination
   influenza for prevention of pneumonia 21
   pneumococcal for prevention of pneumonia 21
vasculitis
   granulomatous 22
   systemic 14
ventilatory
   failure 24
   support, nocturnal, for central sleep apnoea 25

W

weakness, neuromuscular 26
wheeze 4, 6

CURRENT DIAGNOSIS & TREATMENT

in

Rheumatology & musculoskeletal disorders

Edited by
Michael Doherty

Series editors
Roy Pounder
Mark Hamilton

A QUICK Reference for the Clinician

Contributors

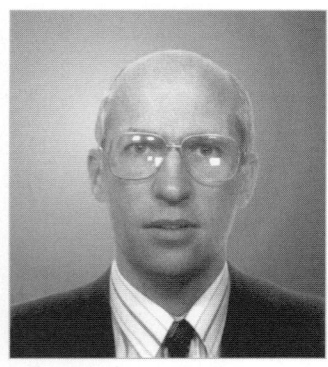

EDITOR

M Doherty

Dr Michael Doherty is Reader and Consultant in Rheumatology at Nottingham and current editor of Annals of the Rheumatic Diseases. He has a strong interest in undergraduate and postgraduate education, and his current research centres on clinical, epidemiological, and genetic aspects of osteoarthritis.

REFEREES

Dr Cyrus Cooper
MRC Environmental Epidemiology Unit
Southampton General Hospital
Southampton, UK

Dr Michael Shipley
Department of Rheumatology
Middlesex Hospital
London, UK

AUTHORS

ACUTE CRYSTAL SYNOVITIS
Dr Michael Doherty
Rheumatology Unit
Nottingham City Hospital
Nottingham, UK

ANKYLOSING SPONDYLITIS
Dr Andrei Calin
Royal National Hospital for Rheumatic Diseases
Bath, UK

ARTHRITIS, PSORIATIC
Professor Verna Wright
Rheumatology and Rehabilitation Research Unit
University of Leeds
Leeds, UK

ARTHRITIS, RHEUMATOID
Dr Chris Deighton
Department of Rheumatology
City Hospital
Nottingham, UK

ARTHRITIS, SEPTIC
Dr Vivienne Weston
Microbiology and Public Health Laboratory
Queen's Medical Centre
Nottingham, UK

Dr Adrian Jones
Rheumatology Unit
City Hospital
Nottingham, UK

GOUT
Dr Diana Macfarlane
Consultant Rheumatologist
Homeopathic Hospital
Tunbridge Wells, UK

MYOSITIS, INFLAMMATORY
Professor David Isenberg
Department of Medicine
University College Hospital
London, UK

OSTEOARTHRITIS
Dr Adrian Jones
Rheumatology Unit
City Hospital
Nottingham, UK

Dr Michael Doherty
Rheumatology Unit
Nottingham City Hospital
Nottingham, UK

POLYMYALGIA RHEUMATICA AND GIANT-CELL ARTERIES
Dr Brian Hazleman
Department of Rheumatology
Addenbrooke's Hospital
Cambridge, UK

SYSTEMIC LUPUS ERYTHEMATOSUS
Dr Richard Powell
Clinical Immunology Unit
Queen's Medical Centre
Nottingham, UK

SYSTEMIC SCLEROSIS
Professor Carol M Black
Department of Rheumatology
Royal Free Hospital
London, UK

VASCULITIS, SYSTEMIC
Dr David Carruthers
Department of Rheumatology
Queen Elizabeth Hospital
Birmingham, UK

Dr David Scott
Department of Rheumatology
Norfolk and Norwich Hospital
Norwich, UK

Contents

2 Acute crystal synovitis

4 Ankylosing spondylitis

6 Arthritis, psoriatic

8 Arthritis, rheumatoid

10 Arthritis, septic

12 Gout

14 Myositis, inflammatory
   dermatomyositis
   polymyositis

16 Osteoarthritis

18 Polymyalgia rheumatica and giant-cell arteritis

20 Systemic lupus erythematosus

22 Systemic sclerosis
   diffuse cutaneous disease
   limited cutaneous disease

24 Vasculitis, systemic
   large-artery vasculitis (giant-cell arteritis, Takayasu's arteritis)
   medium-artery vasculitis (Kawasaki's disease, polyarteritis nodosa)
   medium- or small-artery vasculitis (Churg–Strauss vasculitis, microscopic polyangiitis, Wegener's granulomatosis)
   small-vessel vasculitis (essential mixed cryoglobulinaemia, Henoch–Schönlein purpura, leucocytoclastic cutaneous vasculitis)

26 Index

Acute crystal synovitis M. Doherty

Diagnosis

Symptoms
- Usual sites are knee or wrist for pseudogout and first metatarsophalangeal joint, mid- or hindfoot, knee, or wrist for gout.
- Usually, only one or a few joints are involved; polyarticular attacks are rare.
- Symptoms develop rapidly, often becoming maximal within 4–12 h of onset.

Severe pain: 'worst ever'.
Stiffness, tenderness, swelling.
Fever and systemic upset: particularly with large- or multiple-joint involvement.

Signs
Overlying erythema: later desquamation.
Tense effusion, increased warmth, marked joint-line and periarticular tenderness, restricted movement with stress pain: i.e. florid synovitis.
Lymphangitis, local lymphadenopathy.
Pyrexia: possible confusion, especially in elderly patients.
Turbid or blood-stained aspirated fluid: high cell count, >95% polymorphs.
Red hot joint: i.e. periarticular and articular inflammation; always suggests crystals or sepsis.

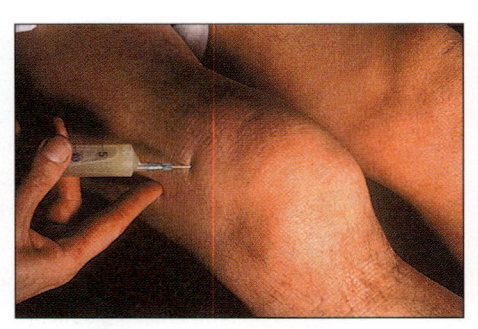

Turbid synovial fluid aspirated from acute knee synovitis due to gout.

Investigations

Diagnostic: synovial fluid analysis
Compensated polarized light microscopy: usual method of crystal identification: monosodium urate crystals: strong (negative) birefringence, needle-shaped, 2–25 µm long, easily identified;
calcium pyrophosphate dihydrate crystals: weak (positive) birefringence, rhomboid, 2–10 µm long, difficult to identify;
other crystals (cholesterol, oxalate, injected steroid) rare.
Gram stain and culture: essential to exclude sepsis.

Supportive but non-diagnostic
Radiography: to detect chondrocalcinosis (pseudogout); osteophyte, sclerosis, cysts, joint-space narrowing (pseudogout, gout); para-articular erosion (gout); although characteristic, such changes are not always present.
ESR, CRP measurement: usually raised.
Serum uric acid measurement: often but not always raised in gout.

Disease associations
- These should be considered after diagnosis and acute management.

Urea, creatinine measurement: for renal impairment in primary or secondary gout.
Lipoprotein measurement, liver function tests: in primary and alcohol-associated gout.
Metabolic screening: calcium, alkaline phosphatase, ferritin, magnesium; if patient is <55 years or has polyarticular chondrocalcinosis (pseudogout).

Complications
Cluster attacks: one attack triggers attacks at other sites.
Joint rupture: with associated soft-tissue inflammation.
Nerve entrapment: due to acute soft-tissue swelling (most often median nerve).

Differential diagnosis
Septic arthritis: sepsis usually superimposes on abnormal, previously symptomatic joint. Other crystal synovitis.
- Acute crystal synovitis and septic arthritis may coexist.
- More than one crystal type may be present ('mixed crystal deposition').

Aetiology

Causes of primary gout
Inherited renal undersecretion of uric acid (in most patients).
Inherited overproduction of uric acid (rare).
Inherited crystal nucleation or growth-promoting tissue factors.
Obesity, excess alcohol intake (mainly beer).

Causes of secondary gout
Chronic diuretic treatment.
Chronic renal impairment.
Lead poisoning (in 'moonshine' drinkers).

Causes of pseudogout
Sporadic isolated chondrocalcinosis, pyrophosphate arthropathy (osteoarthritis subset).
Familial predisposition (unusual).
Metabolic predisposition (rare): haemochromatosis, hypomagnesaemia, hyperparathyroidism, hypophosphatasia.

Triggering factors
Local trauma, intercurrent acute illness, surgery, initiation of drug treatment, e.g. allopurinol (gout), thyroxine (pseudogout), parenteral fluids, joint lavage.
- 'Shedding' of preformed (previously asymptomatic) crystals initiates acute attack.

Epidemiology
- Crystal synovitis is the most common cause of acute monoarthritis in middle-aged and elderly patients.
- More men than women present with gout aged <65 years (mainly primary).
- As many men as women present with gout aged >65 years (mainly secondary).
- Patients with pseudogout are predominantly elderly, with as many men as women.
- Pseudogout is rare in patients <55 years (suggests familial or metabolic predisposition).

Treatment

Diet and lifestyle
- No special precautions are necessary.

Pharmacological treatment

Intra-articular steroids
- Steroids are indicated for problematic attacks (large joints, polyarticular involvement, elderly ill patient) or if oral agents are contraindicated.
- They usually reduce synovitis within 24–48 h.
- The dose should be varied according to joint size; doses listed here are for the knee.

Standard dosage	Methylprednisolone 40 mg.
	Triamcinolone hexacetonide 20 mg.
	Triamcinolone acetonide 40 mg.
Contraindications	Coexistent sepsis.
Special points	Aseptic technique and single-dose vial should be used.
Main drug interactions	None.
Main side effects	Facial flushing, local skin or fat atrophy (mainly fluoridated steroids), exacerbation of pain (temporary), sepsis (rare).

Oral NSAIDs
- Simple analgesics (e.g. paracetamol, co-proxamol) may be effective with other treatments, but quick-acting NSAIDs are generally preferred (see Gout *for further details*).

Colchicine
- Colchicine is effective in any crystal synovitis, but it should be used only for very resistant attacks because of toxicity.

Standard dosage	Colchicine 1 mg, then 0.5 mg orally every 6 h until pain controlled or side effects develop (maximum, 8 mg).
Contraindications	Renal or hepatic impairment, dehydration.
Special points	Never given parenterally; not to be given again within 7 days.
Main drug interactions	None.
Main side effects	Severe nausea, vomiting, watery diarrhoea.

Non-pharmacological treatment

Local physical measures
- The following are the first line of treatment and must be done early.

Aspiration: to reduce intracapsular hypertension (often temporary).

Local heat or cold: may ameliorate pain and swelling.

Resting support (possibly with splintage): to ease symptoms.

Elevation: to reduce oedema.

Early rehabilitation (active movement, mobilization, graded exercise): to maintain muscle and range of movement.

- Prolonged immobilization should be avoided: regular passive movement should punctuate assisted rest.

Lavage
- Lavage is indicated for the following:

Florid, large joint synovitis unresponsive after 48 h to aspiration, steroid injection, and oral medications.

Large loculated effusion (inhibiting effective aspiration).

Coexistent sepsis.

Treatment aims
To relieve pain.
To reduce intra-articular hypertension.
To avoid muscle wasting or capsular restriction.

Prognosis
- Acute attacks resolve spontaneously, even without treatment, within 1–3 weeks.
- Although prolonged florid synovitis is potentially detrimental, most episodes settle with no apparent resulting damage.
- Incomplete recovery of muscle strength or bulk is the most common problem.

Follow-up and management
- Long-term interventions should be instituted only after an acute attack of gout has settled.
- Metabolic screening for pseudogout should be undertaken if appropriate.
- Patients with associated chronic pyrophosphate arthropathy should be advised about alteration of adverse mechanical factors, reduction in obesity, appropriate exercise, and use of symptomatic agents.

Key references
Arie E, Doherty M: Crystal associated rheumatic disease: current management considerations. *Drugs* 1989, **37**:566–576.

Doherty M: Crystal arthropathies: calcium pyrophosphate dihydrate. In *Rheumatology*. Edited by Klippel JH, Dieppe PA. London: Mosby, 1994 7.13.1–7.13.12.

Wallace SL, Singer JZ: Therapy in gout. *Rheum Dis Clin North Am* 1988, **14**:441–457.

Ankylosing spondylitis — A. Calin

Diagnosis

Symptoms
- Symptoms are manifest in >90% of patients, usually beginning during the third decade, although some patients present in their teens and a few in their 30s.
- Onset is insidious.

Back pain and stiffness: worse in morning, improving with exercise, deteriorating with rest.

Peripheral joint symptoms: in 40%; affecting particularly shoulders, hips, knees.

Fatigue.

Uveitis and other stigmata of the spondylarthropathies: e.g. related to psoriatic spondylitis, reactive arthropathy, enteropathic arthritis.

Signs
- Signs may be nonexistent or minimal.

Decreased mobility of lumbar spine, reduced chest expansion, poor mobility of cervical spine.

Decreased mobility of hips and shoulders, knee synovitis, achilles tendinitis, dactylitis, psoriasis, psoriatic nail change.

Evidence of uveitis: during active attack.

Increasing stoop: with disease progression.

Anaemia of chronic disease: particularly in patients with peripheral joint involvement.

Investigations
Radiography of pelvis: reveals sacroiliitis (sacroiliac change may be minimal, moderate, or severe), juxta-articular sclerosis and erosions, lumbar spine changes, calcification, cervical spine involvement.

ESR, plasma viscosity, CRP measurement: raised values in 50% of patients; laboratory changes may be absent even in severely ill patients.

Complications
Hip deterioration: ~20% of patients who develop the disease in their teens or early 20s need one or two new hips within 15 years of disease onset.

Knee involvement: occasionally results in need for total knee replacement.

Deteriorating vision: resulting from persistent uveitis.

Spinal fracture: can occur as a result of osteoporotic changes associated with spinal fusion; resulting spinal-cord injury can be catastrophic.

Cauda equina syndrome: rare.

Differential diagnosis
Reactive arthropathy (Reiter's disease), psoriatic arthropathy, inflammatory bowel disease.

Nonspecific back pain (much more common): radiography differentiates the two.

Other causes of peripheral joint disease with coincidental back pain.

Aetiology
- Ankylosing spondylitis is the result of interplay between HLA B27 and other genes and environmental triggers.
- Environmental triggers probably include agents recognized in other forms of reactive arthropathy (e.g. *Chlamydia* spp., ureaplasma, *Campylobacter*, *Shigella*, *Yersinia*, and *Salmonella* spp., and other Gram-negative organisms).

Epidemiology
- Ankylosing spondylitis occurs in 0.5% of the population in communities where HLA B27 is prevalent (northern Europe, United States, Asia, Central America).
- The male:female ratio is 2.5:1 overall, 3:1 in teenagers, and 1.5:1 with onset in the late 20s.

Treatment

Diet and lifestyle
- Exercise is of paramount importance.
- Attention to posture throughout the day and night is essential.
- Hydrotherapy and physiotherapy are needed as an initial introduction to a lifelong exercise programme.
- Patients and family members must understand the concept of treatment, and literature should be available describing the precise exercise programme needed.
- Patients should avoid smoking.

Pharmacological treatment
- NSAIDs are needed by 80% of patients.

Standard dosage	Indomethacin 75 mg slow release once daily; dose and frequency titrated against patient's needs.
Contraindications	Active peptic ulcer disease, indomethacin intolerance (alternative NSAID should be tried); caution in elderly patients, those on anticoagulants, and those with past history of gastrointestinal bleed or perforation.
Main drug interactions	Warfarin and other anticoagulants.
Main side effects	CNS disturbance, gastrointestinal problems.

- Sulphasalazine may be useful in patients with peripheral joint involvement but appears to have little effect on spinal disease.

Treatment aims
To allow a good night's sleep.
To decrease morning stiffness (pharmacological treatment).
To enable patient to follow the important exercise programme
To maintain good function and posture.

Prognosis
- Outcome is determined by genetic and environmental factors.
- Although the disease does not burn out, most patients can follow a normal social, family, and professional life.
- Up to 10% of patients have relentless progression, with deteriorating posture and spinal fusion, needing spinal surgery.
- Patients with early age of onset and lower educational or social status may be at most risk of severe disease.

Follow-up and management
- After the patient has become stable, visits every 6–12 months to the rheumatologist suffice.
- For patients with severe disease, specialist inpatient management is appropriate.
- For disease flares, readmission may be appropriate.

Patient support
National Ankylosing Spondylitis Society, 5 Grosvenor Crescent, London SW1X 7ER, tel 0171 235 9585.

Key references
Calin A, Edmunds L, Kennedy LG: Fatigue in ankylosing spondylitis – why is it ignored? *J Rheumatol* 1993, **20**:991–995.

Gran JT, Husby G: The epidemiology of ankylosing spondylitis. *Semin Arthritis Rheum* 1993, **22**:319–334.

Kirwan J *et al.*: The course of established ankylosing spondylitis and the effects of sulphasalazine over 3 years. *Br J Rheumatol* 1993, **32**:729–733.

Arthritis, psoriatic — V. Wright

Diagnosis

Symptoms and signs

Any form of psoriasis or a history compatible with psoriasis.

Skin lesions: possibly years after arthritis (family history of psoriasis may be suggestive).

Peripheral polyarthritis: frequently symmetrical; may be indistinguishable from rheumatoid arthritis, involving small joints of hands and feet, wrists, ankles, knees, and elbows.

Inflammatory oligoarthritis: mainly lower limbs, asymmetrical.

Inflammatory involvement of distal interphalangeal joints: nearly always with psoriatic nail changes.

Asymmetrical spondylitis and sacroiliitis, insertion enthesopathy, e.g. of Achilles tendon, plantar fascia, musculotendinous insertions around pelvis.

Mutilating arthritis: with telescoping of fingers and toes (rare).

Dactylitis: 'sausage' digits.

- Rheumatoid nodules and other extra-articular features are absent.

Investigations

Blood tests: rheumatoid factor absent; biochemical response to active disease similar to rheumatoid arthritis; ESR or plasma viscosity best guide to activity; cytidine deaminase not helpful.

Radiography: shows asymmetrical small joint changes, tendency to ankylosis, osteolysis with pencil-in-cup deformity, whittling terminal phalanges (especially hallux); enthesitis; asymmetrical sacroiliitis and syndesmophytes.

Complications

Amyloidosis, exfoliation of skin: rare.

Differential diagnosis

Rheumatoid arthritis.
Reactive (Reiter's) disease.

Aetiology

- Psoriatic arthritis has a genetic component: HLA B27 positive in 71% of patients with psoriatic spondylitis, 32% in distal joint group.
- It may be triggered by trauma.

Epidemiology

- 5–8% of patients with psoriasis have psoriatic arthritis.
- The male:female ratio is equal, but more men have the distal-joint and spondylitic forms.
- Juvenile psoriatic arthritis is rare; it is found in similar groups to adults.

Classification

Classic psoriatic arthritis: involving predominantly distal interphalangeal joints of hands and feet, in 5% of patients.
Arthritis mutilans: with sacroiliitis, in 5%.
Symmetrical polyarthritis: resembling rheumatoid arthritis but with negative serum rheumatoid factor, in 15%.
Asymmetrical, pauci-articular, small joint involvement: with 'sausage' digits, in 70%.
Ankylosing spondylitis: with or without peripheral arthritis, in 5%.

Associated features

Palmar-plantar pustulosis: sternoclavicular hyperostosis, chronic sterile multifocal osteomyelitis, hyperostosis of spine and peripheral arthritis.
Eye lesions: conjunctivitis in 20% of patients; iritis in 7%.
Oedema: unilateral.
HIV infection: exacerbates psoriatic but not rheumatoid arthritis.
Keratoderma blenorrhagica of Reiter's disease: may develop into psoriasis vulgaris.

Treatment

Diet and lifestyle
- Activity should be encouraged.
- No special diet is necessary.

Pharmacological treatment

Principles
For psoriasis (simple cases): dithranol or coal tar (*see* Psoriasis *for further details*).
For arthritis (simple cases): NSAIDs, analgesics.
For severe cases: second-line treatment according to severity of each system.

Second line for arthritis alone

Standard dosage	Sulphasalazine 1 g twice daily. Sodium aurothiomalate 10 mg i.m. test dose, then 50 mg increase weekly to 1 g, then spaced out to monthly maintenance.
Contraindications	*Sulphasalazine:* hypersensitivity to sulphonamides or salicylates. *Sodium aurothiomalate:* pregnancy, lactation, renal or hepatic disease, history of blood dyscrasias, exfoliative dermatitis, or SLE; caution in elderly patients, urticaria, eczema, colitis.
Special points	*Sulphasalazine:* full blood count initially and monthly for first 3 months, liver function tests also monthly for first 3 months. *Sodium aurothiomalate:* urine test for protein before injection, skin inspection for rash; full blood count and urine checks monthly. Antimalarials, e.g. chloroquine, hydroxychloroquine, can also be used.
Main drug interactions	*Sodium aurothiomalate:* aspirin.
Main side effects	*Sulphasalazine:* nausea (dose must be reduced), reversible azoospermia, bone-marrow suppression. *Sodium aurothiomalate:* proteinuria, bone-marrow suppression, dermatitis.

Second line for arthritis and skin involvement
- Treatment should be given under specialist supervision.

Standard dosage	Methotrexate, azathioprine, etretinate, or cyclosporin A.
Contraindications	*Methotrexate:* liver damage, excess alcohol intake, pregnancy. *Azathioprine:* pregnancy. *Etretinate:* hepatic and renal impairment, pregnancy. *Cyclosporin:* renal impairment.
Special points	*Methotrexate:* regular blood tests (full blood count, liver function).
Main drug interactions	*Methotrexate:* NSAIDs, co-trimoxazole, phenytoin, retinoids, diuretics. *Azathioprine:* allopurinol, rifampicin. *Etretinate:* anticoagulants, methotrexate. *Cyclosporin:* angiotensin-converting enzyme inhibitors, NSAIDs.
Main side effects	*Methotrexate:* bone-marrow suppression, liver damage, nausea and vomiting, stomatitis. *Azathioprine:* bone-marrow suppression. *Etretinate:* fetal malformation, cheilosis, hypercholesterolaemia. *Cyclosporin:* impaired renal function, nausea.

Treatment aims
To relieve pain and stiffness.
To achieve full functional capacity.
To prevent progression of arthritis.
To minimize skin lesions.

Prognosis
- Prognosis is usually good.
- A few patients are disabled.

Follow-up and management
- A few patients need regular review.
- Second-line drugs need blood monitoring.

Orthopaedic guidelines
- Psoriatic arthritis has the same indications as other arthropathies.
- It has no more infective complications than other diseases.
- Physicians should liaise with medical, physiotherapy, and occupational therapy staff.
- Early postoperative mobilization is advised.

Key references
Arnett FC *et al.*: Psoriasis and psoriatic arthritis associated with human immune deficiency virus infection. *Rheum Dis Clin North Am* 1991, **17**:59–78.

Gladman DD *et al.*: Longitudinal study of clinical and radiological progression in psoriatic arthritis. *J Rheumatol* 1990, **17**:809–812.

Helliwell PS *et al.*: A re-evaluation of the osteoarticular manifestation of psoriasis. *Br J Rheumatol* 1991, **30**:339–345.

Oriente CB *et al.*: Psoriasis and psoriatic arthritis. Dermatological and Rheumatological Co-Operative Clinical Papers. *Acta Venereol (Stockholm)* 1989, **Suppl 146**:69–71.

Arthritis, rheumatoid — C. Deighton

Diagnosis

Symptoms
Painful, swollen, warm joints, with morning stiffness and impaired function: onset usually insidious, sometimes rapid; characteristically in hands or feet, occasionally monoarticular, most often in a knee; often accompanied by tiredness.

Signs

Articular
Warm, tender, swollen joints: decreased range of movement; peripheral joints most often affected; characteristic symmetry of involvement; proximal interphalangeal, metacarpophalangeal, wrist, and metatarsophalangeal joints usually affected.

Extra-articular
Bursitis: e.g. olecranon.

Tenosynovitis.

Nodules: extensor surfaces.

Serositis: e.g. pleurisy.

Keratoconjunctivitis sicca: secondary Sjögren's syndrome.

Vasculitis, scleritis.

Fibrosing alveolitis.

Investigations
- No single diagnostic test is available; the diagnosis relies on some or all of the following:

ESR, CRP, plasma viscosity measurement: for evidence of inflammation.

Immunology: rheumatoid factor positivity (not essential for diagnosis).

Radiography: initially shows periarticular osteoporosis, followed by erosions around affected joint.

Blood count: for anaemia of chronic disease, thrombocytosis.

Serum immunoglobulin measurement: for polyclonal gammopathy.

- In addition, the duration of morning stiffness, level of functional impairment, and number of inflamed joints must be monitored in established disease.

Complications
- The following occur in patients with established disease and global decline in function or severe systemic malaise.

Widespread active synovitis.

Septic arthritis.

Systemic rheumatoid disease.

Iatrogenic problems: e.g. NSAIDs and anaemia, gold and renal impairment.

Atlanto-axial subluxation.

Non-Hodgkin's lymphoma.

Amyloidosis.

Differential diagnosis
Seronegative spondarthritis.

Reactive arthritis: gastrointestinal or sexually acquired.

Viral arthritis: e.g. rubella, hepatitis B virus infection.

Septic polyarthritis: e.g. staphylococcal or gonococcal infections.

Crystal polyarthritis: e.g. gout.

Generalized nodal osteoarthritis: may have inflammatory component.

SLE.

Aetiology
- The cause of rheumatoid arthritis is unknown, but the following have a role:

Genetic factors: subtypes of HLA DR4 and DR1.

Hormonal factors: remission during pregnancy; contraceptive pill protects from disease.

Epidemiology
- Rheumatoid arthritis is a significant disease that affects 1–2% of the population.
- It is a chronic disease, with high prevalence and low incidence.
- It is a modern disease, with little evidence to indicate its presence >400 years ago.
- The female:male ratio is 3:1.

Treatment

Diet and lifestyle
- Activity should be encouraged, but heavy work intensifies joint inflammation.
- Physiotherapy, taught exercise, and 'joint protection' are helpful to maintain strength and function.

Pharmacological treatment

NSAIDs
- The response is variable and idiosyncratic; if one drug fails, another from a different group may be worth trying.
- The most commonly used drugs are diclofenac, ibuprofen, indomethacin, and naproxen.

Standard dosage	Depends on drug used.
Contraindications	Caution in peptic ulceration, asthma, renal impairment, pregnancy, and elderly patients.
Special points	No influence on disease progression.
Main drug interactions	Diuretics, warfarin.
Main side effects	Dyspepsia, altered bowel habit, renal impairment, fluid retention.

Second-line agents
- These are increasingly started early in the disease process, particularly in patients who do not respond to NSAIDs or who respond partially but have evidence of active disease.

Standard dosage	Sulphasalazine 2 g daily, with gradual build-up over 4 weeks. Methotrexate 2.5–15 mg orally once weekly (not daily).
Contraindications	*Sulphasalazine:* sulphonamide and salicylate hypersensitivity. *Methotrexate:* pregnancy, liver disease.
Special points	*Sulphasalazine:* full blood count every 2 weeks for 2 months, monthly for 2–3 months, then 3-monthly; liver function test at onset, monthly for 3 months, then 3-monthly. *Methotrexate:* full blood count monthly, U&E and liver function test 3-monthly; close monitoring in renal impairment; alcohol and NSAIDs should be avoided.
Main drug interactions	*Sulphasalazine:* warfarin, co-trimoxazole. *Methotrexate:* co-trimoxazole, trimethoprim, phenytoin.
Main side effects	*Sulphasalazine:* nausea, vomiting, rashes, reversible azoospermia. *Methotrexate:* nausea, diarrhoea, rash, pulmonary hypersensitivity, blood dyscrasias.

Other options
Gold (oral or i.m.)
Hydroxychloroquine.
Penicillamine.
Local steroids.
Systemic steroids: either induction before or adjunctive to second-line agents in poorly controlled disease.
Immunosuppressants: for severe articular or extra-articular disease.

Treatment aims
To decrease pain and symptoms and signs of inflammation.
To prevent progression of irreversible joint damage.
To monitor for and treat extra-articular manifestations.
To restrict disability and handicap.

Other treatments
Physiotherapy: during active disease.
Occupational therapy.
Surgery: synovectomies, arthroplasty, arthrodesis, tendon repair; for painful joints (particularly at night), functionally restricted joints, and joints that do not respond to other treatments.

Prognosis
- The prognosis is very variable.
- Poor prognostic markers include female sex, insidious onset, high-titre rheumatoid factor, low educational achievement, persistently raised ESR or CRP, and extra-articular manifestations.

Follow-up and management
- Second-line treatment must be monitored regularly.
- Stable disease needs occasional assessment for progressive functional decline.
- Active disease needs regular follow-up to consider modifying the various treatment options.
- Care should be shared between primary care and hospital services.

Key references
Anonymous: Slow-acting antirheumatic drugs. *Drug Ther Bull* 1993, **31**:17–20.
Harris ED: Rheumatoid arthritis. Pathophysiology and implications for treatment. *N Engl J Med* 1990, **332**:1277–1289.
Hazes JMW, Silman AJ: Review of UK data on the rheumatic diseases – 2. Rheumatoid arthritis. *Br J Rheumatol* 1990, **29**:310–312.

Arthritis, septic
V. Weston and A. Jones

Diagnosis

Symptoms
- Symptoms and signs are more difficult to interpret in the presence of pre-existing joint disease and may be muted in immunosuppressed or elderly patients.
- Polyarticular infection occurs in 10–15% of patients.

Pain: most consistent feature; typically progressive; may be worse at night; with pre-existing joint disease, change or exacerbation of pain is an important warning sign.

Loss of function, limp: possibly presenting feature in children.

Fever: possibly only manifestation, particularly in elderly patients.

Signs
Swelling and local tenderness, pain and restriction of movement: most marked in previously fit younger patients.

Local erythema: possibly but often less marked than in crystal synovitis.

Fever: although temperature normal in up to one-third of patients.

Confusion: possibly prominent feature in elderly patients.

Investigations
- Most investigations are nonspecific, and results may be normal; a high index of suspicion is necessary to make the diagnosis.
- Adequate specimens must be obtained for microbiological examination before starting antimicrobial treatment.

Synovial fluid analysis: Gram film positive in 50% of patients; culture positive in 75%; presence of leucocytes not diagnostic; crystals may coexist with sepsis.

Blood cultures: positive in 50%.

Urogenital swabs: should be obtained if gonococcal infection suspected.

Plain radiography: usually unhelpful in early stages of infection.

Leucocyte or Tc radioisotope scanning, MRI: more sensitive, but treatment should not depend on or be delayed by these investigations.

Complications
Death: in up to 15%, especially elderly, immunosuppressed, and rheumatoid arthritis patients.

Loss of function of joint.

Loss of prosthesis.

Osteomyelitis: from direct spread.

Differential diagnosis
Acute flare of inflammatory joint disease.
Crystal synovitis.
Haemarthrosis.

Aetiology
- Pathogens depend on age and predisposing factors; most infections are due to *Staphylococcus aureus* and streptococci; in children <5 years, *Haemophilus influenzae* type b has been an important pathogen; gonococcal infection appears to be in decline but should be considered in sexually active patients.
- Spread is usually haematogenous; joint disease or blunt trauma may act to localize blood-borne pathogens.
- Direct inoculation during surgery, injection, or trauma occurs but is unusual.
- Risk factors include extremes of age, previous joint disease, diabetes mellitus, immunosuppression, prosthetic joint material, and corticosteroids.

Epidemiology
- The incidence of septic arthritis is unknown but is estimated to be 3–10 in 100 000 population.

Treatment

Diet and lifestyle
- No special precautions are necessary.

Pharmacological treatment

General principles
- A possible septic arthritis is a medical emergency and should be urgently referred to a specialist rheumatologist or orthopaedic surgeon.
- High-dose antibiotics are given i.v. for at least 2 weeks, then orally for at least a further 4 weeks, depending on the clinical response and presence of prosthesis.
- Antibiotics should be started only after appropriate specimens for culture have been obtained.
- Initially, a 'best guess' choice of antibiotics is used, based on the most probable pathogen, patient's age, and sensitivities of pathogen; treatment is later tailored by the results of the Gram stain and culture.

Possible 'best-guess' regimen
Child <5 years: cefotaxime and flucloxacillin.

Child >5 years, adult: flucloxacillin (with benzylpenicillin if gonococcal infection likely).

Immunosuppressed, prosthetic-joint patient: cefotaxime and flucloxacillin.

Specific drugs

Standard dosage	Flucloxacillin 4–8 g i.v. daily.
	Benzylpenicillin 4.8–9.6 g i.v. daily.
	Cefotaxime 3–6 g i.v. daily.
Contraindications	Hypersensitivity.
Special points	Full blood count needed twice weekly.
	Aminopenicillin can be used instead of phenoxymethyl-penicillin for oral treatment.
Main drug interactions	None.
Main side effects	Rash, hypersensitivity reaction (rare), neutropenia (after prolonged treatment), diarrhoea.

Treatment aims
To prevent septicaemia or osteomyelitis.
To preserve joint function.
To resolve infection.

Other treatments
- Repeated medical aspiration with adequate drainage may be associated with better outcome than surgical drainage.
- Surgery is indicated for the following:
Inability to drain medically.
Failure to settle on antibiotic or medical management.
Osteomyelitis.
Prosthetic joints (surgical drainage, debridement, or removal).

Prognosis
- The overall mortality is 15%.
- The prognosis is worse if treatment is delayed, in elderly patients with Gram-positive infection, and in patients with predisposing joint or systemic disease.
- Infection of prosthetic material carries a particularly poor prognosis; revision or removal of the prosthesis is a common outcome.

Follow-up and management
- Patients with infected prostheses may need long-term suppressive antibiotic treatment, although, in most, revision surgery is delayed rather than prevented.

Key references
Broy SB, Schmid FR: A comparison of medical drainage (needle aspiration) and surgical drainage (arthrotomy or arthroscopy) in the initial treatment of infected joints. *Clin Rheum Dis* 1986, **12**:501–522.

Cooper C, Cawley M: Bacterial arthritis in an English health district: a 10 year review. *Ann Rheum Dis* 1986, **45**:458–463.

Hendrix RW, Fisher MR: Imaging of septic arthritis. *Clin Rheum Dis* 1986, **12**:459–487.

Shaw BA, Kasser JL: Acute septic arthritis in infancy and childhood. *Clin Orthop* 1990, **257**:212–225.

Gout   D. Macfarlane

Diagnosis

Symptoms
Acute pain in a single joint: usually base of great toe; often starting at night; self-limiting but tendency to recur.
Mild systemic disturbance, with irritability and low-grade fever.
Polyarticular attacks: in 5–10% of patients (50% of elderly patients).
Chronic asymmetrical polyarthritis: after repeated acute attacks.

Signs
Swollen, shiny, red, tender joints.
Desquamation: as attack subsides.
Tophi in helix of ear, elbow, and over small joints of hands and feet: in severe cases.
Olecranon bursitis: 'boozer's elbow'; common.

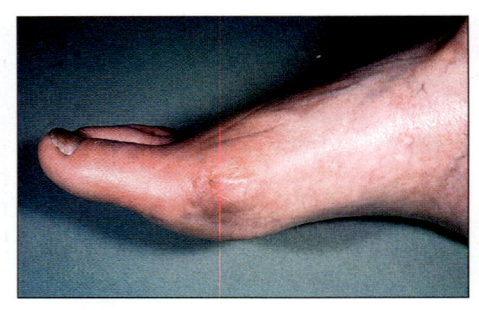

Acute gout in big toe.

Investigations
Polarized light microscopy: needle-shaped, negatively birefringent crystals in synovial fluid from the affected joint are diagnostic.
Serum uric acid measurement: concentration usually raised but may fall to normal during acute attack.
Full blood count: to exclude secondary cause, e.g. lymphoproliferative disorder.
ESR measurement: rate may be raised during acute attack.
Creatinine measurement: renal failure may result from or be caused by hyperuricaemia.
Fasting lipids measurement: hyperlipidaemia common.
Urinary urate excretion measurement: differentiates overproducers from underexcretors (while on low-purine diet).
Radiography: may show characteristic para-articular punched-out erosions without accompanying osteoporosis around joints in patients with chronic arthritic gout.

Complications
Prolongation of acute attack: by incorrect use of allopurinol.
Gastrointestinal bleeding: due to high-dose NSAIDs.
Renal impairment: due to drug interference with renal cortical blood flow.

Differential diagnosis
Acute gout
Septic arthritis.
Cellulitis.
Pyrophosphate arthritis ('pseudogout').

Chronic tophaceous gout
Rheumatoid arthritis.
Septic arthritis.
Hyperlipidaemia with xanthomata.

Non-gout
Painful bunion with asymptomatic hyperuricaemia.

Aetiology
- Gout is often precipitated by overindulgence, surgery, or intercurrent illness.
- Primary gout may be caused by a genetic predisposition to overproduction or underexcretion of urate or failure to inhibit crystallization in tissues.
- Secondary gout may be caused by diuretics (particularly in older women), renal impairment, diet (high purine intake coupled with obesity), high cell turnover (malignant disease), alcohol excess, or heavy-metal poisoning, especially lead (saturnine gout).

Epidemiology
- Gout is particularly prevalent in middle-aged men, post-menopausal women, and patients with renal failure.

Treatment

Diet and lifestyle
- Most patients with gout should lose weight.
- Alcohol intake should be moderated because alcohol inhibits urate excretion by the kidney and is often associated with high energy intake.
- Consumption of meat and shellfish should be restricted because they are high in purines, which produce uric acid.

Pharmacological treatment

For acute attack

Standard dosage	Rapidly acting NSAID, e.g. indomethacin or diclofenac 100 mg initially, followed by 50 mg 3 times daily until attack starts to subside, then reduced dose. Colchicine 0.5 mg 4 times daily, reduced as attack subsides.
Contraindications	*Indomethacin:* peptic ulcer, anticoagulants, renal impairment. *Colchicine:* hypersensitivity.
Special points	*Colchicine:* can be used for longer to prevent recurrence at 0.5 g twice daily. Alternatives for resistant or difficult cases include intra-articular or oral steroids.
Main drug interactions	*Indomethacin, diclofenac:* warfarin.
Main side effects	*Indomethacin, diclofenac:* indigestion, gastric bleeding, headache, nausea, dizziness (worse with indomethacin). *Colchicine:* nausea, diarrhoea.

For hyperuricaemia

- Treatment can be considered between attacks if the serum urate concentration remains raised.
- Allopurinol is indicated for recurrent attacks of gout, chronic tophaceous gout, renal impairment due to hyperuricaemia, induction of chemotherapy, and asymptomatic hyperuricaemia (>0.7 mmol/L).

Standard dosage	Allopurinol 100 mg initially, gradually increased by 100 mg intervals according to urate concentrations to 300–900 mg daily.
Contraindications	Acute gout, hypersensitivity.
Special points	Lower dose in renal failure to prevent build up of metabolites; additional prophylactic NSAID or colchicine for first 3 months to prevent multiple attacks of gout.
Main drug interactions	Azathioprine.
Main side effects	Rash.

Treatment aims
To control inflammation during acute attack.

To prevent recurrent acute attacks and chronic gouty arthritis by lowering serum urate concentrations.

Prognosis
- The prognosis is excellent; with modern hypouricaemic treatment, most patients are effectively cured.

Follow-up and management
- Patients are usually followed up by the GP, who should monitor serum urate concentrations to adjust the dose of hypo-uricaemic treatment and to ensure compliance.
- Referral to a specialist is indicated if the diagnosis is in doubt, response to treatment is poor, or drug sensitivity develops.

Key references
Cohen MG, Emmerson BJ: Gout. In *Rheumatology* vol 7. Edited by Klippel JH, Dieppe PA. St Louis: Mosby, 1994, pp 12.1–12.16.

Myositis, inflammatory
D.A. Isenberg

Diagnosis

Symptoms
Weakness: principally affecting proximal muscles in arms and legs; 15–30% of these patients have associated arthralgias, Raynaud's phenomenon, or myalgia.

Interstitial lung disease, pulmonary hypertension, ventilatory failure, heart block or arrhythmias, dysphagia: unusual, severe manifestations.

Skin rashes.

- Patients with dermatomyositis, especially men aged >45 years, may have an accompanying tumour, causing various symptoms, e.g. weight loss.

Signs
Muscle wasting: principally of proximal muscles.

Loss of muscle reflexes: in late-stage disease.

Heliotrope rash: lilac discoloration around eyelids.

Gottron's papules: small raised reddish plaques over knuckles.

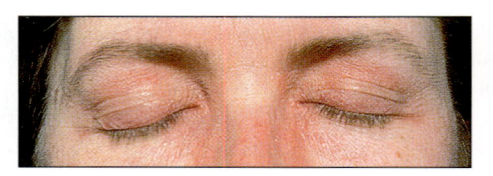

Erythematous rash: over face, upper chest, and arms, usually on extensor surfaces.

Classic heliotrope rash on the eyelids of a patient with dermatomyositis.

Investigations

Key investigations
Creatine kinase measurement: concentration 5–30 times upper limit of normal but not disease-specific; concentrations higher in many patients with muscular dystrophy.

Electromyography: to check for insertional irritability and small polyphasic potentials.

Muscle biopsy: needle or open surgical technique; classic changes are inflammation, with mononuclear cell infiltrate composed mainly of lymphocytes (some macrophages and plasma cells), with muscle-fibre necrosis, and, in chronic cases, replacement of muscle fibres by fat and fibrous tissue; changes often patchy, and up to 20% of patients may have relatively normal appearance.

Other investigations
Measurement of other enzymes: e.g. aldolase and transaminases; concentrations may be raised.

24-h urine creatine excretion measurement: may be high but less specific than raised creatine kinase.

Myoglobin measurement: appears to reflect disease activity.

Autoantibody analysis: weak positive antinuclear antibody reaction in 60–80% of patients with myositis; antibodies to transfer RNA synthetase enzymes have been found to be virtually disease-specific, notably the anti-Jo-1 antibody.

Complications
Interstitial lung fibrosis, arthritis, Raynaud's phenomenon: in patients with Jo-1 antibody.

Cardiac or respiratory failure: rare; caused by rapidly progressive myositis.

Underlying neoplasm: muscle disease often intractable until tumour identified and treated.

Recurrent falls and danger of major internal trauma: caused by an unusual, steroid-resistant form of myositis, associated with inclusion bodies.

Differential diagnosis
Muscular dystrophy.
Osteomalacia.
Rhabdomyolysis.
Drug-induced inflammatory disease (including D-penicillamine).

Aetiology
- Inflammatory muscle diseases are part of the family of autoimmune rheumatic diseases.
- Causes include the following:

Hormonal component.
Immunogenetic predisposition: HLA B8 and DR3 associated with myositis, principally in whites; DR3 linked to Jo-1 antibody.
Environmental factors: increased risk of developing myositis at different times of year found in one study.
Viruses, e.g. Picorna viruses and retroviruses: may be triggering factors; link between myositis and HIV has been suggested.

Epidemiology
- The annual incidence of myositis is 5 in one million population.
- The prevalence is 5–8 in 100 000.
- The female:male ratio is 2–3:1 overall and 9:1 in patients with an associated autoimmune rheumatic disease.

Factors suggesting malignancy
Dermatomyositis in male patients.
Age >45 years.
Weight loss.
Poorer than expected response to treatment.
Absence of autoantibodies.
Unexplained historical, physical, or laboratory abnormalities.

Dermatomyositis or polymyositis?

Dermatomyositis
Onset: childhood to old age.
Skin rash, microvascular injury.
Perifascicular atrophy common.
Endomysial infiltration less common.
Surrounded and invaded fibres less than in polymyositis.
Anti-Jo-1 in 5%, other antisynthetases at least as much as in polymyositis.

Polymyositis
Onset: adulthood.
No skin rash or microvascular injury.
Perifascicular atrophy uncommon.
Endomysial infiltration common.
Surrounded and invaded fibres frequent.
Anti Jo-1 in 30%.

Treatment

Diet and lifestyle
- Exercise and activity are limited during the inflammation.
- No special diet is necessary.

Pharmacological treatment

Corticosteroids
- After the diagnosis has been established, treatment should be initiated quickly.

Standard dosage	Prednisolone 1 mg/kg daily initially (usually 60–80 mg); continued until creatine kinase returned to near normal (usually 1–3 months); then reduced to 5–10 mg daily over following 3 months.
Contraindications	Severe osteoporosis.
Main drug interactions	None.
Main side effects	Osteoporosis, increased risk of infection, diabetes, hypertension.

Other immunosuppressants
- These are indicated in patients who have not shown a response to high-dose steroids after 1 month or who cannot tolerate them.

Standard dosage	Azathioprine 2–3 mg/kg. Methotrexate up to 15 mg weekly.
Contraindications	*Methotrexate:* abnormal liver function, major renal disease, porphyria.
Main drug interactions	*Methotrexate:* many analgesics and antibacterials.
Main side effects	Bone-marrow suppression, liver damage.

Other options
- Oral or occasionally i.v. cyclophosphamide has been used in severely affected patients, occasionally combined with steroids and methotrexate or azathioprine.
- Reports of the use of cyclosporin in myositis are conflicting, and it is not widely used in this disease.
- Intravenous gammaglobulin may be used.

Treatment aims
To control disease as soon as possible.
To maintain reasonable degree of mobility.
To reduce treatment to smallest dose needed after 3–4 months of aggressive therapy to avoid side effects (e.g. intercurrent infection or osteoporosis).

Other treatments
Total lymph-node irradiation and thoracic duct drainage in severe cases.
Physiotherapy and hydrotherapy.

Prognosis
- ~20% of patients recover fully.
- 10–20% die as a direct result of the disease or as a consequence of its treatment.
- Most patients are left with some muscle weakness.
- Patients who respond most slowly to initial treatment have the poorest prognosis.

Follow-up and management
- Patients must be followed for several years.
- Regular clinical examination, creatine kinase measurement, and formal muscle strength testing are needed.
- Judicious use of physiotherapy and hydrotherapy help to keep the range of joint movement normal and to maintain muscle power.
- If patients fail to respond to conventional treatment, the original biopsy should be re-examined for evidence of inclusion-body myositis (such patients often fail to respond to immunosuppression); further biopsy should be considered to exclude the possibility of another cause, e.g. rhabdomyolysis, and to check for evidence of type II fibre atrophy, associated with an excess of corticosteroids.

Key references
Dalakas MC: Polymyositis, dermatomyositis, and inclusion-body myositis. *N Engl J Med* 1992, **325**:1487–1498.

Sigurgeirsson B *et al.*: Risk of cancer in patients with dermatomyositis or polymyositis. *N Engl J Med* 1992, **326**:363–367.

Targoff IN: Polymyositis and dermatomyositis: adult onset. In *Textbook of Rheumatology.* Edited by Maddison P *et al.* Oxford: Oxford University Press, 1993, pp 794–821.

Osteoarthritis — A. Jones and M. Doherty

Diagnosis

Symptoms
- Many patients are asymptomatic.
- Women have more symptoms than men.
- Symptoms occur more frequently in large, weight-bearing joints.
- They are often phasic and are not always progressive; muscle weakness and psychological status are often better predictors of symptoms or functional impairment than structural damage.

Pain: typically on use.
Stiffness after inactivity: 'gelling' common.
Functional impairment: particularly of gait; a major problem.

Signs
- Signs are often discordant with symptoms.

Bony swelling, deformity, crepitus, restriction of movement: bony swelling may be marked in interphalangeal joints (Heberden's and Bouchard's nodes).
Joint-line tenderness.
Local heat, effusion: occasional inflammatory features, particularly in crystal-related osteoarthritis or developing finger nodes.

Investigations
- Osteoarthritis is principally a clinical diagnosis. Often occuring in middle-aged or elderly patients, the question is not usually whether it is present but whether it is the cause of current symptoms; only clinical examination can answer this.

General
Radiography: may show structural change, e.g. loss of joint space (cartilage), osteophytosis, sclerosis, cysts, osteochondral bodies.

Premature osteoarthritis
- Onset occurs before the age of 55 years.

Ferritin measurement: for haemochromatosis.
Calcium, phosphate, alkaline phosphatase measurement: for hyperparathyroidism.
Urine homogentisic acid measurement: if ochronosis suspected.
Lateral spine radiography: for spondyloepiphyseal dysphasia.
Pituitary studies: if acromegaly suspected.

Acute flare
Synovial fluid examination: for sepsis and crystals.

'Locking'
Arthroscopy or MRI: for loose bodies (osteochondral), meniscal lesions.

Complications
Acute crystal synovitis: mainly calcium pyrophosphate crystals.
Septic arthritis.
Loose-body formation.
Avascular necrosis.

Differential diagnosis
- Periarticular lesions may coexist and may be the prime source of symptoms.

Polyarticular osteoarthritis
Inflammatory arthropathies.
Gout.

Poor bone response and destruction
Charcot arthropathy.
Sepsis.

Acute crystal-related oligoarthritic osteoarthritis
Sepsis.
Gout.
Inflammatory arthropathy.

Aetiology
- Osteoarthritis probably has many causes; recognised factors include the following:

Obesity.
Age.
Occupational trauma.
Genetics: nodal osteoarthritis, (spondylo-) epiphyseal dysplasia, type II collagen abnormalities.
Metabolic or endocrine disorders: haemochromatosis, hyperparathyroidism, ochronosis, acromegaly.
Previous joint disease or damage.

Epidemiology
- Osteoarthritis is strongly age-related.
- It is the most common cause of locomotor disability.
- Nodal osteoarthritis may manifest with florid polyarticular disease and Heberden's nodes in menopausal women.

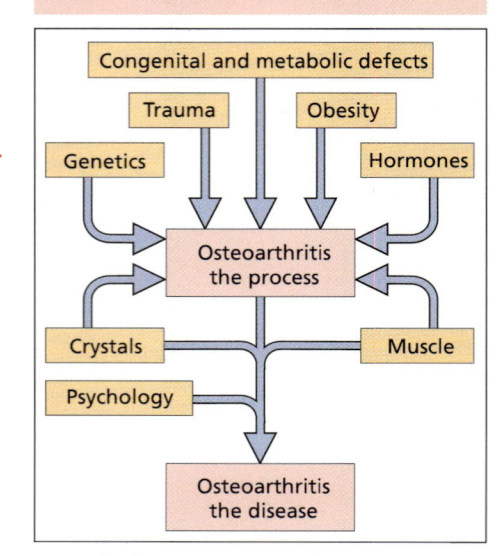

Factors leading to progression of osteoarthritis.

Treatment

Diet and lifestyle
- Patients should be encouraged to take control of the condition.
- Physical activity should be encouraged, e.g. aerobic fitness and muscle strengthening.
- Biomechanical factors, e.g. obesity, varus knee deformity, should be tackled (wedge insoles, shock-absorbing footwear, use of stick).

Pharmacological treatment

Analgesics
- These are often sufficient.
- Compound preparations with opiates may only increase adverse effects, without improving symptom control.

Standard dosage	Paracetamol 1 g every 6 h.
Contraindications	None.
Main drug interactions	None.
Main side effects	Rare, except in overdosage when hepatic failure may ensue.

NSAIDs
- NSAIDs should be tried only if analgesics fail.
- Use should be regularly reviewed.

Standard dosage	Depends on agent; lowest dose needed for benefit.
Contraindications	Active peptic ulceration, hypersensitivity, renal impairment (relative).
Special points	Patients show marked variation in response to different drugs.
Main drug interactions	Warfarin.
Main side effects	Gastrointestinal ulceration, anaemia, renal dysfunction, skin rashes.

Intra-articular steroids
- Local corticosteroids are indicated for short-term relief of inflammatory episodes or coexistent periarticular lesions.

Standard dosage	Depends on agent and joint; in large joints, generally no more than 3-monthly; in small joints, yearly.
Contraindications	Septic arthritis, hypersensitivity (rare).
Special points	Longer-acting steroids provide more benefit.
Main drug interactions	None.
Main side effects	Occasional facial flushing, deterioration of diabetic control.

Topical antirheumatics
- These include NSAIDs and rubifacients.
- Their role is controversial, but they are probably effective.
- Contraindications include sensitive or broken skin.

Treatment aims
To relieve pain.
To maintain functional ability.

Other treatments
Arthroplasty: for patients with persistent pain or marked functional impairment.

Prognosis
- Many patients show phasic symptoms, and some improve with time.
- Symptoms may remain static for years.

Follow-up and management
- Follow-up is usually in a primary care setting.
- The aims are to determine the need for further intervention as a result of deterioration in symptoms or function and to monitor treatment, particularly by NSAIDs to assess the need for continued use and the development of adverse effects.

Key references
Bradley JD et al.: Comparison of an anti-inflammatory dose of ibuprofen, an analgesic dose of ibuprofen, and acetaminophen in the treatment of osteoarthritis of the knee. *N Engl J Med* 1991, **325**:87–91.

Brandt K: The pathogenesis of osteoarthritis. *Rheumatol Rev* 1991, **1**:3–11.

Jones AC, Doherty M: The treatment of osteoarthritis. *Br J Clin Pharmacol* 1992, **33**:357–362.

Polymyalgia rheumatica and giant-cell arteritis
B.L. Hazleman

Diagnosis

Symptoms

Polymyalgia rheumatica
Pain and stiffness: bilateral and symmetrical, affecting neck, shoulder, and pelvic girdles; stiffness usually predominant, particularly severe after rest, and may prevent patient getting out of bed.

Giant-cell arteritis
Headache: in two-thirds or more of patients; severe pain, usually localized in the temple but may be occipital or be less defined and precipitated by brushing the hair.

Pain on chewing: due to claudication of muscles of mastication, in up to two-thirds of patients.

Visual disturbances: in 25%; visual loss evident in <10%.

Signs

Polymyalgia rheumatica
Unimpaired muscle strength: although pain makes interpretation of muscle testing difficult.

Tenderness of involved structures: with restriction of shoulder movement, if diagnosis delayed.

Peripheral synovitis: uncommon and transient.

Giant-cell arteritis
Scalp tenderness: particularly around temporal and occipital arteries; may disturb sleep.

Thickened, tender, and nodular arteries: with absent or reduced pulsation.

Partial or complete visual loss: due to anterior ischaemic optic neuropathy.

Investigations

Baseline clinical investigations
- These are used to make the diagnosis and exclude other diagnoses.

Full blood count.
Biochemical profile.
Protein electrophoretic strip.
Thyroid function test.
Rheumatoid factor test.
Chest radiography.
ESR measurement: rate usually greatly raised, but can be normal.
Acute-phase protein (e.g. CRP) measurement: concentration usually raised.

Specific investigations
Temporal artery biopsy: for suspected giant-cell arteritis, not for polymyalgia rheumatica; findings can be focal, may be normal.

Complications
Visual loss: in up to 10% of patients, permanent blindness in giant-cell arteritis.

Differential diagnosis
Neoplastic disease.
Joint disease: osteoarthritis (particularly of cervical spine), rheumatoid arthritis, connective tissue disease.
Multiple myeloma.
Leukaemia.
Lymphoma.
Muscle disease: polymyositis, myopathy.
Infections: e.g. bacterial endocarditis.
Bone disease: particularly osteomyelitis.
Hypothyroidism.
Parkinsonism.
Functional disorders.

Aetiology
- A distinct prodromal event is often noted, resembling influenza, although viral studies are negative.
- HLA-DR4 is increased in both polymyalgia rheumatica and giant-cell arteritis.
- Lymphocytes in arteritic lesions express the T-cell phenotype, and the CD4- subset predominates.

Epidemiology
- The peak age is 60–75 years.
- The female:male ratio is 3:1.
- The annual incidence of biopsy-positive disease is 6.7 in 100 000 people (16.8 in 100 000 >55years).
- The disease occurs predominantly in northern Europe and northern United States.

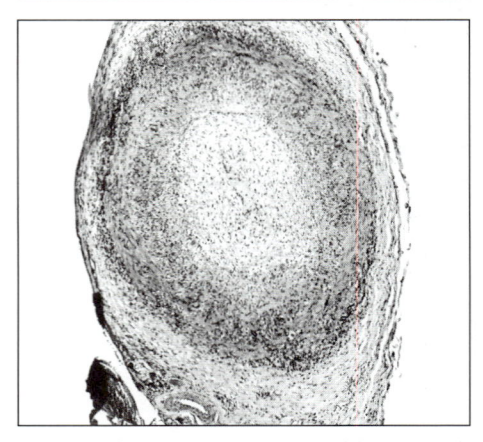

Ecclusion of lumen due to intimal proliferation and inflammation of the media.

Treatment

Diet and lifestyle
- No special precautions are necessary.

Pharmacological treatment
- Patients with giant-cell arteritis should be referred as an emergency to a specialist to arrange a biopsy and to initiate treatment.
- Treatment by a systemic corticosteroid has long been recognised as mandatory in patients with giant-cell arteritis in order to prevent serious vascular complications, particularly blindness.
- Corticosteroids are usually also needed for patients with polymyalgia rheumatica.
- Many patients remain on treatment for years.

For polymyalgia rheumatica

Standard dosage	Prednisolone 10–20 mg initially for 1 month, reduced by 2.5 mg every 2 weeks to 10 mg daily, then 1 mg daily every 2–4 weeks; maintenance dose 5–7 mg daily for 6–12 months; final reduction, 1 mg every 6–8 weeks.
Contraindications	Systemic infections; caution in pregnancy, hypertension, diabetes mellitus, osteoporosis, glaucoma, epilepsy, peptic ulceration.
Special points	In patients who cannot reduce prednisolone dosage because of recurring symptoms or who develop serious steroid-related side effects, azathioprine has been shown to have a modest steroid-sparing effect, and methotrexate may be more effective.
Main drug interactions	Rifampicin, phenylbarbitone, and phenytoin reduce corticosteroid concentrations; anticoagulant dosage may need adjustment; reduced effect of NSAIDs.
Main side effects	Weight gain, oedema, increased intraocular pressure, cataracts, glaucoma, gastrointestinal disturbances, peptic ulceration, diabetes, osteoporosis, skin atrophy.

For giant-cell arteritis without visual symptoms
Prednisolone 20–40 mg daily initially for 8 weeks, reduced by 5 mg every 2 weeks to 10 mg daily; then as for polymyalgia rheumatica.

For giant-cell arteritis with possible or definite ocular involvement
Prednisolone 40–80 mg daily initially for 8 weeks, reduced to 20 mg daily over next 4 weeks; then as for uncomplicated giant-cell arteritis.

Treatment aims
To relieve pain and symptoms.
To reduce the incidence of complications.

Prognosis
- Untreated, patients have prolonged ill health, and up to 20% of those with giant-cell arteritis go blind or develop vascular complications.
- Treated, between one-third and one-half of patients can discontinue treatment after 2 years.

Follow-up and management
- Treatment is monitored clinically and by acute-phase response (ESR, CRP).
- Long-term low-dose maintenance prednisolone ≤3 mg, is sometimes needed.

Key references
Behn AR, Perera T, Myles AB: Polymyalgia rheumatica and corticosteroids: how much for how long? *Ann Rheum Dis* 1983, **42**:374–378.

Krall PL, Mazanec DJ, Wilke WS: Methotrexate for corticosteroid-resistant polymyalgia rheumatica and giant-cell arteritis. *Cleve Clin J Med* 1989, **56**:253–277.

Kyle V, Cawston TE, Hazleman BL: Erythrocyte sedimentation rate and c reactive protein in the assessment of polymyalgia rheumatica/giant cell arteritis on presentation and during follow-up. *Ann Rheum Dis* 1989, **48**:667–671.

Kyle V, Hazleman BL: Treatment of polymyalgia rheumatica and giant cell arteritis. I. Steroid regimens in the first two months. *Ann Rheum Dis* 1989, **48**:658–661.

Kyle V, Hazleman BL: Treatment of polymyalgia rheumatica and giant cell arteritis. II. Relation between steroid dose and steroid associated side effects. *Ann Rheum Dis* 1989, **48**:662–666.

Systemic lupus erythematosus — R.J. Powell

Diagnosis

Symptoms and signs

Tiredness: indicating anaemia.

Polyarthralgias and non-erosive symmetric arthritis: involving predominantly small joints (rarely deforming).

Rashes: photosensitive, discoid, and, less often, classic facial butterfly rash.

Vasculitic lesions of extremities: leading to gangrene of digits.

Oral or pharyngeal ulcers.

Myalgia.

Pleuritic or pericardial pain: indicating serositis.

Epistaxis, bleeding gums, menorrhagia, purpura: symptoms of thrombocytopenia

Visual and auditory hallucinations or epilepsy.

Oedema or hypertension: e.g. nephrotic syndrome or acute nephritic illness.

Alopecia.

Raynaud's phenomenon.

Lymphadenopathy.

Fever.

Livedo reticularis.

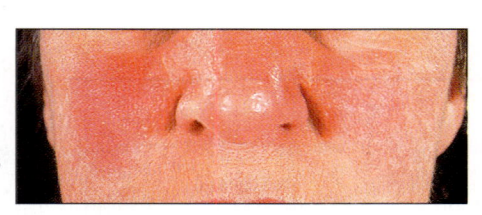

Classic butterfly rash.

Differential diagnosis
Other connective tissue diseases: e.g. rheumatoid arthritis, progressive systemic sclerosis.
Infection.
Malignancy.

Aetiology
- Causes include the following:

Genetic factors and inherited defects of the early components of the classic complement pathway.
Environmental factors: e.g. sunlight
Drugs: e.g. hydralazine, procainamide, phenytoin.

Epidemiology
- The prevalence of SLE in the UK is 45 in 100 000 women, 3.7 in 100 000 men.
- The highest incidence is in the 40–60 year age group.
- SLE is unusual in children.

Investigations

Laboratory tests
- These are useful in the diagnosis of SLE, but no single diagnostic test is available.

Full blood count: may reveal anaemia, leucopenia, neutropenia, lymphopenia, or thrombocytopenia; raised ESR common in active disease; evidence of haemolytic anaemia requires further investigation, e.g. a Coomb's test.

Antinuclear antibody analysis: antibodies found in at least 95% of SLE patients but not disease-specific; antibodies to double-stranded DNA and Sm are relatively disease-specific but do not occur in all patients (~50% and ~5%, respectively); antibodies to Ro, La, and U1 ribonucleoprotein helpful in defining disease subsets and overlap syndromes; positive antiphospholipid antibodies and lupus anticoagulant define patients at risk from major arterial and venous thromboses.

For markers of disease activity or organ involvement

ESR measurement: raised ESR with normal CRP usual except when bacterial infection coexists.

Plasma-complement analysis: low C3 and C4 and raised C3 conversion products indicate activity.

Anti double-stranded DNA antibody analysis: antibodies can rise with disease flares, especially those involving the kidney.

Dipstick testing of urine: for proteinuria and haematuria.

Measurements of renal function and 24-h urine protein loss.

Complications

Severe renal involvement.

Cerebral involvement: infarcts or neuropsychiatric disease.

Infections secondary to immunosuppression.

Major thrombotic events: especially when high-titre antiphospholipid antibodies are present.

Treatment

Diet and lifestyle
- Patients, especially those with photosensitivity, should avoid sunlight and should use high-factor sun screen (ultraviolet A and B).

Pharmacological treatment

Indications
Discoid lupus erythematosus rashes: topical steroids.

Joint and skin involvement: hydroxychloroquine.

Systemic involvement: acute treatment by corticosteriods, introduction of cytotoxic agents, e.g. azathioprine, chlorambucil, methotrexate.

Severe vasculitis (including cerebral and renal involvement): pulse cyclophosphamide and methylprednisolone.

Systemic treatment

Standard dosage	Hydroxychloroquine 200 mg daily. Prednisone 10–40 mg daily and azathioprine 1–2.5 mg/kg daily to allow subsequent steroid reduction. Pulse methylprednisolone 1 g i.v. initially weekly and pulse cyclophosphamide 1 g i.v. weekly until clinical improvement or occurrence of bone-marrow suppression.
Contraindications	Known hypersensitivity, systemic infections.
Special points	*Cyclophosphamide:* infusions must be preceded by a full blood count to check for bone-marrow toxicity, in particular evidence of neutropenia.
Main drug interactions	*Cyclophosphamide:* concurrent allopurinol should be avoided because of enhanced toxicity.
Main side effects	*Hydroxychloroquine:* retinopathy, skin rashes. *Azathioprine:* bone-marrow suppression, gastrointestinal disturbances, liver toxicity. *Cyclophosphamide:* nausea and vomiting, hair loss, haemorrhagic cystitis, premature menopause. *All cytotoxic agents:* teratogenicity (adequate contraception essential).

Treatment aims
To alleviate disease flares.

Prognosis
- Renal and cerebral involvement and the complications of treatment, especially infection, are the major contributors to mortality.
- The survival rate has improved in the past 2 decades and is now ~95% at 5 years.

Follow-up and management
- Prompt treatment of lupus flares is mandatory.
- The use of oral cytotoxic drugs requires monthly blood counts to check for bone-marrow suppression and liver function tests with methotrexate.

Key references
Hopkinson ND, Doherty M, Powell RJ: Clinical features and race-specific incidence/prevalence rates of systemic lupus erythematosus in a geographically complete cohort of patients. *Ann Rheum Dis* 1994, **53**:675–680.

Hopkinson ND, Doherty M, Powell RJ: The prevalence and incidence of systemic lupus erythematosus in Nottingham, UK, 1989–1990. *Br J Rheumatol* 1993, **32**:110–115.

Hughes GRV: *Connective Tissue Diseases* edn 4. Oxford: Blackwell Scientific Publications, 1994.

Tan E et al.: The 1982 revised criteria for the classification of systemic lupus erythematosus. *Arthritis Rheum* 1982, **25**:1271–1277.

Systemic sclerosis — C.M. Black

Diagnosis

Symptoms
- Scleroderma is unlikely in the absence of Raynaud's phenomenon.
- It has two major subgroups of prognostic and therapeutic importance, as follows:

Limited cutaneous disease
- This occurs in 60% of patients.
- It was previously called CREST.
Swollen painful fingers: ulcers possible.
Thick skin on hands.
Calcium deposits.
Swallowing difficulties.

Diffuse cutaneous disease
- This occurs in 40% of patients.
Puffy hands, feet, arms, legs, tight skin.
Weight loss, fatigue.
Muscle and joint pain.
Breathlessness, dry cough, palpitations.
Indigestion, bloating, diarrhoea.

Signs

Limited cutaneous disease
Early (<10 years)
- Distribution is limited to hands, feet, and face.
Sclerodactyly, swollen fingers, microstomia.
Pitting scars, pulp atrophy.
Digital ulcers.
Telangiectasia.
Calcinosis.

Late (>10 years)
Loud pulmonary second sound.
Right heart failure.
Abdominal bloating.
Wasting and other signs of malabsorption.

Diffuse cutaneous disease
Early (<5 years)
Diffusely puffy or sclerosed skin, including truncal changes.
Friction rubs.
Joint contractures.
Muscle weakness.
Digital pits and ulcers.
Basal crepitations, pericardial rub, arrhythmia.

Late (>5 years)
Dry, shiny skin.
Ulcers: atrophic, on fingers or elbows.
Muscle wasting.
Joint contractures.
Cardiac or respiratory failure.

Investigations

Full blood count: to detect anaemia of chronic disease.

U&E and creatinine clearance measurement: to assess renal function.

Autoantibody tests: antinuclear antibodies are positive in 90% of patients; full screen useful to mark subsets of systemic sclerosis or overlap with other disorders.

Nailfold capillary tests (ophthalmoscope or microscopic): useful in 'pre-scleroderma' and early disease; abnormal pattern of vessel drop-out and distortion.

Oesophageal scintiscanning: to detect dysmotility (other 'gut' tests as indicated).

ECG, echocardiography, Doppler ultrasonography: to detect cardiac involvement and to estimate pulmonary artery pressure.

Chest radiography, pulmonary function tests, high-resolution CT: to detect lung involvement; CT best test for presence and extent of early fibrosis.

Electromyography, biopsy: to diagnose muscle disease.

Joint radiography: to detect acro-osteolysis, calcinosis.

Skin biopsy: usually not needed in established disease, best used in early puffy stage for diagnosis or to differentiate systemic sclerosis from fasciitis.

Complications

Hypertensive renal crisis: in diffuse cutaneous disease, usually within first 5 years of disease; in 7–10% of patients.

Pseudo-obstruction: late complication often of limited cutaneous disease; in <5%.

Carcinoma of lung: associated with pulmonary fibrosis.

Differential diagnosis
Eosinophilic fasciitis.
Mixed connective tissue disease.
Overlap syndromes.
Chronic graft-versus-host disease.
Eosinophilic myalgic syndrome.
Vinyl chloride disease.
Toxic-oil syndrome.
Scleromyxoedema.
Scleroedema of Bushke.
Carcinoid syndrome.
Insulin-dependent diabetes mellitus skin changes.
Chronic reflex sympathetic dystrophy.
Idiopathic pulmonary fibrosis.
Primary pulmonary hypertension.
Cardiomyopathies.
Intestinal hypomotility syndromes.

Aetiology
- In most cases, the cause is unknown, but the following may play a role:
Genetic: HLA classes II and III genes (weak association).
Environmental: organic chemicals (e.g. vinyl chloride), epoxy resins, silica, rape-seed oil, drugs (e.g. bleomycin).

Epidemiology
- Systemic sclerosis occurs world wide.
- 12–20 in one million people are affected annually.
- The female:male ratio is 3:1 overall and 10:1 in people of child-bearing age.
- The disease is more severe in non-whites.
- 30–60 years is the usual age of onset.

Treatment

Diet and lifestyle
- Patients should avoid cold and sudden drops in temperature.
- Patients should stop smoking.
- Skin care involves protection and moisturizers (cosmetic cover for telangiectasia).
- Patients should follow a daily exercise programme to prevent, reduce, or delay contractures and to maintain strength and function.

Pharmacological treatment

For Raynaud's phenomenon and vascular insufficiency
- Response can be variable, so more than one drug within a class is worth trying.

Standard dosage	*Calcium antagonists:* e.g. nifedipine 10–40 mg slow release twice daily.
	Angiotensin-converting enzyme (ACE) inhibitors: captopril 6.25–18.75 mg daily; enalapril 5–15 mg daily.
	Enhancers of prostaglandin-I_3 (PGI_3) production: omega-3-marine triglycerides 5 capsules daily.
Contraindications	*Calcium antagonists:* pregnancy; caution in hepatic or renal disease
	ACE inhibitors: pregnancy.
	PGI_3 enhancers: epilepsy, bleeding disorders.
Special points	*ACE inhibitors:* may cause rapid fall in blood pressure.
Main drug interactions	*Calcium antagonists:* antiepileptics, antiarrhythmics.
	ACE inhibitors: must not be given with potassium-sparing diuretics.
	PGI_3 enhancers: anticoagulants.
Main side effects	*Calcium antagonists:* flushing, headache, oedema.
	ACE inhibitors: dry cough, voice change, rashes.
	PGI_3 enhancers: nausea, headaches.

For early diffuse disease
- No drug is of proven efficacy.

Standard dosage	D-Penicillamine 750–1000 mg daily.
	Methotrexate 7.5–15 mg orally weekly.
	Cyclosporin A 2.5–5 mg/kg orally daily.
	Cyclophosphamide 2 mg/kg daily.
	Prednisolone 20 mg on alternate days.
Contraindications	Pregnancy, existing liver and renal disease.
Main drug interactions	Cyclophosphamide with allopurinol, cyclosporin with ACE inhibitors.
Main side effects	Bone-marrow toxicity, renal and liver impairment, alopecia, rashes.

For oesophageal involvement

Standard dosage	*Proton-pump inhibitor:* omeprazole 20 mg daily.
	Prokinetic drug: cisapride 10 mg 3–4 times daily for 12 weeks, taken 30 min before meal or at bed-time.
Contraindications	Pregnancy, breast-feeding.
Special points	*Omeprazole:* can increase bowel colonization.
Main drug interactions	Oral anticoagulants, phenytoin, theophylline.
Main side effects	*Omeprazole:* constipation, headache, diarrhoea.
	Cisapride: abdominal cramps, diarrhoea.

For mid-gut involvement: bacterial overgrowth
- Rotation antibiotics can be used in various combinations, e.g. metronidazole 400–600 mg twice daily, tetracycline 250 mg 3 times daily, erythromycin 250 mg 4 times daily, or ciprofloxacin 500 mg twice daily.
- These should be given for short periods, e.g. 3–4 weeks, with 'holidays' of 1–2 weeks.

Treatment aims
To reduce symptoms.
To halt disease.
To treat complications.
- Systemic sclerosis has no cure.

Other treatments
Lumbar or digital sympathectomy for severe Raynaud's phenomenon with critical ischaemia.
Selective removal of calcinosis.

Prognosis
- The 5-year cumulative survival rate is 34–73%.
- Factors adversely affecting outcome are increasing age, male sex, extent of skin involvement, and lung, heart, and kidney disease.
- For patients with diffuse cutaneous disease, the first 5 years are the most dangerous; with limited cutaneous disease, the most dangerous period is after 10 years, with a risk of pulmonary hypertension and widespread gut disease.

Follow-up and management
- Diffuse disease needs frequent follow-up in the first 4 years, i.e. 3-monthly or more frequently if necessary; hypertensive renal crisis is the greatest risk.
- Limited disease needs yearly follow-up, with attention to late disease complications, i.e. pulmonary hypertension, malabsorption.
- Attention to vascular insufficiency, possible superimposed infections, and changing internal organ involvement permits therapeutic adjustments that can improve quality of life for patients.

Key references
LeRoy EC: Pathogenesis of systemic sclerosis. *Arthritis and Allied Conditions* 1993, **2**:1293–1299.

Medsger TA Jr: Systemic sclerosis (scleroderma), localized forms of scleroderma and calcinosis. *Arthritis and Allied Conditions* 1993, **2**:1253–1292.

Penez M, Kohn SR: Systemic sclerosis. *J Am Acad Dermatol* 1993, **28**:525–547.

Torres MA, Furst DE: Treatment of generalized systemic sclerosis. *Rheum Dis Clin North Am* 1990, **16**:217–241.

Vasculitis, systemic
D.M. Carruthers and D.G.I. Scott

Diagnosis

Symptoms
- Symptoms depend on the size and site of the vessel involved. The following concentrates particularly on primary systemic vasculitis involving small- and medium-sized arteries.

Malaise, weight loss, fever, diffuse myalgia, arthralgia.
Symptoms of any underlying disease or secondary vasculitis: e.g. rheumatoid arthritis, SLE.
Rash.
Epistaxis, nasal crusting, sinusitis: especially in Wegener's granulomatosis.
Chest pain, haemoptysis, dyspnoea, cough, late-onset asthma (normally precedes Churg–Strauss syndrome).
Mouth ulcers, abdominal pain, diarrhoea.
Numbness, weakness.

Signs
Pyrexia, lymphadenopathy, muscle wasting, weakness.
Microscopic haematuria or proteinuria, or both.
Skin purpura, ulcer, infarction.
Nasal crusting or collapse, septal perforation: especially in Wegener's granulomatosis.
Crackles, wheeze, cardiomyopathy, pericarditis: especially in Churg–Strauss vasculitis.
Mononeuritis or mononeuritis multiplex, peripheral neuropathy.
Arthritis: usually of large joints.

Investigations
Urinalysis: most urgent investigation because renal involvement influences prognosis.
Plasma urea and creatinine, 24-h urinary protein and creatinine clearance measurement: to assess renal function.
Full blood count: shows anaemia, leucocytosis (leucocyte count normal or low in vasculitis secondary to rheumatoid arthritis or SLE), eosinophilia (especially in Churg–Strauss vasculitis), thrombocytosis.
ESR, CRP, and liver enzymes (e.g. alkaline phosphatase) measurement: raised values.
Antineutrophil cytoplasmic autoantibody analysis: most useful for diagnosis; diffuse cytoplasmic staining (anti-proteinase III) in 80% of patients with systemic Wegener's granulomatosis, 50% limited Wegener's; perinuclear staining less specific (antimyeloperoxidase) but common in microscopic polyangiitis and idiopathic crescentic glomerulonephritis.
Other autoantibody tests: antinuclear antibody and rheumatoid factor nonspecific; may reflect underlying disease; C3 and C4 usually increased in primary vasculitis, low or normal in vasculitis associated with SLE and rheumatoid arthritis; high levels of cryoglobulins may indicate need for plasma exchange.
Von Willebrand's factor antigen test: measure of vascular damage; also increased in noninflammatory vascular injury (e.g. thrombosis).
Viral studies: for hepatitis B, cytomegalovirus, Epstein–Barr virus.
Chest radiography: shows nodules, fibrosis, infiltrate.
Sinus radiography: shows sinusitis, bone destruction.
Angiography: shows microaneurysms in up to 70% of patients with polyarteritis nodosa; rarely with Wegener's granulomatosis and Churg–Strauss vasculitis.
2-dimensional echocardiography: to exclude vegetations and atrial myxoma.
Biopsy: of kidney, skin, nose, muscle, sural nerve, rectum, or temporal artery.

Complications
Renal failure: acute, especially if diagnosis or treatment delayed, or chronic (<10% of patients dependent on dialysis).
Gangrene or infarction: can lead to amputation or chronic skin ulcer.
Neuropathy: possibly permanent (e.g. footdrop), although 60% improve on treatment.
Subglottic stenosis: leading to tracheostomy.
Nasal collapse: permanent and may necessitate later plastic surgery.
Severe pulmonary haemorrhage: may cause breathlessness; and unexplained anaemia.
Coronary arteritis: may cause myocardial infarction; and heart failure.
Hypertension.

Differential diagnosis
Nonspecific systemic illness
Infection: subacute bacterial endocarditis, other chronic and atypical infections.
Connective tissue disease.
Malignancy: especially myeloproliferative, metastatic disease, multiple myeloma.
Sarcoid, HIV, Goodpastures syndrome.

Vasculopathy and necrotizing granuloma
Lymphomatoid granulomatosis, idiopathic midline granuloma.
Cholesterol atheroembolism.
Cardiac myxoma, antiphospholipid antibody syndrome.

Aetiology
- Causes include the following:

Autoimmune: autoantibodies, e.g. anti-neutrophil cytoplasmic autoantibodies in Wegener's granulomatosis.
Immune complex: particularly secondary vasculitis associated with SLE and rheumatoid arthritis.
Viral infection: e.g. hepatitis B, HIV, cytomegalovirus.
Neoplasms (especially haematological).

Epidemiology
- The annual incidence may be increasing, ~40 in one million being affected each year.
- The male:female ratio is 1.5:1.
- The age range is wide, with an increasing incidence with age in women.

Classification
Large-artery
Giant-cell arteritis, Takayasu's arteritis.

Medium-artery
Polyarteritis nodosa, Kawasaki disease.

Medium- or small-artery
Wegener's granulomatosis, Churg–Strauss vasculitis, microscopic polyangiitis.

Small-vessel
Henoch–Schönlein purpura, essential mixed cryoglobulinaemia, leucocytoclastic cutaneous vasculitis.

- Secondary vasculitis, e.g. infection, drugs, rheumatoid arthritis, SLE, and Sjögren's syndrome, usually involves either medium or small arteries or pure small vessel.

Treatment

Diet and lifestyle
- Patients should take precautions against possible infections because they are often immunosuppressed.

Pharmacological treatment

Steroids
- Steroids are only used alone in patients with small-vessel or large-artery disease (*see* Classification).

Standard dosage	*Continuous:* prednisolone 15–60 mg orally depending on severity and type of vasculitis; usually reducing course. *Pulse:* methylprednisolone 1 g i.v. or 100 mg orally for 3 days; dose and frequency varied according to response.
Contraindications	Infection (e.g. subacute bacterial endocarditis).
Special points	Adrenal suppression may be a problem with long-term treatment.
Main drug interactions	Drugs that induce liver enzymes promote steroid metabolism; prednisolone antagonizes antihypertensive treatment.
Main side effects	Diabetes, hypertension, osteoporosis, mood change, cushingoid appearance.

Immunosuppressants
- Immunosuppressants are indicated for more severe vasculitis, particularly of small or medium artery.

Standard dosage	*Continuous:* cyclophosphamide 2 mg/kg orally daily. *Pulse:* cyclophosphamide 15 mg/kg i.v.; alternatively, 5 mg/kg orally daily for 3 days; dose and frequency vary according to response, renal function, and leucocyte count (measured at 7, 10, and 14 days).
Contraindications	Pregnancy (first trimester especially), uncontrolled infection.
Main drug interactions	None.
Main side effects	Bone-marrow suppression, haemorrhagic cystitis (rare with pulse treatment), nausea, alopecia, infertility.

Combination treatment
Pulse i.v. cyclophosphamide 15 mg/kg and methylprednisolone 1 g 2-weekly for 6 courses (remission induction), then 3-weekly for 2 pulses, then monthly for 3 pulses (maintenance).

Pulse oral cyclophosphamide 5 mg/kg daily and prednisolone 100–200 mg daily for 3 consecutive days; interval between treatments as for pulse i.v. treatment.

Continuous oral cyclophosphamide 2 mg/kg daily and prednisolone 40–60 mg daily; prednisolone reduced to 20 mg daily by month 3, to 10 mg daily by month 6.

- Cyclophosphamide should be withdrawn at 9–12 months.
- Longer treatment or change to azathioprine 2 mg/kg daily is often needed in patients with Wegener's granulomatosis or rheumatoid vasculitis.

Other drugs
Azathioprine: steroid-sparing and immunosuppressive.

Septrin: for localized Wegener's granulomatosis.

Plasmapheresis: for pulmonary haemorrhage and severe renal disease.

Treatment aims
To induce and maintain remission.
To recognise and treat relapses early.
To avoid toxicity and side effects.

Prognosis
- In patients with Wegener's granulomatosis or polyarteritis nodosa, 75% remit and 50% relapse with continuous oral treatment.
- The 2-year survival rate ranges from 10% with no treatment to 80% with cyclophosphamide treatment.
- For patients with small-vessel vasculitis, the prognosis is good.

Follow-up and management
- Long-term follow-up is essential, with regular clinical examination, full blood count, renal function tests (especially urinalysis), and immunology.
- Daily steroids are more often used for large- and small-vessel vasculitis, with reduction in dose when the patient is in remission, aiming for alternate-day treatment.
- Early recognition of relapse is essential.

Key references
Chakravarty K, Scott DGI: Management of systemic vasculitis. *Rheumatol Rev* 1992, **1**:81–99.

Gross WL, Schmitt WH, Caernok E: ANCA associated diseases: a rheumatologist's perspective. *Am J Kidney Dis* 1991, **2**:175–179.

Hoffman G: Wegener's granulomatosis: an analysis of 158 patients. *Ann Intern Med* 1992, **116**:488–498.

Index

A

ACE inhibitors *see* angiotensin-converting enzyme inhibitors
acromegaly 16
algodystrophic syndrome *see* dystrophy, reflex sympathetic
allopurinol for gout 13
alveolitis, fibrosing 8 *see also* fibrosis, pulmonary; lung disease, interstitial
amyloidosis 6, 8
analgesics for psoriatic arthritis 7
angiitis *see* vasculitis
angiotensin-converting enzyme inhibitors for vascular insufficiency 23
anthralin *see* dithranol
antibiotics for bacterial overgrowth in systemic sclerosis 23
anti-inflammatory drugs, nonsteroidal *see* NSAIDs
antirheumatic agents *see* NSAIDs
arteritis
   coronary 24
   giant-cell 18
   temporal *see* arteritis, giant-cell
arthralgia 14, 24
arthritis 14 *see also* polyarthritis
   bacterial *see* arthritis, septic
   degenerative *see* osteoarthritis
   infectious *see* arthritis, septic
   mutilans 6
   postinfectious *see* arthritis, reactive
   psoriatic 6
   pyrophosphate 12
   reactive 8
   rheumatoid 6, 8, 12, 18, 20
   septic 2, 8, 10, 12, 16
   viral 8
arthropathy
   Charcot 16
   inflammatory 16
   neurogenic *see* arthropathy, Charcot
   psoriatic 4
   reactive 4
atheroembolism, cholesterol 24
azathioprine
   for polymyalgia rheumatica 19
   for psoriatic arthritis 7
   for systemic lupus erythematosus 21
   for systemic vasculitis 25

B

bacterial overgrowth in systemic sclerosis 23
Bechterew's disease *see* spondylitis, ankylosing
benzylpenicillin for septic arthritis 11
blood pressure, high *see* hypertension
Bouchard's nodes 16
bowel disease, inflammatory 4
bursitis 8
   olecranon 12

C

calcinosis 22
calcium
   antagonists
      for Raynaud's phenomenon 23
      for vascular insufficiency 23
   pyrophosphate crystals 16
carcinoid syndrome 22
carcinoma of lung 22
cardiac *see* heart
cardiomyopathy 22
cauda equina syndrome 4
cefotaxime for septic arthritis 11
cellulitis 12
chlorambucil for systemic lupus erythematosus 21
chloroquine for psoriatic arthritis 7
Churg–Strauss syndrome 24
ciprofloxacin for bacterial overgrowth in systemic sclerosis 23
cisapride for oesophageal involvement in systemic sclerosis 23
coal tar for psoriatic arthritis 7
colchicine
   for acute crystal synovitis 3
   for gout 13
connective tissue disease 18, 22, 24
corticosteroids
   for acute crystal synovitis 3
   for giant-cell arteritis 19
   for inflammatory myositis 15
   for osteoarthritis 17
   for polymyalgia rheumatica 19
   for rheumatoid arthritis 9
   for systemic lupus erythematosus 21
   for systemic vasculitis 25
CREST 22
crisis, hypertensive renal 22
cyclophosphamide
   for early diffuse systemic sclerosis 23
   for inflammatory myositis 15
   for systemic lupus erythematosus 21
   for systemic vasculitis 25
cyclosporin A
   for inflammatory myositis 15
   for psoriatic arthritis 7
   for systemic sclerosis 23
cytotoxic drugs for systemic lupus erythematosus 21

D

dermatomyositis 14
diclofenac
   for gout 13
   for rheumatoid arthritis 9
dithranol for psoriatic arthritis 7
dysphasia, spondyloepiphesial 16
dystrophy
   reflex sympathetic 22
   muscular 14

E

enalapril
   for Raynaud's phenomenon 23
   for vascular insufficiency 23
endocarditis, subacute bacterial 24
epilepsy 20
epistaxis 24
erythromycin for bacterial overgrowth in systemic sclerosis 23
etretinate for psoriatic arthritis 7

F

fasciitis, eosinophilic 22
fibrosis, pulmonary 22 *see also* alveolitis, fibrosing; lung disease, interstitial
flucloxacillin for septic arthritis 11
Foresteir–Certonciny syndrome *see* polymyalgia rheumatica

G

gammaglobulin for inflammatory myositis 15
Goodpasture's syndrome 24
gout 2, 12, 16
granulomatosis, lymphomatoid 24

Index

H

haematuria 24

haemochromatosis 16

haemoptysis 24

hallucination
  auditory 20
  visual 20

Hamman–Rich syndrome *see* alveolitis, fibrosing

hand shoulder syndrome *see* dystrophy, reflex sympathetic

headache 18

heart
  block 14
  failure 14, 22

Heberden's nodes 16

hydralazine 20

hydroxychloroquine
  for psoriatic arthritis 7
  for rheumatoid arthritis 9
  for systemic lupus erythematosus 21

hyperlipidaemia with xanthomata 12

hyperparathyroidism 16

hypertension 20
  pulmonary 14

hyperuricaemia 12

hypomotility syndrome, intestinal 22

I

ibuprofen for rheumatoid arthritis 9

immunosuppressants
  for inflammatory myositis 15
  for systemic vasculitis 25

indomethacin
  for ankylosing spondylitis 5
  for gout 13
  for rheumatoid arthritis 9

infection
  Haemophilus influenzae 10
  Staphylococcus aureus 10
  Yersinia 4

J

joint disorders *see* arthritis, polyarthritis

K

keratoconjunctivitis sicca 8

keratoderma blenorrhagica 6

L

leukaemia 18

Libman–Sacks disease *see* lupus erythematosus, systemic

livedo reticularis 20

lung
  disease, interstitial 14 *see also* alveolitis, fibrosing; fibrosis, pulmonary
  fibrosis, interstitial 14

lupus
  anticoagulant 20
  erythematosus, systemic 20

lymphadenopathy 24

lymphoma 18
  non-Hodgkin's 8

M

malignancy, myeloproliferative 24

Marie–Streumpell disease *see* spondylitis, ankylosing

methotrexate
  for early diffuse systemic sclerosis 23
  for inflammatory myositis 15
  for polymyalgia rheumatica 19
  for psoriatic arthritis 7
  for rheumatoid arthritis 9
  for systemic lupus erythematosus 21

methylprednisolone
  for acute crystal synovitis 3
  for systemic lupus erythematosus 21
  for systemic vasculitis 25

metronidazole for bacterial overgrowth in systemic sclerosis 23

microstomia 22

myalgia 14, 24

myalgic syndrome, eosinophilic 22

myeloma
  multiple 18, 24
  plasma cell *see* myeloma, multiple

myositis
  inflammatory 14
  multiple *see* polymyositis

myxoma, cardiac 24

N

naproxen for rheumatoid arthritis 9

necrosis, avascular 16

nerve
  compression syndrome *see* nerve entrapment
  entrapment 2

neuropathy 24

nifedipine
  for Raynaud's phenomenon 23
  for vascular insufficiency 23

nonsteroidal anti-inflammatory drugs *see* NSAIDs

NSAIDs
  for acute crystal synovitis 3
  for ankylosing spondylitis 5
  for gout 13
  for osteoarthritis 17
  for psoriatic arthritis 7
  for rheumatoid arthritis 9

O

ochronosis 16

oligoarthritis, inflammatory 6

omega 3 marine triglycerides
  for Raynaud's phenomenon 23
  for vascular insufficiency 23

omeprazole for oesophageal involvement in systemic sclerosis 23

osteoarthritis 16
  crystal-related oligarthritic 16
  nodal 8, 16
  polyarticular 16
  premature 16

osteoarthrosis *see* osteoarthritis

osteomalacia 14

osteomyelitis 10, 18

P

papules, Gottron's 14

penicillamine
  for early diffuse systemic sclerosis 23
  for rheumatoid arthritis 9

poisoning, heavy metal 12

polyarteritis nodosa 24

polyarthralgia 20

polyarthritis 12 *see also* arthritis
  crystal 8
  septic 8

polymyalgia rheumatica 18

polymyositis 18

prednisolone
  for early diffuse systemic sclerosis 23
  for giant-cell arteritis 19
  for polymyalgia rheumatica 19
  for systemic vasculitis 25

prednisone for systemic lupus erythematosus 21

Index

proteinuria 24

proton-pump inhibitors for oesophageal involvement in systemic sclerosis 23

pseudogout 2, 12

pseudo-obstruction 22

pseudopolyarthritis, rhizomelic *see* polymyalgia rheumatica

psoriasis
    arthritic *see* arthritis, psoriatic
    arthropathica *see* arthritis, psoriatic

R

rash
    butterfly 20
    heliotrope 14

Raynaud's phenomenon 14, 20, 22

Reiter's syndrome 4, 6

rhabdomyolysis 14

rheumatism, peri-extra-articular *see* polymyalgia rheumatica

rubifacients for osteoarthritis 17

rupture, joint 2

S

sarcoid 24

scleritis 8

sclerodactyly 22

scleroedema of Bushke 22

scleromyxoedema 22

sclerosis, systemic 22

sepsis 16

Sjögren's syndrome, secondary 8

SLE *see* lupus erythematosus, systemic

sodium aurothiomalate for psoriatic arthritis 7

spondarthritis, seronegative 8

spondylarthritis *see* spondylitis, ankylosing

spondylitis
    ankylosing 4, 6
    rheumatoid *see* spondylitis, ankylosing

stenosis, subglottic 24

steroids *see* corticosteroids

subluxation, atlanto–axial 8

sulphasalazine
    for ankylosing spondylitis 5
    for psoriatic arthritis 7
    for rheumatoid arthritis 9

synovitis
    acute crystal 2, 10, 16
    peripheral 18

T

telangiectasia 22

tenosynovitis 8

tetracycline for bacterial overgrowth in systemic sclerosis 23

trauma, internal 14

triamcinolone for acute crystal synovitis 3

trophi 12

U

uveitis 4

V

vasculitis
    Churg–Strauss 24
    systemic 24

ventilatory failure 14

vinyl chloride disease 22

vision disturbance 18

W

wasting, muscle 14

X

xanthomata 12